DRUGS AFFECTING LIPID METABOLISM

RISK FACTORS AND FUTURE DIRECTIONS

Medical Science Symposia Series

Volume 10

The titles published in this series are listed at the end of this volume.

Drugs Affecting Lipid Metabolism

Risk Factors and Future Directions

Edited by

A.M. Gotto, Jr.
Baylor College of Medicine, The Methodist Hospital, Houston, TX, U.S.A.

R. Paoletti
Institute of Pharmacological Sciences, Milan, Italy

L.C. Smith
Baylor College of Medicine, Houston, TX, U.S.A.

A.L. Catapano
Institute of Pharmacological Sciences, Milan, Italy

and

A.S. Jackson (Managing Editor)
Giovanni Lorenzini Medical Foundation, Houston, TX, U.S.A.

KLUWER ACADEMIC PUBLISHERS
DORDRECHT / BOSTON / LONDON

Fondazione Giovanni Lorenzini, Milan, Italy
Giovanni Lorenzini Medical Foundation, Houston, U.S.A.

A C.I.P. Catalogue record for this book is available from the Library of Congress

ISBN-13: 978-94-010-6625-9 e-ISBN-13: 978-94-009-0311-1
DOI: 10.1007/978-94-009-0311-1

Published by Kluwer Academic Publishers,
P.O. Box 17, 3300 AA Dordrecht, The Netherlands.

Kluwer Academic Publishers incorporates
the publishing programmes of
D. Reidel, Martinus Nijhoff, Dr W. Junk and MTP Press.

Sold and distributed in the U.S.A. and Canada
by Kluwer Academic Publishers,
101 Philip Drive, Norwell, MA 02061, U.S.A.

In all other countries, sold and distributed
by Kluwer Academic Publishers Group,
P.O. Box 322, 3300 AH Dordrecht, The Netherlands.

Table of Contents

VI. Modified Lipoproteins and Lipoprotein Metabolism

VII. The Effects of Omega-3 Fatty Acids on Lipid Metabolism

PREFACE

Even a brief scan of the table of contents of the present volume is enough to disclose the diversity of research interests and opinions in the field of lipidology. It is precisely this diversity that is the strength of our field and that was showcased by the XII International Symposium of DRUGS AFFECTING LIPID METABOLISM (DALM). The papers published here from these proceedings may be divided into three categories: those that define—and refine—our understanding of the clinical benefit of aggressive lipid management, those that develop our knowledge of risk assessment, and those that discuss the genetic, biochemical, and biophysical mechanisms underlying the pathology of coronary heart disease.

On the clinical front, further analysis of the results of the Scandinavian Simvastatin Survival Study (4S) has indicated the cost-effectiveness of therapy in patients with established coronary heart disease. The West of Scotland Coronary Prevention Study (WOSCOPS), whose methodology was described at the DALM XII symposium, has demonstrated in a mostly primary-prevention population what 4S demonstrated for secondary prevention the year before: aggressive lipid-regulating therapy reduces coronary heart disease morbidity and mortality rates without concurrently increasing mortality from noncardiovascular causes. In the future, important considerations will be to develop protocols that maximize benefit in groups underrepresented in traditional clinical research—for example, women and the elderly—and to improve compliance to existing treatment regimens. Furthermore, antioxidant, omega-3 fatty acid, and gene therapies warrant further investigation.

Another important area will be the refinement of risk assessment by identifying new or more sensitive markers for coronary heart disease risk and by developing new modalities for imaging disease. Of particular interest are the roles of triglyceride, insulin resistance, diabetes, and cell apoptosis in the pathology of clinical disease.

Although the clinical benefit of lipid-regulating therapy is clear, the mechanisms underlying that benefit and atherogenesis remain enigmatic. Fortunately, much progress has been made in elucidating basic mechanisms of lipid metabolism, platelet coagulation, smooth muscle cell signaling, and lipoprotein oxidation.

It is hoped that the vigorous exchange of ideas undertaken at DALM XII and represented by the following papers will contribute to a synthesized understanding of the clinical and mechanistic aspects of atherosclerosis and the dyslipidemias. It is through such synthesis that we may expect to develop new therapies for hyperlipidemia, improve existing therapies, and reduce the toll of coronary heart disease.

The Editors

OXIDIZED LDL, ITS RECEPTORS, AND ITS ROLE IN ATHEROSCLEROSIS

Daniel Steinberg
University of California, San Diego, Department of Medicine 0682, 9500 Gilman Drive, La Jolla, California 92093-0682, USA

Introduction

The hypothesis that oxidative modification of low density lipoprotein (LDL) plays a critical role in the atherogenic process is receiving ever-increasing attention from the biomedical community. The National Library of Medicine cited 4 articles relating to "oxidized LDL" in 1985, 53 articles in 1990, and 145 articles in 1994. These papers run the gamut from basic studies of mechanisms involved in LDL oxidation, through animal model experiments testing the efficacy of antioxidants in inhibiting atherogenesis, and on to clinical studies of the effects of antioxidants on susceptibility of LDL to oxidative modification. No attempt will be made here to summarize all of the published information. Instead we shall focus on those aspects on which a consensus is emerging: 1) How oxidized LDL fits into the pathogenesis of the early lesion; 2) The receptors involved in the uptake of oxidized LDL; 3) The recent evidence that these receptors may play a critical role in uptake of damaged and apoptotic cells as well as oxidized LDL; and 4) The possibility that these receptors and oxidized LDL may play a role in the evolution of the plaque, helping to determine whether it will be a primarily fibrotic (i.e. relatively benign) lesion or a lesion with a large necrotic lipid core (i.e. an unstable lesion prone to rupture and thrombosis).

The Role of Oxidized LDL in the Formation of the Fatty Streak Lesion

Over the past two decades, as a result of studies in animal models and studies of the human disease, there has been a convergence of points of view with regard to the unit processes and the sequence of those unit processes leading to formation of a fatty streak. In Figure 1 we have attempted to bring these together in a single scheme. The critical step we are particularly concerned with is step 7, the modification of LDL to a form that can be taken up more avidly by the macrophage and/or the smooth muscle cell. Goldstein et al. [1] were the first to show that chemical modification of LDL--by acetylation--generated a form recognized by a specific macrophage receptor and taken up at a sufficient rate to lead to cholesterol accumulation. The critical finding was that this new receptor (acetyl LDL receptor), unlike the LDL receptor, did not down regulate as the cholesterol content of the

A. M. Gotto, Jr. et al. (eds.), Drugs Affecting Lipid Metabolism, 1–15.

cell increased and thus continued to take up acetyl LDL even when the cholesterol content of the cell was markedly elevated. However, there was no evidence (and there still is none) for the formation of acetyl LDL at a significant rate *in vivo*. Henriksen, Mahoney, and Steinberg [2-4] showed that incubation of LDL with cultured cells *in vitro* led to modifications of its structure and function such that the modified LDL was taken up more avidly by macrophages and taken up to a large extent by way of the acetyl LDL receptor. Later studies showed that the major effect of the incubation with cells was to oxidize the LDL [5,6].

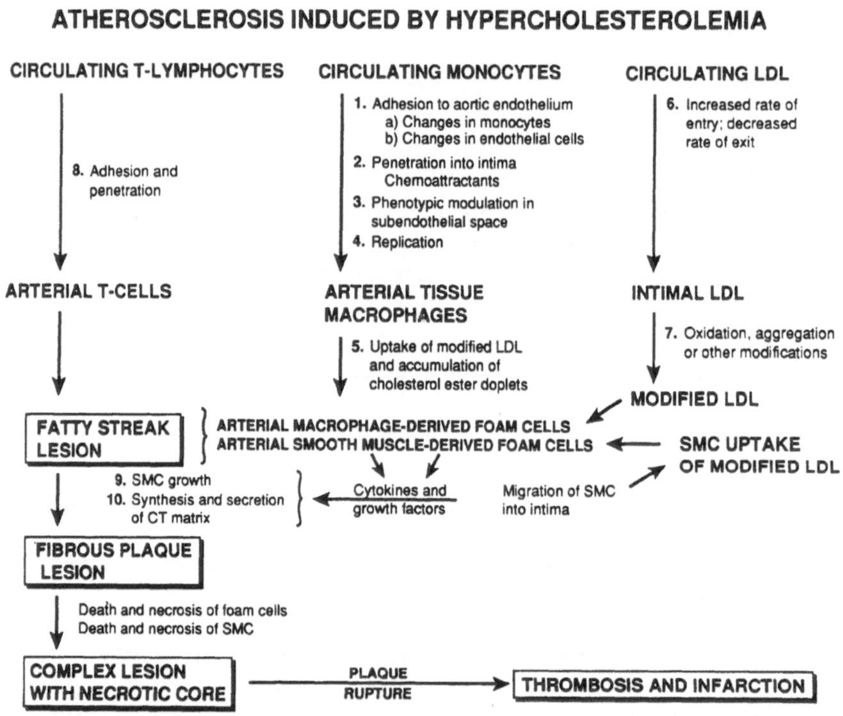

Figure 1. A schematic representation of our current concepts of the pathogenesis of atherosclerosis. (Reproduced by permission from *Drug Treatment Hyperlipidemia*, Basil M. Rifikind, editor, 1991).

Until recently the basis for the generation of foam cells from smooth muscle cells was puzzling. Uptake by way of the LDL receptor cannot lead to significant accumulation of cholesterol, as just discussed, and the acetyl LDL receptor is not normally expressed by smooth muscle cells. Recent studies by Pitas and co-workers [7,8], however, show that smooth muscle cells can be induced to express the acetyl LDL receptor. Thus, foam cell formation from both macrophages and smooth muscle cells may be explained on the same basis.

The acetyl LDL receptor accounts for a large part of oxidized LDL binding and uptake by mouse peritoneal macrophages but cannot account for it all, as shown by early studies on the binding and degradation of oxidized LDL under *in vitro* conditions [9]. Below we will discuss the several new receptors that have been identified as possibly playing a role in oxidized LDL uptake.

Before going on, we should note that oxidative modification is only one of several modifications that could play a role in foam cell formation. Aggregation, whether induced by physical denaturation [10] or by enzyme treatment [11], leads to rapid uptake and that uptake has been shown to occur by phagocytosis. LDL aggregates have been demonstrated in the subendothelial space and it has been shown that this aggregation can occur very rapidly [12]. Immune complexes of LDL can be taken up rapidly, utilizing the Fc receptor pathway. Since autoantibodies against oxidized LDL occur very commonly, such immune complexes may be contributing significantly to oxidized LDL uptake by macrophages in the lesion. While these alternative modifications have not been fully evaluated *in vivo* neither has their participation been ruled out.

Oxidation of LDL not only converts it to a ligand for macrophage scavenger receptors, it also confers on it a large number of biological properties that could in principle be proatherogenic. For example, oxidized LDL is chemotactic for monocytes [13] and for T-cells [14] which are found in lesions, but not for B-cells or neutrophils, which are not. Much of this chemotactic activity seems to be due to lysolecithin generated during the oxidative modification [15]. Even minimally oxidized LDL, studied extensively by Fogelman, Berliner and their co-workers [16], acquires proatherogenic properties even though at this early stage of oxidation it is not a ligand for macrophage scavenger receptors. Such minimally oxidized LDL (MM-LDL) stimulates the release of MCP-1 and of MCSF from cultured endothelial cells [17,18]. A property of oxidized LDL receiving a great deal of attention at the clinical level is its ability to inhibit vasodilatation triggered by NO and by other vasodilators [19-21]. Indeed, the normal vasodilatory response to acetylcholine can be converted to a paradoxical vasoconstriction in the coronary arteries of hypercholesterolemic patients, presumably the result of oxidized LDL in the vessel wall. There are more than a dozen other biological properties of oxidized LDL that could be proatherogenic but we will not try to review them all. Only a small number of these have been critically tested to determine their importance *in vivo*.

The Effectiveness of Antioxidants in Animal Models of Atherosclerosis

The oxidative modification hypothesis is strongly supported by a large number of studies in animal models of atherosclerosis using various antioxidant compounds. As listed in Table 1, more than 20 studies have been published, using LDL receptor-deficient rabbits, cholesterol-fed rabbits, cholesterol-fed nonhuman primates, cholesterol-fed hamsters, and apoE-deficient mice. Most of the studies have been done using probucol as the antioxidant but others have utilized diphenylphenylenediamine (DPPD), butylated hydroxytoluene

Table 1. Antioxidants in animal models of atherosclerosis.

		Result	Reference
Probucol in LDL-R deficient rabbits:			
Carew et al., 1987		+	[23]
Kita et al., 1987		+	[54]
Mao et al., 1991		+	[55]
Daugherty et al., 1991		±	[56]
Fruebis et al., 1994		+	[22]
Morel et al., 1994		+	[57]
Probucol analogues in LDL-R deficient rabbits:			
Mao et al., 1991		+	[58]
Fruebis et al., 1994		-	[22]
Probucol in C-fed rabbits:			
Stein et al., 1989		-	[59]
Daugherty et al., 1989		+	[60]
Prasad et al., 1994		+	[61]
Other antioxidants in rabbits:			
DPPD	Sparrow et al., 1992	+	[62]
BHT	Björkhem et al., 1991	+	[63]
Vitamin E	Prasad et al., 1993	+	[64]
	Morel et al., 1994	-	[57]
	Kleinveld et al., 1995	-	[65]
	Fruebis et al., 1995	-	[66]
Antioxidants in rodents:			
Probucol in hamsters	Parker et al., 1995	+	[67]
Vitamin E in hamsters	Parker et al., 1995	+	[67]
DPPD in apoE-deficient mice	Tangirala et al, 1995	+	[68]
Antioxidants in nonhuman primates:			
Probucol	Sasahara et al., 1994	+	[69]
Vitamin E	Verlangieri and Bush, 1992	±	[70]

"Meta-analysis": 15+ 2± 5-

(BHT), or vitamin E. Several of the papers included trials of more than one agent. Overall there have been 17 positive results and 5 negative (2 using vitamin E, 1 using probucol, and 2 using analogs of probucol that were less effective antioxidants than probucol itself). Since several different antioxidants have been shown to be effective, it seems reasonable to ascribe the inhibition of lesion progression to the property they share in common, i.e. their antioxidant property. On the other hand, a large fraction of the studies done have been done with probucol and probucol has additional biological effects that could contribute significantly to its antiatherogenic potential. Fruebis et al. [22] studied a close structural analog of probucol comparing it with probucol itself. The analog was a very effective antioxidant, albeit not quite as effective as probucol itself under the conditions used. The analog caused a three-fold increase in diene conjugation lag time, but gave no detectable inhibition of lesion progression. Probucol prolonged lag time more than 9-fold and, as in the original studies of Carew et al. [23], inhibited lesion formation by about 50%. Unfortunately, in only a few studies has the change in diene conjugation lag time been explicitly measured. Consequently it is difficult to say what the relationship is between the level of protection afforded LDL against oxidation *ex vivo*, on the one hand, and the extent of protection against atherogenesis, on the other hand. Much more experimental work needs to be done along these lines. It might be mentioned here that many of the clinical papers comparing LDL samples from different patients with respect to their susceptibility to oxidation report differences in diene conjugation lag time as small as 30 or 40%, yet they imply that these small differences may explain differences in CHD risks. Yet if the animal studies are indicative, antioxidants may need to prolong diene conjugation lag time many-fold before we can expect to see antiatherogenic effects. At this point we cannot even be certain that there will be a good correlation between the level of protection afforded to LDL against oxidation *ex vivo* and the extent of protection against lesion progression *in vivo*. For example, we know that antioxidants can play a role in intracellular metabolism and that their antiatherogenic potential may relate to such intracellular roles in addition to the direct protection of the LDL particle they reside in. We may need to develop new ways of assessing antioxidant activity at the cellular level before we can properly assess the value of this or that antioxidant intervention.

Receptors for Oxidized LDL

Scavenger Receptor A (Acetyl LDL Receptor)

As mentioned above, competition between oxidized LDL and acetylated LDL suggested very early on that part of the uptake of oxidized LDL by mouse peritoneal macrophages would be attributable to the same receptor that recognizes acetyl LDL [9]. This was conclusively demonstrated in the laboratory of Dr. Monty Krieger, where the acetyl LDL receptor was cloned [24,25] and where it was shown that cells transfected to express the acetyl LDL receptor also bound and took up oxidized LDL (albeit with a lower affinity than for acetyl LDL). More recently it has been shown that peritoneal macrophages from mice in which the SRA has been "knocked out" by gene targeting take up and degrade oxidized

LDL at a reduced rate compared to that seen in wild-type macrophages (T. Kodama, personal communication). Some residual binding and uptake were seen, showing again that more than one receptor is involved.

CD36

Endemann et al. [26], using expression cloning, showed that the mouse homolog of human CD36 could bind and mediate the uptake of oxidized LDL and Nicholson et al. [27] showed that human CD36 also binds oxidized LDL. Studies by Nozaki et al. in the laboratory of Dr. Y. Matsuzawa [28] showed that monocyte/macrophages from patients with a rare mutation leading to complete deficiency in CD36 expression, both on monocytes and platelets, take up and degrade oxidized LDL at only about 60% the rate seen in normal wild-type monocyte/macrophages. This establishes that CD36 and its mouse homolog are potentially important in the uptake of oxidized LDL.

Macrosialin and Its Human Homolog, CD68

Ottnad et al. [29] partially purified from mouse peritoneal macrophages a 94-97 kD protein that bound oxidized LDL with high affinity on ligand blots. Earlier this year Ramprasad et al. [30] purified this protein to near homogeneity and were able to identify it as macrosialin on the basis of amino acid sequences of several tryptic peptides derived from it. Macrosialin was first characterized by Smith and Koch on the basis of its reactivity with a monoclonal antibody generated against mouse peritoneal macrophages [31]. It was subsequently characterized by studies in the laboratory of Dr. Siamon Gordon [32] and cloned by Holness et al. [33]. It is a heavily glycosolated membrane protein found predominantly in the late endosomal fraction with only minor amounts in the lysosomal fraction and in the plasma membrane [34]. Its function remains uncertain. Possibilities that have been considered include protection of endosomal/lysosomal membranes against enzymatic self digestion or a role in antigen presentation. The fact that macrosialin and CD68 bind oxidized LDL with high affinity in a ligand blot and the fact that they also bind phosphatidylserine liposomes suggest a role in uptake of oxidized LDL. How can that be reconciled, however, with a very low level of expression on the plasma membrane?

Macrosialin is a member of the lamp family (lysosomal membrane associated proteins). Some other members of this family, like macrosialin, are found predominantly in lysosomes or endosomes but exchange very rapidly with other membrane compartments, including the plasma membrane. This has been particularly well studied by Lippincott-Schwartz and Fambrough in the case of LEP 100 [35]. Fukuda has pointed out that even though a very small percentage of a lamp protein is on the plasma membrane at any one time, it can nevertheless play a role in cell adhesion [36]. Our preliminary studies confirm the findings of Rabinowitz and Gordon in that only a very small percentage of macrosialin is expressed on the plasma membrane of resident mouse peritoneal macrophages. On the other hand, macrophages elicited by intraperitoneal injection of thioglycollate broth show a marked increase in the total amount of macrosialin expressed, as reported by Rabinowitz and Gordon [32], and using these elicited macrophages we have been able to demonstrate surface expression of the protein. We did this using a monoclonal antibody specific for macrosialin (generously provided by Dr. R.P. DaSilva and Dr. S. Gordon of Oxford University) and also by using biotinylation of plasma membrane proteins followed by immunoprecipitation. The precipitating antiserum was prepared against a synthetic peptide representing the C-terminal cytoplasmic tail of macrosialin. Thus, our preliminary studies suggest that macrosialin may play a role as an oxidized LDL receptor but careful kinetic studies remain to be carried out.

Fc Receptor

Using expression cloning, Stanton et al. [37] cloned the FcγRII-B2 receptor from a mouse macrophage library. However, they later reported that antibodies directed against this Fc receptor failed to inhibit the uptake and degradation of oxidized LDL by mouse peritoneal macrophages [26]. We have made similar observations in this laboratory (G. Sambrano and D. Steinberg, unpublished results). We have also shown that the binding of oxidized red blood cells to mouse peritoneal macrophages is inhibited by oxidized LDL but not inhibited by an antibody against the FcγRII-B2 receptor [38]. As a positive control we showed that the antibody did inhibit the binding of opsonized RBC. Thus at this point it seems unlikely that the Fc receptor is directly involved in the binding and uptake of oxidized LDL or oxidatively damaged cells by mouse peritoneal macrophages.

SR-B1

This receptor, cloned from a mutant line of Chinese hamster ovary cells by Acton et al. [39], has over 30% homology with human CD36. It is almost identical to the human CLA-1 receptor [40]. It was initially selected and studied because of its ability to bind acetyl LDL but it also bound oxidized LDL, maleylated bovine serum albumin, and native LDL. Further studies showed, however, that its affinity for high density lipoprotein (HDL) was the highest of all and that it facilitated the transfer of cholesterol esters from bound HDL to the interior of the transfected cells without any internalization of the apoprotein [41]. Its tissue distribution--almost exclusively in liver, adrenal and ovary--showed that it was almost certainly an HDL receptor involved in the selective uptake of HDL cholesterol esters, a previously well-described phenomenon in rats *in vivo* and in several different kinds of cultured cells *in vitro* [42]. Whether the ability of this receptor to bind oxidized LDL (and other lipoproteins) is functionally important or not remains to be established. At the moment its limited tissue distribution, namely, in cells that use cholesterol for steroid hormone or bile acid synthesis, suggests that it may not play an important scavenger receptor role (i.e. a role in uptake of modified lipoproteins or damaged cells).

Others?

Dr. Oswald Quehenberger in our laboratory has used expression cloning using Xenopus oocytes to determine whether there are additional receptors for oxidized LDL on mouse macrophages [43]. Screening was based on specific binding of 125I-OxLDL to Xenopus oocytes previously injected with mRNA. This screening yielded 5 clones, only one of which has been sequenced thus far. That turned out to be acylCoA: cholesterol acyltransferase. Current studies are directed at determining whether this protein is actually itself expressed on the plasma membrane or whether it induces changes in the metabolism of the cell such that a receptor for oxidized LDL is expressed on the plasma membrane at a higher level.

What Function or Functions of the So-Called Scavenger Receptors Accounts for their Persistence During Evolution?

The acetyl LDL receptor is highly conserved across mammalian species; proteins with similar biological properties have been described all the way back to Drosophila [44]. The persistence of this receptor (or these receptors) cannot be accounted for on the basis of a role in the atherogenic process. Clearly there cannot be any genetic pressures, either positive or negative, based on a disease that only occurs in humans and which does not take any toll until after the child-bearing years. In thinking about the possible vital functions of these receptors we asked ourselves what ligands there might be that resembled LDL to the point that they might share common receptor-binding domains. Well, the plasma membrane of cells is similar in structure to LDL. Both consist of a phospholipid layer (in the case of a plasma membrane, a bilayer) in which proteins are embedded. Oxidative damage to either of them leads to the formation of hydroperoxy fatty acids; degradation of the fatty acid chains with the generation of aldehydes and other lower molecular weight fragments; linkage of aldehydic products to lysine amino groups; and cross linking of lipid to lipid and of lipid to protein, both intramolecularly and intermolecularly. In other words, it is quite conceivable that some common structural domains may be generated both in an oxidatively damaged LDL and in an oxidatively damaged plasma membrane. We chose the simplest cell model, the red blood cell (RBC), to test this hypothesis. Sambrano et al. [38] showed that nonopsonized, washed human RBC showed almost no binding to mouse peritoneal macrophages until those RBC were subjected to oxidative damage. That damage was inflicted by incubating for 90 minutes with a mixture of copper and ascorbic acid. The key point was that the binding of oxidized RBC (Ox-RBC) was almost completely prevented by competition with oxidized LDL (OxLDL) whereas there was no significant competition by either acetyl LDL or native LDL. Further studies by Sambrano [45] confirmed the earlier findings of Schroit et al. [46] and the findings of Schlegel et al. [47], that this binding is probably attributable to recognition of an excess of phosphatidylserine on the outer leaflet of the membrane. The binding of OxRBC and the binding of OxLDL are both inhibited by phosphatidylserine-rich liposomes but not by phosphatidylcholine-rich liposomes. Thus it was striking to find that phosphatidylserine-rich liposomes bound specifically to the 94-97 kDA membrane protein that had been shown previously to bind oxidized LDL as well [29]. This finding is one of the pieces of evidence implicating macrosialin as playing a role in recognition of damaged cells as well as oxidatively damaged LDL. However, much remains to be done before it can be concluded that macrosialin does indeed play this kind of role.

CD36, on the other hand, clearly plays a role both in recognition of oxidized LDL and in recognition of damaged cells. Above we have briefly summarized the evidence for the binding of oxidized LDL to CD36. Hall et al. [48] have shown that apoptotic cells bind to CD36 which, in association with the vitronectin receptor and thrombospondin, leads to their phagocytosis. Evidently apoptotic cells can be recognized and taken up by at least two quite separate mechanisms. Thus, apoptotic cells are taken up by elicited peritoneal macrophages by a mechanism dependent upon phosphatidylserine appearance on the external leaflet of the plasma membrane whereas the same apoptotic cells are taken up by bone marrow-derived macrophages by a mechanism linked to CD36 and the vitronectin receptor [49] As pointed out by Savill et al. [50] it is understandable that there might be redundancy in a system as important as the system for clearing apoptotic cells before they can become necrotic and aggravate the inflammatory processes.

Is There a Role for Oxidized LDL and Oxidized LDL Receptors in Advanced Lesions and in the Fatal Thrombosis?

The pioneering work of Paris Constantinides [51] and the beautiful recent work of Michael Davies [52] has established that 80% or more of myocardial infarctions are the result of a thrombosis developing at the site of a ruptured plaque. Surprisingly, the lesions most likely to be the site of a fatal thrombosis tend not to be the very highly stenotic lesions but rather lesions at about 50% stenosis. These unstable lesions are characterized by a large necrotic, lipid-rich pool; the predominantly fibrotic lesions containing less lipid are more stable. The triggering event appears to be an erosion of or rupture of the thin fibrous cap that separates the underlying lipid pool from the lumen. The plaque is rich in tissue factor and other prothrombogenic factors and the exposure of blood to these factors presumably triggers the thrombosis. The thrombus may then extend into the lumen and become totally occlusive. It is generally assumed that the lipid pool is the result of necrosis of lipid-laden foam cells although explicit evidence for this is limited. What determines whether a lesion matures into a predominantly fibrous--and therefore "safe"--lesion or into a lesion with a large lipid pool--and therefore an "unsafe" lesion? One possibility is that it rests on the extent to which apoptotic foam cells are taken up before they can spill their content. In that case the receptors we have been studying, because they can participate in uptake of oxidized LDL and generation of foam cells, may have a second and critical function in determining the direction of the evolution of the plaque. If lipid-laden cells enter the apoptotic program and are efficiently phagocytosed by surrounding macrophages (or other cells) the development of the lipid pool can at least be deferred (see Figure 2). This buying of time may be very valuable because the lipid from the foam cells would have at least the possibility of being mobilized out of the lesion over time in a nondamaging way. If, on the other hand, a lipid-laden cell enters the apoptotic program but fails to be phagocytosed, the cell has a high probability of going on to eventually become necrotic and to spill its content, contributing to the build up of the necrotic lipid pool. This is one way in which the "oxidized LDL receptors" may be important in the late history of the lesion, i.e. by determining the kind of lesion that is going to develop. Additionally, as emphasized by Peter Libby and his colleagues [53], the probability that the fibrous cap will be eroded and eventually rupture may be increased by metalloproteases secreted by the macrophage and by other lytic enzymes that can contribute to the weakening of the fibrous cap.

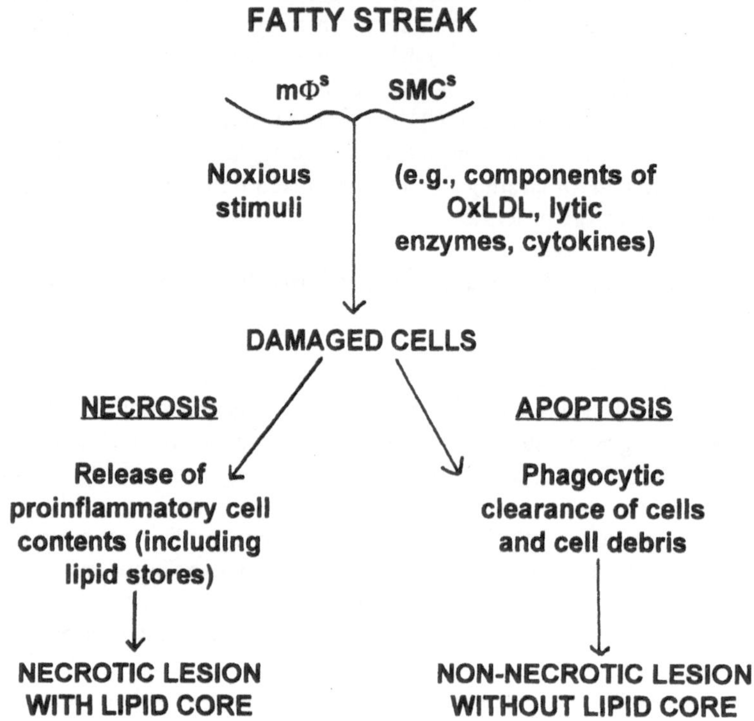

Figure 2. A schematic representation of how an optimally operating apoptotic "scavenger" system might favor the formation of a predominantly fibrotic lesion rather than a predominantly necrotic lesion.

Summary

The oxidative modification hypothesis for atherogenesis rests on a strong scientific base and has been validated in a number of animal models of atherosclerosis. The receptors that recognize oxidatively modified LDL--at least some of them--have an alternative and probably more important function in the recognition of damaged and apoptotic cells. Atherosclerotic lesions contain a large number of apoptotic cells and the fate of these cells may influence the direction in which a developing plaque evolves. If lipid-laden cells undergo necrosis, one is more apt to develop a lesion rich in lipid and therefore at higher risk for rupture and terminal thrombosis. On the other hand, if the receptors involved in recognizing apoptotic cells function properly and engulf the dying cell before its content can be spilled, perhaps one is more likely to develop a more predominantly fibrotic lesion, i.e. a "safe" lesion.

References

1. Goldstein JL, Ho YK, Basu SK, Brown MS. Binding site on macrophages that mediates uptake and degradation of acetylated low density lipoprotein, producing massive cholesterol deposition. Proc Natl Acad Sci USA 1979;76:333-37.
2. Henriksen T, Mahoney EM, Steinberg D. Enhanced macrophage degradation of low density lipoprotein previously incubated with cultured endothelial cells: Recognition by receptors for acetylated low density lipoproteins. Proc Natl Acad Sci USA 1981;78:6499-503.
3. Henriksen T, Mahoney EM, Steinberg D. Interactions of plasma lipoproteins with endothelial cells. Ann N Y Acad Sci 1982;401:102-16.
4. Henriksen T, Mahoney EM, Steinberg D. Enhanced macrophage degradation of biologically modified low density lipoprotein. Arteriosclerosis 1983;3:149-59.
5. Steinbrecher UP, Parthasarathy S, Leake DS, Witztum JL, Steinberg D. Modification of low density lipoprotein by endothelial cells involves lipid peroxidation and degradation of low density lipoprotein phospholipids. Proc Natl Acad Sci USA 1984;81:3883-87.
6. Morel DW, DiCorleto PE, Chisolm GM. Endothelial and smooth muscle cells alter low density lipoprotein in vitro by free radical oxidation. Arteriosclerosis 1984;4:357-64.
7. Pitas RE. Expression of the acetyl low density lipoprotein receptor by rabbit fibroblasts and smooth muscle cells. Up-regulation by phorbol esters. J Biol Chem 1990;265:12722-27.
8. Pitas RE, Friera A, McGuire J, Dejager S. Further characterization of the acetyl LDL (scavenger) receptor expressed by rabbit smooth muscle cells and fibroblasts. Arterioscler Thromb 1992;12:1235-44.
9. Sparrow CP, Parthasarathy S, Steinberg D. A macrophage receptor that recognizes oxidized low density lipoprotein but not acetylated low density lipoprotein. J Biol Chem 1989;264: 2599-604.
10. Khoo JC, Miller E, McLoughlin P, Steinberg D. Enhanced macrophage uptake of low density lipoprotein after self-aggregation. Arteriosclerosis 1988;8:348-58.
11. Heinecke JW, Suits AG, Aviram M, Chait A. Phagocytosis of lipase-aggregated low density lipoprotein promotes macrophage foam cell formation. Sequential morphological and biochemical events. Arterioscler Thromb 1991;11:1643-51.
12. Nievelstein PF, Fogelman AM, Mottino G, Frank JS. Lipid accumulation in rabbit aortic intima 2 hours after bolus infusion of low density lipoprotein. A deep-etch and immunolocalization study of ultrarapidly frozen tissue. Arterioscler Thromb 1991;11:1795-1805.
13. Quinn MT, Parthasarathy S, Fong LG, Steinberg D. Oxidatively modified low density lipoproteins: A potential role in recruitment and retention of monocyte/macrophages during atherogenesis. Proc Natl Acad Sci USA 1987;84:2995-98.
14. McMurray HF, Parthasarathy S, Steinberg D. Oxidatively modified low density lipoprotein is a chemoattractant for human T lymphocytes. J Clin Invest 1993;92:1004-1008.
15. Quinn MT, Parthasarathy S, Steinberg D. Lysophosphatidylcholine: A chemotactic factor for human monocytes and its potential role in atherogenesis. Proc Natl Acad Sci USA 1988;85: 2805-2809.
16. Berliner JA, Schwartz DS, Territo MC, et al. Induction of chemotactic cytokines by minimally

oxidized LDL. Adv Exp Med Biol 1993;351:13-18.
17. Cushing SD, Berliner JA, Valente AJ, et al. Minimally modified low density lipoprotein induces monocyte chemotactic protein 1 in human endothelial cells and smooth muscle cells. Proc Natl Acad Sci USA 1990;87:5134-38.
18. Rajavashisth TB, Andalibi A, Territo MC, et al. Induction of endothelial cell expression of granulocyte and macrophage colony-stimulating factors by modified low-density lipoproteins. Nature 1990;344:254-57.
19. Kugiyama K, Kerns SA, Morrisett JD, Roberts R, Henry PD. Impairment of endothelium-dependent arterial relaxation by lysolecithin in modified low-density lipoproteins. Nature 1990;344:160-62.
20. Harrison DG, Ohara Y. Physiologic consequences of increased vascular oxidant stresses in hypercholesterolemia and atherosclerosis: Implications for impaired vasomotion [see comments]. Am J Cardiol 1995;75:75B-81B.
21. Anderson TJ, Meredith IT, Yeung AC, Frei B, Selwyn AP, Ganz P. The effect of cholesterol-lowering and antioxidant therapy on endothelium-dependent coronary vasomotion [see comments]. N Engl J Med 1995;332:488-93.
22. Fruebis J, Steinberg D, Dresel HA, Carew TE. A comparison of the antiatherogenic effects of probucol and of a structural analogue of probucol in low density lipoprotein receptor-deficient rabbits. J Clin Invest 1994;94:392-98.
23. Carew TE, Schwenke DC, Steinberg D. Antiatherogenic effect of probucol unrelated to its hypocholesterolemic effect: Evidence that antioxidants in vivo can selectively inhibit low density lipoprotein degradation in macrophage-rich fatty streaks and slow the progression of atherosclerosis in the Watanabe heritable hyperlipidemic rabbit. Proc Natl Acad Sci USA 1987;84:7725-29.
24. Kodama T, Reddy P, Kishimoto C, Krieger M. Purification and characterization of a bovine acetyl low density lipoprotein receptor. Proc Natl Acad Sci USA 1988;85:9238-42.
25. Kodama T, Freeman M, Rohrer L, Zabrecky J, Matsudaira P, Krieger M. Type I macrophage scavenger receptor contains alpha-helical and collagen-like coiled coils. Nature 1990;343:531-35.
26. Endemann G, Stanton LW, Madden KS, Bryant CM, White RT, Protter AA. CD36 is a receptor for oxidized low density lipoprotein. J Biol Chem 1993;268:11811-16.
27. Nicholson AC, Frieda S, Pearce A, Silverstein RL. Oxidized LDL binds to CD36 on human monocyte-derived macrophages and transfected cell lines. Evidence implicating the lipid moiety of the lipoprotein as the binding site. Arterioscler Thromb Vasc Biol 1995;15:269-75.
28. Nozaki S, Kashiwagi H, Yamashita S, et al. Reduced uptake of oxidized low density lipoproteins in monocyte-derived macrophages from CD36-deficient subjects. J Clin Invest 1995;96:1859-65.
29. Ottnad E, Parthasarathy S, Sambrano GR, et al.. A macrophage receptor for oxidized low density lipoprotein distinct from the receptor for acetyl low density lipoprotein: partial purification and role in recognition of oxidatively damaged cells. Proc Natl Acad Sci USA 1995;92:1391-95.
30. Ramprasad MP, Fischer W, Witztum JL, Sambrano GR, Quehenberger O, Steinberg D. The 94- to 97-kDa mouse macrophage membrane protein that recognizes oxidized low density lipoprotein and phosphatidylserine-rich liposomes is identical to macrosialin, the mouse homologue of human CD68. Proc Natl Acad Sci USA 1995;92:9580-84.
31. Smith MJ, Koch GL. Differential expression of murine macrophage surface glycoprotein antigens in intracellular membranes. J Cell Sci 1987;87:113-19.

32. Rabinowitz SS, Gordon S. Macrosialin, a macrophage-restricted membrane sialoprotein differentially glycosylated in response to inflammatory stimuli [published erratum appears in J Exp Med 1992 Jan 1;175(1):309]. J Exp Med 1991;174:827-36.
33. Holness CL, da Silva RP, Fawcett J, Gordon S, Simmons DL. Macrosialin, a mouse macrophage-restricted glycoprotein, is a member of the lamp/lgp family. J Biol Chem 1993; 268:9661-66.
34. Rabinowitz S, Horstmann H, Gordon S, Griffiths G. Immunocytochemical characterization of the endocytic and phagolysosomal compartments in peritoneal macrophages. J Cell Biol 1992;116:95-112.
35. Lippincott-Schwartz J, Fambrough DM. Cycling of the integral membrane glycoprotein, LEP100, between plasma membrane and lysosomes: Kinetic and morphological analysis. Cell 1987;49:669-77.
36. Fukuda M. Lysosomal membrane glycoproteins. Structure, biosynthesis, and intracellular trafficking. J Biol Chem 1991;266:21327-30.
37. Stanton LW, White RT, Bryant CM, Protter AA, Endemann G. A macrophage Fc receptor for IgG is also a receptor for oxidized low density lipoprotein. J Biol Chem 1992;267:22446-51.
38. Sambrano GR, Parthasarathy S, Steinberg D. Recognition of oxidatively damaged erythrocytes by a macrophage receptor with specificity for oxidized low density lipoprotein. Proc Natl Acad Sci USA 1994;91:3265-69.
39. Acton SL, Scherer PE, Lodish HF, Krieger M. Expression cloning of SR-BI, a CD36-related class B scavenger receptor. J Biol Chem 1994;269:21003-21009.
40. Calvo D, Vega MA. Identification, primary structure, and distribution of CLA-1, a novel member of the CD36/LIMPII gene family. J Biol Chem 1993;268:18929-35.
41. Acton S, Rigotti A, Landschulz KT, Xu S, Hobbs HH, Krieger M. Identification of scavenger receptor SR-BI as a high density lipoprotein receptor [see comments]. Science 1996;271:518-20.
42. Steinberg D. A docking receptor for HDL cholesterol esters [comment]. Science 1996;271: 460-61.
43. Green S, Steinberg D, Quehenberger O. Cloning and expression in Xenopus oocytes of a mouse homologue of the human acylcoenzyme A:cholesterol acyltransferase and its potential role in metabolism of oxidized LDL. Biochem Biophys Res Comm 1996;218:924-29.
44. Abrams JM, Lux A, Steller H, Krieger M. Macrophages in drosophila embryos and L2 cells exhibit scavenger receptor-mediated endocytosis. Proc Natl Acad Sci USA 1992;89:10375-79.
45. Sambrano GR, Steinberg D. Recognition of oxidatively damaged and apoptotic cells by an oxidized low density lipoprotein receptor on mouse peritoneal macrophages: Role of membrane phosphatidylserine. Proc Natl Acad Sci USA 1995;92:1396-400.
46. Schroit AJ, Tanaka Y, Madsen J, Fidler IJ. The recognition of red blood cells by macrophages: Role of phosphatidylserine and possible implications of membrane phospholipid asymmetry. Biol Cell 1984;51:227-38.
47. Schlegel RA, Prendergast TW, Williamson P. Membrane phospholipid asymmetry as a factor in erythrocyte-endothelial cell interactions. J Cell Physiol 1985;123:215-18.
48. Hall SE, Savill JS, Henson PM, Haslett C. Apoptotic neutrophils are phagocytosed by fibroblasts with participation of the fibroblast vitronectin receptor and involvement of a mannose/fucose-specific lectin. J Immunol 1994;153:3218-27.
49. Fadok VA, Savill JS, Haslett C, et al. Different populations of macrophages use either the vitronectin receptor or the phosphatidylserine receptor to recognize and remove apoptotic

cells. J Immunol 1992;149:4029-35.
50. Savill J, Fadok V, Henson P, Haslett C. Phagocyte recognition of cells undergoing apoptosis. Immunol Today 1993;14:131-36.
51. Constantinides P. Experimental Atherosclerosis. Amsterdam: Elsevier, 1965:1p.
52. Davies MJ. Anatomic features in victims of sudden coronary death. Coronary artery pathology. Circulation 1992;85:I19-24.
53. Libby P. Molecular bases of the acute coronary syndromes. Circulation 1995;91:2844-50.
54. Kita T, Nagano Y, Yokode M, et al. Probucol prevents the progression of atherosclerosis in Watanabe heritable hyperlipidemic rabbit, an animal model for familial hypercholesterolemia. Proc Natl Acad Sci USA 1987;84:5928-31.
55. Mao S, Yates MT, Rechtin AE, Jackson RL, Sickle WA. Antioxidant activity of probucol and its analogues in hypercholesterolemic watanabe rabbits. J Med Chem 1991;34:298-302.
56. Daugherty A, Zweifel BS, Schonfeld G. The effects of probucol on the progression of atherosclerosis in mature watanabe heritable hyperlipidaemic rabbits. Br J Pharmacol 1991; 103:1013-18.
57. Morel DW, de la Llera-Moya M, Friday K. Treatment of cholesterol-fed rabbits with dietary vitamins E and C inhibits lipoprotein oxidation but not development of atherosclerosis. Am Inst Nutri 1994;2123-30.
58. Mao S, Yates M, Parker R, Chi E, Jackson R. Attenuation of atherosclerosis in a modified strain of hypercholesterolemic watanabe rabbits with use of a probucol analogue (MDL 29,311) that does not lower serum cholesterol. Arterio and Thromb 1991;11:1266-75.
59. Stein Y, Stein O, Delplanque B, Fesmire JD, Lee DM, Alaupovic P. Lack of effect of probucol on atheroma formation in cholesterol-fed rabbits kept at comparable plasma cholesterol levels. Atherosclerosis 1989;75:145-55.
60. Daugherty A, Zweifel BS, Schonfeld G. Probucol attenuates the development of aortic atherosclerosis in cholesterol-fed rabbits. Br J Pharmacol 1989;98:612-18.
61. Prasad K, Kalra J, Lee P. Oxygen free radicals as a mechanism of hypercholesterolemic atherosclerosis: Effects of probucol. International J Angiology 1994;3:100-12.
62. Sparrow CP, Doebber TW, Olszewski J. Low density lipoprotein is protected from oxidation and the progression of atherosclerosis is slowed in cholesterol-fed rabbits by the antioxidant N,N'-diphenyl-phenylenediamine. J Clin Invest 1992;89:1855-91.
63. Björkhem I, Henriksson-Freyschuss A, Breuer O, Diczfalusy U, Berglund L, Henriksson P. The antioxidant butylated hydroxytoluene protects against atherosclerosis. Arterio and Thromb 1991;11:15-22.
64. Prasad K, Kalra J. Oxygen free radicals and hypercholesterolemic atherosclerosis: Effect of vitamin E. Am Heart Journal 1993;125:958-73.
65. Kleinveld HA, Hak-Lemmers H, Hectors M, de Fouw NJ, Demacker P, Stalenhoef A. Vitamin E and fatty acid intervention does not attenuate the progression of atherosclerosis in watanabe heritable hyperlipidemic rabbits. Arterio Thromb and Vasc Biol 1995;15:290-97.
66. Fruebis J, Carew TE, Palinski W. Effect of vitamin E on atherogenesis in LDL receptor-deficient rabbits. Atherosclerosis 1995;117:217-24.
67. Parker RA, Sabrah T, Cap M, Gill BT. Relation of vascular oxidative stress, a-Tocopherol, and hypercholesterolemia to early atherosclerosis in hamsters. Arterio, Thromb and Vasc Biol 1995;15:349-58.
68. Tangirala RK, Casanada F, Miller E, Witztum JL, Steinberg D, Palinski W. Effect of the antioxidant N,N'-Diphenyl 1,4-Phenylenediamine (DPPD) on atherosclerosis in apoE-deficient mice. Aterio,Thromb and Vasc Biol 1995;15:1625-30.

69. Sasahara M, Raines EW, Chait A, et al. Inhibition of hypercholesterolemia-induced atherosclerosis in the nonhuman primate by probucol. I. Is the extent of atherosclerosis related to resistance of LDL to oxidation? J Clin Invest 1994;94:155-64.
70. Verlangieri AJ, Bush MJ. Effects of d-a-tocopherol supplementation on experimentally induced primate atherosclerosis. J Am Coll Nutri 1992;11:131-38.

DRUGS PROTECTING THE ARTERIAL WALL

Franco Bernini*, Alberto Corsini, Stefano Bellosta, Elena Donetti, Maurizio Soma, and Rodolfo Paoletti
Institute of Pharmacology and Pharmacognosy, University of Parma, Via delle Scienze, 43100 Parma, Italy and Institute of Pharmacological Sciences, University of Milan, Via Balzaretti 9, 20133 Milan, Italy

Introduction

Two key events in the atherogenic cascade are the deposition of lipids, mainly cholesterol esters, and migration and proliferation of arterial smooth muscle cells (SMC) [1-5].

Migration and proliferation of arterial myocytes are a second key prerequisite process leading to vascular occlusion in both atherosclerosis and restenosis after angioplasty [4]. Animal models of vascular injury have shown that an arterial lesion is followed by proliferation of the medial SMC, many of which migrate to the intima and further proliferate to form a neointimal lesion [2,6]. Recent findings have elucidated that SMC constitute approximately 90-95% of the cellular component of an atherosclerotic lesion in a young adult and an average of 50% of advanced atherosclerotic plaque [1,5,7]. In addition, vascular myocytes contribute to the lesion by synthesis of extracellular matrix and can accumulate lipids and become foam cells [5,8,9]. Accumulation of cholesterol within the vessel wall appears to be a consequence of an imbalanced cholesterol influx-efflux. There is compelling evidence supporting the concept that the lipids deposited in the atherosclerotic lesions are mostly derived from modified LDL [1,2,10-12]. Macrophages are the main lipid-loaded cells in the lesion. The mechanism by which they accumulate lipoprotein cholesterol and develop into foam cells depends mainly on receptor-mediated processes, involving the so-called "scavenger receptor" that recognizes chemically and biologically modified low density lipoprotein (LDL), such as acetyl LDL and oxidized LDL [13,14]. The scavenger receptor, unlike the LDL receptor, escapes feed-back regulation, and the result is a massive accumulation of cholesterol in cells. This sterol accumulates in macrophages in esterified form by a process involving the enzyme acyl-coenzyme A-cholesterol acyltransferase (ACAT), which catalyzes cholesterol esterification in the cytoplasm [15].

Thus, the elucidation of the factors affecting all the above phenomena affords new entry points for selective interference and inhibition of the process of atherogenesis.

Several drugs are able to antagonize or prevent the first stages of lesion formation, among them calcium antagonists and vastatins, the well-known plasma lipid (LDL) lowering

A. M. Gotto, Jr. et al. (eds.), Drugs Affecting Lipid Metabolism, 17–26.

drugs, antioxidants, and angiotensin-converting enzyme (ACE) inhibitors.

Direct Arterial Effect of Calcium Antagonists

The calcium antagonists show several important antiatherosclerotic activities *in vitro* and *in vivo*. In *in vitro* models these drugs protect cells against cholesterol deposition and control their proliferation. In addition the matrix synthesis by SMC is reduced. In *in vivo* models calcium antagonists protect against lesions induced by cholesterol feeding, endothelial injury and experimental calcinosis [16].

The antiatherosclerotic effect of calcium antagonists does not involve a reduction of plasma cholesterol or blood pressure suggesting a direct effect on the arterial wall [16]. In a series of animal experiments the influence of calcium antagonists on calcium deposition within the vessel wall and on the development of artificially induced atherosclerosis proved to be favorable [17-19]. While the efficacy of calcium antagonists as coronary and peripheral vascular dilators can be accounted for in terms of their inhibitory effects on calcium influx throughout the voltage-sensitive calcium channels, their ability to act as antiatherosclerotic agents is less understood. Several calcium-dependent processes contribute to the atherogenesis, including lipid infiltration and oxidation, endothelial injury, action of chemotactic and growth factors, and smooth muscle cell migration and proliferation.

An *in vivo* model for the study of SMC in the carotid walls of rabbits has been used in our laboratory. To characterize the antiatherogenic activity of the new calcium antagonist lacidipine, we studied the effect of this drug on the atherosclerotic response of the hypercholesterolemic rabbit carotid artery 14 days after perivascular manipulation of the vessel. This model, described by Booth et al. [20], allows direct following, *in vivo*, and independently of other factors, of the effect of a drug on arterial myocyte proliferation in normotensive hypercholesterolemic rabbits. The use of lacidipine, a lipophilic dihydropyridine, clearly indicates the possibility to use this, and similar, calcium antagonists as protective agents against lesions to the arterial walls (Table 1).

The availability of quantitative procedures to assess in man the thickening of the carotid arterial walls in pathological conditions, also opens the way for clinical studies leading to the protection of the carotid artery in the presence of one or more major risk factors and not only in hypertensive patients.

Calcium antagonists may also affect cellular cholesterol metabolism and deposition. Data from our laboratory indicate that lacidipine, like verapamil, inhibits the enzyme acylcoenzyme A-cholesterol acyltransferase (ACAT), and affects intracellular cholesterol homeostasis by preventing acetyl LDL-cholesterol esterification [21]. Nifedipine has no effect on cholesterol esterification in macrophages (Table 2). Verapamil is known to have a major effect on cellular lipid metabolism by inhibiting cholesterol hydrolysis in lysosomes [22]. This action indirectly reduces cholesterol esterification, but paradoxically leads to a reduction in the free-to-esterified cholesterol ratio, due to the accumulation in lysosomes of cholesterol esters transported by lipoproteins. In cells stimulated by 25-hydroxycholesterol [23], and in cholesteryl ester-preloaded cells, verapamil has less effect and becomes inactive in cell-free homogenate [24,25]. Data obtained in our laboratory indicate that this is not the case for lacidipine, which appears to act by directly inhibiting ACAT activity. Moreover, lacidipine may inhibit ACAT activity *in vivo* in rabbit aorta (Bernini et al., manuscript in preparation).

Table 1. Effect of lacidipine (3 mg/kg/day) on proliferative lesions induced by perivascular manipulation of hypercholesterolemic normotensive rabbit carotid arteries.

Treatment	I:M	SD	% of Control	p
Control	0.56	0.11	--	--
Sham	0.03	0.02	5	--
Lacidipine	0.32	0.10	57	0.01

I:M, intimal:medial tissues ratio; SD, standard deviation; p value, lacidipine versus control treatment. Data from [26].

Table 2. Effects of lacidipine, verapamil, and nifedipine on the cholesterol esterification in mouse peritoneal macrophages.

Drugs (μM)	[^{14}C]oleate Incorporation into Cholesteryl Ester (ng/mg cell protein x h)
Basal	54.9
Control + AcLDL (50 μg/ml)	1555.2
Lacidipine 50 + AcLDL	6.6
Verapamil 50 + AcLDL	10.2
Nifedipine 50 + AcLDL	1399.2

acLDL = acetyl low-density lipoproteins. Data from [21].

Direct Arterial Effects of Vastatins

The 3-hydroxy-3-methylglutaryl coenzyme A (HMG-CoA) reductase inhibitors (vastatins) are potent pharmacological agents that are active in reducing plasma total and LDL cholesterol levels in subjects with primary hypercholesterolemia [27,28]. Recent studies in animals and humans [28] have documented a reduction in the severity of arterial lesions and cardiovascular diseases after treatment with lovastatin or simvastatin. The anti-atherosclerotic effect of these drugs has been linked to their hypolipidemic properties [29-

31], suggesting that the hypolipidemic effect is the main mechanism for preventing the development of atherosclerosis.

A number of other effects, however, could be contributory to explain vastatins antiatherosclerotic properties. The increased understanding of the mechanisms of atherogenesis suggests several targets other than modifying the concentrations of circulating lipids [1-3,32]. Vastatins competitively inhibit intracellular synthesis of mevalonate, a precursor of nonsterol compounds (such as geranylgeraniol and farnesol) involved in several cell function and proliferation [33,34]. Hence it is conceivable that vastatins can directly affect major events occurring in the arterial wall during atherogenesis, independently of their lipid lowering effect. In our laboratory we utilized "*in vitro*" and "*in vivo*" models to investigate this possibility.

Our results demonstrate that treatment of cultured arterial myocytes with vastatins inhibits proliferation in a dose-dependent manner. This effect is overcome by simultaneous exposure of SMC to exogenous mevalonate (Table 3). One critical end product of mevalonate is cholesterol that, in proliferating cells, is required for cell membrane formation [35,36]. It is unlikely, however, that inhibition of cholesterol synthesis explains the actions of fluvastatin and simvastatin on SMC proliferation. In fact, cells were stimulated to growth by exposure to a medium containing 10% fetal calf serum which provides an exogenous source of cholesterol. Thus, inhibition of cell proliferation by vastatins likely resulted from inhibition of production of one or more isoprenoids intermediates of mevalonate metabolism. Recently, several proteins that are involved in growth factor signal transduction have been shown to be lipid-modified by the covalent attachment of mevalonate-derived isoprenoid group (prenylation) such as geranylgeraniol or farnesol [33,35,37-41]. Function and localization of these proteins are dependent on their covalent modification by these specific lipids [33,37-40,42]. Vastatins inhibit the biosynthesis of these two isoprenoids; one possible mechanism by which fluvastatin and simvastatin inhibit cell growth may be the interference with signaling pathways that require prenylated proteins. The fact that geranylgeraniol can, under these experimental conditions, partially prevent vastatin-induced inhibition of cell growth in the absence of other prenyl intermediates suggests that proteins modified by this isoprene (rather than, or in addition to, those that have been farnesylated) are responsible for inducing cell proliferation. The characterization of some of these proteins, such as nuclear lamin B [43], ras protein [44], and heterotrimeric and low molecular weight guanine nucleotide-binding proteins [45], provides new insights into the link between the mevalonate pathway, signal transduction, and cell cycle progression.

In our hands vastatins also inhibit fibrinogen-induced SMC migration suggesting a direct relationship between the mevalonate synthetic pathway and this cellular process (Table 4).

In accordance with "*in vitro*" observations, *in vivo* data showed that vastatins decreased neointimal proliferation in normocholesterolemic rabbits without affecting plasma cholesterol levels, albeit with different potencies.

Several vastatins have been tested in our laboratory in order to establish if they directly affect neointimal formation in the carotid arteries of normocholesterolemic rabbits independently of the lowering of plasma cholesterol concentration. For this purpose, we have used a scheme for the drug-treatment regimen that did not modify the plasma cholesterol level in normolipemic rabbits. Intimal thickening was induced by inserting a flexible extra-arterial collar around the common carotid artery.

Table 3. Ability of mevalonate and its derivatives to prevent cell growth inhibition by vastatins.

Addition	Concentration (μM)	Cells (% of control)
Simvastatin	3.5	27
Simvastatin + Mevalonate	10	50
	50	92
	100	100
Simvastatin + Farnesol	0.1	48
	1	58
	5	63
	10	87
Simvastatin + Geranylgeraniol	0.1	57
	1	64
	5	82
Simvastatin + Squalene	10	39
Fluvastatin	3.5	7
Fluvastatin + Mevalonate	100	99
Fluvastatin + Geranylgeraniol	5	73

Data are from [46,47].

Rabbits pretreated with vastatins, resulted in the inhibition of hyperplasia (Table 5) and in fewer layers of intimal cells. The inhibition of SMC proliferation induced by vastatins was totally abolished by local infusion of mevalonate.

We recently proposed the involvement of the mevalonate pathway on intracellular cholesterol homeostasis in macrophages [26]. Fluvastatin and simvastatin, inhibited cholesterol esterification induced by acetylated LDL in mouse peritoneal macrophages (Table 6). The evaluation of fluvastatin enantiomers demonstrated the stereospecificity of drug action, with most of the inhibitory effect associated to the antipode with the highest inhibitory activity on HMG-CoA reductase. Mevalonate and geranylgeraniol prevented the inhibitory effect of vastatins, further supporting the view that the effects of these drugs were due to their primary action on HMG-CoA reductase.

Table 4. Effect of vastatins on the fibrinogen-induced migration of rat aortic myocytes.

Addition	Concentration (μM)	SMC Migration (cells per HPF)
None	--	38.9 ± 4.1
Simvastatin	1	27.8 ± 3.2*
	2	23.3 ± 2.6**
	3	20.2 ± 1.5**
	5	8.0 ± 2.0**
Fluvastatin	1	23.6 ± 3.0**
	2	21.5 ± 4.1**
	3	15.2 ± 2.6**
	5	6.7 ± 2.0**

* $p < 0.05$; ** $p < 0.01$ (Student's t-test). Data are from [47].

Table 5. Effect of different vastatins on intimal thickening induced by perivascular manipulation of rabbit carotid arteries after 2 weeks.

Treatment	I/M (mean)	SD	Percent of Control	p
Positive Control	0.36	0.04	--	--
Sham	0.03	0.02	3	--
Lovastatin	0.24	0.03	67	0.001
Simvastatin	0.20	0.03	56	0.001
Fluvastatin	0.17	0.03	47	0.001

I/M, intimal/medial layer ratio; SD, standard deviation. Data are from [48].

Table 6. Effect of mevalonate and geranylgeraniol on the inhibition of cholesterol esterification induced by fluvastatin in murine macrophages.

Addition	[^{14}C]-oleate Incorporation into Cholesteryl Ester (pmol/mg cell protein x h)	Control (%)
AcLDL (50 μg/mL)	6537 ± 239	100
Fluvastatin 1 μM	3398 ± 109**	52
+ Mevalonate 10 μM	4576 ± 181**	70
+ Mevalonate 50 μM	5992 ± 230*	92
+ Mevalonate 100 μM	6340 ± 66	97
+ Geranylgeraniol 1 μM	3704 ± 162**	57
+ Geranylgeraniol 5 μM	4576 ± 68**	70
+ Geranylgeraniol 10 μM	6428 ± 126	98

* $p < 0.05$; ** $p < 0.001$ (Student's t-test). Data are from [49].

Consistent with their effect on cholesterol esterification, both simvastatin and fluvastatin, reduce cellular content of esterified as well as of total cholesterol. Our results show that HMG-CoA reductase inhibitors can inhibit, at least "*in vitro,*" the esterification of excess cholesterol delivered to macrophages by modified LDL through their primary action on HMG-CoA reductase activity and suggests that the mevalonate synthetic pathway may be involved in the control of this cellular event. This effect might contribute to the direct antiatherosclerotic activity of vastatins.

The inhibition of cholesterol esterification as well as the reduction of total cholesterol content of cell, as reported for fluvastatin and simvastatin, is a likely explanation for the reduction in macrophage area observed in atherosclerotic lesions of cholesterol-fed rabbits. The above preclinical studies indicate that even vastatins may act directly on the arterial walls.

In conclusion, calcium antagonists and HMG-CoA reductase inhibitors may exert a direct antiatherosclerotic effect on the arterial wall. This activity, which affects major processes involved in the formation of atherosclerotic lesions, is linked most probably to local effects and could translate into a more significant prevention of cardiovascular disease.

References

1. Wissler RW. Update on the pathogenesis of atherosclerosis. Am J Med 1991;91(1B):1B-3S-

1B-9S.
2. Ross R. The pathogenesis of atherosclerosis: A perspective for the 1990s. Nature 1993;362: 801-809.
3. Schwartz CJ, Valente AJ, Sprague EA. A modern view of atherogenesis. Am J Cardiol 1993; 71:9B-14B.
4. Ip JH, Fuster V, Badimon L, Badimon J, Taubman MB, Chesebro JH. Syndromes of accelerated atherosclerosis: Role of vascular injury and smooth muscle cell proliferation. J Am Coll Cardiol 1990;15:1667-87.
5. Katsuda S, Boyd HC, Fligner C, Ross R, Gown AM. Human Atherosclerosis. III. Immunocytochemical analysis of the cell composition of lesions of young adults. Am J Pathol 1992;140:907-14.
6. Clowes AW, Clowes MM, Fingerle J. Regulation of smooth muscle cell growth injured artery. J Cardiovasc Pharmacol 1989;14:S12-S15.
7. Wissler RW, Vesselinovitch D, Komatsu A. The contribution of studies of atherosclerotic lesions in young people to future research. Ann NY Acad Sci 1990;598:418-34.
8. Schwartz SM, Campbell GR, Campbell JH. Replication of smooth muscle cells in vascular disease. Circ Res 1986;58:427-44.
9. Stary HC, Chandler AB, Glagov S, et al. A definition of initial, fatty streak, and intermediate lesions of atherosclerosis. A report from the Committee on Vascular Lesions of the Council of Atherosclerosis, American Heart Association. Arterioscl Thromb 1994;14:840-56.
10. Badimon JJ, Fuster V, Chesebro JH, Badimon L. Coronary atherosclerosis. A multifactorial disease. Circulation 1993;87(II):II-3-II-16.
11. Brown MS, Goldstein JL. A receptor-mediated pathway for cholesterol homeostasis. Science 1986;232:34-47.
12. Steinberg D, Parthasarathy S, Carew T, Khoo J, Witztum J. Beyond cholesterol. Modifications of low-density lipoprotein that increase its atherogenicity. New Engl J Med 1989;320:915-24.
13. Brown MS, Goldstein JL. Lipoprotein metabolism in the macrophage: implications for cholesterol deposition in atherosclerosis. Ann Rev Biochem 1983;52:223-61.
14. Kurihara Y, Matsumoto A, Itakura H, Kodama T. Macrophage scavenger receptors. Curr Opin Lipidol 1991;2:295-300.
15. Brown MS, Ho YK, Goldstein JL. The cholesteryl ester cycle in macrophage from cells: continual hydrolysis and re-esterification of cytoplasmic cholesteryl esters. J Biol Chem 1980; 255:9344-52.
16. Raiteri M, Corsini A, Soma MR, et al. Antiatherosclerotic drugs: A critical assessment. In: Catapano AL, Gotto AM, Jr., Smith LC, Paoletti R, editors. Drugs Affecting Lipid Metabolism. Dordrecht, The Netherlands: Kluwer Academic Publishers, 1993:317-31.
17. Schmitz G, Hankovitz J, Kovacs EM. Cellular processes in atherogenesis: Potential targets of calcium channel blockers. Atherosclerosis 1991;88:109-32.
18. Fronek K. Calcium antagonists and experimental atherosclerosis. Cardiovasc Drug Rev 1990; 8:229-37.
19. Scheneider W, Kober G, Roebruck P, et al. Retardation of development and progression of coronary atherosclerosis: A new indication for calcium antagonists? Eur J Clin Pharmacol 1990;39:S17-S23.
20. Booth RGF, Martin JF, Honey AC, Hassall DG, Beesley JE, Moncada S. Rapid development of atherosclerotic lesions in the rabbit carotid artery induced by perivascular manipulation. Atherosclerosis 1989;76:257-68.
21. Bernini F, Corsini A, Raiteri M, Soma MR, Paoletti R. Effects of lacidipine on experimental

models of atherosclerosis. J Hypertens 1993;11(3):S61-S66.
22. Bernini F, Catapano AL, Corsini A, Fumagalli R, Paoletti R. Effects of calcium antagonists on lipids and atherosclerosis. Am J Cardiol 1989;64:129I-134I.
23. Brown MS, Dana SE, Goldstein JL. Cholesterol ester formation in cultured human fibroblasts. J Biol Chem 1975;250:4025-27.
24. Bernini F, Bellosta S, Didoni G, Fumagalli R. Calcium antagonists and cholesteryl ester metabolism in macrophages. J Cardiovasc Pharmacol 1991;18(10):S42-S45.
25. Stein O, Stein Y. Effect of verapamil on cholesteryl ester hydrolysis and reesterification in macrophages. Arteriosclerosis 1987;7:578-84.
26. Soma MR, Donetti E, Seregni R, et al. Effect of lacidipine on fatty and proliferative lesions induced in hypercholesterolemic rabbits. Br J Pharmacol 1996;117: in press.
27. Hunninghake DB. HMGCoA reductase inhibitors. Curr Opin Lipidol 1992;3:22-28.
28. Zhu BQ, Sievers RE, Sun YP, Isenberg WM, Parmley WW. Effect of lovastatin on suppression and regression of atherosclerosis in lipid-fed rabbits. J Cardiovasc Pharmacol 1992;19:246-55.
29. Kobayashi M, Ishida F, Takahashi T, et al. Preventive effect of MK-733 (simvastatin), an inhibitor of HMGCoA reductase, on hypercholesterolemia and atherosclerosis induced by cholesterol feeding in rabbits. Japan J Pharmacol 1989;49:125-33.
30. Blankenhorn DH. Blood lipids and human atherosclerosis regression: The angiographic evidence. Curr Opin Lipidol 1991;2:2324-29.
31. Watanabe Y, Ito T, Shiomi M, et al. Preventive effect of pravastatin sodium, a potent inhibitor of 3-hydroxy-3-methylglutaryl coenzyme A reductase, on coronary atherosclerosis and xanthoma in WHHL rabbits. Biochim Biophys Acta 1988;960:294-302.
32. Cleland JG, Krikler DM. Modification of atherosclerosis by agents that do not lower cholesterol. Br Heart J 1993;69:S54-S62.
33. Maltese WA. Posttranslational modification of proteins by isoprenoids in mammalian cells. FASEB J 1990;4:3319-28.
34. Habenicht AJR, Glomset JA, Ross R. Relation of cholesterol and mevalonic acid to the cell cycle in smooth muscle and Swiss 3T3 cells stimulated to divide by platelet-derived growth factor. J Biol Chem 1980;255:5134-40.
35. Goldstein JL, Brown MS. Regulation of the mevalonate pathway. Nature 1990;343:425-430.
36. Chen HW. Role of cholesterol metabolism in cell growth. Fedn Proc 1984;43:126-30.
37. Glomset JA, Gelb MH, Farnsworth CC. Prenyl proteins in eukaryotic cells: A new type of membrane anchor. TIBS 1990;15:139-42.
38. Sinensky M, Lutz RJ. The prenylation of proteins. Bioessays 1992;14:25-31.
39. Casey PJ. Biochemistry of protein prenylation. J Lipid Res 1992;33:1731-40.
40. Casey PJ, Moomaw JF, Zhang FL, Higgins JB, Thissen JA. Prenylation and G protein signaling. In: Anonymous Recent Progress in Hormone Research. Academic Press Inc., 1994:215.
41. Farnsworth CC, Gelb MH, Glomset JA. Identification of geranylgeranyl-modified proteins in HeLa cells. Science 1990;247:320-22.
42. Feussner G. HMG CoA reductase inhibitors. Curr Opin Lipidol 1994;5:59-68.
43. Farnsworth CC, Wolda SL, Gelb MH, Glomset JA. Human lamin B contains a farnesylated cysteine residue. J Biol Chem 1989;264:20422-29.
44. Casey PJ, Solsky PA, Der CJ, Buss JE. p21ras is modified by a farnesyl isoprenoid. Proc Natl Acad Sci USA 1989;86:8323-27.
45. Glomset JA, Farnsworth CC. Role of protein modification reactions in programming

interactions between ras-related GTPases and cell membranes. Ann Rev Cell Biol 1994;10: 181-205.

46. Corsini A, Mazzotti M, Raiteri M, et al. Relationship between mevalonate pathway and arterial myocyte proliferation: in vitro studies with inhibitors of HMG-CoA reductase. Atherosclerosis 1993;101:117-25.
47. Corsini A, Raiteri M, Soma MR, Bernini F, Fumagalli R, Paoletti R. Pathogenesis of atherosclerosis and the role of drug intervention: Focus on HMG-CoA reductase inhibitors. Am J Cardiol 1995;76:21A-28A.
48. Soma MR, Donetti E, Parolini C, et al. HMG CoA reductase inhibitors: In vivo effects on carotid intimal thickening in normocholesterolemic rabbits. Arterioscl Thromb 1993;13:571-78.
49. Bernini F, Didoni G, Bonfadini G, Bellosta S, Fumagalli R. Requirement for mevalonate in acetylated LDL induction of cholesterol esterification in macrophages. Atherosclerosis 1993; 104:19-26.

APOPTOSIS IN VASCULAR DISEASE: RELEVANCE AND REGULATION

Martin R Bennett
Unit of Cardiovascular Medicine, Department of Medicine, Addenbrooke's Hospital, Cambridge CB2 2QQ, United Kingdom

Introduction

Cell death has long been recognized within the vessel wall, in particular, in disease states such as atherosclerosis. Indeed, in humans, there is extensive pathological evidence of cell death in atherosclerotic plaques, with areas of obvious cell fragmentation and cell debris, particularly around the lipid core [1,2]. High rates of cell death are also evident in animal models of atherosclerosis, such as pigs fed a cholesterol-rich diet, particularly if accompanied by balloon catheter injury [3,4]. Traditionally, cell death has been considered to be due to a toxic insult, for example, as a reaction to free radical generation or oxidized lipids. However, more recently, death in cells of the vessel wall has been shown to occur by apoptosis [5-9], a mode of death considered to be more highly regulated or programmed. This short review attempts to outline some current concepts regarding apoptotic cell death, and its relevance and regulation in vascular disease.

Apoptosis, Necrosis, and Programmed Cell Death

For the purposes of consistency, it is important to define what we mean by each of the terms, apoptosis, necrosis, and programmed cell death. Apoptosis defines a type of cell death distinct from necrosis on the basis of characteristic morphological features. Specifically, these features are condensation of nuclear chromatin, at first around the inner face of the nuclear membrane, and then clumping of the chromatin; loss of cell-cell contact with cell shrinkage; fragmentation of the cell with formation of membrane-bound processes and vesicles containing fragments of nuclear material or organelles, which then become apoptotic bodies, and, in some instances, are phagocytosed by adjacent cells. The whole process occurs with minimal disruption of membrane integrity, or release of lysosomal enzymes, with consequently little inflammatory reaction. In addition, organelle structure and function appear to be maintained until late into the process.

In contrast, necrosis actually describes the morphological stigmata of a cell when it has passed the point of no return, i.e. when it has committed to die. However, the more common usage of the term necrosis now, in particular in contradistinction to an apoptotic

A. M. Gotto, Jr. et al. (eds.), Drugs Affecting Lipid Metabolism, 27–34.

mode of cell death, is to describe cell death characterized by cell swelling without the chromatin condensation seen in apoptosis, organelle dysfunction early in the process, loss of membrane integrity, and release of lysosomal enzymes with consequent inflammation. Apoptosis can also be distinguished from necrosis by typical electrophoresis patterns of DNA. Apoptosis is frequently associated with the activation of a nonlysosomal Ca^{2+}, Mg^{2+}-dependent endonuclease [10], which cleaves DNA into high molecular fragments at first, and then later into oligonucleosomal fragments of 180 bp. In contrast, DNA fragmentation in necrotic death is random, and appears as a smear of genomic DNA on a gel.

Although the terms are frequently used synonymously, programmed cell death and apoptosis are not interchangeable. Programmed cell death has been used in the literature to describe death in at least three different situations: (1)Cell death occurring at defined times in embryogenesis. This is clearly "physiological" cell death and initiated by a specific genetic program. (2) Cell death occurring in adult organisms during regression of a variety of hyperplastic tissues, in particular, the hormone-dependent regression of breast or uterine tissues. Death in this instance is also a physiological response, but the factor triggering death may be intrinsic or exogenous, for example removal of a trophic stimulus. (3) Cell death occurring after application of a noxious stimulus, whether it be physical chemical or biological, or occurring in a pathological tissue as a result of the disease process. Clearly, cell death under these circumstances is not physiological, or "programmed," as death is a response to the stimulus. However, although the trigger to cell death occurring in all three instances may be different, death may occur via the same morphological pattern, and by using the same pathway. While death occurring in a programmed fashion is frequently by apoptosis, this is not always the case [11].

Although we can define apoptosis and necrosis by morphological criteria, and this is probably the most discriminative method, the boundaries between the modes of cell death frequently become blurred, and there is evidence that the same stimulus can induce both morphological forms at different concentrations, (see [12] for example), or even simultaneously, and features of necrosis may be the end-product of an apoptotic mode of death seen earlier in the time-course of death [13]. The simultaneous occurrence of both forms of cell death, or the occurrence of both forms at different time-points after the same stimulus, has meant that it is most important to have a biochemical marker for apoptosis which is not seen in necrosis. Unfortunately, no such marker exists. The early identification of genes activated in apoptosis such as TRPM-2/SGP-2, polyubiquitin, TGF beta-1, c-*fos*, c-*myc*, or transglutaminase lead to the idea that expression of a single gene product could be used a marker for apoptosis. However, although individual genes are activated in some cell types following some stimuli, there is no consistency between cell types, or even within the same cell type following a different inducer of apoptosis. Potentially of more use is the identification that cleavage of a specific substrate, poly(ADP-ribose)polymerase (PARP) may be a marker for apoptotic death [14-16], particularly if, as has been proposed, the enzymes mediating the cleavage are conserved as part of a final common path of all apoptotic deaths. Whether all apoptosis is accompanied by PARP cleavage, and whether PARP cleavage only occurs in apoptosis has not yet been established however.

There are of course, other methods for detecting apoptosis. One of the early criteria which defined this form of cell death was that it was dependent upon new protein synthesis, and new gene transcription. However, this is again not universally found, and frequently inhibitors of protein synthesis induce apoptosis, implying that apoptosis in some tissues is dependent upon a labile inhibitor. For example, the apoptosis induced by a serine protease isolated from cytotoxic granules of natural killer cells is not inhibited by cycloheximide [17] and apoptosis can actually be induced by both actinomycin D and cycloheximide in HL-60 cells [18]. In fact, the emerging picture is that apoptosis is regulated by the interactions of many pro- and antiapoptotic gene products simultaneously, and whether a cell undergoes apoptosis or not upon inhibition of protein synthesis or new gene transcription depends upon the relative concentrations of each agent, the presence of trophic or survival factors, and cell-cell relationships (see [19] for review). Thus, inhibition of protein synthesis in any one cell type may promote or inhibit apoptosis dependent upon the expression and half life of the gene products critical for death of that cell type.

Apoptosis in Animal Models of Vascular Disease and Atherosclerosis

There have been a number of recent reports of apoptosis in cells of the vessel wall, in both animal models and in specimens from human atheromatous plaques and normal vessels [7-9,20]. In summary, these studies have shown cells to be present in the ballooned rat and mouse carotid artery model of injury that stain positive in the terminal UTP nick end-labelling (TUNEL) reaction (a measure of DNA breaks), have suggestive electron microscopic features of apoptosis, and bright nuclear staining with propidium iodide. Similarly, cells with the same characteristics have been demonstrated in atherectomy tissues from human plaques, and to a lesser extent from normal human vessels, and appear to be both macrophages and vascular smooth muscle cells (VSMCs). Apoptosis of human VSMCs derived from both atheromatous plaques and normal vessels has also been demonstrated *in vitro* [6,21]. However, while this data indicates that apoptosis occurs in the atherosclerotic plaque *in vivo*, and the ability to undergo this form of cell death is maintained *in vitro*, does it tell us any more? In particular, does the fact that death of cells in the vessel wall occurs via an apoptotic morphology indicate the stimulus to cell death, or the genetic pathway by which cells die, or even whether the death is "programmed"or in some way physiological?

Although atherosclerosis is undoubtedly a pathological process, cell death in atherosclerosis may still perform a physiological role. In many tissues, apoptosis is seen as an inevitable accompaniment to cell proliferation, as a method of maintaining cell number and tissue architecture [22]. Although the role of cell proliferation in atherosclerosis is controversial [23-25], apoptosis may be seen as the counterpoint to cell proliferation in this situation. Indeed, Virchow's original description of atherosclerosis described the process as depending upon first the replication of cells in the plaque and then the death of these same cells: "Thus, we have here an active process which really produces new tissues, but then hurries on to destruction in consequence of its own development." Thus, the presence of cell death in the plaque may be part of a tissue response in an attempt to maintain cell number or architecture [26].

More difficult to establish is the mechanism of cell death of VSMCs and macrophages in atherosclerotic plaques. A multitude of stimuli have been identified which induce apoptosis, initiating the death of specific cells. These include cytokines such as TGF-β, TNF-α, IFN-λ, IL-1 etc., which are all present in atherosclerotic plaques, and receptors such as the Fas ligand. These cytokines or receptors converge on second messenger pathways to mediate apoptosis in a manner similar to those signalling cell proliferation, and frequently the same signalling pathways signal both processes. Similarly, many of the down-stream gene products which regulate apoptosis, such as proto-oncogenes and tumour suppressor genes, are mediators of both apoptosis and cell proliferation (see [19,27] for reviews). Although much of the signalling pathways leading to apoptosis are not yet characterized, some of the mediators of apoptosis of VSMCs are known, at least *in vitro*.

Genes Regulating Apoptosis of VSMCs

Apoptosis of VSMCs can be promoted by deregulated expression of the proto-oncogene c-*myc* [5,28]. c-Myc at physiological levels is capable of inducing apoptosis of VSMCs, and overexpression of the gene product is not required [5]. For example, cells expressing constant levels of c-*myc* undergo apoptosis upon removal of serum from the culture conditions, a situation in which c-*myc* expression is normally rapidly shut off in VSMCs [29]. Thus the signal for apoptosis is the inability to suppress c-*myc* expression upon removal of survival factors, or upon induction of growth arrest [5]. The same part of the c-*myc* protein which promotes proliferation also promotes apoptosis [5,30], and this function of c-*myc* is seen as requiring dimerization with Max and DNA binding [30]. Thus constant expression of c-*myc* drives both proliferation and apoptosis simultaneously, and growth arrest is not required for apoptosis of VSMCs [31]. Indeed, apoptosis induced by c-*myc* occurs in all phases of the cell cycle [32].

How c-*myc* induces apoptosis of VSMCs is unknown. Some studies have found that induction of c-*myc* target genes are necessary for apoptosis [33], but few c-*myc* target genes have been identified. However, we have recently demonstrated that c-*myc*-induced apoptosis of VSMCs may be regulated by p53 [28]. Coexpression of mutant p53 (which sequesters wild type p53 function) suppresses c-*myc*-induced apoptosis, and conversely, overexpression of wild-type p53 augments c-*myc* action. Whether c-*myc* -induced death is actually dependent upon p53 is more difficult to establish, and will await the results of studies performed on p53 null animals. C-*myc*-induced death can also be blocked by co-expression of the proto-oncogene *bcl*-2, which can also prevent apoptosis of normal VSMCs in low serum, both human and rat [6,28]. Whether *bcl*-2, or *bcl*-2 family members (of which there are an increasing number) regulate apoptosis of VSMCs *in vivo* is more debatable. VSMCs express low levels of *bcl*-2 *in vitro* and *in vivo* [6,28,34], although this is not universally found [7,35], but only when *bcl*-2 was overexpressed could effects on VSMC apoptosis be demonstrated [6,28].

Survival Cytokines

Another key regulator of apoptosis of VSMCs appears to be the presence of survival cytokines. Many cell types require the constant presence of survival factors to prevent apoptosis. Examples include serum-deprived fibroblasts [36], FGF-deprived endothelial cells [37-38], cytokine-deprived T-lymphocytes [39], IL-6-deprived M1 leukaemia cell lines [40], and neurotropic growth factor-deprived neurones in the developing embryo [22]. VSMCs cultured in low serum undergo apoptosis, which can be partially prevented by the presence of IGF-1 and, to a lesser extent, PDGF [6,32]. These agents do not act as mitogens under these circumstances. Indeed, IGF-1 is a very weak mitogen of VSMCs, and VSMCs which do not require PDGF to undergo mitosis (for example, VSMCs expressing deregulated c-*myc*) are still rescued frcm apoptosis by provision of this cytokine [32]. The same concentrations of each agent which promote proliferation also protect against apoptosis [6], but the relative efficacies of the two actions, and the ability to protect against death when cells no longer require the agent for proliferation (i.e. postcommitment point) [32], argues that different signalling pathways exist for each agent to induce proliferation or protect against cell death. Although both IGF-1 and PDGF are present in the normal vessel wall and the atherosclerotic plaque, low concentrations of survival factors may induce apoptosis in the deeper regions of the plaque.

Role of Apoptosis in Vessel Wall Homeostasis

Like the mediators of apoptosis in the vessel wall, the role of apoptosis *in vivo* in the vessel is only speculative. There is increasing evidence that apoptosis is the method whereby endothelial cells are lost from the lumenal surface. Whether apoptosis plays a similar role in regulating vascular smooth muscle cell number physiologically is unknown. The identification that different mediators may regulate both proliferation and apoptosis simultaneously, and also differentially regulate both processes independently however, suggests a mechanism by which vessel wall mass can be maintained. Indeed, regulation of apoptosis *per se* may be responsible for changes in vessel wall mass irrespective of changes in rate of cell proliferation. In an elegant study using neonatal lambs, it has been recently shown that apoptotic rates govern VSMC number and vessel calibre during physiological arterial remodelling after changes in blood flow, and changes in apoptotic rates alone are sufficient to mediate profound changes in vessel wall mass, irrespective of changes in cell proliferation [41]. Presumably, remodelling during atherogenesis or in hypertension may also be mediated by coordinated action of cell proliferation and apoptotic cell death.

The role of apoptosis in the response to vessel injury, or in atherogenesis, is also unknown. So far, apoptotic VSMCs have been demonstrated in the ballooned rat and mouse carotid arteries after injury, particularly after 7-15 days, but is no longer present after re-endothelialization [9,20]. Similarly, apoptotic VSMCs and macrophages have been demonstrated in atherectomy specimens from human coronary and peripheral plaques, with a higher incidence of apoptosis in specimens from restenotic tissues, but apoptosis was also present to a lesser extent in nonatherosclerotic arteries [7-9]. While it is arguable how much apoptosis is occurring in atherogenesis, as the labelling indices in all three studies appear to be remarkably high in a tissue with little proliferative activity, evidence from these studies and unpublished data from many sources indicates that apoptosis is occurring in atherosclerotic plaques. One can speculate that apoptosis of VSMCs in critical regions of the plaque predisposes to plaque rupture and thus subsequent thrombosis, or that apoptosis of macrophages removes potentially damaging cells from the plaque, promoting plaque stability. In addition, apoptosis of VSMCs may occur in the profound changes in arterial calibre observed during atherogenesis, or in the atrophy of the media below a plaque. At present, we lack information on the location, frequency, and time-course of apoptosis in any of these pathological entities. However, the observation from animal studies of atherogenesis that rates of cell proliferation and cell death are regulated independently *in vivo* [3,4], and also *in vitro* [28] suggests that therapy aimed at cell death is potentially a very attractive target.

Conclusions

The most critical question still to be answered is the role of apoptosis in vessel wall homeostasis and disease. So far, the anatomical location of apoptotic cells within the plaque, the types of cells involved, or the disease entities in which apoptosis has been identified give no clue even as to whether apoptosis is promoting plaque stability or rupture. Furthermore, we lack good models of apoptosis in the vessel wall, with reproducible levels of VSMC apoptosis, in which we can test the *in vivo* activity of pro- or antiapoptotic cytokines or gene products. However, the prospect of mediators of apoptosis distinct from those regulating cell proliferation offer the prospect of controlling vessel wall mass via the direct induction or repression of apoptosis. While it unlikely the that VSMCs possess apoptotic machinery which is unique to these cells, local delivery of pro- or antiapoptotic molecules could profoundly regulate vessel wall architecture.

Acknowledgements

MRB is supported by a British Heart Foundation Clinical Scientist Research Fellowship.

References

1. Garratt KN, Edwards WD, Kaufmann UP, Vlietstra RE, Holmes DRJ. Differential histopathology of primary atherosclerotic and restenotic lesions in coronary arteries and saphenous vein bypass grafts: Analysis of tissue obtained from 73 patients by directional atherectomy. J Am Coll Cardiol 1991;17(2):442-48.
2. Arbustini E, Grasso M, Diegoli M, et al. Coronary atherosclerotic plaques with and without thrombus in ischemic heart syndromes: A morphologic, immunohisto-chemical, and biochemical study. Am J Cardiol 1991;68:36B-50B.
3. Thomas WA, Reiner JM, Florentin FA, Lee KT, Lee WM. Population dynamics of arterial smooth muscle cells. V. Cell proliferation and cell death during initial 3 months in atherosclerotic lesions induced in swine by hypercholesterolemic diet and intimal trauma. Exp

Mol Pathol 1976;24(3):360-74.
4. Thomas W, Kim D, Lee K, Reiner J, Schmee J. Population dynamics of arterial cells during atherogenesis. XIII. Mitogenic and cytotoxic effects of a hyperlipidaemic (HL) diet on cells in advanced lesions in the abdominal aortas of swine fed an HL diet for 270-345 days. Exp Mol Pathol 1983;39:257-70.
5. Bennett MR, Evan GI, Newby AC. Deregulated c-*myc* oncogene expression blocks vascular smooth muscle cell inhibition mediated by heparin, interferon-λ, mitogen depletion and cyclic nucleotide analogues and induces apoptotic cell death. Circ Res 1994;74:525-36.
6. Bennett MR, Evan GI, Schwartz SM. Apoptosis of human vascular smooth muscle cells derived from normal vessels and coronary atherosclerotic plaques. J Clin Invest 1995;95:2266-74.
7. Isner J, Kearney M, Bortman S, Passeri J. Apoptosis in human atherosclerosis and restenosis. Circulation 1995;91:2703-11.
8. Geng Y, Libby P. Evidence for apoptosis in advanced human atheroma: Colocalization with interleukin-1β converting enzyme. Am J Path 1995;147: 251-66.
9. Han D, Haudenschild C, Hong M, Tinkle B, Leon M, Liau G. Evidence for apoptosis in human atherosclerosis and in a rat vascular injury model. Am J Path 1995;147:267-77.
10. McConkey DJ, Hartzell P, Nicotera P, Orrenius S. Calcium-activated DNA fragmentation kills immature thymocytes. FASEB J 1989;3:1843-49.
11. Schwartz LM, Smith SW, Jones ME, Osborne BA. Do all programmed cell deaths occur via apoptosis? Proc Natl Acad Sci U S A 1993;90(3):980-84.
12. Dypbukt JM, Ankarcrona M, Burkitt M, et al. Different prooxidant levels stimulate growth, trigger apoptosis, or produce necrosis of insulin-secreting RINm5F cells. The role of intracellular polyamines. J Biol Chem 1994;269(48):30553-60.
13. Ledda-Columbano G, Coni P, Curto M, et al. Induction of two different modes of cell death, apoptosis and necrosis, in rat liver after a single dose of thioacetamide. Am J Path 1991;139:1099-1109.
14. Gu Y, Sarnecki C, Aldape R, Livingston D, Su M. Cleavage of poly(adp-ribose) polymerase by interleukin-1-beta converting-enzyme and its homologs TX and nedd-2. J Biol Chem 1995;270:18715-18.
15. Tewari M, Quan L, O' Rourke K, et al. Yama/cpp32-beta, a mammalian homolog of ced-3, is a crma-inhibitable protease that cleaves the death substrate poly(adp-ribose) polymerase. Cell 1995;81:801-809.
16. Nicholson D, Ali A, Thornberry N, et al. Identification and inhibition of the ICE/ced-3 protease necessary for mammalian apoptosis. Nature 1995;376:37-43.
17. Shi L, Kraut RP, Aebersold R, Greenberg AH. A natural killer cell granule protein that induces DNA fragmentation and apoptosis. J Exp Med 1992;175(2):553-66.
18. Martin SJ, Lennon SV, Bonham AM, Cotter TG. Induction of apoptosis (programmed cell death) in human leukemic HL-60 cells by inhibition of RNA or protein synthesis. J. Immunol. 1990;145(6):1859-67.
19. Bennett MR, Evan GI. The molecular basis of apoptosis. Heart Failure 1994;9:199-212.
20. Bochatonpiallat M, Gabbiani F, Redard M, Desmouliere A, Gabbiani G. Apoptosis participates in cellularity regulation during rat aortic intimal thickening. Am J Path 1995;146:1059-64.
21. Bjorkerud S, Bjorkerud B, Joelsson M. Structural organization of reconstituted human arterial smooth muscle tissue. Arterioscler Thromb 1994;14(4):644-51.
22. Raff MC. Social controls on cell survival and cell death. Nature 1992;356 (6368):397-400.

23. Strauss BH, Umans VA, van Suylen RJ, et al. Directional atherectomy for treatment of restenosis within coronary stents: Clinical, angiographic and histologic results. J Am Coll Cardiol 1992;20(7):1465-73.
24. Pickering JG, Weir L, Jekanowski J, Kearney MA, Isner JM. Proliferative activity in peripheral and coronary atherosclerotic plaque among patients undergoing percutaneous revascularization. J Clin Invest 1993;91(4):1469-80.
25. O'Brien ER, Alpers CE, Stewart DK, et al. Proliferation in primary and restenotic coronary atherectomy tissue. Implications for antiproliferative therapy. Circ Res 1993;73(2):223-31.
26. Virchow R. Cellular pathology as based upon physiological and pathological histology. vol ed 2. Birmingham, AL: Classics of Medicine Library, 1858:361.
27. Whyte M, Evan G. The last cut is the deepest. Nature 1995;376:17-18.
28. Bennett MR, Evan GI, Schwartz SM. Apoptosis of rat vascular smooth muscle cells is regulated by p53 dependent and independent pathways. Circ Res 1995;77: 266-73.
29. Bennett MR, Littlewood TD, Hancock DC, Evan GI, Newby AC. Downregulation of the c-*myc* proto-oncogene - a signal for vascular smooth muscle cell arrest? Biochem J 1994;302:701-709.
30. Amati B, Littlewood T, Evan G, Land H. The c-*myc* protein induces cell cycle progression and apoptosis through dimerisation with Max. 1993; in preparation.
31. Harrington E, Fanidi A, Evan G. Oncogenes and cell death. Curr Opin Genet Dev 1994;4:120-29.
32. Harrington EA, Bennett MR, Fanidi A, Evan GI. c-Myc induced apoptosis in fibroblasts is inhibited by specific cytokines. EMBO J 1994;13:3286-95.
33. Packham G, Cleveland JL. Ornithine decarboxylase is a mediator of c-Myc-induced apoptosis. Mol Cell Biol 1994;14(9):5741-47.
34. Hockenbery DM, Zutter M, Hickey W, Nahm M, Korsmeyer SJ. Bcl2 protein is topographically restricted in tissues characterized by apoptotic cell death. Proc Natl Acad Sci U S A 1991;88(16):6961-65.
35. Leszczynski D, Zhao Y, Luokkamaki M, Foegh ML. Apoptosis of vascular smooth muscle cells. Protein kinase C and oncoprotein Bcl-2 are involved in regulation of apoptosis in non-transformed rat vascular smooth muscle cells. Am J Pathol 1994; 145(6):1265-70.
36. Evan GI, Wyllie AH, Gilbert CS, et al. Induction of apoptosis in fibroblasts by c-*myc* protein. Cell 1992;69:119-128.
37. Araki S, Shimada Y, Kaji K, Hayashi H. Apoptosis of vascular endothelial cells by fibroblast growth factor deprivation. Biochem Biophys Res Commun 1990;168 (3):1194-200.
38. Araki S, Simada Y, Kaji K, Hayashi H. Role of protein kinase C in the inhibition by fibroblast growth factor of apoptosis in serum-depleted endothelial cells. Biochem Biophys Res Commun 1990;172(3):1081-85.
39. Migliorati G, Pagliacci C, Moraca R, Crocicchio F, Nicoletti I, Riccardi C. Interleukins modulate glucocorticoid-induced thymocyte apoptosis. Int J Clin Lab Res 1992;21(4):300-3.
40. Lotem J, Sachs L. Regulation of leukaemic cells by interleukin 6 and leukaemia inhibitory factor. Ciba Found Symp 1992;167:80-88.
41. Cho A, Courtman D, Langille L. Apoptosis (programmed cell death) in arteries of the neonatal lamb. Circ Res 1995;76:168-75.

MECHANISM OF ATHEROSCLEROTIC CALCIFICATION

Kristina Boström and Linda L. Demer
Division of Cardiology, UCLA School of Medicine, 10833 LeConte Ave., CHS 47-123, Los Angeles, California 90095, USA

Introduction

Arterial calcification associated with atherosclerosis has long been regarded as a progressive, passive end-stage process of questionable significance. This impression developed despite careful studies by early pathologists demonstrating that arterial calcification was a common phenomenon and contained several features suggesting an organized underlying mechanism. The common occurrence of arterial calcification has been confirmed by improved methods of detection, and its significance in clinical scenarios is becoming more apparent. Vascular calcification may microscopically appear as calcified, acellular mineral deposits or as foci of ectopic bone formation, known as ossification. The acellular, calcified matrix may be a precursor lesion to ossification. Subsets of cells from the artery media are capable of osteoblastic differentiation. These cells may be derived from multipotent mesenchymal cells and be one of many subsets capable of responding differently to a multitude of stimuli. Better understanding of medial artery wall cells and the steps leading to induction of artery wall calcification will provide us with better tools to control clinical calcification and its consequences.

Clinical Significance of Arterial Calcification

Development of improved methods to detect vascular calcification such as ultrafast computed tomography (CT) and intravascular ultrasound have made it possible to relate arterial calcification to clinical disease. Calcification is common. Ninety percent of patients with coronary artery disease have calcified lesions and 80% of clinically significant lesions are calcified [1]. Calcification is not only part of complex plaques in severe atherosclerosis but is a progressive process which begins as early as the second and third decades of life [2,3] and therefore may precede narrowing of vessels [4]. It has been identified as a strong positive predictive factor for clinically significant atherosclerosis, increasing the risk of death, ischemic heart disease including myocardial infarction and heart failure, systolic hypertension, and serious complications of interventional procedures and surgery [1,5-9].

The clinical consequences caused by arterial calcification may occur by several

A. M. Gotto, Jr. et al. (eds.), Drugs Affecting Lipid Metabolism, 35–42.

mechanisms. One is plaque rupture. Deposition of calcium mineral in the atherosclerotic plaque creates an interface between the calcium deposits and softer plaque elements where solid shear stress is highly concentrated [8,10,11]. During coronary angioplasty, plaque rupture occurs along this interface making coronary calcification the most important risk factor for plaque dissection. The same mechanism may account for spontaneous plaque rupture and would account for the increased risk of myocardial infarction and mortality in patients with coronary calcification [1,6].

Deposition of calcium mineral also increases aortic rigidity which may lead to significant cardiovascular consequences including ischemia, left ventricular hypertrophy, heart failure, and stroke [1,12-16]. Ischemia results from aortic rigidity; cardiac perfusion depends on diastolic coronary flow which depends on diastolic aortic pressure and reverse aortic flow. Calcification decreases the aortic compliance so that less blood volume is stored in the aorta at the start of diastole and less elastic recoil is generated to drive reverse flow to the coronaries. Therefore, coronary perfusion becomes significantly impaired [17] and the insufficient blood flow through the coronary inlets may lead to cardiac ischemia independent of coronary stenosis. Coronary insufficiency and ischemia have been reproduced in the absence of coronary stenosis, in animals with artificially imposed chronic aortic rigidity, but not controls [9]. Consequently, aortic calcification may aggravate ischemia, hypoxemia, and ventricular dysfunction resulting from myocardial infarction [6] as well as clinical coronary artery disease [18].

Heart failure, another severe consequence of aortic rigidity, develops as a result of the increased cardiac work necessary to overcome the increased outflow impedance in a calcified, rigid aorta [19]. In animal studies, aortic rigidity increases the energy cost to the heart for maintaining adequate flow, doubles the oxygen requirement for a given stroke volume, and limits reserve capacity [20]. Insertion of noncompliant grafts in patients with a subsequent acute increase in aortic rigidity, was found to produce left ventricular hypertrophy, systolic hypertension, diastolic hypotension, and decreased coronary flow. In some cases, this resulted in fatal heart failure which was attributed to loss of the "Windkessel effect," i.e. aortic compliance and elastic recoil [13]. The physiology of the Windkessel effect is comparable to aortic balloon counterpulsation used clinically to support cardiac function.

Aortic rigidity largely determines systolic blood pressure [21], and a calcified aorta will therefore increase the risk for systolic hypertension. Isolated systolic hypertension is a significant, independent risk factor for cardiovascular morbidity and mortality including stroke [22,23].

Compensatory arterial enlargement preserves vessel lumen in early atherosclerosis [1]. As the disease progresses, this process fails, and stenosis results. Calcification may be the limiting factor. Intravascular ultrasound imaging has revealed that calcified coronary segments are more likely to be stenotic, have less compensatory enlargement relative to plaque area and are more likely to require treatment [24]. Autopsy studies indicate that calcification nearly always colocalizes with atherosclerosis. However, when angiographic and ultrafast CT results are compared, coronary calcification often occurs in areas without any evidence of stenosis. This suggests that calcification precedes failure of compensatory enlargement, contrary to the impression that it is end-stage. If vascular calcification were prevented, and compensatory enlargement allowed to proceed indefinitely, stenosis and its clinical consequences might never occur.

Histopathology of Arterial Calcification

The pathology of atherosclerosis and vascular calcification was extensively studied in early atherosclerosis research [25,26]. Most commonly, vascular calcification was seen as a well-defined calcified matrix without any obvious bone architecture. However, it was soon recognized that in addition to these calcium mineral deposits, the artery wall is the most common site of ectopic ossification. True formation of osteoid and fully formed bone was described already in 1863 when Virchow described the mineral component in calcified arteries as "an ossification, and not a mere calcification; ... we see ossification declare itself in precisely the same manner as when an osteophyte forms on the surface of bone ... [1]". Following Virchow's report, several investigators reported similar findings. Extensive searches for bone formation in atherosclerotic vessels were made by Mönckeberg who reported ten positive cases of about 100 cases [26]. Poscharissky examined 31 vessels and found bone tissue in four of them [26]. Foci of bone formation were widespread and affected arteries included the aorta, the coronary arteries, the axillary artery and all the major arteries in the lower extremities.

Vascular calcification occurs in either intima or media. Ossification associated with atherosclerosis is usually found at the base of the atherosclerotic plaque, in the intima immediately adjacent to the luminal side of the fragmented internal elastic lamina. Intimal calcification may appear to be at the outer edge of the artery wall due to thinning of the media. Where bone tissue is well developed with distinct trabeculae, areas imitating marrow cavities may be present. Large, dilated capillaries, blood sinuses and in some cases, many cells of bone-marrow type may be encountered in these spaces (Figure 1), giving an impression of true red marrow. In other cases, the marrow cavities contain numerous fat cells imitating fatty bone marrow (Figure 2).

Similar to the foci of bone, foci of cartilage of embryonal type has also been encountered in calcified arteries. Such areas are made up of large polygonal or spheroidal cells, sometimes grouped with varying amounts of intercellular substance.

The calcified matrix appears to be intimately related to ossification; in fact, several of the early investigators interpreted calcified matrix together with "young connective tissue" to be a prerequisite for ossification [25,26]. It appeared to them that resorption of calcified matrix was an essential stage in the production of bone tissue which was usually accompanied by deposition of osteoid tissue, corresponding in extent and conformation to the areas previously occupied by calcification. They describe giant cells localized to concavities in the calcium mineral apparently engaged in resorbing. We have observed similar multinucleated osteoclast-like cells in calcified coronary artery specimens and it may be that these cells represent the link between calcification and ossification. Specific stimuli, such as the presence of calcium mineral may induce the formation of osteoclast-like cells that in turn induce differentiation of osteoblast precursors able to use the calcified matrix for formation of bone tissue. However, it remains to be determined if this connection is viable.

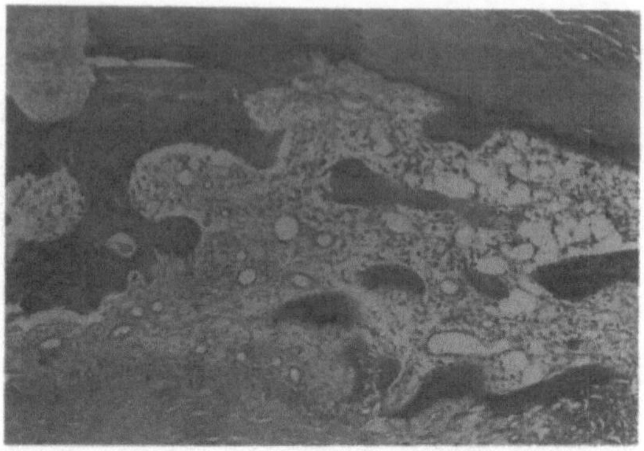

Figure 1: Human atherosclerotic plaque containing bone trabeculae and areas resembling red bone marrow.

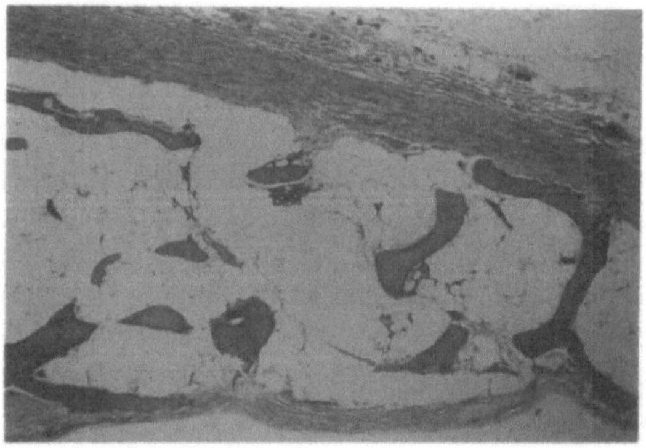

Figure 2: Human atherosclerotic plaque containing bone trabeculae and fat cells resembling fatty bone marrow.

Vascular Cells in Arterial Calcification

To account for the findings of multiple ectopic tissues in atherosclerotic arteries, we hypothesize that multipotent embryonic cells are present in the artery wall. Such cells may be capable of responding to different stimuli present in the atherosclerotic plaque and to start differention into the ectopic tissues found in the artery wall. It has already been proposed that developmental mechanisms are involved in arterial pathologic processes [27, 28]. Arterial calcification may be a very interesting example thereof. Embryonic osteogenesis occurs by one of two models: endochondral ossification or intramembranous ossification. In endochondral ossification, occurring in the growth plate of long bone and recurring in adult fracture repair, bone forms on and replaces a cartilage scaffold. In intramembranous ossification, bone replaces primitive connective tissue. Both models may be applicable to the artery wall where areas of endochondral ossification have been compared to the ossification front in long bones [25,26] and proliferation of dedifferentiated smooth muscle cells is part of the response to endothelial injury.

Several studies support the concept that progenitor cells for osteoblasts are undifferentiated mesenchymal cells residing in connective tissue or imported on microvessels [29]. Evidence suggests that osteoprogenitor cells in the artery wall are derived from the neural crest [30]. Multipotential neural crest cells migrate from along both sides of the notochord to anterior structures. During migration, they lose potential and each eventually commits to one of several mesenchymal lineages: pericytes, osteoblasts, chondroblasts, fibroblasts, smooth muscle cells, adipocytes, melanocytes, or neural cells. It has been postulated that some neural crest-derived cells retain multipotentiality in the adult [31,32].

Calcifying vascular cells (CVC), a subpopulation of adult aortic medial cells has been identified by our laboratory to undergo osteoblastic differentiation *in vitro* [33,34]. CVC share many feature with microvascular pericytes. Pericytes, but not endothelial cells, are derived from the neural crest [35]. They are believed to be immature mesenchymal progenitor cells located in the subendothelial basement membrane in microvessels. As with CVC, they form calcifying nodules *in vitro*, and they can differentiate into osteoblasts in the periosteum. Similarly, CVC may serve as progenitor cells in larger vessels *in vivo* and undergo osteoblastic differentiation in response to various stimuli such as injury of the endothelium or presence of vascular calcium deposits formed by other processes.

Epithelial cells induce mesenchymal differentiation through a coordinated, reciprocal expression of bone morphogenetic proteins (BMPs) when embryological calcified tissue is formed [36]. BMPs are potent osteogenic differentiation factors, that induce bone formation when injected into skeletal muscle *in vivo* [1]. They also mediate embryonic development of the thoracic aorta [37] and are chemotactic for monocytes *in vivo* [38]. It is possible that injured or altered vascular endothelial cells express BMPs which in turn would induce osteoblastic differentiation of underlying intimal and/or medial cells. Our previous finding of mRNA for BMP-2 in endarterectomy specimen by *in situ* hybridization is consistent with this hypothesis [33].

Bone mineral is formed extracellularly, not secreted by cells. The active aspect is the secretion of matrix vesicle and the specialized matrix, osteoid. Each provides a nidus for crystal formation at low calcium/phosphate concentrations, and factors in osteoid matrix regulate crystal growth. Osteoid calcifies ~10 days after secretion, at ~1 μ from the secretory cell. Both matrix vesicles and most components of osteoid have been demonstrated in human atherosclerosis [1,39] and in calcified human valves [40,41], including collagen I, matrix Gla protein, osteonectin, and osteocalcin [40,42-44]. Ossification appears to require microvascular invasion, which may explain its location at the lesion base near vasa vasorum ingrowth.

Conclusion

Multipotentiality in the artery wall is potentially a very important concept. Not only may this give an explanation for the mechanism of arterial calcification but it may also contribute to the understanding of major medical problems such as hypertension. It is possible that different cell populations exist in the artery wall, cell populations that may respond differently to various stimuli and that may exist in different proportions in genetically different individuals. Clarification of the events leading to arterial calcification is an important step in clarifying the roles and characteristics of pluripotent artery wall cells.

References

1. Demer LL, Watson KE, Boström K. Mechanism of calcification in atherosclerosis. Trends Cardiovasc Med 1994;4:45-49.
2. Cornhill JF, Herderick EE, Stary HC. Topography of human aortic sudanophilic lesions. Monogr Atherosclerosis 1990;15:13-19.
3. Hirsch D, Azoury R, Sarig S, Kruth HS. Colocalization of cholesterol and hydroxyapatite in human atherosclerotic lesions. Calcif Tissue Int 1993;52:94-98.
4. Rumberger JA, Schwartz RS, Simons DB, Sheedy III PF, Edwards WD, Fitzpatrick LA. Relation of coronary calcium determined by electron beam computed tomography and lumen narrowing determined by autopsy. Am J Cardiol 1994;73: 1169-73.
5. Detrano RC, Wong ND, Tang W, et al. Prognostic significance of cardiac cinefluoroscopy for coronary calcific deposits in asymptomatic high risk subjects. J Am Coll Cardiol 1994;24:354-58.
6. Mitchell JR, Adams JH. Aortic size and aortic calcification: A necropsy study. Atherosclerosis 1977;27:437-46.
7. Pearson AC, Guo R, Orsinelli DA, Binkley PF, Pasierski TJ. Transesophageal echocardiographic assessment of the effect of age, gender, and hypertension of thoracic aortic wall size, thickness, and stiffness. Am Heart J 1994;128:344-52.
8. Fitzgerald PJ, Ports TA, Yock PG. Contribution of localized calcium deposits to dissection after angioplasty. An observational study using intravascular ultrasound. Circulation 1992;86:64-70.
9. Ohtsuka S, Kakihana M, Watanabe H, Sugishita Y. Chronically decreased aortic distensibility causes deterioration of coronary perfusion during increased left ventricular contraction. J Am Coll Cardiol 1994;24:1406-14.
10. Lee RT, Loree HM, Cheng GC, Lieberman EH, Jaramillo N, Schoen FJ. Computional structural analysis based on intravascular ultrasound imaging before in vitro angioplasty: Prediction of plaque fracture locations. J Am Coll Cardiol 1993;21:777-82.
11. Cheng GC, Loree H M, Kamm RD, Fishbein MC, Lee RT. Distribution and circumferential stress in ruptured and stable atherosclerotic lesions. A structural analysis with histopathological correlation. Circulation 1993;83:1179-87.
12. Nakashima T, Tanikawa J. A study of human aortic distensibility with relation to atherosclerosis and aging. Angiology 1971;22:477-90.
13. Maeta H, Hori M. Effects of a lack of aortic "Windkessel": Properties of the left ventricle. Jpn Circ J 1985;49:232-37.
14. Bouthier JD, DeLuca N, Safar ME, Simon AC. Cardiac hypertrophy and arterial distensibility

in essential hypertension. Am Heart J 1985;109:1345-52.
15. Katz AM. Cardiomyopathy of overload: A major determinant of prognosis on congestive heart failure. N Engl J Med 1990;332:100-110.
16. Franklin SS, Weber MA. Measuring hypertensive cardiovascular risk: The vascular overload concept. Am Heart J 1994;128:793-803.
17. Bogren HG, Mohiaddin RH, Klipstein RK, et al. The function of the aorta in ischemic heart disease: A magnetic resonance and angiographic study of aortic compliance and blood flow patterns. Am Heart J 1989;118:234-47.
18. Stefanadis C, Wooley CF, Bush CA, Koibash AJ, Boudoulas H. Aortic distensibility abnormalities in coronary artery disease. Am J Cardiol 1987;58:1300-1304.
19. Kim SY, Hinkamp TJ, Jacobs WR, Lichtenberg RC, Posniak Y, Pifaree R. Effect of an inelastic synthetic vascular graft on exercise hemodynamics. Ann Thorac Surg 1995;59:981-89.
20. Kelly RP, Tunin R, Kass DA. Effect of reduced aortic compliance on cardiac efficiency and contractile function of in situ canine left ventricle. Circ Res 1992;71: 490-502.
21. O'Rourke M. Arterial stiffness, systolic blood pressure, and logical treatment of arterial hypertension. Hypertension 1990;15:339-47.
22. Kannel WB, Wolf PA, McGee DL, Dawber TR, McNamara P, Castelli WP. Systolic blood pressure, arterial rigidity and risk of stroke. Am Med Assoc 1982;245:1225-29.
23. Garland C, Barrett-Connor E, Suarez L, Criqui MH. Isolated systolic hypertension and mortality after age 60 yrs. Am J Epidemiol 1983;118:365-76.
24. Mintz GS, Painter JA, Pichard AD, et al. Atherosclerosis in angiographically "normal" coronary artery reference segments: and intravascular ultrasound study with clinical correlations. J Am Coll Cardiol 1995;25:1479-85.
25. Bunting CH. The formation of true bone with cellular (red) marrow in a sclerotic aorta. J Exper Med 1906;8:365-76.
26. Buerger L, Oppenheimer A. Bone formation in sclerotic arteries. J Exper Med 1908;10:354-67.
27. Schwartz SM, Heimark RL, Majesky MW. Developmental mechanisms underlaying pathology of arteries. Physiol Rev 1990;70:1177-1209.
28. Majesky MW, Giachelli CM, Reidy MA, Schwartz SM. Rat carotid neointimal smooth muscle cells reexpress a developmentally regulated mRNA during repair of arterial injury. Circ Res 1992;71:759-68.
29. Owen M. The origin of bone cells. Int Rev Cytol 1970;28:213-38.
30. Hood LC, Rosenquist TH. Coronary artery development in the chick: Origin and deployment of smooth muscle cells, and the effects of neural crest ablation. Anat Rec 1992;234:291-300.
31. Stemple DL, Anderson DJ. Lineage diversification of the neural crest: *In vitro* investigations. Dev Biol 1993;159:12-23.
32. Bronner-Fraser M, Fraser SE. Cell lineage analysis reveals multipotency of some avian neural crest cells. Nature 1988;335:161-64.
33. Boström K, Watson KE, Horn S, Wortham C, Herman IM, Demer LL. Bone morphogenetic protein expression in human atherosclerotic lesions. J Clin Invest 1993;91:1800-1809.
34. Watson K, Boström K, Ravindranath R, Lam T, Norton B, Demer LL. TGF-ß1 and 25-hydroxycholesterol stimulate osteoblast-like vascular cells to calcify. J Clin Invest 1994;93:2106-13.
35. LeLievre CS, LeDouarin NM. Mesenchymal derivatives of the neural crest: Analysis of chimaeric quail and chick embryos. J Embryol Exp Morph 1975;34:125-54.

36. Vainio S, Karavonova I, Jowett A, Thesleff I. Identification of BMP-4 as a signal mediating secondary induction between epithelial and mesenchymal tissues during early tooth development. Cell 1993;75:45-58.
37. Lyons KM, Hogan BL, Robertson EJ. Colocalization of BMP-7 and BMP-2 RNAs suggests that these factors cooperatively mediate tissue interactions during murine development. Mech Dev 1995;50:71-83.
38. Cunningham NS, Paralkar V, Reddi AH. Osteogenin and recombinant bone morphogenetic protein 2B are chemotactic for human monocytes and stimulate transforming growth factor beta 1 mRNA expression. Proc Natl Acad Sci 1992; 89:11740-44.
39. Ikeda T, Shirasawa T, Esaki Y, Yoshiki S, Hirokawa K. Osteopontin mRNA is expressed by smooth muscle-derived foam cells in human atherosclerotic lesions of the aorta. J Clin Invest 1993;92:2814-20.
40. Kim KM. Calcification of matrix vesicles in human aortic valve and aortic media. Fed Proc 1976;35:156-62.
41. O'Brien ER, Garvin MR, Stewart DK, et al. Osteopontin is synthesized by macrophage, smooth muscle, and endothelial cells in primary and restenotic human coronary atherosclerotic plaques. Arterioscler Thromb 1994;14:1648-56.
42. Shanahan CM, Cary NRB, Metcalfe JC, Weissberg PL. High expression of genes for calcification-regulating proteins in human atherosclerotic plaques. J Clin Invest 1994;93:2393-2402.
43. Rekhter MD, Zhang K, Narayanan AS, Phan S, Schork MA, Gordon D. Type I collagen gene expression in human atherosclerosis. Am J Pathol 1993;143:1634-48.
44. Fleet JC, Hock JM. Identification of osteocalcin in mRNA in nonosteoid tissue of rats and human by reverse transcription-polymerase chain reaction. J Bone Miner Res 1994;9:1565-73.

HMG-CoA REDUCTASE INHIBITORS IN THE CONTROL OF LIPID METABOLISM IN MACROPHAGES

Franco Bernini*, Stefano Bellosta, Monica Canavesi, and Remo Fumagalli
*Institute of Pharmacology and Pharmacognosy, University of Parma, Via delle Scienze, 43100 Parma, Italy and Institute of Pharmacological Sciences, Via Balzaretti 9, University of Milan, Italy

Modified low density lipoproteins (LDL), like acetylated LDL (AcLDL), deliver to macrophages, after lysosomal degradation, large amounts of unesterified cholesterol which stimulates the activity of the microsomal enzyme acyl-CoA:cholesterol acyltransferase (ACAT) with subsequent intracellular accumulation of esterified cholesterol [1]. This process may induce lipid accumulation in the arterial wall, a major event of atherogenesis [2].

Several compounds have been reported to reduce cholesterol esterification in cells. Some act directly by inhibiting ACAT activity [3], others indirectly by reducing lipoprotein degradation and their cholesteryl ester hydrolysis in the lysosomes [4,5], by slowing down intracellular cholesterol movement [6,7] or inhibiting scavenger receptor expression and cellular influx of modified lipoproteins [8,9]. Depending on the mechanism involved each agent may have different effects on cellular cholesterol content, localization, and on esterified-to-free-form ratio. ACAT inhibitors may increase free cholesterol content of the plasma membrane, with minor effect on total cellular cholesterol [10]. Free cholesterol accumulation in lysosomes is observed with compounds active on intracellular cholesterol movement [6,7]. Accumulation of cholesteryl esters in these organelles is achieved with agents inhibiting the activity of lysosomal enzymes [4,5]. Finally, a decrease of total cellular cholesterol is observed with compounds inhibiting the expression of scavenger receptors [9].

Recently it was reported that vastatins are able to inhibit cholesterol esterification and deposition induced by AcLDL in human macrophages [11] and mouse peritoneal macrophages (MPM) [12] (Table 1). Since this inhibition did not occur in cell-free homogenates nor in cholesterol preloaded cells, but was observed only when vastatins were simultaneously incubated with AcLDL, it was concluded that these drugs are not direct inhibitors of ACAT. Results obtained in our laboratory showed that inhibition of cholesterol esterification in MPM by vastatins could be fully reversed by exogenous mevalonate or by geranylgeraniol (a mevalonate metabolite), and took place in the presence of an excess of exogenous cholesterol [12]. These results provided the first evidence that the mevalonate pathway plays an essential role in the process of esterification of excess cholesterol delivered to macrophages by modified LDL.

A. M. Gotto, Jr. et al. (eds.), Drugs Affecting Lipid Metabolism, 43–47.

Table 1. Effect of vastatins on free, esterified, and total cholesterol content in MPM incubated with acLDL.

Vastatins (μM)	Cellular Cholesterol (μg/mg cell prot.)		
	Free	Esterified	Total
Basal	24.6	2.1	26.7
AcLDL (50 μg/ml)	37.0	30.9	67.9
AcLDL + Fluvastatin 0.5	36.4	19.8	56.2
AcLDL + Fluvastatin 1	41.9	15.3	57.2
AcLDL + Fluvastatin 5	40.6	8.8	49.4
AcLDL + Simvastatin 0.5	38.8	24.1	62.9
AcLDL + Simvastatin 1	39.8	23.3	63.1
AcLDL + Simvastatin 5	37.7	9.0	46.7

Recently, we also repeated these data in human macrophages incubated with oxidized LDL (manuscript in preparation), confirming that vastatins do not affect esterification by preventing the intracellular formation of substrate for ACAT (i.e. cholesterol), but rather by inhibiting the formation of nonsterol mevalonate product(s).

Inhibition of cholesterol esterification by another vastatin, lovastatin, has been reported in the CaCo-2 intestinal cell line [13]. Inhibition of intestinal ACAT activity has also been reported in rabbits given simvastatin [14]. In these cells the action of the drug is apparently linked to a mechanism different from that exerted in macrophages, since the inhibitory effect was not prevented by the addition of mevalonate [13], and involved a direct inhibition of ACAT activity as tested in cell-free systems [13,15]. Fellermann et al. [16] showed that mevinolin failed to inhibit cholesterol esterification in enterocytes in the presence of high concentrations of exogenous mevalonate. In these experiments the large amount of mevalonate supplied to cells produced sufficient cholesterol substrate to directly stimulate ACAT activity. These experiments demonstrate that mevinolin did not inhibit esterification of endogenous-derived cholesterol, but did not provide any information on the involvement of mevalonate product(s) on esterification of lipoprotein-derived cholesterol.

More recently in our laboratory we showed that HMG-CoA reductase inhibitors reduce "*in vitro*" cholesterol accumulation elicited by AcLDL in mouse peritoneal macrophages by inhibiting the endocytosis of these lipoproteins by cells [17].

Inhibition ^{125}I acLDL degradation (Table 2) and fluorescent DI-acLDL internalization offered direct evidence for this conclusion. As mentioned above the inhibition by vastatins of AcLDL-induced cholesterol esterification in human macrophages was previously reported by Kempen et al. [11]. These authors reported a slight not statistically significant effect of these drugs on AcLDL degradation, and concluded that the inhibitory effect of vastatins on cholesterol esterification could not be attributed to a decrease in receptor-mediated uptake or degradation of AcLDL. The reasons for this discrepancy are not clear. A species difference is possible; however, the results reported by Kempen et al. indicating a net reduction of total cellular cholesterol content in human macrophages, are consistent with our observations. In any case, our results do not exclude additional mechanisms (such as an interference with the intracellular cholesterol trafficking) [11], that may contribute to the ability of vastatins to reduce cholesterol esterification.

Table 2. Effect of fluvastatin and fluvastatin plus mevalonate derivatives on ^{125}I-AcLDL degradation in mouse peritoneal macrophages.

	^{125}I-AcLDL degraded (μg/mg cell prot.)
Control	32000 ± 871
Fluvastatin 5 μM	18000 ± 1590[a]
Fluvastatin 5 μM + Mevalonate 100 μM	32700 ± 1435[b]
Fluvastatin 5 μM + Geranylgeraniol 10 μM	33000 ± 1875[b]

[a] $p < 0.05$ versus control; [b] $p < 0.01$ versus fluvastatin alone.

The mechanism involved in fluvastatin action on AcLDL endocytosis needs clarification. The effect is not related to a decreased expression of the scavenger receptors since no decrease of cellular binding at 4° C could be detected. Although we cannot exclude an inhibitory effect of vastatins on the endocytosis of other ligands, the effect on AcLDL seems not due to a nonspecific depression of cellular endocytotic functions since in the condition in which AcLDL degradation was reduced, a slight but significant increase of native LDL degradation was observed (Table 3). Our results show that the inhibition by fluvastatin of AcLDL catabolism is reversed by mevalonate and its isoprenoid derivative geranylgeraniol (Table 2). This result suggests the involvement of nonsterol products of the mevalonate pathway in AcLDL endocytosis.

Interestingly, data from our laboratory indicate that the effects of fluvastatin are more pronounced in cholesterol-loaded cells. This result may be explained by the lower HMG-CoA reductase activity in cholesterol rich cells as compared to unloaded cells [18]. This observation suggests the possibility that the mevalonate pathway in the arterial lesions may represent a selective target for pharmacological intervention. In conclusion, vastatin inhibition of AcLDL endocytosis might affect foam cells formation and have beneficial effects on atheroma generation not only by reducing plasma cholesterol levels, but also by directly acting on the arterial wall.

Table 3. Comparison of fluvastatin effect on ^{125}I-AcLDL and ^{125}I-LDL degradation in MPM.

	Control	Drug (5 μM)
	^{125}I-LPs degraded (μg/mg cell prot.)	
^{125}I-AcLDL (40 μg/ml)	30172 ± 186	21093 ± 131*
^{125}I-LDL (40 μg/ml)	1992 ± 112	2498 ± 178*

*p < 0.01 versus control.

References

1. Brown MS, Goldstein JL, Krieger M, Ho YK, Anderson RGW. Reversible accumulation of cholesteryl esters in macrophages incubated with acetylated lipoproteins. J Cell Biol 1979;82: 597-613.
2. Ross R. The pathogenesis of atherosclerosis: A perspective for the 1990s. Nature 1993;362: 801-809.
3. Sliskovic DR, White AD. Therapeutic potential of ACAT inhibitors as lipid lowering and anti-atherosclerotic agents. Trends Pharmacol Sci 1991;12:194-99.
4. Goldstein JL, Brown MS, Ho YK, Innerarity TL, Mahley RW. Cholesteryl ester accumulation in macrophages resulting from receptor-mediated uptake and degradation of hyper-cholesterolemic canine b-very low density lipoproteins. J Biol Chem 1980;255:1839-48.
5. Bernini F, Catapano AL, Corsini A, Fumagalli R, Paoletti R. Effects of calcium antagonists on lipids and atherosclerosis. Am J Cardiol 1989;64:129I-134I.
6. Liscum L, Faust JR. The intracellular transport of low density lipoprotein-derived cholesterol is inhibited in Chinese hamster ovary cells cultured with 3-b-[2-(diethylamino)ethoxy]androst-5-en-17-one. J Biol Chem 1989;264:11796-806.
7. Butler JD, Blanchette-Mackie J, Goldin E, et al. Progesterone blocks cholesterol translocation from lysosomes. J Biol Chem 1992;267:23797-805.
8. Bottalico LA, Wager RE, Agellon LB, Assoian RK, Tabas I. Transforming growth factor-β1 inhibits scavenger receptor activity in THP-1 human macrophages. J Biol Chem 1991;266: 22866-71.
9. Geng Y-J, Hansson GJ. Interferon-τ inhibits scavenger receptor expression and foam cell formation in human monocyte-derived macrophages. J Clin Invest 1992;89:1322-30.
10. Xu X-X, Tabas I. Lipoprotein activate acyl-coenzyme A: cholesterol acyltransferase in macrophages only after cellular cholesterol pools are expanded to a critical threshold level. J Biol Chem 1991;266:17040-48.
11 Kempen HJM, Vermeer M, de Wit E, Havekes LM. Vastatins inhibit cholesterol ester accumulation in human monocyte-derived macrophages. Arteriosel Thromb 1991; 1:146-53.
12. Bernini F, Didoni G, Bonfadini G, Bellosta S, Fumagalli R. Requirement for mevalonate in acetylated LDL induction of cholesterol esterification in macrophages. Atherosclerosis 1993; 104:19-26.
13. Kam N, Albright E, Mathur S, Field F. Effect of lovastatin on acyl-CoA: cholesterol O-acyltransferase (ACAT) activity and the basolateral-membrane secretion of newly synthesized

by CaCo-2 cells. Biochem J 1990;272:427-33.
14. Ishida F, Sato A, Iizuka Y, Kitani K, Sawasaki Y, Kamei T. Effects of MK-733 (simvastatin), an inhibitor of 3-hydroxy-3-methylglytaryl coenzyme A reductase, on intestinal acylcoenzyme A: cholesterol acyltransferase activity in rabbit. Biochim Biophys Acta 1989;1004:117-23.
15. Ishida F, Sato A, Iizuka Y, Kamei T. Inhibition of acyl coenzyme A: cholesterol acyltransferase by 3-hydroxy-3-methylglutaryl coenzyme A reductase inhibitors. Chem Pharm Bull 1989;37: 1635-36.
16. Fellermann K, Reimann FM, Herold J, Stange EF. Mevinolin, a competitive inhibitor of hydroxymethylglutaryl coenzyme A reductase, suppresses enterocyte esterification of exogenous but not endogenous cholesterol. Biochim Biophys Acta 1992;1165:78-83.
17. Bernini F, Scurati N, Bonfadini G, Fumagalli R. HMG-CoA reductase inhibitors reduce acetyl LDL endocytosis in mouse peritoneal macrophages. Arterioscl Thromb Vasc Biol 1995;15: 1352-58.
18. Goldstein JL, Brown MS. Regulation of the mevalonate pathway. Nature 1990;343:425-30.

ANTIOXIDANTS AND CARDIOVASCULAR RISK

Paul Nestel[1], Mavis Abbey[2], and Michio Suzukawa[3]
[1]Baker Medical Research Institute, Commercial Road, Prahran, Melbourne, Australia 3181, [2]CSIRO Division Of Human Nutrition, Kintore Avenue, Adelaide, Australia 5000, and [3]1st Department of Medicine, National Defense Medical College, Tokorozawa, Saitama, Japan

Introduction

The role of antioxidants in preventing coronary heart disease (CHD) is being substantiated through a better understanding of the biochemical, physiological, and pathological pathways induced by free radical damage. This is clearly a factor in atherogenesis, lipoprotein damage, endothelial dysfunction, and myocardial ischemia. The main challenges are to establish causality more clearly and to show protection through well-designed intervention trials.

A common initiator is oxidation of a polyunsaturated fatty acid (PUFA) in a lipoprotein or cell membrane leading to an unstable molecule with a highly reactive oxygen species. An unstable radical, so formed, can propagate the process by attacking further PUFA until eventually more stable compounds such as aldehydes are formed. By this time damage to a membrane might have occurred. Inside a low density lipoprotein (LDL) for instance, the protein may also become damaged (apoprotein B), so that the entry of LDL into an artery is no longer controlled, and excess LDL cholesterol is deposited within macrophages in the artery, producing the foam cell of an early plaque.

Defense mechanisms against free radical attack comprise typically vitamin E, beta-carotene and other lipid soluble antioxidants (e.g. ubiquinol-10) which are carried within the core of the LDL, and water soluble antioxidants such as vitamin C. However only vitamin E is present in multiple molecules for each LDL particle. That is not the case for β-carotene or ubiquinol. The vitamins scavenge, quench, and stabilize the free oxygen species, such as superoxide and hydroxyls.

Several epidemiological studies, published recently [1,2] suggest that women and men who obtain the highest amounts of vitamin E from dietary supplements, experienced fewest new clinical CHD events. Further, plasma concentrations of alpha-tocopherol (vitamin E) are inversely correlated with CHD events and mortality across populations [3]. The evidence for β-carotene and vitamin C is weaker. However in a large study of 25,800 people, among 123 who developed myocardial infarction, those who smoked and had a heart attack had shown the lowest plasma carotenoid levels (β-carotene and possibly also

A. M. Gotto, Jr. et al. (eds.), Drugs Affecting Lipid Metabolism, 49–56.

lycopene) [4]. The EURAMIC trial (Europe and Israel) confirmed the link between low β-carotene concentrations (in adipose tissue, a surrogate of dietary intake) and myocardial infarction in smokers [5]. In a recent follow-up report this association was related to PUFA consumption.

Oxidized lipoproteins, LDL, as well as other atherogenic lipoproteins, affect adversely several key atherogenic processes. These include the attraction of circulating monocytes from blood into artery (these are the precursors of foam cells), increased delivery of lipoprotein cholesterol into macrophage foam cells, and release of growth factors and cytokines which induce the proliferative and inflammatory phase of the plaque. Moreover oxidized LDL oppose the release of endothelium-derived relaxing factor and thus encourage coronary artery constriction.

Other classes of antioxidants have also been shown recently to be associated with reduced coronary heart disease. These include the polyphenols such as flavones and isoflavones which are widely spread through the plant kingdom. Indeed we are on the threshold of major discoveries of potent, naturally occurring antioxidants. Some of the well-known protection of vegetarians against CHD and possibly other degenerative diseases may be due more to eating plant foods than to avoiding animal-derived foods. Cross-sectional epidemiological studies have frequently shown strong inverse correlations between consumption of fruits and vegetables and CHD [6]. These are found in green and colored vegetables, tea, soybeans, sesame seeds, cruciferous vegetables, etc. The Japanese paradox is probably related to their dietary protection in the face of continuing high risks posed by the high prevalence of smoking and hypertension. Green tea is one of the richest sources of antioxidants and soybeans contain substantial amounts of genistein and other antioxidants. We have shown that adding genistein to LDL *in vitro* protects strongly against oxidants. Consequently Japanese excrete far more flavenoids in urine than do Finns [7]. This of course reflects also, inversely, the differing incidences of CHD.

Wine has attracted much attention and the polyphenols in red wine are potent antioxidants, when consumed in moderate amounts [8] or when added to LDL *in vitro* as we have shown. The picture is still confused; apparently alcohol is required simultaneously to allow the polyphenols to become absorbed. White wine with its lower polyphenol content is less effective.

Further examples of the apparent protective effect of these polyphenols have come from a prospective study of elderly Dutch people [9] where those who consumed the most flavenoids from tea, onions, and apples, sustained the fewest heart attacks. The French paradox, that is the apparently low rate of CHD despite relatively high intake of dairy fats from cheese, has been attributed to their high intake of fruits, vegetables, nuts, vegetable oils, and possibly wine [6].

Supplementing with vitamin E (between 200 mg and 1000 mg daily) protects LDL from becoming oxidized. β-carotene and vitamin C are less effective. We have shown this in long term trials (3-6 months) in which the enrichment of LDL with alpha-tocopherol was inversely correlated with the likelihood of LDL being oxidized [10]. Others have reported similar findings [11], and protection against LDL oxidizability (*in vitro*) has been reported at intakes as low as 25IU daily, although effectiveness rises linearly with higher consumption

[12].

Because low β-carotene intakes associate with heart attacks in smokers we examined the potential benefit of food supplements rich in β-carotene and vitamin C on LDL oxidizability in smokers [13]. Our objective was to evaluate the effect of daily supplementation with foods high in vitamin C and β- carotene on plasma vitamin levels and oxidation of low density lipoprotein (LDL) in cigarette smokers. Fifteen normolipidemic male cigarette smokers who did not usually take vitamin supplements ate during the study a polyunsaturated fatty acid rich diet which provided 36% of energy as fat; they also drank a vitamin-free drink daily for 3 weeks followed by a further 3 weeks when they consumed daily supplements of orange juice (145 mg vitamin C) and carrot juice (16 mg β-carotene). Prior to supplementation, these smokers had plasma β-carotene and vitamin C concentrations which were lower than normal. The vitamin-rich supplements raised plasma levels of ascorbic acid (1.6-fold) and β-carotene (2.6-fold). Malondialdehyde, one end-product of oxidation, was lower in copper oxidized LDL (measured *in vitro*) after vitamin supplementation (65.7 ± 2.0 and 57.5 ± 2.9 µmol/g LDL protein before and after supplementation respectively, $P < 0.01$). The lag time before the onset of LDL oxidation was not affected by antioxidant supplementation. Therefore in habitual cigarette smokers, antioxidant vitamins, which can be feasibly provided from food, partly protected LDL from oxidation despite a diet enriched in polyunsaturated fatty acids.

Since PUFA have from 2-6 double bonds (linoleic acid to docosahexaenoic acid in fish), they are vulnerable to oxidation. We tested the oxidizability of LDL from people eating polyunsaturated or monounsaturated oils. PUFA-rich LDL were indeed more readily oxidized [14], so that the best mix of dietary fat should contain only modest amounts of linoleic acid-rich oils, no more than Australians and Americans are currently eating (on average 6-7% of total energy). Oleic acid-enriched LDL were less vulnerable to oxidation. Other workers have reported similar data [15] and have shown that small, dense LDL which commonly occur in hyperlipidemia and in subjects with CHD, are particularly prone to oxidation especially if rich in linoleic acid.

We also isolated LDL from individuals who had been taking fish oil for some time and found that those LDL were particularly susceptible to oxidation. In *in vitro* studies we found that such LDL were oxidized by macrophages which led to a rapid uptake of cholesterol-rich LDL into those potential foam cells. This led to three sets of studies in which we explored the relationship between fish oil and LDL oxidation and the potential of prevention with vitamins. The effect of fish oil and corn oil supplementation on low density lipoprotein (LDL) oxidation was examined in 20 treated hypertensive subjects [16]. The randomized double-blind crossover study consisted of two 6-week interventions with a highly purified fish oil (4 g/day containing 3.4 g n-3 fatty acids) or corn oil (4 g/day). Fish oil supplementation significantly (-24%, $P < 0.01$) reduced plasma triglyceride; however LDL-cholesterol was higher (+6%, $P < 0.01$ compared to corn oil) but LDL particles were larger ($P < 0.01$ compared to baseline) after fish oil. LDL size was inversely correlated with plasma triglyceride ($P < 0.001$) both before and after fish oil supplementation, and positively correlated with high density lipoprotein cholesterol ($P < 0.01$). Fish oil reduced lag time before onset of copper-induced LDL oxidation (-25%, $P < 0.001$) and increased production of thiobarbituric acids-reactive substances (TBARS) 3-4 fold. Corn oil had no significant effect on lag time, oxidation rate or TBARS production. Consumption of fish oil increased macrophage uptake of copper-oxidized LDL and of macrophage-modified LDL. Corn oil was without effect. We conclude that from the standpoint of atherosclerosis, n-3 fatty acids adversely raise the susceptibility of LDL to copper-induced and macrophage-mediated oxidation which however can be prevented with supplemental vitamin E as shown in our following studies.

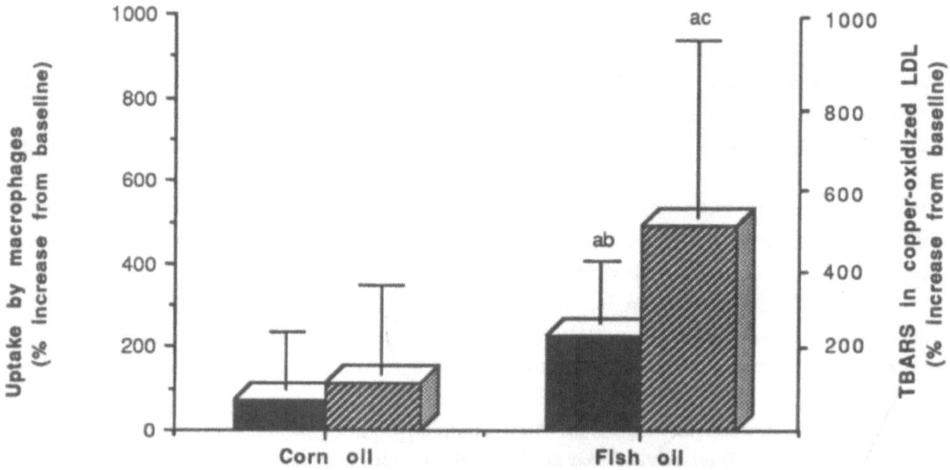

Figure 1. Effect of corn oil and fish oil supplementation on uptake of macrophage-oxidized LDL by macrophages (solid bars) and TBARS generated in the medium by macrophage-mediated LDL oxidation (hatched bars). [^{3}H]CE-LDL (10 μg/ml) separated from plasma at baseline and after corn oil and fish oil supplementation were incubated with monolayers of J774 macrophages in Ham's F-10 medium. After 24 hours incubation, uptake of macrophage-oxidized [^{3}H]CE-LDL by J774 macrophages and TBARS generated in medium during incubation were measured. (Values are expressed as percent of baseline and represent means $\pm$ SD(n = 20). [a]significant ($P < 0.01$) compared to baseline, [b]significant ($P < 0.01$) compared to corn oil, [c]significant ($P < 0.05$) compared to corn oil.

These results indicate that dietary supplementation with n-3 fatty acids increases the oxidizability of LDL which may counteract some of the beneficial effects of fish oil which relate to the risk of developing atherosclerosis. Consumption of adequate amounts of antioxidants such as vitamin E should be considered to minimize these adverse effects.

We investigated possible mechanisms through which the capacity of n-3 fatty acid-enriched macrophages to oxidize low density lipoprotein (LDL) may be enhanced, and the value of antioxidant vitamins in preventing this. Macrophages were enriched with n-3 fatty acids (eicosapentaenoic acid, docosapentaenoic acid, and docosahexaenoic acid) following incubations with fish oil [17]. These macrophages produced large amounts of TBARS in medium containing metals and showed enhanced capacity to oxidize LDL (3-4 fold increase compared to control cells) and to accumulate the modified LDL. Antioxidants, either as vitamin E-enriched macrophages or as vitamin C in the medium, inhibited this increased capacity to oxidize LDL.

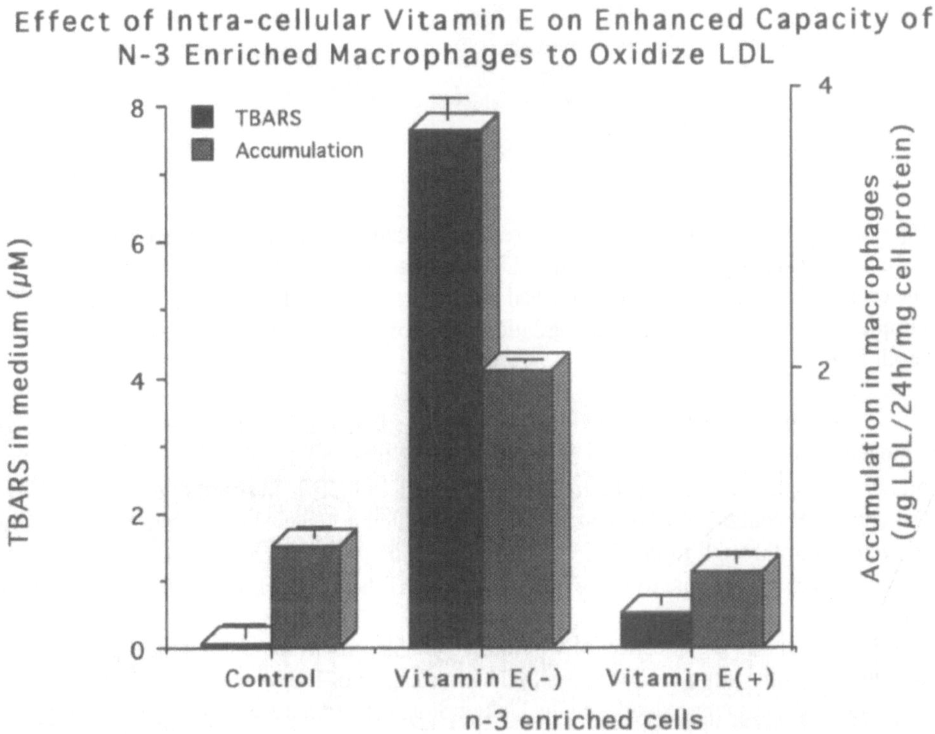

Figure 2. Effects of enrichment of macrophages with vitamin E on enhanced capacity of n-3 fatty acid-enriched macrophages to oxidize LDL. Fish oil fatty acids were added to macrophages with or without vitamin E (1 μM). The cells were washed after incubation for 24 hours, and then [^{3}H]CE-LDL in macrophages were measured. Values represent means ± SD (n = 4).

Finally, we tested LDL from subjects eating normal diets to determine whether adding vitamin E *in vitro* at the time when the LDL were exposed to macrophages, would protect the LDL against oxidation [18]. Macrophages have the capacity to oxidize lipoproteins (especially when the fatty acids of either the lipoproteins or the cells are highly unsaturated), and can then take up such modified lipoproteins through the scavenger receptor.

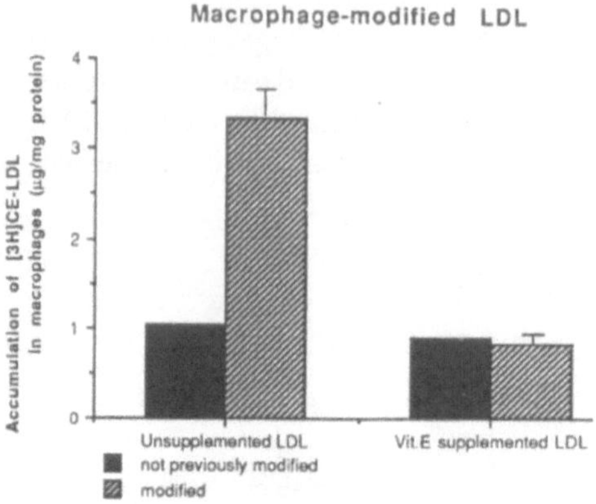

Figure 3. As shown in Figure 3 in the absence of vitamin E enrichment, more [^{3}H]CE-LDL accumulated in macrophages when the LDL had been modified through preincubation with the cells in Ham's F10 than when they had not been conditioned. However, with vitamin E-supplemented [^{3}H]CE-LDL, accumulation was not increased through preincubation and modification.

In vitro supplementation of vitamin E, when taken together with *in vivo* supplementation with the vitamin strongly suggests that additional vitamin E, either in the diet or as supplement, may be desirable with diets rich in PUFA. In the above *in vitro* study, the vitamin E content of LDL was raised 4-fold which is achievable with supplementation *in vivo*, if not through foods. This may be analogous to the recent EURAMIC study [19] which showed β-carotene to protect smokers against heart attack when PUFA intake was high.

This raises the question of whether vegetable oils which are rich in PUFA should contain additional vitamin E, that is should fortification of PUFA margarines with vitamin E, occur? First, recommendations in the United States (National Research Council) suggest that for each gram of linoleic acid in the diet, there should be approximately 0.4 mg of alpha-tocopherol. Studies carried out in Australia show that Australians probably eat about 0.66 mg vitamin E for every gram of linoleic acid [20]. The US recommendation is based on their RDAs which is not the same as an optimal ratio. Some authorities suggest that there should be at least 1mg of vitamin E for each gram of linoleic acid (EPA) and more for docosahexaenoic acid (DHA) obtained from fish oil. Higher amounts of vitamin E would also be needed to cover increased alpha-linolenic acid consumption.

It should be remembered that tocopherols are a family of compounds and that they have differing bioavailabilities and differing biological activities; that is they are not absorbed equally nor are they equally effective. Further, there are three asymmetric carbons leading to several stereoisomers. The most potent is alpha-tocopherol in which each of those carbons faces in the same direction (so called RRR alpha-tocopherol) [21]. Vitamin E taken in capsule form usually contains a mix of synthetic tocopherols containing only a proportion of the most active alpha-tocopherol, and all of them esterified as acetates, which require hydrolysis in the small intestine.

It would be very difficult to make a clear recommendation at the present time about the need to fortify PUFA margarines and oils with vitamin E, over and above the amounts naturally present. It should be remembered in this context that the alpha-tocopherol content of oils varies substantially, with safflower and sunflower oil for instance containing substantially more than cotton seed, soybean, or olive oils. The only clear case for adding vitamin E would be to restore the vitamin level to that which would be obtained from a sunflower or safflower oil full fat margarine. The reason for this being, that many people derive much of their dietary vitamin E from PUFA-rich oils and margarines. With such a high proportion of individuals now taking vitamin E supplements as well, it is unclear whether there is any lack of vitamin E intake to cover current PUFA consumption. Although olive oil contains relatively little alpha-tocopherol, it does contain a variety of other potent antioxidants [22].

Finally, before we can make a decision on fortification, we will need to establish a stronger link between dietary antioxidants and cardiovascular disease prevention. Important areas that still need to be researched in the future are suggested as follows:

- Confirm *in vitro* studies *in vivo*
- Establish *in vivo* role of oxidized LDL
- Develop tests for *in vivo* oxidant status
- Define optimal antioxidant status
- Develop strategies for antioxidant status
- Study pharmacokinetics of nutrient antioxidants
- Modify food technologies to retain antioxidants in processing, to improve release of food antioxidants, and to define need and strategy for fortification.

References

1. Stampfer MJ, Hennekens CH, Manson J-AE, Colditz GA, Rosner B, Willett WC. Vitamin E consumption and the risk of coronary disease in women. N Eng J Med 1993;328:1444-49.
2. Knekt P, Reunanen A, Jarvinen R, Seppanen R, Heliovara M, Aromaa A. Am J Epidemiol 1994;139:1180-89.
3. Gey KF, Puska P, Jordan P, Moses UK. Inverse correlation between vitamin E and mortality from ischemic heart disease in cross-cultural epidemiology. Am J Clin Nutr 1991;53:326-40S.
4. Street DA, Comstock GW, Salkeld RM, Schüep W, Klag MJ. Serum antioxidants and myocardial infarction: Are low levels of cartenoids and α-tocopherol risk factors for myocardial infarction? Circulation 1994;90:1154-61.
5. Kardinaal AFM, Kok FJ, Ringstad J, et al. Antioxidants in adipose tissue and risk of myocardial infarction: The EURAMIC study. Lancet 1993;342:1379-84.
6. Renaud S, de Lorgeril M. Wine, alcohol, platelets, and the French paradox for coronary heart disease. Lancet 1992;339:1523-26.
7. Adlercreutz H, Markkanen H, Watanabe S. Plasma concentrations of phyto-oestrogens in

Japanese men. Lancet1 993;342:1209-10.
8. Furham B, Lavy A, Aviram M. Consumption of red wine with meals reduces the susceptibility of human plasma and low-density lipoprotein to lipid peroxidation. Am J Clin Nutr 1995;61:549-54.
9. Hertog MGL, Feskens EGM, Hollman PCH, Katan MB, Kromhout D. Dietary antioxidant flavenoids and risk of coronary heart disease: The Sutphen Elderly Study. Lancet 1993;342:1007-11.
10. Abbey M, Nestel PJ, Baghurst PA. Antioxidant vitamins and low density lipoprotein oxidation. Am J Clin Nutr 1993;58:525-32.
11. Jialal I, Fuller CJ, Huet BA. The effect of α-tocopheral on LDL oxidation. A dose-response study. Arterioscler Thromb Vasc Biol 1995;15:190-98.
12. Princen HMG, van Duyvenvoorde W, Buytenhek R, et al. Supplementation with low doses of vitamin E protects LDL from lipid peroxidation in men and women. Arterioscler Thromb Vasc Biol 1995;15:325-33.
13. Abbey M, Noakes M, Nestel PJ. Dietary supplementation with orange and carrot juice in cigarette smokers lowers oxidation products in copper-oxidized low-density lipoproteins. J Am Diet Assoc 1995;95:671-75.
14. Abbey M, Belling GB, Noakes M, Hirata F, Nestel PJ. Oxidation of low density lipoproteins: intraindividual variability and the effect of dietary linoleate supplementation. Am J Clin Nutr 1993;57:391-98.
15. Reaven P, Parthasarathy S, Grasse BJ, Miller E, Steinberg D, Witzum JL. Effects of oleate-rich and linoleate-rich diets on the susceptibility of low density lipoprotein to oxidative modification in mildly hypercholesterolemic subjects. J Clin Invest 1993;91:668-76.
16. Suzukawa M, Abbey M, Howe PRC, Nestel PJ. Effects of fish oil fatty acids on low density lipoprotein size, oxidizability, and uptake by macrophages. J Lipid Res 1995;36:473-84.
17. Suzukawa M, Abbey M, Clifton P, Nestel PJ. Enhanced capacity of n-3 fatty acid-enriched macrophages to oxidize low density lipoproteins. Mechanisms and effects of antioxidant vitamins. Atheroslerosis; in press.
18. Suzukawa M, Abbey M, Clifton P, Nestel PJ. Effects of supplementing with vitamin E on the uptake of low density lipoprotein and the stimulation of cholesteryl ester formation in macrophages. Atherosclerosis 1994;110:77-86.
19. Kardinaal AFM, Aro A, Kark JD, et al. Association between β-carotene and acute myocardial infarction depends on polyunsaturated fatty acid status: the EURAMIC study. Arterioscler Thromb Vasc Biol 1995;15:726-32.
20. Baghurst KI, Record SJ, Syrette J, Baghurst PA, Powis G, Worsley T, Crawford D. What are Australians eating - results from the 1985 and 1990 Victorian Nutrition Surveys 1993. Deakin University, Victoria.
21. Acuff RV, Thredford SS, Hidiroglou NN, Papas AM, Odom TA. Relative bioavailability of RRR- and all-rac-α-tocopheryl acetate in humans: Studies using deuterated compounds. Am J Clin Nutr 1994;60:397-402.
22. Visioli F, Bellomo G, Montedoro GF, Galli C. Low density lipoprotein oxidation is inhibited in vitro by olive oil constituents. Atherosclerosis 1995;117:25-32.

NATURAL ANTIOXIDANTS FROM THE DIET AND PROTECTION FROM CORONARY HEART DISEASE

Francesco Visioli and Claudio Galli
Institute of Pharmacological Sciences, University of Milan, Via Balzaretti, 9, 20133 Milan, Italy

Introduction

Uncontrolled production of free radicals in biological systems is involved in the onset of a series of pathological conditions. In particular, the development of the arterial lesions in the atherosclerotic disease might be exacerbated by free radical-induced oxidation of low density lipoprotein (LDL); interest in dietary antioxidants is therefore related to their potential protective effects against this type of process. In addition to antioxidant vitamins (vitamin E and β carotene), several other compounds in the diet are of potential interest. Flavonoids, present in foods and beverages of plant origin, appear to be protective against coronary heart disease (CHD), and the presence of antioxidants in red wine may partly explain the lower incidence of CHD in populations in which wine consumption is part of the diet. Recent findings from our laboratory demonstrate that olive oil constituents effectively inhibit LDL oxidation *in vitro*, suggesting that the intake of such antioxidants might play a role in the observed lower incidence of CHD in the Mediterranean countries, where olive oil is the major component of the dietary fats.

This chapter outlines the recent evidence that correlates natural antioxidant intake with protection from free radical-mediated diseases and discusses the role of olive oil in such processes.

Interest in free radicals and antioxidants has greatly increased in the last decade, due to the growing evidence that oxidative processes, resulting in chemical and functional modifications of lipoproteins, are involved in the onset of the arterial lesions in the atherosclerotic disease and that these processes may be controlled by antioxidants. The formation and progression of the arterial lesions appear, in fact, to be facilitated by enhanced deposition of oxidatively modified (LDL), and their recognition by the macrophage scavenger receptor leads to uncontrolled accumulation of cholesterol ester-laden foam cells in the arterial wall [1]. Following these pioneer observations, a number of studies have been devoted to elucidate the steps involved in the oxidation of LDL in various models of oxidation; to evaluate the chemical markers and the functional alterations of the oxidized LDL; to establish whether measurements of the *ex vivo* susceptibility of LDL to oxidation

A. M. Gotto, Jr. et al. (eds.), Drugs Affecting Lipid Metabolism, 57–67.

are predictive of the *in vivo* progression of the arterial lesions; and finally to develop new approaches for assessing oxidative processes *in vivo*. Several studies have indeed produced evidence that enhanced lipid/lipoprotein oxidation occurs in patients at risk for coronary heart disease (CHD), whereas, on the other side, a high intake of antioxidants appears to be protective against CHD. Various reviews have appeared in this area [1,2].

Natural Antioxidants

Interest in natural antioxidants from foods and beverages results from progress in the identification of factors present in the diet as micronutrients (including vitamins, trace minerals and several other compounds) with antioxidant activity, as well as from data of epidemiological and controlled studies showing lower incidence of CHD in population groups on diets rich in or in groups supplemented with antioxidant vitamins [3-8]. In addition to vitamins, other nonessential nutrients present in the diet are endowed with antioxidant and other activities of biological interest. Among these, the flavonoids represent a very large class of compounds, present in various types of foods and beverages of plant origin, and widely studied from the point of view of their biological activities. Flavonoids have been shown to inhibit carcinogen-induced tumors in rats [9], and colonic cell proliferation in vitro [10]. In addition, some compounds inhibit various types of oxidative reactions [11-13], including the oxidative modification of LDL [14]. Of the various types of activities of flavonoids, the antioxidant properties are the most widely studied and characterized, so that they are considered somewhat the prototypes of natural antioxidants. However, they are also able to inhibit several cellular enzymes like ATPase, phospholipase, and lipoxygenase [15]. These observations have led to claims of potential pharmacological applications of flavonoids in areas such as inflammation and allergic diseases, but their use as drugs appears rather unpractical.

Flavonoids in foods and beverages have been repeatedly estimated, over the years, but the methodology available in the early studies has not allowed accurate determinations. Calculated intakes of flavonoids reported in the literature and generally quoted are in the order of several hundred milligrams, up to almost one gram/day [16], but recent determinations resulted in more conservative estimations, in the order of few tens of mg/day [17]. These amounts appear, however, to exceed those of antioxidant vitamins such as carotenoids and tocopherols. Data on the flavonoid and polyphenol contents of foods and beverages is still scarce, but available analyses indicate fruits and vegetables as the foods with the highest content of such compounds (Table 1).

The average daily intake of natural antioxidants varies according to dietary habits in different population groups, and the upper and lower limits of daily flavonoids consumption in different populations have been estimated to be included within the 2.6 mg/d-68.2 mg/d range [18]. An inverse association between flavonoids intake and mortality from CHD has been reported [18,19], suggesting that high amounts of flavonoids and phenols in the diet may effectively protect LDL against free radical attack. An obvious unresolved question concerns the bioavailability of these complex molecules following oral intake. Available data, still obtained with somewhat unreliable methodologies, suggest that they are indeed absorbed, although the quantitative aspects and the possible metabolic modifications occurring during absorption have not been established.

Table 1. Average contents of total flavonoids in selected foods and beverages.

Lettuce	14
Onion	347
Endive	46
Broad Beans	45
Celery	130
Tomato	8
Broccoli	102
Kale	321
Brussel Sprouts	7
Apple	36
Red Wine	20
Black Tea	36
Apple Juice	3

Values are expressed as mg/kg. Adapted from reference [18].

Attention to the possible protective effects of dietary components, with respect to diseases such as CHD, is generally elicited by epidemiological observations in population groups with different incidence of the disease and different dietary habits. A debated paradox in the epidemiology of CHD, based on comparisons of fat consumption in different countries, is that observed in the French population which has a low incidence of cardiovascular events in spite of a diet high in saturated fat [20-22]. As partial explanation of this discrepancy, a protective effect due to high intake of natural antioxidants, provided by red wine in particular, has been proposed. Additional experimental evidence of a beneficial effects on the cardiovascular system provided by red wine components include inhibiton of platelet activity and restenosis in animals, in which wine and grape juice were tested [23]. These effects resemble those observed in humans that where supplemented with antioxidant vitamins [24]. There is however still some controversy concerning the significance of the observed effects of wine consumption on oxidative parameters in relation to protection from CHD.

Mediterranean Diet

The concept that the type of food was one of the factors responsible for the lower incidence of cardiovascular events in the Mediterranean basin, compared to other geographical areas, was initially proposed on the basis of studies (the Seven Countries Study) showing an inverse correlation between certain dietary components, e.g. saturated fat, which are low in the Mediterranean diet, and CHD [25]. The term "Mediterranean diet" describes the food patterns found in Greece, southern Italy, and Crete in the mid-1950s. In spite of the variations among different countries, certain characteristics were common. Plant foods, including grains, cereals, legumes, fresh fruit, and vegetables were major components, whereas red meat (beef and lamb) and eggs were consumed in low amounts when compared to countries from the central and northern parts of Europe. Fish and poultry intake were moderate and alcohol was consumed as wine with meals. Total fat intake of such diet ranged from 25% to 35% of energy from one area to another, and saturated fat yielded only 7-8% of energy [26]. Since then, the Mediterranean diet has changed for the worst. Meat and dairy products (especially milk) consumption has increased as has the incidence of CHD. Still, olive oil remains the typical dietary fat, being employed mainly uncooked in salad dressings. A diet enriched in the monounsaturated oleic acid, the major fatty acid in olive oil, at the expense of saturated oils, lowers plasma LDL [27-29]. The effects of dietary fatty acids on plasma levels of the protective high density lipoproteins (HDL) are complex. All classes of fatty acids, saturates (SAT), monounsaturates (MUFA), and polyunsaturates (PUFA), when replacing carbohydrates in the diet, raise HDL levels to different extents: MUFA increase HDL levels more than PUFA [30,31]. In addition to the advantageous effects of diets with a high MUFA content on lipoprotein levels, oleate-enriched LDL is also more resistant to oxidative modification than linoleate-enriched LDL, and this lowers its potential atherogenicity [32-35]. Thus, most of the helpful effects of the Mediterranean diet on the incidence of CHD have been so far attributed to the favorable fatty acid profile, i.e. a high MUFA-PUFA/SAT ratio, provided by olive oil.

It has been shown, however, that LDL from olive oil-fed rats is more resistant to oxidation than that obtained from triolein-fed rat plasma [36]. These data suggest that some dietary components of olive oil other than the triglyceride fraction can contribute to the observed protection from cardiovascular disease.

Olive Oil

Olive oil is the dietary fat of choice in the Mediterranean area. The world production of olive oil reached ~ 2,000,000 tons during the 1991-92 season and its consumption is increasing in the United States, Canada, Russia, and Japan, while remaining relatively constant in the European Community. Olive oil, as compared to other vegetable oils, has a peculiar fatty acid composition. The monounsaturated oleic acid is the most abundant fatty acid (56.0-84.0%), while linoleic acid ranges from 3.0 to 21.0% [37]. In addition to its unique fatty acid composition, olive oil is rich in minor components, responsible for its fruity flavor and taste. It should be mentioned that olive oil is the only vegetable oil that is obtained from *whole fruits*, through physical pressure, rather than from *seeds* and thus it retains all the organoleptic properties of olives. Actually, most of these minor components, some of which are listed in Table 2, can be employed to identify the area of production of each batch of oil, thus guaranteeing its genuineness [38-40].

Table 2. Minor components of olive oil.

Hydrocarbons
Nonglyceride Esters
Tocopherols
Carotenoids
Aliphatic Alcohols
4-methyl Sterols
Sterols
Hydroxy- and Dihydroxyterpenic Alcohols
Phospholipids
Phenolic Compounds (50-800 mg/Kg)
Chlorophyls
Glycolipids
Aldehydes
Ketons
Esters

Adapted from reference [37].

Furthermore, the concentration of the phenolic fraction (up to 800 mg/Kg oil) in the oil can predict its stability to oxidation [41-43]. Hydroxytyrosol, in particular, endowes the oil with resistance to rancidity [42,39,44]. It is noteworthy that "extra-virgin" olive oil, obtained by pressure on the olive paste and with a low concentration of free fatty acids (acidity lower than 1%, as requested by the current regulations), is much richer in phenolic compounds than refined oils, e.g. "plain" olive oil, that are obtained by neutralization of acidity from oils that exceeds the given limits. In turn, the more abundant the phenolic fraction, the higher the quality of the oil and vice versa. As a consequence, consumption of "extra virgin" rather than plain olive oils is recommended.

The beneficial effects on cardiovascular events of a diet in which olive oil is the predominant fat component have been discussed above. A higher consumption of olive oil has also been recently found to be significantly correlated to a lower risk of breast cancer [45]. The mean daily intake of olive oil in countries of the Mediterranean basin varies between few Kg/capita/year (e.g. France) to ~15 Kg/capita/year (Greece). In areas where olive oil consumption is maximal, the daily intake is in the order of 50 gr/day, providing a calculated intake of about 25 mg phenols/day [46]. This amount, as total daily intake, corresponds to the total flavonoid intake that has been associated with a lower incidence of CHD [19].

It is noteworthy that the continuous washing of the olive paste during the milling process yields high amounts of "waste water", a byproduct that is currently discarded while it contains appreciable amounts of phenols that from the olive paste end up in the waste acqueous material according to their partition coefficient. Recent findings from our laboratory showed that waste waters have powerful (in the ppm range) antioxidant activity [47] and might be recovered and employed in preservative chemistry.

The growing interest in natural antioxidant chemistry and the increasing popularity of the Mediterranean diet now gaining ground in the USA and in Japan led us to investigate the potential antioxidant effects of molecules that have been isolated and purified from extra-virgin olive oil. Our goal was to further elucidate the potential beneficial role of olive oil, based on the biological properties of its minor components in cardiovascular protection. To do this, we tested the antioxidant activity of olive oil-derived phenols by employing oxidation of low density lipoprotein as a model of lipoprotein alteration and by measuring various indices of lipid peroxidation and protein modification. Part of the results are summarized in this chapter.

We have measured levels of vitamin E and PUFA in LDL, as markers of oxidatively induced losses of oxidizable substrates, and levels of the thiobarbituric acid-reacting substances (TBARS) and of the lipid peroxides (LOOH), as indices of the formation of oxidation products. A newly proposed index of lipid oxidation is the measurement of a recently discovered family of bioactive compounds derived, in humans, from arachidonic acid through cyclooxygenase-independent free radical-mediated peroxidation of this substrate which includes prostaglandin-like compounds (F_2-isoprostanes). These molecules are formed *in situ* on phospholipids and are subsequently released preformed [48]. Levels of circulating isoprostanes increase during oxidative stress, e.g. in smokers [49], and could therefore be considered as a marker of an ongoing oxidative process. F_2-isoprostanes are also generated in LDL exposed to chemical oxidation [50].

Incubation of human LDL with the potent oxidant agent $CuSO_4$5 μM resulted in the typical reduction of Vitamin E, which completely disappeared from the samples at 30 minutes. Preincubation of LDL with two of the most representative olive oil phenols, i.e. oleuropein (OE, not shown) or hydroxytyrosol (HT) 10^{-5} M before oxidation was initiated, prevented the depletion of α tocopherol (80%protection) at 30 minutes, when compared to oxidized samples (Table 3). At 3 and 6 hours of incubation with $CuSO_4$ several markers of lipid oxidation were markedly elevated (Table 4).

Table 3. Vitamin E levels in LDL 30 min after incubation with 5 μM $CuSO_4$ (oxidized) and in samples preincubated with HT. From reference [46].

	nmoles / mg LDL	% of controls
Control	5.6 ± 0.5	100
Oxidized	0	0
10^{-6} M HT	1.7 ± 0.2	30
10^{-5} M HT	3.9 ± 0.4	70
10^{-4} M HT	4.7 ± 0.5	84

Table 4. Vitamin E, linoleic, and arachidonic acids, TBARS, lipoperoxide, and isoprostane levels in LDL incubated for 3 and 6 hours with $CuSO_4$ in the presence of HT.

	$-CuSO_4$	$+CuSO_4$	+HT	$-CuSO_4$	$+CuSO_4$	+HT
	3 Hours			6 Hours		
VE[1]	100	0	59	100	0	38
LA[1]	100	87	100	100	67	100
AA[1]	100	52	100	100	30	97
TBARS[2]	0	100	6	0	100	7
LOOH[2]	0	100	13	0	100	28
8-epi-$PGF_{2\alpha}$[3]	5	24	9	6	27	12

Values are expressed as: [1]Percentages of levels in nonoxidized ($-CuSO_4$) LDL; [2] Percentages of levels in $CuSO_4$ (5 μM) oxidized LDL; [3]ng/mg protein. HT (hydroxytyrosol) was preincubated at 10^{-5} M, 1 hour before addition of $CuSO_4$. VE, vitamin E; LA, linoleic acid; AA, arachidonic acid; TBARS, thiobarbituric acid reactive substances; LOOH, lipoperoxides. Data from references [46] and [51].

The protective effect on the loss of vitamin E, although smaller, was detectable until termination of the experiment (six hours). Possibly, olive oil phenols protected the natural antioxidant pool in LDL from oxidation, thus retarding the onset of massive lipid peroxidation. The loss in vitamin E preceeded, in fact, that of the long chain oxidizable fatty acids, i.e. those of the polyunsaturated class. Levels of fatty acids with four or more double bonds, such as arachidonic, eicosapentaenoic, and docosahesaenoic acids decreased more markedly than those of the dienoic linoleis acid. After six hours of incubation with $CuSO_4$, PUFAs levels, as compared to their initial values, were as follows: linoleic acid 68%, arachidonic acid 32%, eicosapentaenoic acid 28% (not shown), and docosahexaenoic acid 25% (not shown). Preincubation of the LDL samples with OE or HT prevented the loss of PUFAs and maintained their levels close to basal throughout the experiment.

Both TBARS and LOOH levels rose rapidly after the addition of copper sulphate to the LDL samples, whereas preincubation with OE or HT 10^{-5} M inhibited the rise in both indices of lipid peroxide formation and kept their levels close to control values. F_2-isoprostanes were increased in LDL exposed to chemical oxidation [51], but pretreatment with HT (10 μM) markedly reduced the accumulation of these products, strengthening the evidence that such molecules are markers of lipid peroxidation. In addition, $CuSO_4$-induced oxidative modification of the LDL protein moiety was markedly reduced by pretreatment with olive oil phenols, as indicated by a reduced formation of 4-HNE-lysine and MDA-lysine adducts [46] (Table 5). The observed protective effect toward protein modification might play an important role, given that recognition of LDL, either native or modified, by their receptors involves protein-to-protein interactions. Preservation of protein integrity might thus reduce the LDL fraction (i.e. oxidized) that is taken up by the macrophage scavenger receptor.

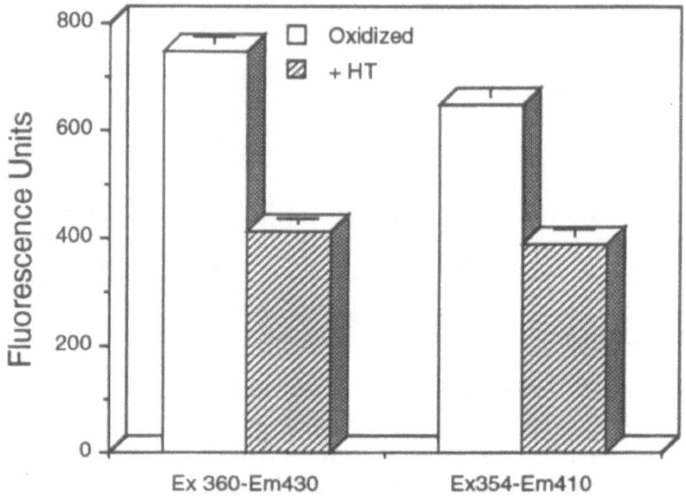

Figure 1. Accumulation of 4-hydroxynonenal-lysine and MDA-lysine adducts in $CuSO_4$ oxidized LDL at 2 hours incubation. HT (hydroxytyrosol) was preincubated at 10^{-5} M, 1 hour before oxidation. Values are arbitrary units of fluorescence at E_x360-E_m430 abd E_x354-E_m410. From reference 47.

General Considerations and Future Perspectives

The beneficial effects of a high intake of dietary antioxidants on pathological conditions that are at least in part triggered by an uncontrolled production of free radicals, such as atherosclerosis, is now well assessed. Increasing the daily intake of fresh fruits and vegetables is thus recommendable. While most of the beneficial effects of the Mediterranean diet have been so far attributed to the peculiarity of its lipid profile (high monounsaturates and low saturates), our investigations suggest that natural antioxidants derived from the major fat component of such diet (olive oil) might contribute to the observed protection from CHD. The potent (10^{-5} M) antioxidant activity exhibited *in vitro* by olive oil phenols indicates, in fact, that these compounds might block oxidation of LDL, one of the risk factors for atherosclerosis. Striving for a higher quality, phenols-rich, olive oil seems therefore appropriate because such oil would provide more dietary antioxidants with the everyday diet. The exact mechanism of action of flavonoids and polyphenols is still under investigation [52-54], but data not reported here suggest that hydroxytyrosol acts both as a free radical scavenger and as a metal ion chelator [46]. A major point that still needs to be addressed is whether olive oil-derived phenols exert their antioxidant activity *in vivo* too. The metabolic fate of flavonoids and phenols in humans is still a matter of investigation. Whereas part of the ingested compounds is degraded by the intestinal flora, another portion can be absorbed in an essentially unchanged form [16]. Further investigations in this direction are underway in our laboratory, and could eventually add weight to the current opinion that part of the beneficial effects of the Mediterranean diet are due to its high content in antioxidants.

Acknowledgements

This work has been partly supported by Contract 93.02710.CT06 of CNR. We thank Professors GF Montedoro and FF Vinceri for the supply of hydroxytyrosol and waste waters extracts, respectively. Mr. Flavio Giavarini assisted with the mass spectrometry assay of isoprostanes.

References

1. Steinberg D, Parthasarathy S, Carew TE, et al. Beyond cholesterol. Modifications of low-density lipoprotein that increases its atherogenicity. N Engl J Med 1989;320:915-24.
2. Steinberg D. Clinical trials of antioxidants in atherosclerosis: Are we doing the right thing? Lancet 1995;346:36-38.
3. Briviba K, Sies H. Nonenzymatic antioxidant defense systems. In: Frei B, editor. Natural antioxidants in human health and disease. Academic Press, 1994: 107-28.
4. Bors W, Heller W, Michel C, et al. Flavonoids as antioxidants: determination of radical-scavenging efficiencies. Methods Enzymol 1990;186:343-55.
5. Rimm EB, Stampfer MJ, Ascherio A, et al. Vitamin E consumption and the risk of coronary heart disease in men. N Engl J Med 1993;328:1450-56.
6. Stampfer MJ, Hennekens CH, Manson JE, et al. Vitamin E consumption and the risk of coronary heart disease in women. N Engl J Med 1993;328:1444-49.
7. Gey KF, Puska P, Jordan P, et al. Inverse correlation between plasma vitamin E and mortality from ischemic heart disease in cross-cultural epidemiology. Am J Clin Nutr 1991;53:326S-34S.
8. Hodis HN, Mack WJ, LaBree L, et al. Serial coronary angiographic evidence that antioxidant vitamin intake reduces progression of coronary artery atherosclerosis. JAMA 1995;273:1849-54.
9. Deschner EE, Ruperto J, Wong G, et al. Quercetin and rutin as inhibitors of azoxymethanol-induced colonic neoplasia. Carcinogenesis 1991;7:1193-96.
10. Ranelletti FO, Ricci R, Larocca LM, et al. Growth-inhibitory effect of quercetin and presence of type-II estrogen-binding sites in human colon cancer cell lines and primary colorectal tumors. Int J Cancer 1992;50:486-92.
11. Robak J, Gryglewski RJ. Flavonoids are scavengers of superoxide anion. Biochem Pharmacol 1988; 37:83-88.
12. Husain SR, Cillard J, Cillard P. Hydroxy radical scavenging activity of flavonoids. Phytochemistry 1985;26:2489-92.
13. Takahama U. Inhibition of lipoxygenase-dependent lipid peroxidation by quercetin: mechanism of antioxidative function. Phytochemistry 1985;24:1443-46.

14. De Whalley CV, Rankin SM, Hoult JRS, et al. Flavonoids inhiibit the oxidative modification of low density lipoproteins. Biochem Pharmacol 1990;39:1743-49.
15. Das DK. Naturally occurring flavonoids: structure, chemistry, and high performance liquid chromatography methods for separation and characterization. Meth Enzymology 1994;34:410-20.
16. Kühnau J. The flavonoids. A class of semi-essential food components: Their role in human nutrition. Wld Rev Nutr Diet 1976;24:117-91.
17. Hertog MGL, Hollman PCH, Katan MB, et al. Intake of potentially anticarcinogenic flavonoids and their determinants in adults in The Netherlands. Nutr Cancer 1993;20:21-29.
18. Hertog MGL, Kromhout D, Aravanis C, et al. Flavonoid intake and long-term risk of coronary heart disease and cancer in the Seven Countries Study. Arch Intern Med 1995;155:381-86.
19. Hertog MLG, Feskens EJM, Katan MB, et al. Dietary antioxidant flavonoids and risk of coronary heart disease: The Zutphen Elderly Study. Lancet 1993;342:1007-11.
20. Frankel ED, Kanner J, German JB, et al. Inhibition of oxidation of human low-density lipoprotein by phenolic substances in red wine. Lancet 1993;341:454-57.
21. Maxwell S, Cruickshank A, Thorpe G. Red wine and antioxidant activity in serum. Lancet 1994;344:193-94.
22. Whitehead TP, Robinson D, Allaway S, et al. Effect of red wine ingestion on the antioxidant capacity of serum. Clin Chem 1995;41:32-35.
23. Demrow HS, Slane PR, Folts JD. Administration of wine and grape juice inhibits in vivo platelet activity and thrombosis in stenosed canine coronary arteries. Circulation 1995;91:1182-88.
24. DeMaio SJ, King SB, Lembo NJ, et al. Vitamin E supplementation, plasma lipids and incidence of restenosis after percutaneous transluminal coronary angioplasty (PTCA). J Am Coll Nutr 1992;11:68-73.
25. Keys A. Coronary heart disease in seven countries. Circulation 1970;41(1):1-211.
26. Willet WC, Sacks S, Trichopoulou A, et al. Mediterranean diet pyramid: A cultural model for healthy eating. Am J Clin Nutr 1995;61:1402S-1406S.
27. Mattson FH, Grundy SM. Comparison of effects of dietary saturated, mono-unsaturated, and polyunsaturated fatty acids on plasma lipids and lipoproteins in man. J Lipid Res 1985;26:194-202.
28. Grundy SM. Comparison of monounsaturated fatty acids and carbohydrates for lowering plasma cholesterol. N Engl J Med 1986;314:745-48.
29. Grundy SM, Denke MA. Dietary influences on serum lipids and lipoproteins. J. Lipid Res. 1990;31:1149-72.
30. Mensink RP, Katan MB. Effect of dietary fatty acids on serum lipids and lipoproteins. Arterioscl Thromb 1992;12:911-19.
31. Hegsted DM, Ausman LM, Johnson JA, et al. Dietary fat and serum lipids: An evaluation of the experimental data. Am J Clin Nutr 1993;57:875-83.
32. Reaven P, Parthasarathy S, Grasse BJ, et al. Feasibility of using an oleate-rich diet to reduce the susceptibility of low-density lipoprotein to oxidative modification in humans. Am J Clin Nutr 1991;54:701-706.
33. Parthasarathy S, Khoo JC, Miller E, et al. Low density lipoprotein rich in oleic acid is protected against oxidative modification: Implications for dietary prevention of atherosclerosis. Proc Natl Acad Sci USA 1990;87:3894-98.
34. Bonanome A, Pagnan A, Biffanti S, et al. Effect of dietary monounsaturated and polyunsaturated fatty acids on the susceptibility of plasma low density lipoproteins to oxidative modification. Arterioscler Thromb 1992;12:529-33.

35. Reaven P, Parthasarathy S, Grasse BJ, et al. Effects of oleate-rich and linoleate-rich diets on the susceptibility of low density lipoprotein to oxidative modification in mildly hypercholesterolemic subjects. J Clin Invest 1993;91:668-76.
36. Scaccini C, Nardini M, D'Aquino M, et al. Effect of dietary oils on lipid peroxidation and on antioxidant parameters of rat plasma and lipoprotein fractions. J Lipid Res 1992;33:627-33.
37. Tiscornia E, Forina M, Evangelisti F. Composizione chimica dell'olio d'oliva e sue variazioni indotte dal processo di rettificazione. La Rivista Italiana delle sostanze grasse 1982;59:519-56.
38. Roncero AV. Phenolic products in olive oil and their influence on the oil characteristics. Rev Fr Corps Gras 1978;25:21-26.
39. Olias JM, Perez AG, Rios JJ, et al. Aroma of virgin olive oil: Biogenesis of the "green" odor notes. J Agric Food Chem 1993;41:2368-73.
40. Montedoro GF, Servili M, Baldioli M, et al. Simple and hydrolyzable compounds in virgin olive oil. 3. Spectroscopic characterizations of the secoiridoid derivatives. J Agric Food Chem 1993;41:2228-34.
41. Chimi H, Rahmani H, Cillard J, et al. Autooxydation des huiles d'olive: role des composes phenoliques. Rev Franc Corps Gras 1990;11/12:363-67.
42. Papadopoulos G, Boskou D. Antioxidant effect of natural phenols on olive oil. JAOCS 1991;68:669-71.
43. Tsimidou M, Papadopoulos G, Boskou D. Phenolic compounds and stability of virgin olive oil-Part 1. Food Chemistry 1992;45:141-44.
44. Montedoro GF, Servili M, Baldioli M, et al. Simple and hydrolyzable phenolic compounds in virgin olive oil. 1. Their extraction, separation, and quantitative and semiquantitative evaluation by HPLC. J Agric Food Chem 1992;40(9):1571-76.
45. Martin-Moreno JM, Willett WC, Gorgojo L, et al. Dietary fat, olive oil intake and breast cancer risk. Int J Cancer 1994;58:774-80.
46. Visioli F, Bellomo G, Montedoro GF, et al. Low density lipoprotein oxidation is inhibited in vitro by olive oil constituents. Atherosclerosis 1995;117:25-32.
47. Visioli F, Vinceri FF, Galli C. "Waste waters" from olive oil production are rich in natural antioxidants. Experientia 1995;51:32-34.
48. Morrow JD, Hill KE, Burk RF, et al. A series of prostaglandins F_2-like compounds are produced in vivo in humans by a non-cyclooxygenase, free radical-catalyzed mechanism. Proc Natl Acad Sci USA 1990;87:9383-87.
49. Morrow JD, Frei B, Longmire AW, et al. Increase in circulating products of lipid peroxidation (F_2-isoprostanes) in smokers. N Engl J Med 1995;332:1198-1203.
50. Lynch SM, Morrow JD, II LJR, et al. Formation of non-cyclooxygenase-derived prostanoids (F_2-isoprostanes) in plasma and low density lipoprotein exposed to oxidative stress *in vitro*. J Clin Invest 1994;93: 998-1004.
51. Salami M, Galli C, De Angelis L, et al. Formation of F_2-isoprostanes in oxidized low density lipoprotein: inhibitory effect of hydroxytyrosol. Pharm Res 1995;31:275-79.
52. Torel J, Cillard J, Cillard P. Antioxidant activity of flavonoids and reactivity with peroxy radicals. Phytochemistry 1986;25:383-85.
53. Husain SR, Cillard J, Cillard P. Hydroxyl radical scavenging activity of flavonoids. Phytochemistry 1987;26:2489-91.
54. Afanas'ev IB, Dorozhko AI, Brodskii AV, et al. Chelating and free radical scavenging mechanisms of inhibitory action of rutin and quercetin in lipid peroxidation. Biochem Pharmacol 1989;38:1763-69.

EFFECTS OF LIPID LOWERING DRUGS ON THE *IN VITRO* OXIDIZABILITY OF LIPOPROTEINS IN DIABETES

Ivo De Leeuw, Luc Van Gaal, and Angi Zhang*
*Endocrinology and Metabolic Medicine, *Faculty of Medicine, University of Antwerp, UIA, Universiteitsplein 1 B2610 Antwerp, Belgium*

Introduction

Early and accelerated atherosclerosis is the principal cause of diabetic morbidity and mortality [1]. Dyslipidemia can be an important contributory factor in the pathogenesis of this complication [2]. Most well-controlled insulin-dependent diabetic patients have however near-normal levels of circulating lipids and lipoproteins [3] but despite the absence of dyslipidemia, abnormalities in lipoprotein metabolism and composition have been described [4]. Moreover, chronic hypertriglyceridemia, linked to episodes of bad glycemic control, have been shown to be a risk factor for coronary heart disease in this kind of patients [5].

Oxidized LDL and VLDL are also involved in the formation of the atherosclerotic plaque [6]. In diabetic patients there are a number of factors that promote lipoprotein oxidation, including increased glycation-induced free radical production, altered lipoprotein composition, and decreased antioxidant defense [7]. All these mechanisms can be inhibited in the presence of a perfect and permanent metabolic control, a goal seldom achieved in insulin-dependent diabetic patients. It is indeed typical that in the well-known DCCT study the risk for all complications except the macroangiopathic ones could be reduced with a sustained intensive insulin treatment [8]. Additional therapeutic intervention therefore looks to be necessary. Hypolipidemic drugs are the natural choice, but the mechanism of action of the various categories of agents is very different and the choice is generally dependent on the kind of dyslipidemia present. In the absence of clear lipid changes, it looks logical to take the antioxidant properties into account. Until recently, only probucol has been shown to possess both hypolipidemic and antioxidant properties [9]. In Belgium this drug is, however, not available and it is the purpose of this work to study the effect of a fibrate and two statins on the lipid status of insulin-dependent diabetic patients, without frank dyslipidemia and with an acceptable degree of metabolic control.

EXPERIMENTAL DESIGN

Forty insulin-dependent diabetic patients gave informed consent to participate in the study.

A. M. Gotto, Jr. et al. (eds.), Drugs Affecting Lipid Metabolism, 69–75.

They were randomized in 4 groups of 10 receiving either placebo, simvastatin (20 mg), pravastatin (20 mg), or fenofibrate (200 mg) before bedtime during a period of 6 weeks. Five patients dropped out during the study for various reasons (intercurrent disease, lack of compliance) so that 35 patients (26 men, 9 women) could be considered for the final analysis: placebo, n = 9; pravastatin, n = 10; simvastatin, n = 6; and fenofibrate, n = 10.

The characteristics of the patients are summarized in Table 1. None of the patients took vitamins or antioxidants and were not treated with drugs that can interfere with lipid metabolism or peroxidation. Insulin treatment and diet were maintained constant during the trial period. Fasting blood samples were collected at the start and after 6 weeks treatment.

Table 1. Characteristics of the patient population.

Group	Age (years)	Sex M/F	Duration of diabetes (years)
Placebo (n = 9)	46.0 ± 12.3	6/3	24.2 ± 10.4
Pravastatin (n = 10)	43.5 ± 11.2	8/2	22.7 ± 6.2
Simvastatin (n = 6)	45.0 ± 10.2	4/2	25.5 ± 5.8
Fenofibrate (n = 10)	42.4 ± 13.8	8/2	24.8 ± 12.5

Results are expressed as mean ± SD.

METHODS

The susceptibility to oxidation of low density cholesterol (LDL) and very low density lipoprotein (VLDL) *in vitro* was measured by the method of Zhang [10]. Total cholesterol, high density lipoprotein (HDL)-cholesterol, triglycerides, and HbA1c were measured with classical routine laboratory techniques. Statistical significance was calculated by means of nonparametric tests (Wilcoxon) using the SPSS/PC+ package.

Results

As shown in Table 2 all three drugs could decrease total cholesterol significantly but only fenofibrate could diminish the triglyceride level and increase the HDL-cholesterol. As expected the level of metabolic control measured with HbA1c did not change.

Table 3 shows that the formation of TBARS *in vitro* could only be significantly decreased in the group treated with fenofibrate. A significant prolongation of the lagtime is also only present in this same group. An increase of peroxidation was not observed.

Table 2. Lipid parameters + HbA_1c before and after treatment (mean ± SD).

	Placebo		Pravastatin		Simvastatin		Fenofibrate	
	Start	6 weeks	Start	6 weeks	Start	6 weeks	Start	6 weeks
Cholesterol (mg/dl)	211 ± 31	222 ± 37	217 ± 35	181 ± 29*	209 ± 31	180 ± 14*	250 ± 45	202 ± 34**
HDL (mg/dl)	67 ± 19	69 ± 18	59 ± 17	63 ± 25	77 ± 8	77 ± 12	55 ± 18	64 ± 23*
TG (mg/dl)	90 ± 44	93 ± 58	123 ± 110	97 ± 90	83 ± 37	66 ± 34	117 ± 63	88 ± 44*
HbA_1c (%)	8.9 ± 1.4	8.8 ± 1.2	7.8 ± 0.7	7.8 ± 0.9	8.6 ± 1.4	8.6 ± 1.2	9.4 ± 2.1	9.1 ± 2.5

*$p < 0.05$; when compared with pretreatment values. **$p < 0.01$; when compared with pretreatment values.

Table 3. The effect of the three drugs on non-HDL lipoprotein oxidizability (mean ± SD).

	Placebo (n = 9)		Pravastatin (n = 9)		Simvastatin (n = 6)		Fenofibrate (n = 10)	
	Start	6 weeks	Start	6 weeks	Start	6 weeks	Start	6 weeks
TBARS formation (nmol MDA equivalent/mg non-HDL cholesterol)								
0 min	0.0 ± 0.0	0.0 ± 0.0	0.0 ± 0.0	0.0 ± 0.0	0.0 ± 0.0	0.0 ± 0.0	0.0 ± 0.0	0.0 ± 0.0*
30 min	0.9 ± 0.3	0.7 ± 0.3	1.2 ± 0.5	1.0 ± 0.4	1.2 ± 0.5	1.3 ± 0.2	1.2 ± 0.3	1.0 ± 0.3*
60 min	3.1 ± 2.5	2.6 ± 1.8	3.5 ± 1.5	2.7 ± 1.3	3.0 ± 0.9	3.1 ± 1.5	5.5 ± 3.7	3.2 ± 2.5*
90 min	20.2 ± 15.7	20.7 ± 15.4	30.1 ± 16.2	23.1 ± 17.7	23.7 ± 12.0	25.2 ± 19.0	32.0 ± 20.1	18.5 ± 18.9*
120 min	47.1 ± 14.2	45.5 ± 15.7	59.6 ± 17.7	49.5 ± 12.3	54.8 ± 17.1	57.4 ± 20.4	56.9 ± 18.2	41.8 ± 26.8*
150 min	63.0 ± 11.2	59.3 ± 7.3	70.1 ± 21.0	66.0 ± 11.5	69.7 ± 12.7	67.8 ± 17.5	69.8 ± 16.6	57.8 ± 21.3*
180 min	68.5 ± 14.6	63.3 ± 7.8	76.8 ± 22.2	72.6 ± 14.5	73.8 ± 12.8	73.3 ± 17.6	74.2 ± 15.9	65.9 ± 15.9*
Fluorescence								
Lagtime (min)	99 ± 4	103 ± 13	94 ± 7	95 ± 11	108 ± 13	112 ± 14	94 ± 19	107 ± 17**
Slope	0.108 ± 0.018	0.111 ± 0.016	0.109 ± 0.010	0.121 ± 0.008	0.129 ± 0.024	0.129 ± 0.035	0.091 ± 0.021	0.082 ± 0.017

*$p < 0.05$, when compared with pretreatment value. **$p < 0.01$, when compared with pretreatment value.

Discussion

This study confirms the well-known cholesterol-lowering effect of statins [11] in insulin-dependent diabetic patients. Fibrates however can also decrease the cholesterol levels significantly, even if their HMG-CoA inhibiting properties are less pronounced [12]. Their main pharmacological activities consist in decreasing the endogenous synthesis of triglycerides in the liver [13] and the activation of VLDL lipolysis by promoting the action of lipoprotein lipase [14]. This mechanism permits a significant decrease of the circulating levels of triglycerides and a concomitant increase of HDL-cholesterol, not obtained with a monotherapy with statins. This essential difference between the hypolipidemic action of statins and fibrates has also been described in nondiabetic patients by Nakandakare and colleagues [15] and Farnier et al.[16]. Since recent observations have suggested that triglyceride-rich lipoproteins even in normolipidemic insulin-dependent diabetic patients can increase the accumulation of esterified cholesterol in THP-1 macrophages [17] the effect on triglycerides could play a major role in the prevention of early atherosclerosis in this kind of patients.

This effect of fibrates on the composition of circulating lipoprotein particles is most probably the explanation of our observation that, in contrast to statins and placebo, fenofibrate can decrease the formation of TBARS and increase the lagtime during *in vitro* induced oxidation of non-HDL lipoproteins. Indeed, it looks as if the fatty acids associated with triglycerides might be more prone to oxidation than those associated with cholesterol [18]. Moreover, the number of very atherogenic small dense LDL particles is determined by the triglyceride level [19] and strongly related to their oxidative susceptibility [20]. It has been found that there is an increased prevalence of these particles in diabetics and patients with coronary heart disease [21,22]. During the treatment of hypertriglyceridemia with other fibrates (ciprofibrate, clofibrate) this abnormal LDL subfraction distribution could however been normalized and the oxidizability significantly decreased [23,24]. Therefore the data obtained with fenofibrate are in accordance with previous findings and the mechanisms, although not directly proven, are most probably similar. It is also noteworthy to report that pravastatin [25] has no effect on LDL size and that in contrast to fenofibrate, simvastatin [26] increased the polyunsaturated fatty acid content of lipoproteins, increasing the substrate for oxidation.

In conclusion one can propose that statins and fibrates are useful drugs for the treatment of hypercholesterolemia in insulin-dependent diabetic patients but in the presence of combined hyperlipidemia or in the absence of frank dyslipidemia, fibrates could offer some supplementary advantages in the prevention of atherosclerosis.

References

1. Panzram G. Mortality and survival in type 2 (non-insulin dependent) diabetes mellitus. Diabetologia 1987;30:123-31.
2. Howard BV. Lipoprotein metabolism in diabetes mellitus. J Lipid Res 1987;28:613-28.
3. Brown WV. Lipoprotein disorders in diabetes mellitus. Medical clinics of North America

1994;78:143-61.

4. Taskinen MR. Quantitative and qualitative lipoprotein abnormalities in diabetes mellitus. Diabetes 1992;41(2):12-7.
5. Laakso M, Pyörälä K, Sarlund H, Voutilainen E. Lipid and lipoprotein abnormalities associated with coronary heart disease in patients with insulin-dependent diabetes mellitus. Arteriosclerosis 1986;6:679-84.
6. Bierman EL. Atherogenesis in diabetes. Arterioscler Thromb 1992;12:647-56.
7. Rabini RA, Fumelli P, Galassi R, et al. Increased susceptibility to lipid oxidation in low-density lipoproteins and erythrocyte membranes from diabetic patients. Metabolism 1994;43:1470-74.
8. The DCCT Study. The effect of intensive treatment of diabetes on the development and progression of long term complications in insulin dependent diabetic patients. N Engl J Med 1993;329:977-86
9. Reaven PD, Parthasarathy S, Beltz WF, Witztum JL. Effect of probucol dosage on plasma lipid and lipoprotein levels and on protection of low-density lipoprotein against in vitro oxidation in humans. Arterioscler Thromb 1991;111:266-75.
10. Zhang A, Vertommen J, Van Gaal L, De Leeuw I. A rapid and simple method for measuring the susceptibility of low-density-lipoprotein and very-low-density-lipoprotein to copper-catalyzed oxidation. Clin Chim Acta 1994;227:159-73.
11. Brown MS, Goldstein JL. A receptor-mediated pathway for cholesterol homeostasis. Science 1986;232:34-47.
12. Berndt J, Gaumert R, Still J. Mode of action of the lipid lowering agents clofibrate and BM15 075, on cholesterol biosynthesis in rat liver. Atherosclerosis 1978;30:147-52.
13. Shepherd J. Mechanism of action of fibrates. Postgrad Med J 1993;69(suppl):S34-S41.
14. Nikkila EA, Huttunen JK, Ehnholm C. Effect of clofibrate on postheparin plasma triglyceride lipase activities in patients with hypertriglyceridaemia. Metabolism 1977;26:179-87.
15. Nakandakare E, Garcia RC, Rocha JC, Sperotto G, Oliveira HCF, Quintao ECR. Effects of simvastatin, bezafibrate and gemfibrozil on the quantity and composition of plasma lipoproteins. Atherosclerosis 1990;85:211-7.
16. Farnier M, Bonnefous F, Debbas N, Irvine A. Comparative efficacy and safety of micronized fenofibrate and simvastatin in patients with primary type IIA or IIb hyperlipidemia. Arch Intern Med 1994;154:441-49.
17. Georgopoulos A, Kafonek SD, Raikhel I. Diabetic postprandial triglyceride-rich lipoproteins increase esterified cholesterol accumulation in THP-1 macrophages. Metabolism 1994;43:1063-72.
18. Berliner JA, Territo M, Navab M, et al. Minimally modified lipoproteins in diabetes. Diabetes 1992;41(2):74-76.
19. Slyper AH. Low-density lipoprotein density and atherosclerosis. unravelling the connection. JAMA 1994;272:305-308.
20. de Graaf J, Hak-Lemmers HL, Hectors MC, Demacker PN, Hendriks JC, Stalenhoef AFH. Enhanced susceptibility to in vitro oxidation of the dense low density lipoprotein subfraction in healthy subjects. Arterioscler Thromb 1991;11:298-306.
21. Chait A, Brazg RL, Tribble D. Susceptibility of small, dense low-density lipoprotein to oxidative modification in subjects with the atherogenic lipoprotein phenotype, pattern B. Am J Med 1993;94:350-56.
22. Watts GF, Mandalia S, Brunt JNH, Slavin BM, Coltart DJ, Lewis B. Independent associations between plasma lipoprotein subfraction levels and the course of coronary artery disease in the

St. Thoma's atherosclerosis regression study (STARS). Metabolism 1993;42:1461-67.

23. Bruckert E, Dejager S, Chapman MJ. Ciprofibrate therapy normalises the atherogenic low-density lipoprotein subspecies profile in combined hyperlipidemia Atherosclerosis 1993;100:91-102.

24. de Graaf J, Hendriks JC, Demacker PN, Stalenhoef AFH. Identification of multiple dense LDL subfractions with enhanced susceptibility to in vitro oxidation among hypertriglyceridemic subjects. normalization after clofibrate treatment. Arterioscler Thromb 1993;13:712-19.

25. Zambon S, Cortella A, Sartore G, Baldo-Enzi G, Manzato E, Crepaldi G. Pravastatin treatment in combined hyperlipidemia, Effect on plasma lipoprotein levels and size. Eur J Clin Pharmacol 1994;46:221-24.

26. Agheli N, Jacotot B. Effect of simvastatin and fenofibrate on the fatty acid composition of hypercholesterolaemic patients. Br J Clin Pharmacol 1991;32:423-28.

CYTOKINE REGULATION OF ARTERIAL CHOLESTEROL TRAFFICKING

Kenneth B. Pomerantz and David P. Hajjar*
Departments of Medicine and Biochemistry, Cornell University Medical College, New York, New York 10021, USA*

Introduction

The mechanisms by which cellular cholesterol content is regulated continues to be the subject of intense research. Brown and Goldstein first showed that cellular cholesterol content is regulated by cholesterol itself [1]. Now, there is substantial evidence indicating that cholesterol content is also regulated by cytokines and intracellular second messengers. In this review, we focus on how signal transduction processes may regulate cholesterol processing in cells comprising the arterial wall.

Transmembrane Signal Transduction Mechanisms

There are at least three major cell surface receptor pathways, including nonreceptor tyrosine kinases, receptor tyrosine kinases, and G-protein-coupled receptors, outlined in Figure 1.

NONRECEPTOR TYROSINE KINASES

Non-receptor kinases, of which *src* is the parent member, are membrane receptors which possess kinase activity, but do not engage ligand. There are at least nine other members of this family, and detailed information on the role of these kinases in signal transduction is reviewed elsewhere [2]. Cell surface receptors which interact with nonreceptor tyrosine kinases include those for IL-2, IL-7, G-CSF, growth hormone, prolactin, Fcγ, and certain adhesion molecules, including CD-2, and CD-18.

RECEPTOR TYROSINE KINASES

Receptor tyrosine kinases are those receptors whose typical configuration includes an extracellular ligand-binding region which confers ligand specificity, a transmembrane domain, and a cytoplasmic domain that possesses intrinsic protein tyrosine kinase activity. Internal sequences which exhibit SH-2 and SH-3 homologies are important and necessary for recognition of specific downstream effectors. Ligands for receptor tyrosine kinases

A. M. Gotto, Jr. et al. (eds.), Drugs Affecting Lipid Metabolism, 77–93.

include those for EGF, PDGF, FGF, and the neurotrophins. This area has also been reviewed elsewhere [3].

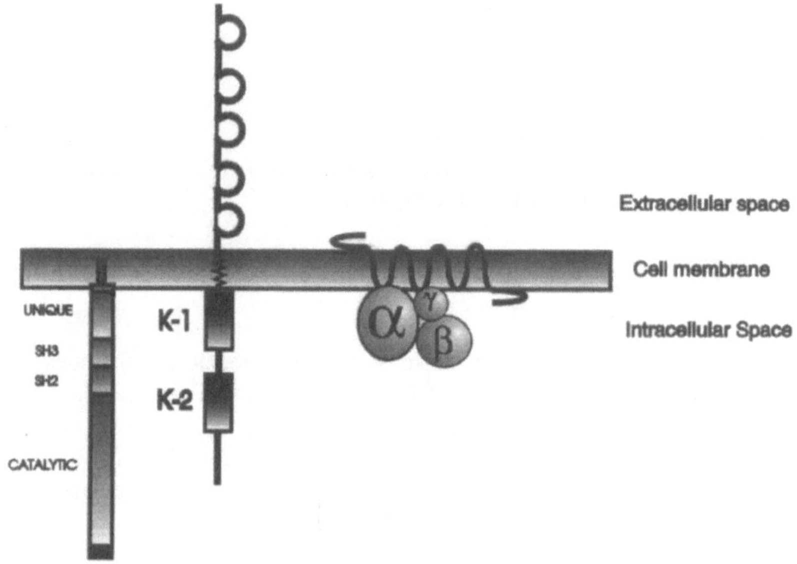

Figure 1. Structural and functional relationships between signal transducing receptors. *Nonreceptor tyrosine kinases* include src, fyn, and lyn, and are tethered to the cell membrane by myristoylation. These proteins have cysteine-rich domains which possess tyrosine phosphorylation sites (called SH-1, and SH-2 domains). *Receptor tyrosine kinases* include those for PDGF, EGF, and FGF. These receptors have an extracellular ligand-specific domain, a transmembrane domain, and a variable number of SH-2 domains which possess intrinsic kinase activity. Receptor-ligand interaction results in receptor, dimerization of these receptors, autophosphorylation, and phosphorylation of other effectors, leading to their subsequent activation. *G-protein-coupled receptors* possess a seven-transmembrane motif which allow for both specificity of ligand binding and specificity for G-protein interaction. Inactive heterotrimeric G-protein α subunits contain GDP, and are noncovalently associated with a regulatory $\beta\gamma$ subunit, which upon receptor-ligand interaction, results in GDP-GTP exchange, subunit dissociation, and activation of downstream signals.

G-PROTEINS AND G-PROTEIN-COUPLED RECEPTORS

Receptors containing the classical seven-membrane spanning domain interact with a family of guanine nucleotide-binding proteins, collectively known as heterotrimeric G-proteins. Receptors which interact with heterotrimeric G-proteins include those for acetylcholine, endothelin, thrombin, bradykinin, angiotensin II, and a variety of others. The diversity of receptor-G-protein interaction is highlighted elsewhere [4]. Briefly, heterotrimeric G-proteins exist as a complex of a catalytic Gα subunit (of which 18 are known), and a βγ regulatory subunit. There are also 5 β and 7 γ isoforms. Upon receptor activation, the Gα subunit dissociates from its βγ heterodimer, and elicits the activation of numerous downstream effects as described below.

INTRACELLULAR DOWNSTREAM SIGNALLING

Receptor ligand interaction elicits a series of downstream intracellular events which amplify and modulate the effect of specific receptor activation, and is highlighted in Figure 2. Briefly, downstream effectors of cell surface receptor activation result in an ordered sequence of molecular events leading to cyclic AMP formation, calcium flux, eicosanoid production, and the stimulation of a kinase cascade leading to alterations in cytoskeletal rearrangements and gene transcription. However, it is important to note here that these distinct signalling pathways have a number of converging points, including the activation of PKC, PLC isozymes, MEKK activation, and eicosanoid production. For the purposes of this review, we focus on the role of cyclooxygenase products, and how they may modulate cholesterol trafficking.

CYCLOOXYGENASE METABOLISM AND REGULATION OF CYTOKINE ACTION

As introduced above, a major consequence of PLA_2 and PLC activation is eicosanoid synthesis. Thus, PDGF [5], IL-1 [6], thrombin [7], and others stimulate eicosanoid synthesis. Endothelial and smooth muscle cells synthesize mainly PGI_2, $PGF_{2\alpha}$, PGE_2, 15-, 12- and 5-HETEs, and epoxyeicosatetraenoic acids (EETs), whereas inflammatory cells generate primarily PGE_2, leukotrienes, and a variety of HETEs. The mechanisms by which cyclooxygenase activity is regulated have recently been the subject of intense research, and are summarized in Figure 3.

Cyclooxygenase products such as PGI_2 and PGE_1 mediate signal transduction either by increasing cyclic AMP [8], after binding to G-protein-coupled receptors coupled to Gαs or by increasing intracellular calcium levels via G-protein-coupled receptor activation of calcium release [9]. Cyclic AMP in turn inhibits MAPK activity [10] and PDGF synthesis [11], and thus antagonizes growth factor-induced DNA synthesis and cell proliferation. In contrast to cyclooxygenase products, LTB_4 mediates phorbol ester-induced TNF gene expression [12]. This aspect of eicosanoid biochemistry becomes important since cholesterol trafficking is in part regulated by eicosanoids and other second messengers.

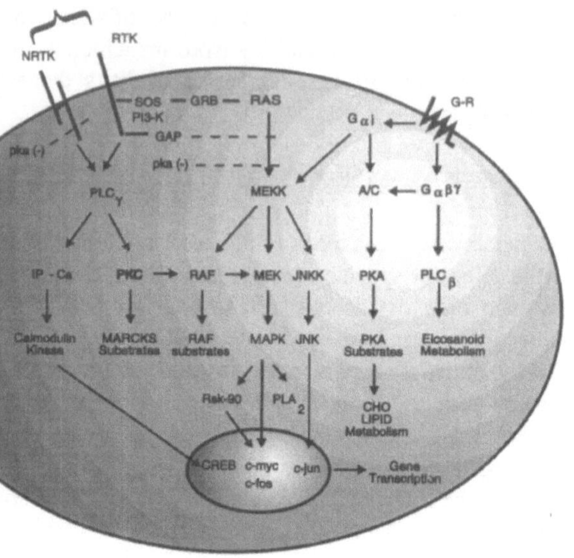

Figure 2. Downstream signals of cell membrane receptor activation - convergence of downstream signals. Activation of *nonreceptor tyrosine kinases (NRTK)* promotes tyrosine phosphorylation, specific binding (through SH domains), and subsequent activation of PLCγ, PI-3-kinase, and p21ras. Similarly, activation of *receptor tyrosine kinases* promotes the activation of the same effectors. PLC isozyme activation results in liberation of IP_3, which promotes calcium release, which regulates calcium-dependent control of gene transcription through the activation of calmodulin-dependent protein kinase (CLM-KINASE) and subsequent binding of CREB to its 5'-promotor binding sites. The other major PLC product, diacylglycerol can stimulate PKC activity, whose major substrates include proteins which regulate cytoskeletal elements, known as myristoylated alanine-rich C kinase substrates (MARCKS). Activation of p21ras elicits a phoshorylation cascade of serine/threonine kinases, which include MEKK, which in turn phosphorylates and hence activates Raf and MEK. Raf can also be activated by PKC. RAF, in addition to MEKK, can activate MEK, whose principal substrate is MAPK (also known as ERK's 1 and 2). MAPK substrates include c-myc and c-fos (a nuclear transcription factor), $cPLA_2$ (responsible for arachidonic acid release), and Rsk-90 (important in initiating protein synthesis). MEKK also phosphorylates a putative kinase responsible for activation of JNK, whose substrate is c-jun (a transcription factor important in initiating mitogenesis). Downstream effectors of *Gα subunits* include PLCβ, adenylate cyclase, phosphodiesterase, and potentially PLA_2. Specifically, Gαs stimulates adenylate cyclase activity, while the pertussis toxin-sensitive G-proteins Gαi1-3 inhibits adenylate cyclase activity. G11, G14, and G16 all stimulate PLCβ. In addition, Gαi may crosstalk to stimulate MEKK. Interestingly, βγ heterodimer may also directly activate PLA_2, PLCβ, and adenylate cyclase. By either mechanism, cyclic AMP modulates the activity of cyclic AMP-dependent protein kinase (PKA). PKA substrates are diverse, and are important in the control of both carbohydrate and lipid metabolism. In addition, PKA will downregulate the activity of src and p21ras. Thus, the major mechanism modulating the mitogenic effects of cytokine stimulation is activation of PKA. Finally, PLA_2 and PLC activation also leads to eicosanoid synthesis.

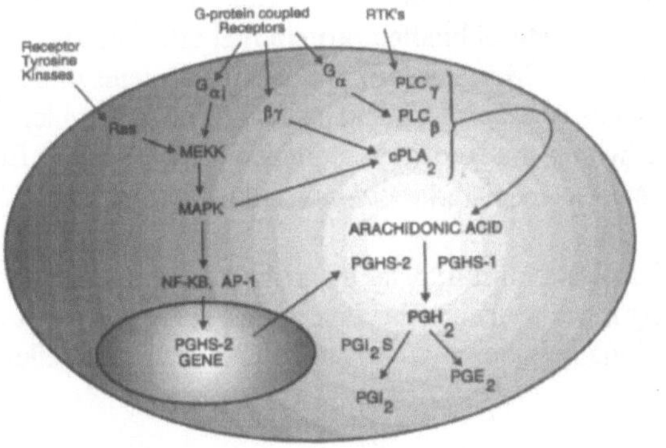

Figure 3. Regulation of eicosanoid synthesis. Activation of G-protein-coupled receptors promote arachidonic acid release directly by activating PLA_2 or PLC-β isozymes. Gαi may also activate $cPLA_2$ after activating MEKK. Activation of receptor and nonreceptor tyrosine kinases activate PLC-γ or PLA_2 by activating MEKK. Arachidonic acid is converted to cyclooxygenase products by a constitutively expressed PGHS-1, and by upregulation of PGHS-2 following activation of MEKK. PGHS-2 expression thus significantly enhances total eicosanoid output.

Regulation of Cholesterol Metabolism by Cytokines and Growth Factors: Role of Second Messengers

Cellular cholesterol levels is regulated by the processes controlling delivery, metabolism, and efflux. Cholesterol delivery is mediated by the LDL receptor, and a number of scavenger receptors which recognize modified forms of LDL. Once internalized, LDL-derived cholesteryl esters (CE) are hydrolyzed by lysosomal (acid) CE hydrolase (ACEH); liberated free cholesterol then enters a pool of cellular free cholesterol derived from *de novo* synthesis by HMG-CoA reductase. Free cholesterol is in equilibrium with its storage form of cytoplasmic CE as a result of continuous esterification by acyl CoA-cholesterol acyltransferase (ACAT), and subsequent hydrolysis by cytoplasmic (neutral) CE hydrolase (NCEH). Otherwise, free cholesterol is used by the cell for membrane biogenesis, stored in the cytoplasm or translocated to the cell membrane for net efflux, which is mediated principally by HDL. However, cholesterol trafficking is also governed by second messengers, as summarized in Table 1, and detailed here.

LDL RECEPTOR (LDL-R)

The expression of the LDL-R is negatively regulated by cholesterol. Briefly, the promotor region of the LDL-R gene contains 16 base-pair repeats [13]. Repeat "3" possesses SP-1 binding sites that augment LDL-R gene transcription independently of sterols. Importantly, Repeat "2" inhibits the activity of Repeat 3, but only in the presence of sterols [14]. The mechanism by which this occurs is unclear. Either cholesterol may directly bind to Repeat 3 or it may bind to a nuclear sterol binding protein that interferes with Sp-1 activation of LDL-R gene transcription [14]. More recently, a cluster of proteins of 59-68 kDa have been identified as a sterol-responsive element binding protein (SREBP), which binds to a 10-base pair SRE-1 imbedded within the Repeat 2 sequence [15]. Thus, SREBP and Sp-1 may cooperate to mediate steroid-mediated repression transcription of the LDL-R gene.

Table 1. Regulation of cholesterol trafficking by growth factors and cytokines. The control of cholesterol trafficking is cell specific. The data in this Table summarize what is presently known regarding cytokine regulation of cholesterol delivery, intracellular trafficking, and efflux.

Cells	Cytokine	Effector	Response
Smooth Muscle Cells	PDGF	LDL-R,SRA-I ACEH, NCEH HMG-CoA-Reductase	Increase
	bFGF, TGF-β	LDL-R	
	TNF	SRA	
Monocyte/ Macrophage	TGF-β, TNF,LPS, IFN-γ, ADP, Fibrinogen, Fibronectin	SRA	Decrease
	GM-CSF,M-CSF	SRA	Increase
	GM-CSF	LDL-R	
	M-CSF	ACEH, NCEH, CD36	
HEP-G2 Cells	IL-1β, EGF, TNF	LDL-R	Increase

The expression of LDL receptor is subject to regulation by cytokines and second messengers. PDGF [16], basic FGF [17], EGF [18], and IL-1β [19] stimulate LDL-receptor activity through at least two mechanisms. Firstly, PDGF increases LDL-receptor activity by either releasing the LDL-R gene from cholesterol-induced suppression [20], or by stimulating LDL-receptor expression independently of cellular cholesterol levels. However, the importance of ambient free cholesterol levels in cytokine-treated cells becomes evident owing to observations that IL-1 and TNF, which could not override transcriptional inhibition of the LDL-R by LDL-derived cholesterol [19]. These results also suggest that free cholesterol levels may be the determining factor in LDL-R expression. In any case, the mechanisms by which cytokines stimulate LDL receptor expression has been partially elucidated. In monocytes, the role of PKC in mediating cytokine induction of the LDL receptor is unclear since PKC activation either stimulated [21] or inhibited [22] LDL-receptor expression. In smooth muscle cells, basic FGF stimulated LDL-receptor expression by a PKC-dependent mechanism [17]. However, agents which stimulate cyclic AMP synthesis, such as PGI_2 reduce LDL-receptor expression [23], even though a cyclic AMP-responsive element in the LDL-R promotor is not identifiable [24]. Finally, the mechanism by which EGF stimulates LDL receptor expression may be due to activation of tyrosine kinases, since EGF-induction of LDL receptor expression can be inhibited by gentisin, but not PKC inhibitors [18]. Taken together these observations suggest that cytokines may stimulate LDL-R expression independently of PKC and PKA. They implicate MAPK cascade in upregulating LDL expression, which is PKA-inhibitable by interfering with ras function. These results support the premise that under quiescent conditions, the LDL receptor is downregulated, and, under conditions of activation or inflammation, LDL receptor activity can be enhanced.

SCAVENGER RECEPTORS

Scavenger receptors are membrane proteins that mediate the endocytosis of modified lipoproteins, such as acetylated LDL (aLDL)[25] and oxidized LDL (oxLDL) [26]. There are two classes of scavenger receptors. The class A receptors include the type I and II macrophage scavenger receptors, termed SR-AI and SR-AII. SR-AI and SR-AII are homotrimeric membrane proteins composed of glycosylated monomers of 453 or 349 amino acids, respectively [27,28], and are derived from alternatively spliced mRNA products of a single gene. The SR-AI receptor contains extra cysteine-rich sequence of 110 amino acids, while the cysteine-rich sequence is absent from the SR-AII receptor and is replaced by a 6-amino acid C-terminus. The class A receptors bind modified LDL, fucoidin, polyguanosinic acid, and carrageenan. Class B scavenger receptors include CD36, which binds oxidized LDL and maleylated albumin, but not fucoidin or other polyanions [29]. Class C scavenger receptors include a novel receptor recently cloned from Drosophilia, which exhibits ligand binding specificities similar to that of SR-As, but has a unique primary sequence [30].

From the context of LDL metabolism, the most highly studied scavenger receptor is the SR-A receptor. The scavenger receptor is not downregulated by cholesterol [31], and can incorporate CE in modified LDL unimpeded by rising intracellular free cholesterol levels. However, scavenger receptor expression is also regulated by cytokines. In the macrophage, the scavenger receptor is downregulated by LPS [32], TNF [33], IFN-γ [34], and platelet products [35]. The mechanisms by which these ligands reduce scavenger receptor expression are unknown. PKC has been ruled out since PKC activation either has no effect [36] or stimulates the scavenger receptor [37]. However, leukotrienes or HETEs have been implicated in scavenger receptor activation since lipoxygenase inhibitors reduce scavenger receptor activity [38]. In contrast to macrophages, smooth muscle cells do not normally express a scavenger receptor, but it can be transiently induced by PDGF [39] and phorbol esters [40]. These observations suggest that quiescent macrophages are the principal scavengers of modified forms of LDL under basal conditions. Thus, under inflammatory conditions, scavenger-receptor-mediated clearance of modified LDL by the macrophage will be determined by the identity and concentrations of cytokines present in the extracellular milieu. However, smooth muscle cells may assume this capacity under inflammatory conditions. These results imply that smooth muscle cells and macrophages can become "foam cells" under atherogenic conditions.

Importantly, there is now evidence demonstrating that the class A scavenger receptor is also capable of signalling. Scavenger-receptor-mediated signalling is complex, and may be due in part to disparate effects of ligands and their constituents on postreceptor signalling. For example, fucoidan stimulated urokinase expression in a PKC-dependent manner [41]. However, oxidized LDL decreased PGI_2 formation in endothelial cells by a mechanism independent of PLC [42], and decreased inducible nitric oxide activity in macrophages [43]. However, these effects are not mimicked by oxidized lipids present in oxidized LDL. Lysophosphatidylcholine can increase steady state mRNA levels for PDGF [44] and ICAM-1 expression in endothelial cells [45]. The fatty acid peroxidation products of linoleic acid, such as 9-hydroxyoctadecadienoic acid (9-HODE) and 2,4-decadienal and 2-octenal, can stimulate IL-1β release from mononuclear cells [46]. Interestingly, hydroxy-acids of linoleate stimulate MAPK activity, c-fos, c-jun-, c-myc RNA expression, and hence, proliferation in smooth muscle cells [47]. These observations appear significant since not only do cytokines mediate expression of the scavenger receptor but pure ligands of the scavenger receptor, and secondary ligands released from the metabolism of oxidized LDL, can signal to affect cell function. Furthermore, the role of the scavenger receptor is further complicated by the fact that CD36, a class B scavenger receptor which is an adhesion molecule [48] that can bind oxidized LDL [49], may be responsible for a significant portion of LDL CE uptake [50]. CD36 is present on monocytes, and can be upregulated by exposure to cytokine-activated endothelial cells [51]. Thus, the metabolism of oxidized LDL by the macrophage will ultimately depend on the degree of cytokine "tone". Since cytokines reduce SR-AI expression, but upregulate CD36 expression, the net uptake of oxidized LDL by macrophages may be unchanged. However, the biological effects of oxidized LDL may ultimately depend upon the degree of oxidation of the LDL, and the identity of the oxidated lipid species released following oxidized LDL degradation. This concept is supported by observations that minimally modified oxidized LDL stimulates cytokine production, while highly oxidized LDL is cytotoxic [52]. Finally, signals induced by SRA-1- and CD36 ligation may promote continued cytokine synthesis, which would favor CD36-mediated oxidized LDL incorporation subsequent to foam cell development.

HYDROXYMETHYL GLUTARYL COA REDUCTASE (HMG-COA REDUCTASE)

HMG-CoA reductase is the committed step in cholesterol biogenesis. The promotor region of the HMG-CoA reductase gene contains an NF-1 binding site which stimulates HMG-CoA reductase gene expression [53]. This expression is inhibited by sterols [54]. Importantly, HMG-CoA reductase is also subject to regulation by cytokines. PDGF can increase HMG-CoA reductase expression [55] by a mechanism which regulates phosphorylation.

HMG-CoA reductase is active when dephoshorylated (by HMG-CoA reductase phosphatase), and inactive when the enzyme is phosphorylated (by PKC) [56]. Unfortunately, little is known about distal regulatory mechanisms following PKC activation on HMG-CoA reductase activities in vascular cells. HMG-CoA reductase may also be sensitive to PKA-dependent pathways, since PGI_2, a PGI_2 analog (iloprost) and PGE_1 can reduce HMG-CoA reductase in monocytes [23], presumably through their ability to stimulate cyclic AMP production. Thus, under inflammatory conditions, cytokines may increase free cholesterol levels in part by increasing the expression of HMG-CoA reductase. However, it is unclear if HMG-CoA reductase activity in the vascular wall is actually increased, since elevated plasma levels of cholesterol would serve to downregulate HMG-CoA reductase expression, especially if scavenger receptor activity is high.

HDL Receptor

HDL promotes net cholesterol efflux by absorption of cell membrane cholesterol in a physicochemical manner though protein/lipid interactions at the cell surface [57], and by a receptor-dependent mechanism through its apolipoprotein moieties (Apo-AI, Apo A-II, and C-3) [58,59]. HDL-induced cholesterol flux from the cytoplasm and endoplasmic reticulum to the cell membrane may occur through activation of specific signal transduction processes. The HDL receptor is coupled to PLC by a pertussis-toxin sensitive G-protein [60], which stimulates PKC. Thus, HDL stimulates cholesterol efflux in a PKC- [61] and cyclic AMP- [62] dependent manner. Cyclic AMP-dependent cholesterol efflux may be due in part to its ability to stimulate eicosanoid production [63,64]. However, eicosanoid-independent cholesterol efflux has also been described in lipid-enriched smooth muscle cells [65].

HDL receptor activity is also regulated by cytokines. HDL-R activity is upregulated by IFN-γ [66] and downregulated by PDGF [67] and insulin [68]. Since IFN-γ inhibits [69] and PDGF induces [70] smooth muscle cell proliferation, HDL-receptor activity may be regulated as a function of phenotype (downregulated in proliferating cells, and upregulated in quiescent/differentiated cells), or regulated by loss of cholesterol repression, and not a consequence of direct cytokine regulation of HDL-receptor gene expression. These observations suggest that receptor-dependent and -independent means for regulating cellular cholesterol content may exist to allow for gross- and fine-tuning of intracellular cholesterol levels.

Intracellular Cholesterol Trafficking-Cholesteryl Ester Hydrolases and ACAT

Cholesterol does not regulate the expression of ACEH or NCEH, but, as a substrate, it determines the kinetics of each of these enzymes. However, ACEH and NCEH are clearly regulated by cytokines/growth factors. PDGF stimulates ACEH activity in smooth muscle cells by increasing PGI_2 production [71], and M-CSF increases NCEH and ACEH activities in macrophages [72], thus promoting CE hydrolysis [73]. The mechanism by which growth factors influence CE-hydrolytic activities appear to be due to the generation of second messengers. In arterial smooth muscle cells, ACEH activity is dependent upon cyclic AMP production following stimulation by PGI_2 [74,75]. Similarly, NCEH activity is augmented by PGI_2-dependent processes leading cyclic AMP synthesis and PKA activation [76]. On the other hand, the overwhelming body of evidence suggests that ACAT is regulated essentially by levels of free cellular cholesterol, and not by alterations in second messenger synthesis. Thus, reductions in ACEH will promote CE retention in prelysosomal pools, as occurs in smooth muscle cells [77], while reductions in NCEH activity can promote cholesterol retention in cytoplasmic pools, as occurs in macrophages [78]. However, since net cholesterol content will ultimately depend on the relative levels of LDL and HDL, the relative contribution of second messengers in modulating CE hydrolase activities is unclear. These observations suggest that cytokine stimulation of arterial cells may increase the rate of cholesterol esterification/hydrolysis, while net free cholesterol content will depend on net LDL and HDL concentrations and their respective receptor activities.

Cytokines and Eicosanoids in Context in the Control of Cholesterol Trafficking

Clearly, the influence of cytokines and second messengers is exceedingly complex, and is dependent on the cell type, the type and distribution of cell surface receptors, and the hierarchy of signal transduction pathways in each cell type. In smooth muscle cells, for example, most growth factors, such as PDGF and bFGF can promote cell proliferation, and as a result, stimulate processes important in the net acquisition of free cholesterol, whether derived from *de novo* synthesis or from LDL-receptor or scavenger receptor derived sources. This is depicted in Figure 4A. In contrast, most cytokines reduce cholesterol delivery through the scavenger receptor, but may increase derivitized LDL incorporation though CD36. In addition, the contribution of eicosanoids in modulating cholesterol trafficking in the macrophage may also be complex, since endogenous synthesis and effects of LTB_4 to mediate net cholesterol influx may be antagonized by PGI_2 derived from the macrophage or by PGI_2 derived from adjacent smooth muscle cells and/or endothelium. This is depicted in Figure 4B.

In addition, signal transduction processes elicited by transmembrane signals are diverse, and depend on isoform specific receptors and specific downstream signals. For example, PDGF signalling is dependent upon the ligand isoform (PDGF-AA, PDGF, BB, PDGF-AB), as well as the receptor isoform ($\alpha\alpha$, $\alpha\beta$, or $\beta\beta$). Similarly, each G-protein receptor has at least two, and as many as five isoforms which differ in tissue distribution and ligand binding affinity. In addition, G-protein agonists are known to have diametrically opposite effects on vascular cells. For example, bradykinin and acetylcholine, both G-protein-coupled agonists, are vasodilators whose effects are mediated principally through thegeneration of nitric oxide and prostacyclin. In contrast, thrombin, angiotensin II, and endothelin are also G-protein-coupled agonists which are vasoconstrictors and are potent mitogens. The downstream signals for each of these ligands is unique, and dependent on interactions with specific $G\alpha$, $\beta\gamma$ subunits, as well as specific PLC-β and PKC isoforms. Unfortunately, the specificity of these receptor-G-protein-effector coupling systems are still not fully characterized. Finally, the net effect of cytokine activation will also depend upon

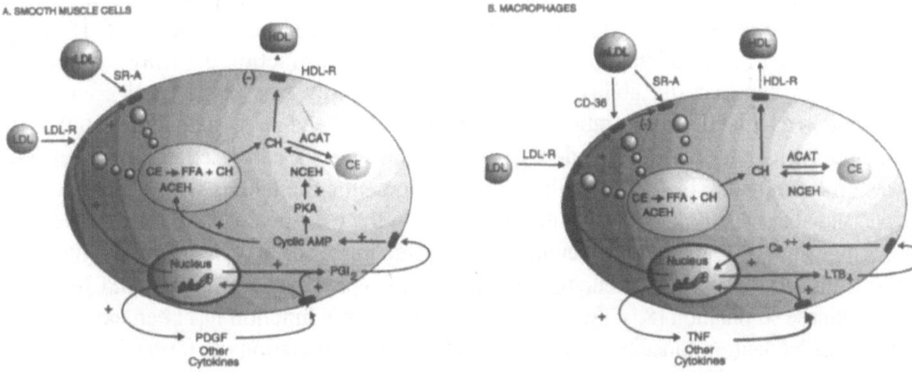

Figure 4. Regulation of cholesterol trafficking by cytokines and growth factors; interactions with second messengers. *Panel A*. Influence of PDGF on cholesterol trafficking in arterial smooth muscle cells. PDGF, the a predominant growth factor generated and released by arterial endothelial and smooth muscle cells, induces the transcription and translation of the LDL- and the scavenger receptors, which allows for LDL and modified LDL delivery of CE. This effect is augmented by PDGF induction of PGI_2 synthesis, which occurs as a results of direct phospholipase activation and nascent synthesis of PGHS-2. PGI_2 then stimulates cyclic AMP formation, and along with PKA activation, stimulates the activities of ACEH, and NCEH, respectively. Since the overall influence of cytokine effect is due in part to magnitude and duration, low levels of cytokine activation may promote CE hydrolysis without allowing for cell-proliferation and or increased CE delivery. *Panel B*. Influence of TNF on cholesterol trafficking in macrophages. TNF, the predominant cytokine generated by macrophages, promotes upregulation of the LDL-receptor, and CD36, and downregulates expression of the SRA scavenger receptor. The macrophage generation of LTB_4 enhances CE accumulation by upregulation of CD36. However, not shown in this panel is the concept that cytokines would also stimulate PGHS-2 expression in the macrophage (as in the arterial smooth muscle cell). However, PGI_2, and PGE_2 are minor products when compared to leukotriene synthesis, and thus may have less impact than in smooth muscle cells to assist in activation of ACEH and NCEH. M-CSF may promote CE clearance by enhancing cyclooxygenase vs lipoxygenase product formation in macrophages, and thus stimulate CE clearance by this method.

two important variables: (1) the strength and duration of ligand interaction, such as the case for FGF receptor action in the regulation of cell phenotype [79], and (2) the influence of multiple cytokine interactions which may serve to either antagonize or synergize each other to promote alterations in cell function. In this regard, there is essentially no information as to how these factors influence cholesterol trafficking in even isolated cells.

Atherosclerosis is characterized by intimal accumulation of CE-laden macrophages and smooth muscle cells. In addition, enhanced growth factor/cytokine production in lesions has been documented [80], while the synthesis of PGI_2 [81] and cyclic AMP [82] are reduced. Thus, in spite of the complexity of the signal transduction pathways elaborated above, it is clear that the ability of cells to maintain low free cholesterol content, is dependent on a high HDL/LDL ratio, low proliferative state, and an intact cellular apparatus that supports cyclic AMP-dependent processes leading to enhanced HDL-dependent cholesterol removal. Thus, at least three novel therapeutic modalities which interact with specific signal transduction pathways may be useful in the treatment of aberrant cholesterol trafficking. First, low molecular weight SH-2 peptide mimetics may be useful in inhibiting signal transduction pathways elicited through nonreceptor tyrosine kinase and receptor tyrosine kinase stimulation [83]. Second, inhibition of p21ras function has been explored by a number of modalities. Since p21ras requires membrane association via farnesylation [84], inhibitors of HMG-CoA reductase [85] and farnesyl transferase [86] may be of use in inhibiting p21ras-dependent pathways leading to MAPK and upregulation of LDL-R and scavenger receptor expression. Calcium channel blockers, useful for the treatment of hypertension, are now being used for the treatment of atherosclerosis since they may stimulate CE hydrolytic activities [87], and PGI_2 synthesis [88]. Importantly, calcium channel blockers also inhibit smooth muscle cell proliferation [89]. It remains to be determined if calcium channel blockers working in concert with the cytokine/eicosanoid "network" can function in a therapeutic setting to mobilize cholesterol and its by-products from the vessel wall to reduce atherosclerosis.

References

1. Goldstein J, Brown M. The low-density lipoprotein pathway and its relation to atherosclerosis. Ann Rev Biochem 1977;46:897-930.
2. Carpenter G. Receptor tyrosine kinases: *src* homology domains and signal transduction. FASEB J 1992;6:3283-89.
3. Bolen J. Signal transduction by the SRC family of tyrosine protein kinases in hemopoietic cells. Cell Growth and Differentiation 1991;2:409-14.
4. Rens-Domiano S, Hamm H. Structural and functional relationships of heterotrimeric G-proteins. FASEB J 1995;9:1059-66.
5. Pomerantz K, Summers B, Hajjar D. Eicosanoid metabolism in cholesterol-enriched smooth muscle cells-II. Evidence for reduced post-transcriptional processing of cyclooxygenase I and reduced cyclooxygenase II gene expression. Biochem 1993; 32:13624-25.
6. Kerr J, Stevens T, Davis G, et al. Effects of recombinant interleukin-1 beta on phospholipase A_2 activity, phospholipase A_2 mRNA levels, and eicosanoid formation in rabbit chondrocytes. Biochem Biophys Res Commun 1989;165:1079-84.
7. Garcia J, Painter R, Fenton J, et al. Thrombin-induced prostacyclin biosynthesis in human endothelium: Role of guanine nucleotide regulatory proteins in stimulus/ coupling responses. J Cell Physiol 1990; 142:186-93.
8. Dembinska-kiec A, Rucker W, Schonhofer P. Effects of PGI_2 and PGI_2 analogs on cAMP levels in cultured endothelial and smooth muscle cells derived from bovine arteries. Naunyn-Schmied Arch Pharm 1980;311:67-70.
9. Goetzl E, An S, Smith W. Specificity of expression and effects of eicosanoid mediators in

normal physiology and human diseases. FASEB J 1995;9:1051-58.
10. Graves LM, Bornfeldt KE, Raines EW, et al. Protein kinase-A antagonizes platelet-derived growth factor-induced signaling by mitogen-activated protein kinase in human arterial smooth muscle cells. Proc Natl Acad Sci U S A 1993;90: 10300-304.
11. Kavanaugh W, Harsh G, Starksen N, et al. Transcriptional regulation of the A and B chain genes of platelet-derived growth factor in microvascular endothelial cells. J Biol Chem 1988;263:8470-72.
12. Horiguchi J, Spriggs D, Imamura K, et al. Role of arachidonic acid metabolism in transcriptional induction of tumor necrosis factor gene expression by phorbol ester. Mol Cell Biol 1989;9:252-58.
13. Mehta K, Brown M, Bilheimer D, et al. The low density receptor in Xenopus laevis. II. Feedback repression mediated by conserved sterol regulatory element. J Biol Chem 1991;266:10415-19.
14. Dawson P, Hofmann S, van de Westhuyzen D, et al. Sterol-dependent repression of low density lipoprotein receptor promotor mediated by 16-base pair sequence adjacent to binding site for transcription factor Sp1. J Biol Chem 1988;263:3372-79.
15. Wang X, Briggs M, Hua X, et al. Nuclear protein that binds sterol regulatory element of low density lipoprotein receptor promoter. II. Purification and characterization. J Biol Chem 1993;268:14497-504.
16. Rechtoris C, Mazzone T. Isoform-specific induction of the low-density lipoprotein receptor gene by platelet-derived growth factor. Amer J Physiol-Cell Physiol 1995; 37:C1033-C1039.
17. Hsu H, Nicholson A, Hajjar D. Basic fibroblast growth factor-induced low density lipoprotein receptor transcription and surface expression. Signal transduction pathways mediated by the bFGF receptor tyrosine kinase. J Biol Chem 1994; 269:9213-20.
18. Graham A, Russell LJ. Stimulation of low-density lipoprotein uptake in hepG2 cells by epidermal growth factor via a tyrosine kinase-dependent, but protein kinase-C-independent, mechanism. Biochem J 1994;298:579-84.
19. Stopeck A, Nicholson A, Mancini F, et al. Cytokine regulation of LDL receptor gene transcription in HEP G2 cells. J Biol Chem 1993;268:17489-94.
20. Mazzone T, Basheeruddin K, Ping L, et al. Relation of growth- and sterol- regulatory pathways for low density lipoprotein receptor gene expression. J Biol Chem 1990;265:5145-49.
21. Auwerx J, Chait A, Wolfbauer G, et al. Involvement of second messengers in regulation of the low-density lipoprotein receptor gene. Mol Cell Biol 1989; 9:2298-2302.
22. Frasier-Scott K, Hatzakis H, Seong D, et al. Influence of natural and recombinant interleukin 2 on endothelial cell arachidonate metabolism: Induction of de novo synthesis of prostaglandin H synthase. J Clin Invest 1988;82:1877-83.
23. Krone W, Klass A, Nagele H, et al. Effect of prostaglandins on LDL receptor activity and cholesterol synthesis in freshly isolated human mononuclear leukocytes. J Lipid Res 1988;29:1663-69.
24. Takagi K, Strauss F. Control of low density lipoprotein receptor gene expression in steroidogenic cells. Can J Physiol Pharmacol 1989;67:968-73.
25. Kodama T, Reddy P, Kishamoto C, et al. Purification and characterization of a bovine acetyl low density lipoprotein receptor. Proc Natl Acad Sci U S A 1988;85: 9238-42.
26. Freeman M, Ekkel Y, Rohrer L, et al. Expression of type I and type II bovine scavenger receptors in Chinese hamster ovary cells: Lipid droplet accumulation and nonreciprocal cross competition by acetylated and oxidized low density lipoprotein. Proc Natl Acad Sci U S A

1991;88:4931-35.

27. Kodama T, Freeman M, Rohrer L, et al. Type I macrophage scavenger receptor contains alpha-helical and collagen-like coiled coils. Nature 1990;343:531-35.

28. Rohrer L, Freeman M, Kodama T, et al. Coiled-coil fibrous domains mediate ligand binding by macrophage scavenger receptor type II. Nature 1990;343:570-72.

29. Acton SL, Scherer PE, Lodish HF, et al. Expression cloning of SR-BI, a CD36- related class b scavenger receptor. J Biol Chem 1994;269:21003-21009.

30. Pearson A, Lux A, Frieger M. Expression cloning of cSR-C1, a class C macrophage-specific scavenger receptor from Drosophila melanogaster. Proc Natl Acad Sci U S A 1995;92:4056-4060.

31. Brown M, Goldstein J. Lipoprotein metabolism in the macrophage: Implications for cholesterol deposition in atherosclerosis. Ann Rev Biochem 1983;52:223-61.

32. Van Lentin B, Fogelman A, Seager J, et al. Bacterial endotoxin selectively prevents the expression of scavenger-receptor activity on human monocyte-macrophages. J Immunol 1985;134:3718-21.

33. Van Lenten B, Fogelman A. Lipopolysacchride-induced inhibition of scavenger receptor expression in human monocyte-macrophages is mediated through tumor necrosis factor-alpha. J Immunol 1992;148:112-16.

34. Fong L, Fong A, Cooper A. Inhibition of mouse macrophage degradation of acetyl-low density lipoprotein by interferon-gamma. J Biol Chem 1990;265: 11751-60.

35. Pomerantz K, Hajjar D. Eicosanoids in regulation of arterial smooth muscle cell phenotype, proliferative capacity, and cholesterol metabolism. Arteriosclerosis 1989; 9:413-29.

36. Jouni Z, McNamara D. Lipoprotein receptors of HL-60 macrophages. Effect of differentiation with tetramyristic phorbol acetate and 1,25-dihydroxyvitamin D3. Arterio and Thromb 1991;11:995-1006.

37. Hayashi K, Dojo S, Hirata Y, et al. Metabolic changes in LDL receptors and an appearance of scavenger receptors after phorbol ester-induced differentiation of U937 cells. Biochim Biophys Acta 1991;1082:152-60.

38. Schroeff J, Havekes L, Weerheim A, et al. Suppression of cholesteryl ester accumulation in cultured human monocyte-derived macrophages by lipoxygenase inhibitors. Biochem Biophys Res Commun 1985;127:366-72.

39. Inaba T, Gotoda T, Shimano H, et al. Platelet-derived growth factor induces c-fms and scavenger receptor genes in vascular smooth muscle cells. J Biol Chem 1992; 267:13107-112.

40. Pitas R. Expression of the acetyl low density lipoprotein receptor by rabbit fibroblasts and smooth muscle cells. J Biol Chem 1990;265:12722-727.

41. Falcone D, McCaffrey T, Vergilio J. Stimulation of macrophage urokinase expression by polyanions is protein kinase C-dependent and requires protein and RNA synthesis. J Biol Chem 1991;266:22726-732.

42. Thorin E, Hamilton CA, Dominiczak MH, et al. Chronic exposure of cultured bovine endothelial cells to oxidized LDL abolishes prostacyclin release. Arterioscler Thromb 1994;14:453-59.

43. Yang XC, Cai BL, Sciacca RR, et al. Inhibition of inducible nitric oxide synthase in macrophages by oxidized low-density lipoproteins. Circ Res 1994;74:318-28.

44. Kume N, Gimbrone MA: Lysophosphatidylcholine transcriptionally induces growth factor gene expression in cultured human endothelial cells. J Clin Invest 1994;93: 907-911.

45. Sugiyama S, Kugiyama K, Ohgushi M, et al. Lysophosphatidylcholine in oxidized low-density lipoprotein increases endothelial susceptibility to polymorphonuclear leukocyte induced

endothelial dysfunction in porcine coronary arteries - role of protein kinase-C. Circ Res 1994;74:565-75.
46. Thomas CE, Jackson RL, Ohlweiler DF, et al. Multiple lipid oxidation products in low density lipoproteins induce interleukin-1 beta release from human blood mononuclear cells. J Lipid Res 1994;35:417-27.
47. Rao G, Alexander R, Runge M. Linoleic acid and its metabolites, hydroperoxy-octadecadienoic acids, stimulate c-fos, c-jun, and c-myc mRNA expression, mitogen-activated protein kinase activation, and growth in rat aortic smooth muscle cells. J Clin Invest 1995;96:842-53.
48. Greenwalt D, Lipsky R, Ockenhouse C, et al. Membrane glycoprotein CD36: A review of its roles in adherence, signal transduction, and transfusion medicine. Blood 1992;80:1105-15.
49. Nicholson AC, Pearce, FS, et al. Oxidized LDL binds to CD36 on human monocyte-derived macrophages and transfected cell lines - evidence implicating the lipid moiety of the lipoprotein as the binding site. Arterioscler Thromb 1995;15: 269-75.
50. Endemann G, Stanton L, Madden K, et al. CD36 is a receptor for oxidized low density lipoprotein. J Biol Chem 1993;268:11811-816.
51. Huh H, Lo S, Yesner L, et al. CD36 induction on human monocytes upon adhesion to tumor necrosis factor-activated endothelial cells. J Biol Chem 1995;270:6267-71.
52. Reid VC, Mitchinson MJ, Skepper JN. Cytotoxicity of oxidized low-density lipoprotein to mouse peritoneal macrophages - an ultrastructural study. J Pathol 1993;171:321-28.
53. Osborne T, Gil G, Goldstein J, et al. Operator constitutive mutation of 3-hydroxy-3-methylglutaryl coenzyme A reductase promoter abolishes protein binding to sterol regulatory element. J Biol Chem 1988;263:3380-87.
54. Gil G, Smith J, Goldstein J, et al. Multiple genes encode nuclear factor 1-like proteins that bind to the promoter for 3-hydroxy-3-methylglytaryl-coenzyme A reductase. Proc Natl Acad Sci U S A 1988;5:8963-67.
55. Habernicht A, Glomset J, Ross R. Relation of cholesterol and mevalonic acid to the cell cycle in smooth muscle and swiss 3T3 cells stimulated to divide by platelet-derived growth factor. J Biol Chem 1980;255:5134-40.
56. Beg Z, Stonik J, Brewer H. Modulation of the enzymic activity of 3-hydroxy-3-methylglutarryl coenzyme A reductase by multiple kinase systems involving reversible phosphorylation: A review. Metabolism 1987;36:900-17.
57. Rothblat G, Mahlberg F, Johnson W, et al. Apolipoproteins, membrane cholesterol domains, and the regulation of cholesterol efflux. J Lipid Res 1992;33:1091-97.
58. Slotte J, Oram J, Bierman E. Binding of high density lipoproteins to cell receptors promotes translocation of cholesterol from intracellular membranes to the cell surface. J Biol Chem 1987;262:12904-907.
59. Vadiveloo P, Fidge N. Studies on the interaction between apolipoprotein A-II-enriched HDL_3 and cultured bovine aortic endothelial (BAE) cells. Biochim Biophys Acta 1990;1045:135-41.
60. Nizih H, Devred D, Martin-Nizard F, et al. Pertussis toxin sensitive G-protein coupling of HDL receptor to phospholipase C in human platelets. Thromb Res 1992; 67:559-67.
61. Dusserre E, Pulcini T, Bourdillon MC, et al. High-density lipoprotein 3 stimulates phosphatidylcholine breakdown and sterol translocation in rat aortic smooth muscle cells by a phospholipase c/protein kinase c- dependent process. Biochem Med Metab Biol 1994;52:45-52.
62. Bernard D, Rodriguez A, Rothblat G, et al. cAMP stimulates cholesteryl ester clearance to high density lipoproteins in J774 macrophages. J Biol Chem 1991;266: 710-16.

63. Pomerantz K, Tall A, Feinmark S, et al. Stimulation of vascular smooth muscle cell prostacyclin and prostaglandin E_2 synthesis by plasma high and low density lipoproteins. Circ Res 1984;54:554-65.
64. Shaknov Y, Larrue J, Perova N, et al. Prostacyclin-mediated efflux from high density lipoproteins as cellular cholesterol acceptors on aortic smooth muscle cells. J Mol Cell Cardiol 1989;21:461-68.
65. Pomerantz K, Hajjar D. High density lipoprotein-induced cholesterol efflux from arterial smooth muscle cell-derived foam cells: Functional relationship of the cholesteryl ester cycle and eicosanoid biosynthesis. Biochem 1990;29:1892-99.
66. Oppenheimer M, Oram J, Bierman E. Upregulation of HDL receptor activity by gamma interferon associated with inhibition of cell proliferation. J Biol Chem 1988; 2630:19318-323.
67. Oppenheimer M, Oram J, Bierman E. Downregulation of high density lipoprotein receptor activity of cultured fibroblasts by platelet-derived growth factor. Arteriosclerosis 1987;7:325-32.
68. Oppenheimer M, Sundquist K, Bierman E. Downregulation of high-density lipoprotein receptor in human fibroblasts by insulin and IGF-1. Diabetes 1989; 38:117-22.
69. Warner S, Friedman G, Libby P. Immune interferon inhibits proliferation and induces 2'-5'-oligoadenylate synthetase gene expression in human smooth muscle cells. J Clin Invest 1989;83:1174-82.
70. Ross R, Glomset J, Kariya B, et al. A platelet-dependent serum factor that stimulates the proliferation of arterial smooth muscle cells in vitro. Proc Natl Acad Sci U S A 1974;71:1207-10.
71. Hajjar D, Marcus A, Hajjar K. Interactions of arterial cells: Studies on the mechanisms of endothelial cell modulation of cholesterol metabolism in co-cultured smooth muscle cells. J Biol Chem 1987;262:6976-81.
72. Inaba T, Shimano H, Gotoda T, et al. Macrophage colony-stimulating factor regulates both activities of neutral and acidic cholesteryl ester hydrolases in human monocyte-derived macrophages. J Clin Invest 1993;92:750-57.
73. Ishii I, Yanagimachi M, Shirai K, et al. Impact of monocyte colony-stimulating factor upon beta- very low density lipoprotein (beta-VLDL) cholesterol metabolism in tetradecanoyl phorbol acetate-derived THP-1 cells. BBA-Lipid Lipid Metab 1994; 1212:278-84.
74. Hajjar D, Weksler B, Falcone D, et al. Prostacyclin modulates cholesteryl ester hydrolytic activity by its effect on cyclic adenosine monophosphate in rabbit aortic smooth muscle cells. J Clin Invest 1982;70:479-88.
75. Hajjar D, Marcus A, Etingin O. Platelet-neutrophil-smooth muscle cell interactions. Inflammatory mediators such as lipoxygenase-derived mono- and di-hydroxy acids activate cholesteryl ester hydrolysis by the cyclic AMP-dependent protein kinase cascade. Biochem 1989;28:8885-91.
76. Khoo JC, Reue K, Steinberg D, et al. Expression of hormone-sensitive lipase messenger RNA in macrophages. J Lipid Res 1993;34:1969-74.
77. Pomerantz K, Hajjar D. Eicosanoid metabolism in cholesterol-enriched arterial smooth muscle cells: Reduced arachidonate release with concomitant decrease in cyclooxygenase products. J Lipid Res 1989;30:1219-31.
78. Ho Y, Brown M, Goldstein J. Hydrolysis and excretion by cytoplasmic cholesterol esters by macrophages: Stimulation by high density lipoproteins and other agents. J Lipid Res 1980;21:391-98.
79. Schlessinger J. Cellular signalling by receptor tyrosine kinases. In: The Harvey Lectures,

1993-1994. New York: Wiley-Liss & Sons, Inc., 1995: 105-124.

80. Ross R, Masuda J, Raines E, et al. Localization of PDGF-B protein in macrophages in all phases of atherogenesis. Science 1990;248:1009-12.

81. Myers S, Russell D, Parks L, et al. Triphasic response of prostacyclin production in rabbit thoracic aorta in early atherosclerosis. Prosta Leuko Essent Fatty Acids 1991; 44:31-36.

82. Yancey PG, St.Clair RW. Mechanism of the defect in cholesteryl ester clearance from macrophages of atherosclerosis-susceptible White Carneau pigeons. J Lipid Res 1994;35:2114-29.

83. Brugge J. New intracellular targets for therapeutic drug design. Science 1993;260: 918-19.

84. Casey PJ. Lipid modifications of G proteins. Curr Opin Cell Biol 1994;6:219-25.

85. Goldstein J, Brown M. Regulation of the mevalonate pathway. Nature 1990;343: 425-30.

86. Vogt A, Qian Y, Blaskovich M, et al. A non-peptide mimetic of Ras-CAAX: Selective inhibition of farnesyltransferase and ras processing. J Biol Chem 1995;270:660-64.

87. Etingin O, Hajjar D. Nifedipine increases cholesteryl ester hydrolytic activity in lipid-laden rabbit arterial smooth muscle cells. A possible mechanism for its antiatherogenic effect. J Clin Invest 1985; 5:1554-58.

88. Nicholson A, Etingin O, Pomerantz K, et al. Dihydropyridine calcium antagonist modulates cholesterol metabolism and eicosanoid biosynthesis in vascular cells. J Cell Biochem 1992;48:393-400.

89. Stein O, Halperin G, Stein Y. Long-term effects of verapamil on aortic smooth muscle cells cultured in the presence of hypercholesterolemic serum. Arteriosclerosis 1987;7:585-92.

STRUCTURE AND FUNCTION OF VASCULAR CELLS IN LESION-PRONE AND -RESISTANT AREAS OF THE AORTA

Yoji Yoshida, Masako Mitsumata, Tetsu Yamane, Mitsuji Okano, Su Wang, Masahiko Kawasumi, and Shigeo Akimoto
Department of Pathology, Yamanashi Medical University, 1110 Shimokato, Tamaho, Yamanashi, 409-38 Japan

Introduction

Careful topographical investigation of human early atherosclerosis has revealed that lesions develop preferentially in the outer lateral walls of bifurcations, and the inner distal walls of curvatures of the arteries. On the other hand, leading edges of flow dividers of branches and outer walls of curvatures are spared lipid deposition [1,2]. Previous investigations of flow profiles on fixed and transparent human arteries showed that the lesion-prone areas were exposed to low mean shear stress induced by turbulence, separation, and/or stagnation of blood flow. The resistant areas against atherosclerosis, were exposed to high laminar shear stress [3,4].

In this paper, we present our findings on structural and functional differences in the endothelial and intimal smooth muscle cells between these two regions of human and rabbit aortas. Also, we describe the effects of laminar shear stress on the vascular cells *in vitro*.

MATERIALS AND METHODS

Inferior mesenteric artery. Human aortas were obtained from 23 autopsy cases with various diseases as the cause of death (hyperlipidemic and/or hypertensive cases were excluded), aged from infancy to 51 years. Both the apex of the flow divider and the proximal lateral wall of the orifice of the artery were investigated electron microscopically and immunohistochemically.

Brachiocephalic trunk. Adult male normo- and hyperlipidemic rabbits, weighing approximately 2 kg, were sacrificed to determine morphological and functional differences in the endothelial cells (EC) between lesion-prone and -resistant areas on the flow divider of the bifurcation of the trunk which is a preferential site of lipid deposition, with immunohistochemical and electron microscopic methods.

Junctional structures between EC were investigated with a freeze-fracture and

A. M. Gotto, Jr. et al. (eds.), Drugs Affecting Lipid Metabolism, 95–101.

replica method (FFR) under an electron microscope. Horseradish peroxidase and ferritin were injected intravenously prior to sacrifice to investigate permeability of EC under an electron microscope.

IN VITRO STUDY

Endothelial cells. Confluent porcine and bovine aortic EC, cultured on polyester sheets in Dulbecco's modified Eagle's medium (DMEM) supplemented with 10% fetal calf serum (FCS), were placed at the bottom of rectangular flow chambers to be exposed to a laminar and unidirectional flow of culture medium (36° C, saturated with 5% CO_2 and 95% air) at a speed which was controlled by the water level of an upper reservoir and a control valve. The fluid was recirculated by a roller pump. Arrow-shaped flow chambers were used to obtain both laminar high speed and stagnation flows in areas B and D, respectively (Figure 1). Static control EC were cultured in the same way as the sheared cells, except they were kept in dishes in an incubator for given experimental periods.

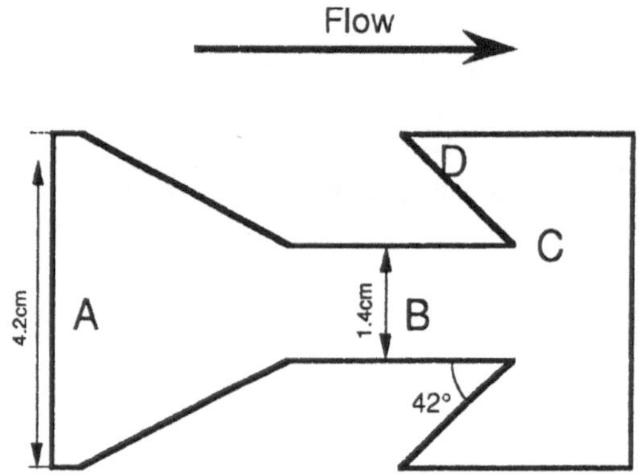

Figure 1. A diagram of an arrow-shaped conduit.

Tight junctions. Anti-ZO-1 and 7H6 [5] (tight junction-related proteins) monoclonal antibodies conjugated with fluorescein isothiocyanate (FITC) were used for histochemical and flow cytometric analysis. Expression of ZO-1 mRNA in EC evoked by the stress was demonstrated with a reverse transcription polymerase reaction (RT-PCR) method. Fine structures of intercellular junctional complexes of EC were investigated by FFR.

Glycosaminoglycans (GAG). Immediately after exposure to shear stress, EC were metabolically labeled with 30 μCi/ml of ^{35}S sulfate in fresh medium for 12 or 24 hours. Conditioned medium (medium fraction), trypsin-extractable substances of cell layers (trypsinated fraction), and a cell pellet (cell fraction) were obtained to detect ^{35}S sulfate GAG. After pronase digestion, GAG were extracted with cetylpyridinium chloride (CPC). Aliquots of pronase digests were treated with chondroitin ABC lyase before CPC precipitation.

Collagen. Immediately after exposure to shear stress, EC were labeled with 50 μCi/ml of ^{3}H proline for 6 hours. Then, medium and cell layer together were collected and homogenized to measure collagens as proteins digestible with bacterial collagenase. Types of collagen were analyzed by fluorography.

Intimal smooth muscle cells (SMC). SMC outgrown from explants of atherosclerotic intima, obtained from rabbits which had been placed on an atherogenic diet for 3 months, were incubated with conditioned media of EC subjected to shear stress in the flow chamber for given periods. The culture medium for the study was DMEM supplemented with 0.1% lipoprotein-deficient rabbit serum (LDS).

To clarify the effects of collagen in the intercellular matrix in the intima, SMC were placed on the top of collagen gels, which had been extracted from bovine fetus skin by a salting-out method and analyzed by sodium dodecyl sulfate polyacrylamide gel (SDS-PAGE), and incubated with DMEM with 10% FCS. Content of cytoplasmic cAMP was measured by a specific radioimmunoassay (RIA) method. Volume percentage of cytoskeletal filaments to whole cytoplasm in SMC was measured by histometry on electron micrographs.

Results

HUMAN INFERIOR MESENTERIC ARTERY

The ratio of intimal thicknesses of the apical to the lateral (A/P) in newborn infants was greater than 1, but in all ages after the second decade, the mean maximal intimal thickness of the lateral wall significantly surpassed that of the apex. Some differences in fine structures of vessel walls in the two regions were recognized before one year of age. Specifically endothelial stress fibers, subendothelial basement membranes, and fibrous structures in the intima were more developed in the apex than in the lateral wall. However, there were no substantial differences in the ultrastructural figures of the intimal SMC of the two regions. In the third and fourth decades, the apical intima, the lesion-resistant area which was covered with flat EC, showed a marked increase in collagen and elastic fibers. Intimal SMC embedded among collagen fibers were contractile in phenotype. In contrast to the apical intima, the upper layer of the lateral intima, the lesion-prone area, had a loose appearance due to the accumulation of intercellular matrix abundant in proteoglycans and a lack of collagen and elastic fibers. Intimal SMC in the mucinous intima were of the synthetic phenotype. EC covering the intima of the lateral wall were sometimes cuboid, filled with synthetic organelles and their basement membranes were thin and fragmented.

After the fourth decade, the lateral mucinous intima exhibited frequent EC denudation, leading to platelet adhesion, the insudation, and accumulation of blood constituents in the subendothelium. Lipid droplets appeared in synthetic SMC in the intima.

Rabbit Brachiocephalic Trunk

Rabbits placed on an atherogenic diet for 2 weeks showed a special geographical pattern of lipid deposition around the bifurcation. The deposition was crescent-shaped on the flow divider, immediately downstream from the leading edge, lesion-resistant area, which covered 170 µm on average from the apex.

The form of EC under SEM varied in relation to the lesion-prone or -resistant area, i.e. the lesion-prone area was covered by ellipsoidal cells, while the resistant was covered by elongated cells. The border between the two regions was clear and sharp. Intact rabbits which had not received an atherogenic diet showed similar forms of EC in these two regions to those of rabbits placed on the atherogenic diet for 2 weeks. Cell shapes were dependent on location but were independent of levels of hyperlipidemia.

Investigation by transmission electron microscopy of intact rabbits revealed that elongated endothelial cells covering the leading edge were most frequently equipped with thick bundles of stress fibers and fewer vacuoles in their cytoplasms and had thick and continuous glycocalyx and subendothelial basement membranes (Figure 2A).

In contrast, ellipsoidal EC covering the lesion-prone area had thicker cytoplasm with many vacuoles, synthetic organelles and mitochondria, but fewer stress fibers (Figure 2B). Glycocalyx was thin and discontinuous. The rabbit aorta has two types of tight junction structure; zonular and macular (Figure 3). The former consists of several layers of long continuous ridges of membrane particles forming a net-like meshwork and the other consists of short ridges barely forming a meshwork. EC in resistant areas were equipped more frequently with well-developed zonular rather than macular tight junctions. Macular type tight junctions were frequently observed between EC in this area. IL-1b and VCAM 1 were observed immunohistochemically in the cytoplasm, even in intact animals.

When the rabbits were injected intravenously with HRP 4 minutes prior to sacrifice or with ferritin 30 minutes before sacrifice, the numbers of vesicles labeled with each tracer were significantly greater in the lesion-prone region than in the resistant region.

In Vitro Study

The effects of intimal matrix on SMC phonotype. Conditioned media of the endothelial cells exposed to 10 dyn/cm^2 for more than 4 hours stimulated collagen synthesis of SMC, particularly of type 3. Therefore, the effects of type of collagen on SMC phenotype and growth rate were examined. The intimal SMC on type 3 collagen gel showed increased numbers of thin filaments in their cytoplasm changing their phenotype from synthetic to contractile. However, those on type 1 collagen gel and in ordinary dishes retained the synthetic phenotype. The growth rate of SMC on type 3 gel was not markedly enhanced, but stationary. On the other hand, the growth rate of SMC on type 1 gel was significantly stimulated as compared to that on plastic dishes.

Concentration of cAMP in the cells was inversely proportional to their growth rate. Responses of the cells to PDGF added to the culture media on day 7 were high in the cells seen in those on type 1 gel or ordinary plastic dishes, but almost no responses were on type

3 gel.

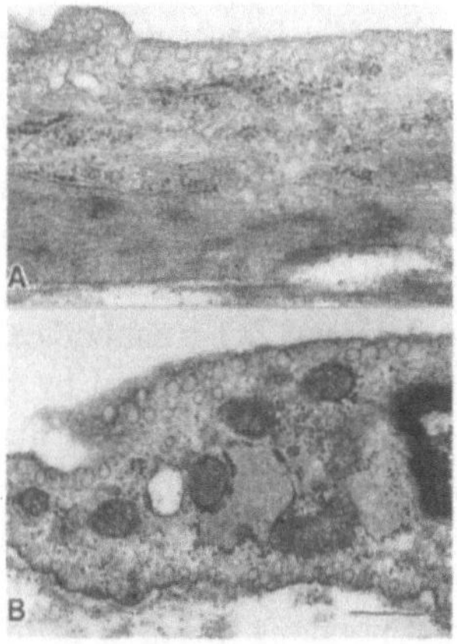

Figure 2. (A) EC covering the leading edge, a lesion-resistant area, on the flow divider of the brachiocephalic bifurcation in a normal rabbit. (B) EC covering a lesion-prone area on the same flow divider. Bar; 400 nm.

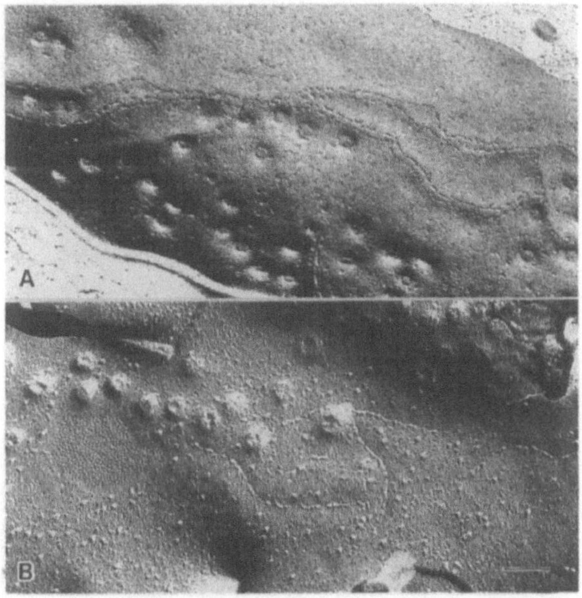

Figure 3. Zonular (A) and macular (B) types of tight junction of EC in the normal rabbit aorta. Bar; 1μm.

Tight junction. Fluorescent immunostaining with anti-ZO-1 and 7H6 monoclonal antibodies was hardly visible in the static cells even after cultivation for 72 hours, but a significant increase in fluorescence was recognized along the cell boundaries in confluent monolayers subjected to 30 dyn/cm^2 for 24 hours. The frequency of stained cells with anti-7H6 antibody increased proportionally with increase in magnitude and duration of shear stress applied. When 30 dyn/cm^2 was applied at the entry of the arrow-shaped conduit, approximately 90 dyn/cm^2 should work on the cells in the narrowest segment, but very low shear stress should apply on the cells in the angle (Figure 1, D) in which the flow stagnated. Under these conditions, the cells in B (Figure 1) showed an elongated form parallel to the flow direction and were strongly stained with 7H6 and ZO-1 antibodies, while those one in the angles showed a polygonal form and were hardly stained by these antibodies after 72-hour exposure (Figure 4). Expression of ZO-1 mRNA was demonstrated by RT-PCR in the sheared cells with 30 dyn/cm^2 after 0.5 hours, but not in the static cells.

Freeze-fracture and replica samples of the junctions between the static cells at confluency showed only some gap junctions, in contrast with cells placed under 30 dyn/cm^2 for 24 hours which developed continuous ridges of membrane particles resembling the macular type of tight junction. They showed increases in length and in number of strands with increases in exposure time to shear stress.

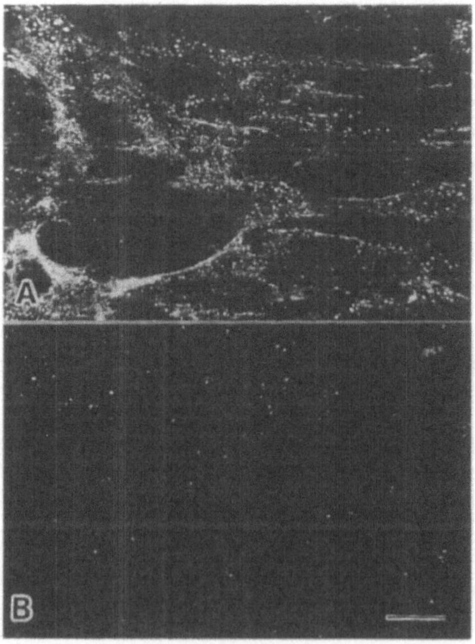

Figure 4. (A) EC which had been subjected to shear stress of 90 dyn/cm^2 for 72 hrs showed clearly 7H6 along cell junctions. Bar; 20μm. (B) Static control EC.

GAGs. EC were exposed to shear stress of 15 or 40 dyn/cm^2 for 24 hours on day 3 after seeding and to ^{35}S sulfate on day 4 for 12 hours. Synthesized GAGs in both medium and trypsin-extractable fractions from EC were significantly (approximately 130%) increased by exposure to shear stress. GAGs increased in the medium fractions induced by shear stress were susceptible to digestion with chondroitin ABC lyase, but those in the trypsinated fractions were not, suggesting that major portions of sulfated GAGs in the medium and on the surface of EC consist of chondroitin or dermatan sulfate and heparan sulfate, respectively.

Collagen. The type IV collagen synthesis of EC was also enhanced by stress in proportion to magnitude and exposure time, but types 1 and 3 were not.

Conclusion

The lesion-resistant areas in the arteries are covered with functionally static endothelial cells characterized with low permeability to blood constituents through both intra- and paracellular pathways, which might be induced by laminar high shear stress.

On the other hand, the lesion-prone areas were covered with activated endothelial cells which might be induced by low shear stress, even in normolipidemic and normotensive individuals. When hyperlipidemia occurs, therefore, lipid can permeate through the endothelial cells into the wall rapidly and easily in the lesion-prone areas to cause development of atherosclerosis.

Acknowledgments

This study was supported in part by grants-in-aid for Scientific Research from the Ministry of Education, Science and Culture and from the Ministry of Health and Welfare of Japan. The authors are grateful to Professors M. Mori, Sapporo Medical University, and S. Tsukita, Kyoto University, Graduate School of Medicine for kindly providing monoclonal antibodies.

We also thank to Mr. T. Iwato, Ms. H. Kunugi, Ms. T. Amano, and Ms. K. Hakii for their excellent technical assistance.

References

1. Ku DN, Giddens DP, Zarins CK, Glagov S. Arteriosclcrosis 1985;5:293-302.
2. Yoshida Y, Wang S, Yamane T, Okano M, Oyama T, Mitsumata M, Suda K, Yamaguchi T, Ooneda G. Acta Med Biol 1990;38[suppl]:1-19.
3. Karino T, Motomiya M. Biorheology 1983;20:119-127.
4. Okano M, Yoshida Y. J Biomech Eng 1992;114:301-308.
5. Zhong Y, Saitoh T, Minase T, Sawada N, Enomoto K, Mori M. J Cell Biol 1993;120:477-483.

ROLE OF ISOPRENOIDS IN THE GROWTH-FACTOR SIGNAL TRANSDUCTION AND THEIR PHARMACOLOGICAL MODULATION

Pierangelo Quarato, Nicola Ferri, Leslaw Rudy*, Rodolfo Paoletti, Remo Fumagalli, and Alberto Corsini
*Institute of Pharmacological Sciences, University of Milan, Via Balzaretti 9, 20133 Milan, Italy and *Department of Pharmacology, School of Medicine, Gdansk, Poland.*

Introduction

It is generally accepted that enhanced growth properties of intimal smooth muscle cells (SMCs) play an important role in the initiation and progression of human atherosclerosis [1-3]. Migration and proliferation of arterial myocytes lead to vascular occlusion in both atherosclerosis and restenosis after angioplasty. Animal models of vascular injury have shown that the appearance of an arterial lesion is followed by proliferation of the medial SMCs, many of which migrate to the intima where they continue to proliferate to form a neointimal lesion [2-4]. Recent findings have indicated that SMCs constitute approximately 90-95% of the cellular component of an atherosclerotic lesion in a young adult and an average of 50% in an advanced atherosclerotic plaque [1,2]. In addition, vascular myocytes contribute to the lesion by synthesizing extracellular matrix; these cells can also accumulate lipids and become foam cells [1,2].

A variety of growth factors participate in the control of SMC growth [5]. These can induce SMC proliferation and are generally not expressed in the normal artery, whereas they are upregulated in atherosclerotic lesions [2]. One of the most studied is platelet-derived growth factor (PDGF) [5]. PDGF is produced by many cells such as endothelial cells, SMCs, and activated monocyte/macrophages [6]. There are three PDGF isoforms denoted PDGF-AA, -AB, and -BB, which are homo- or heterodimers of related A and B polypeptide chains [7]. PDGF binds with high affinity to its receptors [6]. Three possible dimeric receptors can form: $\alpha\alpha$, $\alpha\beta$, and $\beta\beta$: $\alpha\alpha$ binds PDGF-AA, PDGF-AB, and PDGF-BB; $\alpha\beta$ binds PDGF-AB and PDGF-BB; $\beta\beta$ binds only PDGF-BB [6]. In cultured rat SMCs, the PDGF-BB isoform is a potent mitogen whereas PDGF-AA is essentially inactive [2,6,8]. The difference in the effects of PDGF-AA and -BB on DNA and protein synthesis indicates that in SMCs the α receptor mediates cellular hypertrophy (but not hyperplasia) whereas the β-one mediates a mitogenic response [8]. Support for the relevance of these observations in cell culture has come from data demonstrating that PDGF gene expression

A. M. Gotto, Jr. et al. (eds.), Drugs Affecting Lipid Metabolism, 103–110.

is increased in SMCs and in adjacent macrophages in human lesions [2]. Growth factor signal transduction through the PDGF receptor consists of a complex cascade of events [2,6,7,9]. A number of intracellular activities occur rapidly after exposure of a cell to PDGF-BB, including dimerization and autophosphorylation of the PDGF type-β receptor and association and activation of specific proteins [2,6,7,9]. Within the PDGF type-β receptor, several tyrosine residues have been identified, which function as high affinity binding sites for signaling molecules such as p21ras GTPase-activating protein [9].

Recently, several proteins involved in growth factor signal transduction have been shown to be lipid-modified by mevalonate-derived isoprenoids (prenylation), such as farnesylpyrophosphate and geranylgeranylpyrophosphate [10-13]. Function and localization of these proteins are dependent on their covalent modification by these lipids [12]. Mammalian cells synthesize cholesterol and nonsteroidal isoprenoid compounds via a branched pathway in which mevalonate, the product of the reaction catalyzed by HMG-CoA reductase, plays a pivotal role as a precursor for all end-products [10]. While cholesterol seems to be required in the early cell cycle (G_1 phase), mevalonate itself and some of its nonsteroidal derivatives (isoprenoids) are determining factors in cell division and growth regulation [10].

For this reason, inhibition of HMG-CoA reductase, provides a new entry target for pharmacological modulation of SMC proliferation [10,14]. Recently, we provided evidence that simvastatin, a specific competitive inhibitor of HMG-CoA reductase, displayed inhibitory effects on FCS-induced SMC proliferation [15], probably through the inhibition of isoprenoid biosynthesis [14-16].

In the present study we evaluated the effect of simvastatin on growth factor-induced DNA synthesis in rat aortic myocytes and the potential mechanism of its antimitogenic activity.

Materials and Methods

Eagle's Minimum Essential Medium (MEM), trypsin-EDTA, penicillin (10,000 U/ml), streptomycin (10 ng/ml), tricine buffer (1M, pH 7.4), and nonessential amino acid solution (100x) were purchased by GIBCO (Grand Island, New York); fetal calf serum (FCS) was from Labtek (Corsico, Italy); disposable culture flasks and petri dishes were from Corning Glassworks (Corning, New York).

[6-^{3}H]-thymidine (1 mCi/ml) was from Amersham (Bullinghamshire, UK). Trans, trans-farnesol was from Fluka Chemie AG (Buchs, Switzerland); (all-trans)-geranylgeraniol was from Sigma (St. Louis, Missouri). Filters were from Gelman Sciences (Ann Arbor, Michigan).

Simvastatin in the lactone form (Merck, Sharp & Dohme Research Laboratories, Woodbridge, New Jersey) was brought into solution in 0.1 M NaOH (MSD file) to give the active form and the pH was adjusted to 7.4 by adding 0.1 M HCl. Solution was sterilized by filtration.

Cell Cultures

SMCs were cultured according to Ross [17] from the intima-media layers of aortas of male Sprague-Dawley rats (weighing 200-250 g) [12]. Cells were grown in monolayers at 37° C in a humidified atmosphere of 5% CO_2. Cell viability was assessed by tripan blue exclusion.

Experimental Protocol

Cells were seeded at the density of 2.5 x 10^5 myocytes/petri dish (35 mm) and incubated with MEM supplemented with 10% FCS.

Twenty-four hours later the medium was changed to one containing 0.4% FCS (quiescence medium) to stop cell growth and the cultures were incubated for 5 days. When PDGF was investigated, quiescence medium was replaced on the fourth day by one containing 1% PDS (plasma-derived serum). Cells were then cultured with two mitogenic stimuli, 1) PDGF-BB in medium containing 1% PDS and 2) 10% FCS, in the presence or absence of the tested compounds. The incubation was continued for 20 hours before DNA assay.

DNA Synthesis

Relative rates of DNA synthesis were assessed by determination of [6-^{3}H]-thymidine incorporation into trichloroacetic acid (TCA) precipitable material. Cells were pulsed for 2 hours with [6-^{3}H]-thymidine (2 μCi/ml), washed with PBS followed by one wash with 5% (W/V) cold TCA at 4° C (10 min) and one wash with 5% TCA at room temperature. Cells were then dissolved in 1N NaOH, placed in scintillator fluid (Aquasol-Packard, Groningen, The Netherlands) and the radioactivity counted [18]. Protein was measured according to Lowry et al. [19].

Results and Discussion

The effect of simvastatin on DNA synthesis in SMCs was investigated. Simvastatin decreased DNA synthesis dose-dependently, at concentrations ranging between 10 and 40 μM (Figure 1). To further demonstrate that the interference with SMC growth was due to the inhibition of the HMG-CoA reductase activity, we investigated the effect of simvastatin on SMC DNA synthesis in presence of mevalonate or its isoprenoid derivatives. The inhibition of DNA synthesis elicited by simvastatin 40 μM was fully prevented by the addition of mevalonate 100 μM and partially by farnesol 10 μM and geranylgeraniol 5 μM (Figure 2). Similar results were reported when PDGF-BB-induced DNA synthesis was investigated in rat aortic myocytes (Figure 3). These results support the concept that SMCs require mevalonate or some of its nonsterol products, such as farnesol or geranylgeraniol, along with an exogenous source of cholesterol (fetal calf serum), for proliferation.

Cell proliferation is dependent on at least two products synthesized from mevalonate, one of which has been identified as cholesterol [10]. It is unlikely, however, that inhibition of cholesterol synthesis explains the actions of simvastatin on DNA synthesis. In fact, cells were stimulated to grow by exposure to a medium containing 10% fetal calf serum, which provides an exogenous source of cholesterol. Thus it is likely that the decrease of DNA synthesis by statins resulted from an inhibition of production of one or more isoprenoid intermediates of mevalonate metabolism [14,20,21].

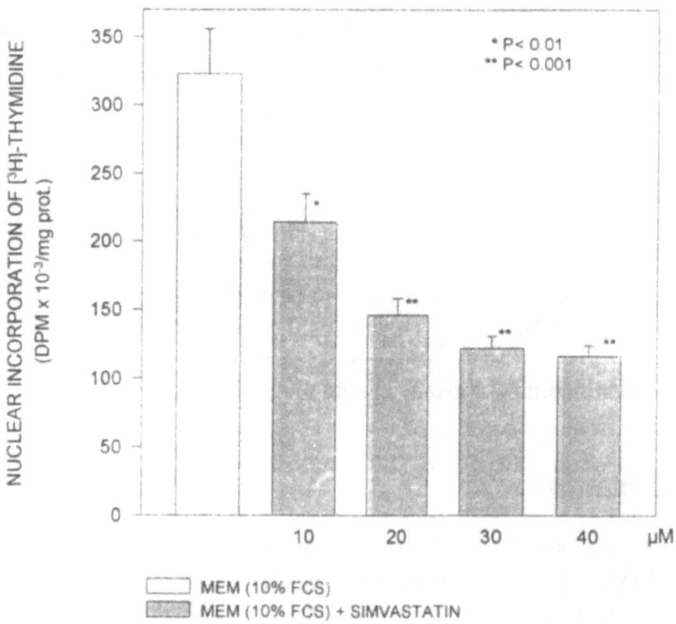

Figure 1. Effect of simvastatin on [^{3}H]-thymidine incorporation by rat aortic myocytes. Cells were seeded at the density of 2.5 x 10^5/dish and incubated with MEM supplemented with 10% FCS; 24 h later the medium was changed with one containing 0.4% FCS to stop cell growth and the cultures were incubated for 120 h. At this time the medium was replaced with one containing 10% FCS and the reported concentration of the tested compound. After 20 h at 37° C, labeled thymidine was then added to the medium and the incubation continued for further 2 h. Each point represents the mean ± SD of triplicate dishes. The mean value of control was 322,863 ± 32,948 DPM/mg prot. Drug versus control: *$P < 0.01$, **$P < 0.001$ (Student's t-test).

A number of proteins that are modified post-translationally by the covalent attachment of mevalonate-derived isoprene groups, such as farnesol or geranylgeraniol, have been identified [10,13]. The characterization of some of these proteins, such as nuclear lamin B, ras proteins, and heterotrimeric and low molecular weight guanine nucleotide-binding proteins, provides new insights into the link between the mevalonate pathway, signal transduction, and cell cycle progression [10,13].

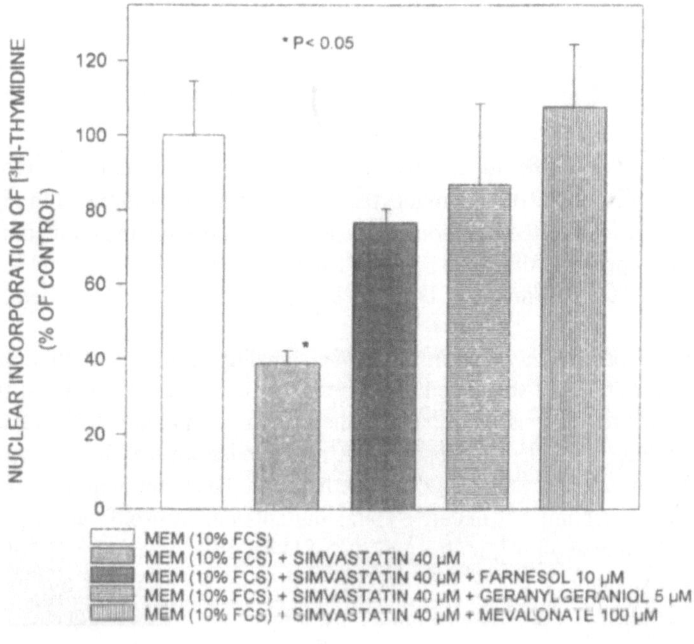

Figure 2. Effect of mevalonate and its derivatives on serum-induced [^{3}H]-thymidine incorporation by simvastatin-treated myocytes. Experimental conditions as in Figure 1. Values are the mean ± SD of triplicates of three different experiments. The mean value of control was 383,039 ± 55,541 DPM/mg prot. Drug versus control: *$P < 0.05$ (Student's t-test).

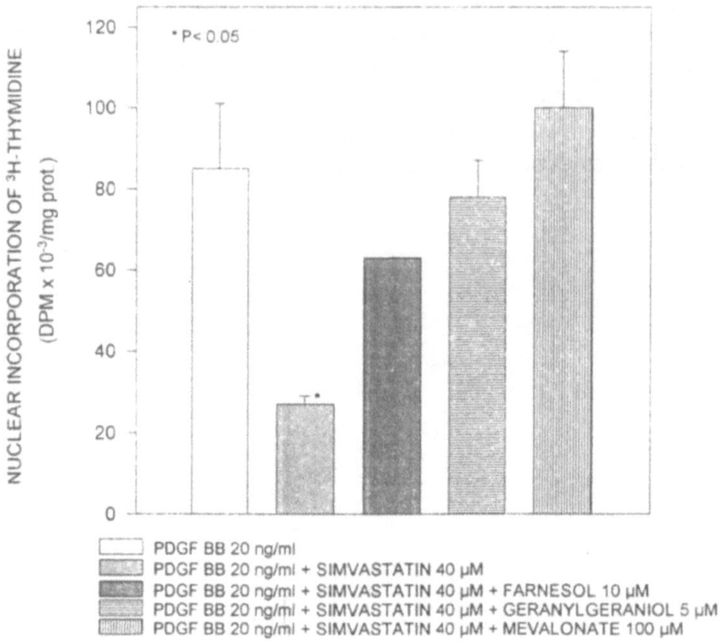

Figure 3. Effect of mevalonate and its derivatives on PDGF-induced [^{3}H]-thymidine incorporation by simvastatin-treated myocytes. Experimental conditions as in Figure 1. 24 hours before adding the tested compounds, cells were cultured in medium containing 1% PDS. Each point represents the mean ± SD of triplicate dishes. The mean value of control was 84,757 ± 16,579 DPM/mg prot. Drug versus control: *$P < 0.05$ (Student's t-test).

Ras, a key protein involved in mitogenic signaling pathways, is thought to be an important mediator of PDGF-stimulated responses [7,8,10,13]. It is known that the activity of p21 ras proteins requires association with the plasma membrane which is facilitated by the farnesyl moiety [13,22]. The observation of an induction of H-ras protooncogene expression in proliferating rat SMCs [23], together with the recent demonstration that the local delivery of transdominant negative H-ras mutants inhibit proliferation after balloon injury of rat carotid artery [24], indicate a role of H-ras as a key transducer of mitogenic signals in vascular myocytes. The fact that geranylgeraniol can, under our experimental conditions, prevent simvastatin-induced inhibition of DNA synthesis, suggests that proteins modified by this isoprene rather than, or in addition to, those that have been farnesylated, are responsible for inducing cell proliferation [4]. Some studies have shown that geranylgeranylated ras proteins support transformation of animal cells [25] and growth of yeast cells [26]. The possibility also exists that authentic garanylgeranylated proteins as those of the rho family [27-29] and rap [30] may compensate for ras in growth factor signal transduction pathway and in the control of cell proliferation. The abundance of data available demonstrates that mitogenic signaling in SMCs is complex and an overlapping of signaling elements can be induced by hormones and growth factors through G-protein serpentine receptors as well as receptor tyrosine kinases [31]. Insights into the mechanism of the mitogenic response of these cells are extremely important in clinical terms, since accelerated growth of SMCs is one of the major features of vascular proliferation disorders, including atherosclerosis and restenosis [2,31].

Our data suggest that mevalonate metabolism and signal transduction are coupled. The most likely explanation is that prenylated proteins are involved in the signal transduction due to several mitogenic stimuli, such as FCS and PDGF-BB [14,22]. Mevalonate pathway, therefore, represents a potential pharmacological target for controlling SMC proliferation, one of the major events involved in the formation of atherosclerotic lesion.

Acknowledgements

This research was partially supported by MURST (Italian government). We thank Dr. Alfred Albers (Merck, Sharp & Dohme) for providing simvastatin. The authors are grateful to Laura Mozzarelli for editorial help.

References

1. Wissler RW. Update on the pathogenesis of atherosclerosis. Am J Med 1991;91(1B):1B-3S-1B-9S.
2. Ross R. The pathogenesis of atherosclerosis: A perspective for the 1990s. Nature 1993;362: 801-809.
3. Clowes AW, Clowes MM, Fingerle J. Regulation of smooth muscle cell growth injured artery. J Cardiovasc Pharmacol 1989;14:S12-S15.
4. Corsini A, Raiteri M, Soma MR, Bernini F, Fumagalli R, Paoletti R. Pathogenesis of atherosclerosis and the role of 3-hydroxy-3-methylglutaryl coenzyme A reductase inhibitors. Am J Cardiol 1995;76:21A-28A.
5. Ross R. Polypeptide growth factors and atherosclerosis. Trends Cardiovasc Med 1991;1:277-82.
6. Bobik A, Campbell JH. Vascular derived growth factors: Cell biology, pathophysiology, and pharmacology. Pharmacol Rev 1993;45:1-42.
7. Claesson-Welsh L. Platelet-derived growth factor receptor signals. J Biol Chem 1994;269: 32023-26.
8. Inui H, Kitami Y, Tani M, Kondo T, Inagami T. Differences in signal transduction between platelet derived growth factor (PDGF) α and β receptors in vascular smooth muscle cells. J Biol Chem 1994;269:30546-52.
9. Zubiaur M, Sancho J, Terhorst C, Faller DV. A small GTP-binding protein, Rho, associator

with the platelet-derived growth factor type-β receptor upon ligand binding. J Biol Chem 1995;270:17221-28.

10. Goldstein JL, Brown MS. Regulation of the mevalonate pathway. Nature 1990;343:425-30.
11. Sinensky M, Lutz RJ. The prenylation of proteins. Bioessays 1992;14:25-31.
12. Casey PJ. Biochemistry of protein prenylation. J Lipid Res 1992;33:1731-40.
13. Glomset JA, Farnsworth CC. Role of protein modification reactions in programming interactions between ras-related GTPases and cell membranes. Ann Rev Cell Biol 1994;10: 181-205.
14. Corsini A, et al. Relationship between mevalonate pathway and arterial myocyte proliferation: In vitro studies with inhibitors of HMG-CoA reductase. Atherosclerosis 1993;101:117-25.
15. Corsini A, Raiteri M, Soma MR, Fumagalli R, Paoletti R. Simvastatin but not pravastatin inhibits the proliferation of rat aorta myocytes. Pharmacol Res 1991;23:173-80.
16. McGuire TF, Xu X-Q, Corey SJ, Romero GG, Sebti SM. Lovastatin disrupts early events in insulin signaling: a potential mechanism of lovastatin's anti-mitogenic activity. Biochem Biophys Res Commun 1994;204:399-406.
17. Ross R. The smooth muscle cell. II. Growth of smooth muscle in culture and formation of elastic fibers. J Cell Biol 1971;50:172-86.
18. Corsini A, Verri D, Raiteri M, Quarato P, Paoletti R, Fumagalli R. Effect of 26-aminocholesterol, 27-hydroxycholesterol and 25-hydroxycholesterol on proliferation and cholesterol homeostasis in arterial myocytes. Arteriosel Thromb Vasc Biol 1995;15:420-28.
19. Lowry OH, Rosebrough NJ, Farr AL, Randall RJ. Protein measurement with the Folin phenol reagent. J Biol Chem 1951;193:265-75.
20. Corsini A, et al. Effect of the new HMG-CoA reductase inhibitor BAY W 6228 on migration, proliferation, and cholesterol synthesis in arterial myocytes. Pharmacol Res 1996; in press.
21. Corsini A, et al. Non-lipid-related effects of 3-hydroxy-3-methylglutaryl coenzyme A reductase inhibitors. Cardiology 1996; in press.
22. Vincent TS, Wulfert E, Merler E. Inhibition of growth factor signaling pathways by lovastatin. Biochem Biophys Res Commun 1991;180:1284-89.
23. Sadhu DN, Ramos KS. Cyclic AMP inhibits c-Ha-ras protooncogene expression and DNA synthesis in rat aortic smooth muscle cells. Experientia 1993;49:567-70.
24. Indolfi C, et al. Inhibition of cellular ras prevents smooth muscle cell proliferation after vascular injury in vivo. Nature Medicine 1995;1:513-15.
25. Cox AD, Hisaka MM, Buss JE, Der CJ. Specific isoprenoid modification is required for function of normal, but not oncogenic, ras protein. Mol Cell Biol 1992;12:2606-15.
26. Trueblood CE, Ohya Y, Rine J. Genetic evidence for in vivo cross-specificity of the CaaX-box protein prenyltransferases, farnesyltransferase and geranylgeranyltransferase-I in Saccharomices cerevisiae. Mol Cell Biol 1993;13:4260-75.
27 Vincent S, Jeanteur P, Fort P. Growth-regulated expression of Rho G, a new member of the ras homolog gene family. Mol Cell Biol 1992;12:3138-48.
28. Olson MF, Ashworth A, Hall A. An essential role for Rho, Rac, and Cdc 42, GTPases in cell cycle progression through G_1. Science 1995;269:1270-72.
29. Vojtek AB, Cooper JA. Rho family members activators of MAP kinase cascades. Cell 1995; 82:527-29.
30. Quarck, et al. Evidence for Rap 1 in vascular smooth muscle cells. Regulation of their expression by platelet-derived growth factor BB. FEBS Lett 1994;342:159-64.
31. Ludwig S, Rapp UR. Cascading towards vascular disorders gene therapy. Nature Medicine 1995;1:513-15.

MODULATION OF THE MEVALONATE PATHWAY IN ATHEROSCLEROSIS AND TUMORS

Roberta Baetta, Elena Donetti, Roberto Seregni, Rodolfo Paoletti, Remo Fumagalli, and Maurizio R. Soma

Institute of Pharmacological Sciences, University of Milan, Via Balzaretti 9, Milan 20133, Italy

Recent findings have gained insights into new physiologic roles for intermediates in the cholesterol synthesis pathway [1]. Mevalonate (MVA) constitutes the basic precursor not only for cholesterol but also for a variety of nonsterol isoprenoids, including farnesyl-pyrophosphate (PPi) and geranylgeranyl-PPi, which are utilized for post-translational modification of a diverse array of cellular proteins, dolichol which is involved in glycosylation synthesis, and polyisoprenoid side chains of ubiquinone and heme-A which play a role in oxidative respiration [1]. These MVA-derived products are requirements for a wide variety of cellular processes such as cell function, growth regulation, DNA replication, and cell cycle progression [1-6]. For more than a decade it has been known that specific 3-hydroxy-3-methyl glutaryl coenzyme A (HMG-CoA) reductase inhibitors, a potent class of hypocholesterolemic drugs, deplete endogenous MVA pools and subsequently arrest cell growth with a concomitant change in cell morphology [7-10].

Therefore, HMG-CoA reductase inhibitors have received increasing attention as pharmacological tools for controlling abnormal cell growth in pathologic situations such as tumors [1,11-13] and atherosclerosis [14,15].

Malignant gliomas are the most common primary brain tumors, accounting for about 15% of all primary brain tumors in humans, and continue to pose major challenges to clinicians and researches. With the mainstay treatment (surgery and radiotherapy) and the adjuvant chemotherapy, the median survival rate is about 1 year [16,17]. Despite recent attempts to improve chemotherapeutic approaches for the treatment of brain tumors, results remain disappointing. The failure of conventional chemotherapy to provide durable, side-effect-free remission against brain tumors has prompted investigators to seek alternative treatment strategies. Carmustine (BCNU) is the chemotherapeutic agent most frequently used for brain tumors, partially due to its ability to cross the blood-brain barrier. Clinical problems in BCNU chemotherapy are related to a variety of factors, such as drugs sensitivity or tumor resistance to drugs, as well as adverse effects on normal tissues [17]. Thus, lowering the BCNU doses without losing its antitumoral efficacy should be beneficial.

C_6 glioma cells exposure to increasing concentrations of either simvastatin or BCNU

A. M. Gotto, Jr. et al. (eds.), Drugs Affecting Lipid Metabolism, 111–118.

resulted in a dose-dependent inhibition of cell growth rate as shown in Figure 1. The concentrations producing 50% inhibition after 48 hours were 5.2 and 9.8 μM for simvastatin and BCNU, respectively. When cells were simultaneously incubated with a subliminal concentration of simvastatin (0.1 μM) and increasing concentrations of BCNU, a strong inhibition of growth rate could be achieved. The simultaneous exposure of cells to simvastatin and BCNU produced a strong synergistic inhibitory effect on cell proliferation as analyzed with the aid of an isobologram (Figure 1). The effect of BCNU and simvastatin on the cell cycle of C_6 proliferating cells was evaluated by cytofluorimetric analysis of DNA cell content (Figure 2). The DNA histograms obtained from cells treated for 24 hours with increasing concentrations of BCNU (0.01 - 10 μM) showed a dose-dependent drug effect on cell cycle distribution, mainly expressed as a decrease in S phase and an accumulation of the cells in G_2-M, particularly at the highest concentrations. The DNA histograms obtained from cells treated for 24 hours with increasing concentrations of simvastatin (0.1 - 10 μM) showed a dose-dependent drug effect on cell cycle distribution (Figure 3). The entry of cells into the S phase progressively decreased. The DNA synthesis inhibition by simvastatin produced an accumulation of cells in G_0-G_1 (presynthetic phase). At concentrations above 1 μM, the G_0-G_1 block was accompanied by a dose-dependent increase of the percentage of cells in G_2-M. This effect (arrest or retardation) was particularly evident since it produced a progressive decrease in G_0-G_1 compartment. Combination of simvastatin and BCNU produced a pronounced retardation of cycling cells in the G_2-M compartment (Figure 2).

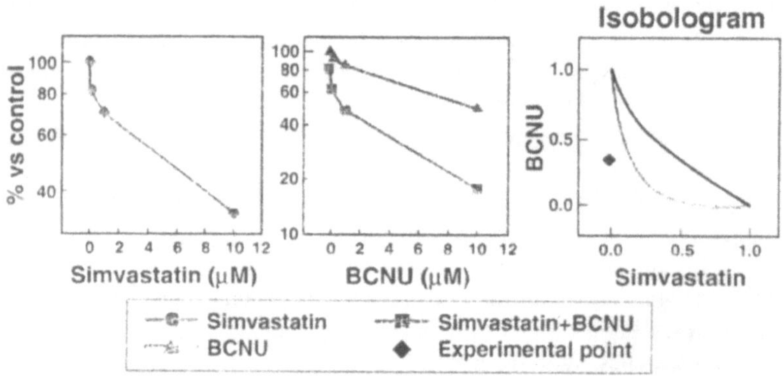

Figure 1. *In Vitro* synergistic interaction between simvastatin (0.1 μM) and BCNU on C_6 glioma cell growth at 48 hours.

To investigate whether the simvastatin-induced G_2-M accumulation was due to a specific block in G_2 or in the M phase, the mitotic index of simvastatin-treated cells (5 and 10 μM) was evaluated on PI-stained cellular suspensions just prior DNA analysis (Figure 4). The number of mitotic cells was 10 times lower in 10 μM simvastatin-treated cells compared to controls, suggesting a specific block of cells in G_2. This effect of simvastatin was prevented and counteracted by mevalonate 100 μM.

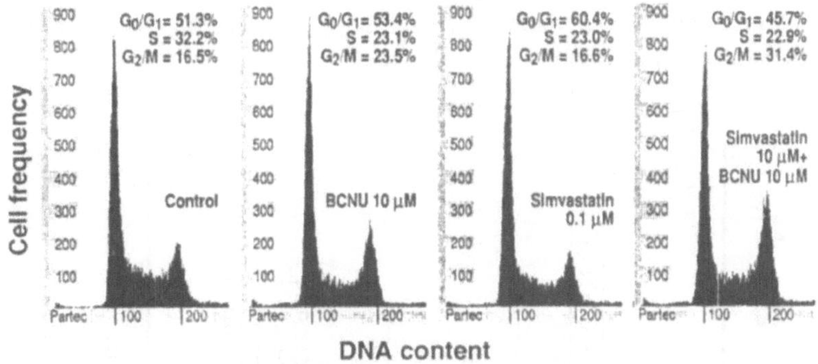

Figure 2. *In vitro* effect of simvastatin and BCNU combination at 24 hours on cell cycle distribution of C_6 exponentially growing cells.

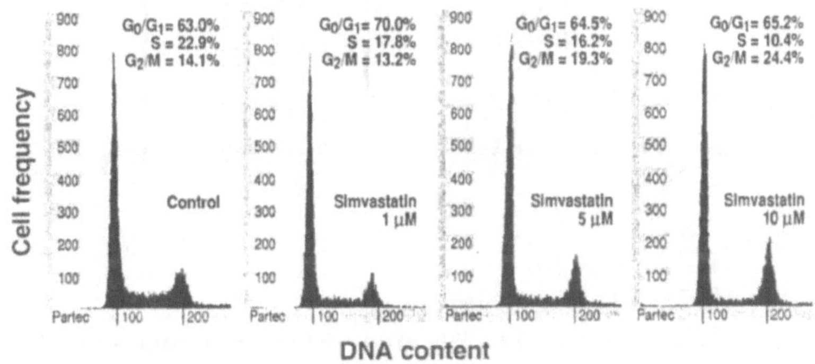

Figure 3. Dose-dependent effect at 24 hours of simvastatin on cell cycle distribution of C_6 exponentially growing cells.

The antiproliferative effects of simvastatin and BCNU alone and in combination were then evaluated in rat brain tumors induced by direct intracerebral injection of C_6 glioma cells. The biparametric (DNA/BrdUrd) cytofluorimetric analysis of nuclear suspensions, obtained by mechanical-enzymatic dispersion of the left brain hemisphere, indicated a significant dose-dependent inhibition of tumor growth rate for both BCNU and simvastatin alone, with ID_{50}s of 8.7 and 61 mg/kg/day, respectively (Figure 5). Simvastatin (25 mg/kg/day) was then tested in combination with BCNU (0.3 and 6.7 mg/kg). Both drug combinations strongly inhibited tumor growth rate. The combination of doses of simvastatin (25 mg/kg/day) and BCNU (0.3 mg/kg), able to inhibit tumor proliferation by about 10% when administered alone, resulted in a significant inhibition of brain tumor growth (about 50%;

$P < 0.05$). To determine whether the inhibitory effect of the BCNU/simvastatin combination was additive or synergistic, we performed the isobologram analysis. We analyzed the combined effect of drug at ID_{50}. The experimental point representing the combined drug effect in the isobologram plots lies below and to the left of the curve joining the doses of the agents that, given alone, have the same effects in the combination, demonstrating a highly synergistic interaction on tumor growth (Figure 5).

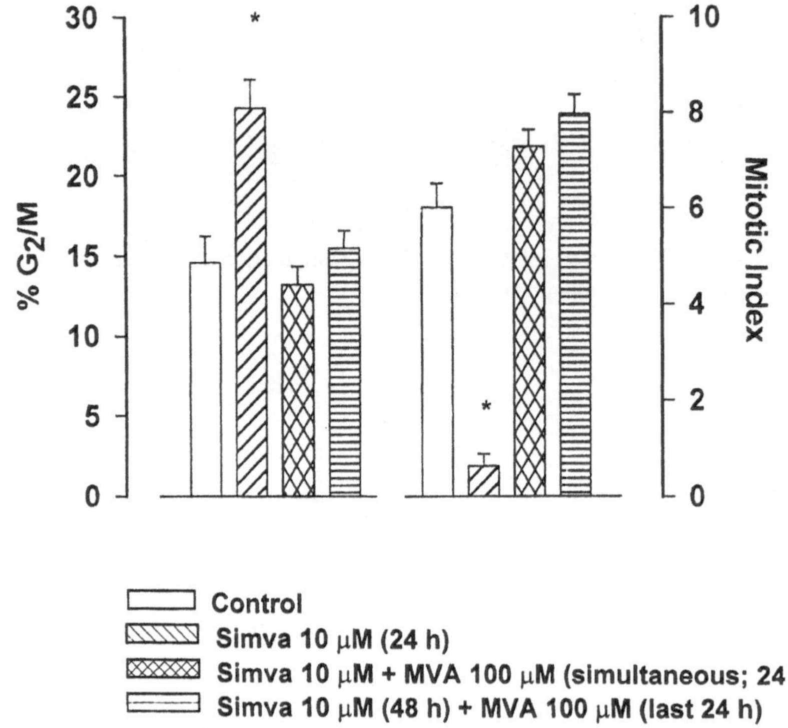

Figure 4. *In vitro* preventing and reverting effect of mevalonate on G_2-M arrest/retardation and mitotic index inhibition by simvastatin.

Drug-treated animals were comparable to the controls with respect to total body weight (Table 1). The myelosuppressive effect of different drug regimens is also reported in Table 1. Simvastatin and BCNU, as single agents at doses of 50 mg/kg/day and 6.7 mg/kg, respectively, decreased white blood cell (WBC) counts and depressed bone marrow LI. This effect was statistically significant only in BCNU-treated rats. Doses of 25 mg/kg/day and 0.3 mg/kg of simvastatin and BCNU, respectively, did not alter either leukocyte counts or LI when given alone, and the combination of the two drugs did not result in any synergistic or additive effect on this parameter.

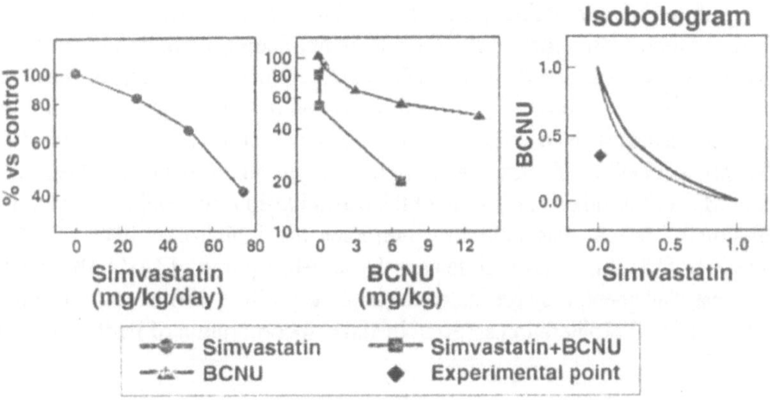

Figure 5. *In vivo* synergistic interaction between simvastatin (25 mg/kg/day) and BCNU on C_6 glioma.

Table 1. Effects of simvastatin and BCNU alone and in combination on rat body weight, WBC, and bone marrow BrdUrd incorporation (LI).

Treatment	Body Weight	WBC[a]	LI Bone Marrow
Control	276 (6)	17 (4)	38 (4)
Simvastatin (25 mg/kg/day)	282 (7)	14 (6)	38 (8)
Simvastatin (50 mg/kg/day)	267 (13)	15 (3)	32 (5)
BCNU (0.3 mg/kg)	284 (22)	13 (3)	41 (6)
BCNU (6.7 mg/kg)	291 (16)	8[b] (1)	25[b] (6)
Simvastatin (25 mg/kg/day) + BCNU (0.3 mg/kg)	255 (11)	12 (4)	35 (3)

[a] WBC was performed with Unopette (Becton Dickinson, San Jose, CA); number of cells x $10^3/mm^3$; [b] $P < 0.05$ versus control

Thus, these data indicate that simvastatin, a potent inhibitor of mevalonate biosynthesis, significantly decreases the proliferation of rat glioblastoma cells (C_6) both *in vitro* and *in vivo*. The drug also shows a strong inhibitory effect on tumor proliferation when combined with BCNU, an antineoplastic agent. These results suggest the possible use of HMG-CoA reductase inhibitors as coadjuvants in antineoplastic brain tumor therapy.

Recently we observed that HMG-CoA reductase inhibitors have also an antiproliferative effect on arterial myocytes *in vitro* and *in vivo* [14,15]. The *in vivo* results are more in accordance with an antiproliferative action of statins than a cholesterol-lowering effect. To assess whether this direct activity of vastatin on intimal hyperplasia was due to inhibition of MVA biosynthesis at the site of the carotid lesion, we evaluated whether or not local infusion of MVA was able to counteract the inhibitory effect of fluvastatin administered i.p. [18]. Local arterial delivery by an Alzet pump of MVA (8 mg/kg/day) at the site of collar placement, fully prevented the inhibitory effect of fluvastatin (5 mg/kg/day) on both I/M and SMC proliferation assessed by direct incorporation of BrdU into replicating DNA (Table 2).

Table 2. Effect of local mevalonate delivery on arterial wall proliferation inhibited by fluvastatin.

	Control	Fluva	Fluva + MVA
Intimal/medial tissue	0.22 $\pm$ 0.04	0.12 $\pm$ 0.05	0.19 $\pm$ 0.05
Labeling index	3.6 $\pm$ 0.3	1.6 $\pm$ 0.4	3.1 $\pm$ 0.3

Fluvastatin and mevalonate treatment, performed as described in the material and methods section, lasted for 5 days. Labeling index represent the percent number of cells that actively incorporated BrDU into replicating DNA. Labeling index was evaluated by immunofluorescence techniques as described in the material and methods section. Parameters from sham-operated rabbits did not change during the study. Values were obtained from 20 serial cross sections per rabbit and are the mean $\pm$ SD from 3 different animals per group.

HMG-CoA reductase inhibitors are well-known agents for treatment of hypercholesterolemia [19]. Several studies have also demonstrated the efficacy of vastatins in reducing the progression and inducing regression of atherosclerosis in animal models [20-22] and human subject [1,23-26]. In all those studies, the antiatherosclerotic effect of vastatins was suggested to be dependent on their lipid lowering properties [20-24,26,27]. In recent years, the development of drugs that inhibit cholesterol synthesis, thus lowering plasma cholesterol levels, has to a large degree, centered on controlling HMG-CoA reductase activity. However, as already mentioned, because mevalonic acid, the product of the enzyme reaction, is the precursor of numerous metabolites, inhibition of HMG-CoA reductase has the potential to result in pleiotropic effects.

Thus, oral administration of HMG-CoA reductase inhibitors significantly and dose-dependently inhibits the neointimal hyperplasia induced by perivascular manipulation of carotid arteries in normocholesterolemic rabbits. This effect is independent of the drug efficacy in lowering cholesterol plasma levels and is obtained in the absence of significant toxicity (evaluated as bone marrow labeling index; data not shown). The data also demonstrate that the mechanism underlying this activity is probably the local inhibition of MVA synthesis by SMCs, as continued infusion of MVA, at the site of lesion induction, fully counteracted the inhibitory effect of the vastatins. Therefore, competitive inhibitors of HMG-CoA reductase merit a serious evaluation as potential clinical agent for simultaneous treating of both hypercholesterolemia and progressive atherosclerosis lesions. Although the former mechanism is now definitively demonstrated in human subjects, the latter still represents a therapeutic potential that deserves large experimental and clinical studies.

References

1. Goldstein JL, Brown MS. Regulation of the mevalonate pathway. Nature 1990;343:425-30.
2. Faust JR, Goldstein JL, Brown MS. Synthesis of ubiquinone and cholesterol in human fibroblast: Regulation of branched pathway. Arch Biochem Biophys 1979;192:86-99.
3. Quesney-Huneeus V, Wiley MH, Siperstein MD. Essential role for mevalonate synthesis in DNA replication. Proc Natl Acad Sci USA 1979;76:5056-60.
4. Habenicht AJR, Glomset JA, Ross R. Relation of cholesterol and mevalonic acid to the cell cycle in smooth muscle and Swiss 3T3 cells stimulated to divide by platelet-derived growth factor. J Biol Chem 1980;255:5134-40.
5. Schmidt RA, Schneider CJ, Glomset JA. Evidence for post-translational incorporation of a product of mevalonic acid into Swiss 3T3 cell proteins. J Biol Chem 1984;259:10175-80.
6. Maltese WA, Sheridan KM. Isoprenoid synthesis during the cell cycle. Studies of 3-hydroxy-3-methylglutaryl-coenzyme A synthase and reductase and isoprenoid labeling in cells synchronized by centrifugal elutriation. J Biol Chem 1988;263:10104-10.
7. Schmidt RA, Glomset JA, Wight TN, Habenicht AJR, Ross R. A study of the influence of mevalonic acid and its metabolites on the morphology of Swiss 3T3 cells. J Cell Biol 1982;95: 144-53.
8. Maltese WA, Sheridan KM. Differentiation of neuroblastoma cells induced by an inhibitor of mevalonate synthesis:relation of neurite outgrowth and acetylcolinesterase activity to changes in cell proliferation and blocked isoprenoid synthesis. J Cell Physiol 1985;125:540-58.
9. Li G, Regazzi R, Roche E, Wollheim CB. Blockade of mevalonate production by lovastatin attenuates bombesin and vasopressin potentiation of nutrient-induced insulin secretion in HIT-T15 cells. Probable involvement of small GTP-binding proteins. Biochem J 1993;289:379-85.
10. Bifulco M, Laezza C, Aloj SM, Garbi C. Mevalonate controls cytoskeleton organization and cell morphology in thyroid epithelial cells. J Cell Physiol 1993;155:340-48.
11. Maltese WA, Defendini R, Green RA, Sheridan KM, Donley DK. Suppression of murine neuroblastoma growth in vivo by mevinolin, a competitive inhibitor of 3-Hydroxy-3-Methylglutaryl-CoenzymeA Reductase. J Clin Invest 1985;76:1748-54.
12. Soma MR, Pagliarini P, Butti G, Paoletti R, Paoletti P, Fumagalli R. Simvastatin, an inhibitor of cholesterol biosynthesis, shows synergistic effect with N,N'-Bis(2-chloroethyl)-N-nitrosourea and beta interferon on human glioma cells. Cancer Res 1992;52:4348-55.
13. Soma MR, Baetta R, de Renzis MR, et al. *In vivo* enhanced antitumor activity of carmustine [*N,N'*-Bis(2-chloroethyl)-*N*-nitrosourea] by simvastatin. Cancer Res 1995;55:597-602.
14. Corsini A, Mazzotti M, Raiteri M, Soma MR, Gabbiani G, Fumagalli R, Paoletti R. Relationship between mevalonate pathway and arterial myocyte proliferation: in vitro studies

with inhibitors of HMG-CoA reductase. Atherosclerosis 1993;101:117-25.
15. Soma MR, Donetti E, Parolini C, et al. HMG-CoA reductase inhibitors: In vivo effects on carotid intimal thickening in normocholesterolemic rabbits. Arterioscl Thromb 1993;13:571-78.
16. Kaye AH, Laidlaw JD. Chemotherapy of gliomas. Curr Opin Lipidol 1992;5:526-33.
17. Paoletti P, Butti G, Knerich R, Gaetani P, Assietti R. Chemothereapy for malignant gliomas of the brain: A review of ten-years experience. Acta Neurochir 1990;103:38-46.
18. Soma MR, Parolini C, Donetti E, Fumagalli R, Paoletti R. Inhibition of isoprenoid biosynthesis and arterial smooth-muscle cell proliferation. J Cardiovasc Pharmacol 1995; 25(4):S20-S24.
19. Grundy SM. HMG-CoA reductase inhibitors for treatment of hypercholesterolemia. New Engl J Med 1988;319:24-33.
20. Kobayashi M, Ishida F, Takahashi T, et al. Preventive effect of MK-733 (Simvastatin), an inhibitor of HMGCoA reductase, on hypercholesterolemia and atherosclerosis induced by cholesterol feeding in rabbits. Japan J Pharmacol 1989;49:125-33.
21. Zhu BQ, Sievers RE, Sun YP, Isenberg WM, Parmley WW. Effect of lovastatin on suppression and regression of atherosclerosis in lipid-fed rabbits. J Cardiovasc Pharmacol 1992;19:246-55.
22. Watanabe Y, Ito T, Shiomi M, et al. Preventive effect of pravastatin sodium, a potent inhibitor of 3-hydroxy-3-methylglutaryl coenzyme A reductase, on coronary atherosclerosis and xanthoma in WHHL rabbits. Biochim Biophys Acta 1988;960:294-302.
23. Hunninghake DB. HMGCoA reductase inhibitors. Curr Opin Lipidol 1992;3:22-28.
24. Brown G, Albers JJ, Fisher LD, et al. Regression of coronary artery disease as a result of intensive lipid-lowering therapy in men with high levels of apolipoprotein B. New Engl J Med 1990;323:1289-98.
25. Kane JP, Malloy MJ, Ports TA, Phillips NR, Diehl JC, Havel RJ. Regression of coronary atherosclerosis during treatment of familial hypercholesterolemia with combined drug regimens. J Am Med Ass 1990;264:3007-12.
26. Blankenhorn DH. Blood lipids and human atherosclerosis regression: The angiographic evidence. Curr Opin Lipidol 1991;2:2324-29.
27. Illingworth DG. HMG CoA reductase inhibitors. Curr Opin Lipidol 1991;2:24-30.

RADIOPHARMACEUTICAL IMAGING OF ATHEROSCLEROSIS

Robert S. Lees, Ann M. Lees, John Lister-James*, and Richard T. Dean*
Boston Heart Foundation, 139 Main Street, Cambridge, Massachusetts 02142 and
**Diatech, Inc., 9 Delta Drive, Londonderry, New Hampshire 03053, USA*

Introduction

One of the major challenges in cardiovascular medicine is the recognition of active, mechanically unstable, atherosclerotic plaque before it causes vascular occlusion by plaque rupture, or plaque hemorrhage [1,2]. Because the bulk of many active plaques is extraluminal, the plaques may not be apparent on coronary angiography [3]. Recently, intravascular ultrasound has made it possible to characterize extraluminal plaque and to at least suspect that it is active and mechanically unstable [4]. However, this highly invasive technique, although promising, is expensive and not applicable to asymptomatic patients.

An important characteristic of unstable plaque, in addition to its mechanical weakness, is its high metabolic activity. Atherosclerotic lesions are unstable when they have a high concentration of foam cells, inflammatory cells, and new thin-walled vasa vasorum in the shoulders of the plaque [4,5]. By contrast, a stable plaque has a thick cap and a large amount of fibrous tissue throughout, which give it mechanical strength. Active plaque is characterized metabolically by several important features. Its permeability to proteins is higher than normal, and it contains considerable amounts of bound plasma proteins including particularly plasma low density lipoprotein (LDL), fibrinogen, and fibrin [6-8]. The endothelium over active plaque is morphologically abnormal and often covered with fibrin and platelets, constituting early mural thrombus [9]. In addition, platelet proteins may be found deep in the wall of unstable lesions along with other blood elements [7,8].

Discussion

We began a quest about 15 years ago to apply the techniques of nuclear medicine to the identification and characterization of unstable plaque. Radiopharmaceutical imaging is attractive for a number of reasons; these include its relatively low cost, minimal invasiveness, and widespread availability. Initially, we attempted to image with ^{111}indium-labeled blood platelets, with the hope that we could detect atheroma by virtue of its mural thrombus [10,11]. Although we devised a method in 1982 for labeling platelets uniformly to high specific activity [10], we found that indium-labeled platelets did not provide the sensitivity

A. M. Gotto, Jr. et al. (eds.), Drugs Affecting Lipid Metabolism, 119–124.

necessary for reliably detecting arterial thrombus.

We therefore switched our focus to LDL, well-characterized plasma proteins that accumulate in high concentration in atherosclerotic lesions [6-8,12,13]. The careful study of Minick and colleagues [14] which showed focal accumulation of cholesterol ester in healing rabbit arterial lesions, led us to postulate that, since the source of the cholesterol ester was LDL, radiolabeled LDL might also accumulate focally in arterial lesions. Following Minick's lead, we adapted the balloon-catheter-deendothelialized healing aortic model, first described in the rat by Baumgartner [15], to the rabbit. This model was ideal for imaging studies, because rabbits are readily imaged and the healing balloon lesions have considerable resemblance to active human atherosclerotic lesions.

Using ^{125}I-labeled LDL, we showed by radioautography that LDL did accumulate focally in healing experimental aortic lesions in rabbits [16]. It is important to note that the rabbits were not hypercholesterolemic and that the success of this model did not depend upon cholesterol feeding. Healing balloon lesions, even those a few cell layers thick, are so metabolically active that they accumulate radiolabeled LDL injected in tracer amounts, e.g. a milligram per rabbit, which allows them to be easily imaged.

Because ^{125}I-LDL was the standard preparation for conducting metabolic studies *in vivo* and *in vitro* at the time, we used it for our first imaging studies [17]. Even with this isotope, whose gamma emission is poorly suited for external imaging, abdominal aortic lesions in the ballooned rabbit [17] were readily visible.

The animal studies were followed by ^{125}I-LDL imaging in humans. We found that human atherosclerotic plaques could also be imaged [18] although the images were not optimal for clinical purposes. The 60-day half-life of ^{125}I is much longer than needed for imaging. Most of the ^{125}I of ^{125}I-LDL ends up in the body's iodide pool, and gives the subject a relatively high dose of gamma irradiation. In addition, while the plasma half-life of LDL is about 2 days in normal subjects, it may be several days longer in hypercholesterolemic patients. The long plasma residence time produced an unacceptably high blood pool background of radioactivity; since the plaques are in the arterial wall, which in turn surrounds the blood in the vessel, the radioactivity of blood and mural lesions were superimposed. This made some lesions difficult to visualize until 40-48 hours after injection of the radiopharmaceutical. This meant that the patient had to return for imaging 2 days after injection, an interval which was impractical for wide clinical application. Thus, a better method for plaque imaging was sought.

The problem of the most suitable radiosiotope was the first one we approached, and the solution was relatively simple. We turned to the most widely used isotope for gamma camera imaging, ^{99m}technetium (^{99m}Tc), a synthetic metastable element which decays to ^{99}Tc by emitting a 140 kev gamma ray that is readily imaged with the gamma scintillation camera. About 70% of clinical nuclear medicine procedures are performed with ^{99m}Tc-labeled radiopharmaceuticals. The isotope, in the form of technetium pertechnetate, is available at low cost in every major hospital and its 6-hour half-life provides low radiation exposure to the patient. With helpful advice from Professors Alan Davison and Alun Jones of MIT and Harvard Medical School [19], we worked out a method for making ^{99m}Tc-labeled LDL [20]. The preparation provided excellent images in rabbits [20] because of the relatively short biological half-life of human LDL in the rabbit (20-21 hours). When we did the corresponding human studies [21], we were able to image human peripheral vascular lesions, but found again that the much longer half-life of LDL in humans and the resulting high blood-pool radioactivity prevented ^{99m}Tc-LDL from being a clinically useful agent, despite the far superior imaging characteristics of ^{99m}Tc in comparison with ^{125}I.

Convinced now that autologous LDL, which in addition to its long residence time in plasma, took about 3 days to isolate and purify from each patient was not a clinically useful radiopharmaceutical, we looked for a more suitable vehicle for targeting ^{99m}Tc to plaques. Fortunately, the primary sequence of apolipoprotein B (apo B), the protein moiety of LDL, had recently been published [22-24]. Because of the remarkably focal nature of LDL accumulation in arterial lesions, we reasoned that one or more specific domains of the apo B sequence must be responsible for directing LDL into arterial lesions. If we could locate such a domain, we could synthesize a short peptide corresponding to that sequence and use it for radiopharmaceutical imaging. Although at that time it was generally believed that short peptides did not have sufficient secondary structure to exhibit biological behavior similar to the proteins after which they were patterned, we began to investigate the structure of apo B with the goal of determining which portion or portions of the molecule caused it to bind focally in arterial lesions. Forgez et al. had already shown [25] that certain portions of the apo B molecule were trypsin-accessible and therefore, presumably on the surface of LDL. We were fairly certain of two relevant facts: 1) that the LDL receptor-binding domain was near the carboxyl terminal end of the apo B molecule [23] and 2) that the LDL receptor could not be the mechanism by which LDL bound to atherosclerotic plaques, since LDL-receptor-negative hypercholesterolemia is characterized by early death from severe atherosclerosis [26]. Therefore, we looked closely at the surface peptides described by Forgez which were closer to the amino terminal end of the molecule, far from the suspected LDL receptor binding domain of apo B.

The surface domain closest to the amino terminus appeared to have the right specifications for a peptide which would bind to arterial lesions. It was amphophilic, with a charged domain and a large lipophilic domain, which might enable it to bind both to the arterial extracellular matrix and to the lipid core of LDL. Therefore, we synthesized an octadecapeptide modeled after that region of the apo B molecule with an amino-terminal tyrosine added to facilitate labeling with ^{125}I. Since this was the fourth synthetic peptide in our series, we named it SP-4. To our delight, experiments in ballooned rabbits showed that ^{125}I-labeled SP-4 accumulated in a focal pattern very similar to the pattern of LDL itself, that is in high concentration at the actively healing edge of rabbit aortic balloon lesions, and nowhere else in the artery [27]. A control peptide, SP-2, modeled after the LDL receptor-binding domain of apo E, had no focal accumulation [27].

Next, a method for labeling SP-4 with ^{99m}Tc had to be developed. Previous methods for labeling proteins with technetium had all been empirical. Pertechnetate was incubated with a protein under reducing conditions and, if one were lucky, the protein became labeled. Little or nothing was known about how proteins bound ^{99m}Tc; therefore, one could neither predict which proteins would label nor optimize the conditions except on a empirical basis. At that point, few defined ligands for ^{99m}Tc had been developed [28] that would allow routine labeling of any protein; peptides had not yet successfully been labeled with technetium by any method. This was the challenge facing the two scientists at Diatech, Inc. (RTD, JLJ) who designed and synthesized several analogs of SP-4 with technetium-binding sequences at either the amino or carboxyl terminus (unpublished). Using uncomplicated labeling methodology, the new compounds were shown to readily bind ^{99m}Tc. Biodistribution studies and imaging studies were then carried out in animals by a number of collaborators using two of the new peptides, P199 and P215 [29-31].

The results were promising. P199 and P215 were tested in a cholesterol-fed, non-balloon-deendothelialized rabbit model of atherosclerosis. Both peptides bound to cholesterol-rich plaques in the rabbit aorta; however, in contrast to labeled LDL, these peptides dissociated to some extent from the lesions after a period of time, usually 30-60 minutes. Despite the transient binding, there was adequate time for the lesions to be imaged; the low-molecular-weight peptides disappeared from the plasma very rapidly, but they entered the lesions even more rapidly. Thus by 20 minutes after injection, the blood pool radioactivity of P199 and P215 was less than 10% of the initial activity [28] while the lesion trapping of the peptide was still maximal. The results indicated the feasibility of testing the peptides in humans.

The initial clinical study, a multicenter trial of ^{99m}Tc-P215 in 27 patients, will be reported elsewhere [manuscript in preparation]. Overall, ^{99m}Tc-P215 allowed better imaging of human atherosclerotic lesions of the human carotid bifurcation than had been possible previously. Nevertheless, the sensitivity of detection of complicated lesions was not as high as desired in this preliminary study.

Meanwhile, we refocused our interest on the original goal for plaque imaging, that of imaging the clotting system components contained within the plaque. Since our original 1982 studies [10,11], a great deal of progress had been made in the biochemistry of thrombosis. The platelet glycoprotein IIbIIIa (GPIIbIIIa) receptor, expressed on the surface of platelets, had been identified as an important high-affinity receptor critically involved in thrombosis and clotting. This receptor is involved in the binding of fibrinogen to activated platelets to produce a thrombus, a finding which triggered the development of a whole class of therapeutic antithrombotic pharmaceuticals [32-34]. It also offered an interesting opportunity for diagnostic imaging. Knowing the structure of molecules which bound to the receptor, we designed GPIIbIIIa receptor-binding peptides and utilized our technetium-labeling technology to produce diagnostic radiopharmaceuticals for imaging that receptor. The first of these agents to be tested clinically, P280, was clearly successful for diagnosing deep vein thrombosis [35]. In addition to continuing studies of venous thrombosis, P280 is now undergoing a clinical trial for diagnosing arterial thrombus. In a pilot study, patients with carotid stenosis are being imaged preoperatively with ^{99m}P280. Early results show encouraging success in identifying unstable carotid plaque with mural thrombus, and the trial is continuing.

In summary, atherosclerotic plaque imaging has progressed significantly over the 15 years since its conception. Both apo B-based and GPIIbIIIa receptor-based radiopharmaceuticals labeled with Tc-99m have been synthesized and used to image atherosclerotic plaque. Although the ideal agent has yet to be found, the results to date suggest that one or both of these methodologic approaches will allow detection and localization of unstable atherosclerotic plaque in the arterial circulation.

Acknowledgements

We are grateful for the research and clinical collaboration of Dr. Jeffrey Borer and his colleagues at New York Hospital/Cornell Medical Center, Drs. Stanley Goldsmith, Shankar Vallabhajosula, Joseph Machak, and their colleagues at Mt. Sinai Hospital, New York, Dr. Pietro Muto and his colleagues at the National Cancer Institute and the University of Naples, among the many investigators who have collaborated with the authors.

References

1. Davies MJ, Thomas AC. Plaque fissuring--the cause of acute myocardial infarction, sudden ischemia death, and crescendo angina. Br Heart J 1985;53:363-73.
2. Fuster V, Stein B, Ambrose JA, et al. Atherosclerotic plaque rupture and thrombosis. Circulation 1990;82(2):47-59.
3. Glagov S, Weisenberg E, Zarins CK, et al. Compensatory enlargement of human atherosclerotic coronary arteries. NEJM 1987;316:1371-75.
4. Hodgson JM, Reddy KG, Suneja R, Nair RN, Lesnefsky, EJ, Sheehan HM. Intracoronary ultrasound imaging: Correlation of plaque morphology with angiography, clinical syndrome and procedural results in patients undergoing coronary angioplasty. JACC 1993;21:35-44.
5. Richardson PD, Davies MJ, Born GVR. Influence of plaque configuration and stress distribution on fissuring of coronary atherosclerotic plaques. Lancet 1989;2:941-44.
6. Smith EB, Staples EM, Dietz HS, Smith RH. Role of endothelium in sequestration of lipoprotein and fibrinogen in aortic lesions, thrombi, and graft pseudo-intimas. Lancet 1979;2:812-16.
7. Kao VC, Wissler RW. A study of the immunohistochemical localization of serum lipoproteins and other plasma proteins in human atherosclerotic lesions. Exp Mol Pathol 1965;4:465-79.
8. MacMillan GC, Adams CWM, Ibrahim MZM. Histochemical identification of plasma proteins in the human aortic intima. J Pathol Bacteriol 1965;89:225.
9. Burrig K-F. The endothelium of advanced arteriosclerotic plaques in humans. Arteriosclerosis and Thrombosis 1991;11:1678-89.
10. Bunting RW, Callahan RJ, Finklestein S, Lees RS, Strauss HW. A modified technique for labeling human platelets with indium-111-oxine using an albumin density-gradient separation. Radiology 1982;145:219-221.
11. Finklestein S, Miller A, Callahan RJ, et al. Imaging of acute arterial injury with 111-indium labeled platelets -- Comparison with scanning electron micrographs. Radiol 1982;145:155-59.
12. Woolf N, Pilkington TRE. The immunohistochemical demonstration of lipoproteins in vessel walls. J Pathol Bacteriol 1965;90:459-63.
13. Walton K, Williamson N. Histological and immunofluorescent studies on the evolution of the human atheromatous plaque. J Atheroscler Res 1968;8:599-624.
14. Minick CR, Stemerman MB, Insull W, Jr. Effect of regenerated endothelium on lipid accumulation in the arterial wall. Proc Natl Acad Sci USA 1977;74:1724-28.
15. Baumgartner HR. Eine neue Methode zur Erzeugung von Thromben durch gezielte uberdehnung der Gefasswand. Z. Gesamte Exp Med 1963;137:227-49.
16. Roberts AB, Lees AM, Lees RS, et al. Selective accumulation of low density liporoteins in

damaged arterial wall. J Lipid Res 1983;24:1160-67.
17. Lees RS, Lees AM, Fischman AJ, Strauss HW. External imaging of active atherosclerosis with ^{99m}Tc-LDL. In: Glagov S, Newman III WP, Schaffer SA, editors. Pathobiology of the human atherosclerotic plaque. New York: Springer-Verlag, 1990:841-51.
18. Lees RS, Lees AM, Strauss HW. Extracorporeal imaging of human atheroslcerosis. J Nucl Med 1983;24:154-56.
19. Jones AG, Orvig C, Trop HS, et al. A survey of reducing agents for the synthesis of tetraphenylarsonium oxytechnetiumbis (ethanedithiolate) from [^{99}Tc] pertechnetate in aqueous solution. J Nucl Med 1980;21:279-81.
20. Lees RS, Garabedian HD, Lees AM, et al. Technetium-99m low density lipoproteins: Preparation and biodistribution. J Nucl Med 1985;25:1056-62.
21. Lees AM, Lees RS, Schoen FJ, et al. Imaging human atherosclerosis with ^{99m}Tc-labeled low density lipoproteins. Arteriosclerosis 1988;8:461-70.
22. Law SW, Grant S, Higuchi K, et al. Human liver apolipoprotein B-100 cDNA: Complete nucleic acids and derived amino acids sequence. Proc Natl Acad Sci USA 1986;83:8142-46.
23. Yang C-Y, Chen SH, Gianturco SH, et al. Sequence, structure, receptor-binding domains and internal repeats of human apolipoprotein B-100. Nature 1986;323:738-42.
24. Knott TJ, Pease RJ, Powell LM, et al. Complete protein sequence and identification of structural domains of human apolipoprotein B. Nature 1986;323:734-38.
25. Forgez P, Gregory H, Young JA, et al. Identification of surface-exposed segments of apolipoprotein B-100 in the LDL particle. Biochem Biophys Res Comm 1986; 140:250-57.
26. Goldstein JL, Hobbs HH, Brown MS. Familial hypercholesterolemia. In: The metabolic and molecular bases of inherited disease. Scriver CR, Beaudet AL, Sly WS, Valle D, editors. New York: McGraw-Hill, 1995:1981-2030.
27. Shih I-L, Lees RS, Chang MY, Lees AM. Focal accumulation of an apolipoprotein B-based synthetic oligopeptide in the healing rabbit arterial wall. Proc Natl Acad Sci USA 1990;87:1436-40.
28. Dean RT, Lister-James J, Lees RS, Lees AM, Vallabhajosula S, Goldsmith SJ. Peptides in biomedical sciences: Principles and practice. In: Martin-Comin J, editor. Radiolabeled Blood Elements. New York: Plenum Press, 1994: 195-99.
29. Vallabhajosula S, Ali KSM, Goldsmith SJ, et al. Evaluation of technetium-99m labeled peptides for imaging atherosclerotic lesions in vivo. J Nucl Med 1993;34 (Suppl):66P.
30. Hardoff R, Zanzonico P, Braegelmann F, et al. Localization of ^{99m}Tc-labeled Apo B synthetic peptide in arterial lesions of an experimental model of spontaneous atherosclerosis. Am J Ther 1995;2:88-99.
31. Lu P, Zanzonico P, Lister-James J, et al. Comparisons in rabbits of Tc-99m-labelled synthetic peptide fragments for imaging of atherosclerotic plaques. J Nucl Med. 1994;34(Suppl):80P.
32. Samanen J, Ali F, Romoff T, et al. Development of a small RGD peptide fibrinogen receptor antagonist with potent antiaggregatory activity in vitro. J Med Chem 1991; 34:3114-3125.
33. Cook NS, Bruttger O, Pally CH, Hagenbach A. The effects of two synthetic glycoprotein IIb/IIIa antagonists, Ro 43-8857 and L-700,462, on platelet aggregation and blleding in guinea-pigs and dogs: evidence that Ro 43-8857 is orally active. Thrombosis and Haemostasis 1993;70:838-47.
34. Mousa SA, Bozarth JM, Forsythe MS, et al. Antiplatelet and antithrombotic efficacy of DMP 728, a novel platelet GPIIb/IIIa receptor antagonist. Circulation 1994;89:3-12.
35. Muto P, Lastoria S, Vaarrella P, et al. Detecting deep venous thrombosis with technetium-99m-labeled synthetic peptide P280. J Nucl Med 1995;36:1384-91.

ANGIOGRAPHIC TRIALS ON PROGRESSION AND REGRESSION OF ATHEROSCLEROSIS BY PLASMA LIPID REDUCTION

Barry Lewis
University of London, 4 Sutcliffe Close, London NW11 6NT, United Kingdom

Introduction

At the time of this review, 24 randomized controlled trials of 26 lipid lowering interventions employing angiographic or ultrasonographic end-points had been reported in full, to assess progression and regression of arterial disease. Among 7 further studies not having randomized control groups, early trials from 1967 showed the feasibility of "regression trials" [1,2]. The first randomized controlled trial appeared in 1983 [3]. Since 1984, numerous trials employing serial coronary angiography have appeared, mostly using quantitative image analysis (QCA); the outcomes have been impressively but by no means absolutely consistent. In general, these studies confirm that atherosclerosis regression induced by lipid lowering in experimental animals [4,5] occurs also in man, though to an anatomically smaller extent. The human trials have provided (i) an affirmative test of the lipid hypothesis, and dietary trials have been consistent with the dietary lipid hypothesis, (ii) evidence that angiographic progression is associated with and is predictive of clinical coronary events, (iii) evidence of mechanisms, e.g. of the association between in-trial lipoprotein levels and progression, (iv) ascertainment of target levels of lipoproteins for lipid-lowering therapy, (v) the means to test new therapies rapidly and economically, and (vi) new insights into preventive strategy.

This information must be seen in the context of other sources of knowledge of atherosclerosis. Unlike clinical outcome trials, in which the end-point is dichotomized, angiographic studies gain statistical power by using a continuously variable endpoint; further, they provide many observations per patient (up to 10 coronary segments may be analyzed). Angiographic trials are comparatively brief, treatment effects becoming established in 2-3 years. Smaller sample size allows closer supervision and better compliance. By contrast, the duration of clinical outcome trials often means that the therapy is in use for many years before results become available. In the case of meta-analyses of such trials, the principle of inclusiveness (needed to minimize selection bias and to permit generalization), carries penalties: results are influenced by obsolete treatments, limiting relevance to current therapy, and trial design may be insufficiently consistent.

A. M. Gotto, Jr. et al. (eds.), Drugs Affecting Lipid Metabolism, 125–136.

Main Results of the Angiographic Trials

CORONARY ARTERIES

Since the choice of endpoint has varied among trials, absolute measurements coming into widespread use only recently, this account is based chiefly on percentage incidence of progression and of regression. In all 6 intervention groups receiving resins alone or in combination with niacin and/or lovastatin, the incidence of progression was substantially lower than in randomized control groups, significantly in 5 [6-11]; and the incidence of regression was higher in all but one. Diminished progression was more common than regression in most trials. Coronary event rates were lower in all treatment groups, significantly so in 3. In the POSCH trials of partial ileal bypass, at 5 years, the incidences of progression were 37% in treated and 65% in control subjects, regression was seen in 12.6% and 4.7%, respectively, and coronary events occurred in 82 and 125 subjects [12].

Three nonpharmacological controlled trials have been completed (Table 1). A moderate lipid-lowering diet was the single intervention in STARS [10]; diet was combined with exercise in HEIDELBERG [13], and LIFESTYLE [14] used a vegetarian diet, exercise, weight loss, stress reduction, and smoking cessation. In all, the incidence of progression was significantly decreased and that of regression significantly increased. In STARS, progression rates were 15% in the diet group and 46% in the control group, and rates of regression were 38% and 4% respectively, while 3 hard coronary events occurred in dieted subjects, 10 in controls. Angina frequency was markedly reduced in the LIFESTYLE intervention group, but in HEIDELBERG there were nonsignificantly more events among treated subjects.

Table 1. Angiographic trials of health-related behavior [10,13,14].

	DESIGN	%Δ LDL-C	%Δ TG	%Δ HDL-C	AMBIENT LDL-C mmol/L	OUTCOME ANGIOGRAPHIC CHANGE Progression Tr	Progression C	Regression Tr	Regression C	CV EVENTS Tr	CV EVENTS C
LIFESTYLE (vegetarian diet, weight loss, exercise, ✗smoking, ✗stress)	41 CHD QCA 15 m	-37	+22	-3	2.46	18	53 (% pts)	82	42	angina frequency -91%	+165%
STARS (27%en fat P:S 0.8, high-fibre diet)	75 CHD QCA 39 m	-16	-20	0	4.19	15	46 ($p<0.02$) % pts	38	4 ($p<0.02$)	3	10 ($p<0.05$)
HEIDELBERG (diet, [AHA III] + exercise)	92 CHD QCA 12 m	-8	-24	+3	3.85	23	48 ($p<0.001$) % pts	32	17 ($p<0.001$)	6	4

Four statin trials were reported fully at the time of this review [15-18]. Progression was significantly reduced in three based on QCA, and in the fourth when based on a visual score (with a favorable nonsignificant trend using QCA). The incidence of regression was increased by treatment, significantly in two trials. Coronary event rates showed a trend to reduction by treatment in all, but only in the large pravastatin trial was this marked (55 versus 93 events) and significant [17].

In two trials, multiple drugs and diet were employed. In SCRIP [19], the larger and longer study (which included intervention against nonlipid risk factors) progression was decreased and regression increased, the former significantly and the latter almost so. Coronary events were significantly reduced. By contrast, HARP [20] reported nonsignificant reductions in progression and in events. Nonrandomized trials of clofibrate [21] and fenofibrate [22] suggested reduction of progression; and uncontrolled LDL apheresis studies recorded regression in heterozygous familial hypercholesterolemia (FH) [23,24]. A further trial in FH [25] compared two treatments; there were no significant differences between the angiographic effects of LDL apheresis plus simvastatin (which lowered levels of LDL and Lp(a)), and the effects of simvastatin and colestipol (which lowered LDL only).

Femoral Arteries

Change in femoral arteries was the endpoint in 5 controlled trials [3,26-29]. Reduced progression was seen in two and increased regression in three. In CLAS [27] favorable angiographic effects were commoner in native coronary arteries and saphenous vein grafts than in femoral arteries of the same patients.

Carotid Arteries

Four ultrasonographic trials have indicated that lipid lowering favorably affects the intimomedial thickness (IMT) of carotid arteries [29-32]. In two, IMT decreased in the treatment group and increased in the controls. In a third, based on a population sample [29], the rate of increase of IMT was considerably reduced, but in the fourth, progression was significantly reduced only in the common carotid.

Angiographic Effects of Lipid Lowering and Clinical Coronary Events

The magnitude of the regression of human atherosclerosis induced by lipid lowering is small; understandably reservations have been expressed as to its clinical relevance. However, many trials [12,8, (both intervention groups), 10, (both intervention groups), 14,18,19,33] show a favorable angiographic outcome to be associated with significant reduction in coronary or cardiovascular event rates. In MARS [15], CCAIT [16], and MAAS [17] coronary events were nonsignificantly reduced. In HARP [20] neither angiographic changes nor event rates changed significantly. That favorable coronary angiographic change is *predictive* of reduced clinical event rates is also evident. Long-term follow-up in POSCH [12] and CLAS [33] showed angiographic effects at 2-3 years to predict event rates in the subsequent 6 years.

This was also evident in FATS [8], when fortuitous angiography was predictive in events in the territory of the progressing coronary segments; this was discernable, too, in the NHLBI trial [6] (though the numbers were small). The relation between angiographic change during lipid-lowering therapy, and reduction in coronary events, is further discussed in the final section.

Associations Between In-Trial Variables and Coronary Angiographic Progression

LIPOPROTEIN CONCENTRATIONS

Biochemical and other observations were made repeatedly during many angiographic trials; this afforded the opportunity to seek relationships between angiographic change and mean concentrations of lipoproteins. Several such relationships are shown in Table 2.

Table 2. Correlations between lipoprotein concentrations and coronary angiographic progression [6-10,15,16,19,22,26,34,35].

	Serum Chol: HDL-C Ratio	LDL-C	LDL3-C	HDL-C (Negative)	Triglyceride or VLDL-C	Lp(a)	ApoB	ApoC-III
LEIDEN	✔							
NHLBI	✔				✔ and IDL			
FATS		✔		✔		✔	✔	
CLAS					✔			✔ (in HDL)
UCSF-SCOR		✔						
STARS		✔	✔ (multivariate)			✔	✔	
Hahmann et al.		✔						
MARS	✔				✔ (univariate)			✔ (in VLDL+LDL)
SCRIP		✔						
CCAIT		✔		✔				

Not all measurements were made in all trials, and entry criteria in some may have attenuated the likelihood of detecting associations by truncating the range of certain variables. Nevertheless there is a consistent positive association between in-trial LDL cholesterol levels and progression. LDL subclasses were measured only in STARS; multivariate analysis revealed the strongest independent lipoprotein predictor of progression to be the concentration of LDL_3 or small dense LDL [34]. Less consistently, progression has been found to be associated with the serum cholesterol:HDL cholesterol ratio, and with triglyceride or VLDL-cholesterol levels. In FATS and STARS it was also associated with Lp(a) concentration.

To achieve regression and for secondary prevention it has been held that LDL cholesterol levels should be reduced to 2.5 mmol/L. Such levels were achieved in CLAS [7], LIFESTYLE [14], and MARS [15], and were approached in the colestipol-lovastatin group of FATS [8]. In STARS [10] mean LDL cholesterol level of subjects showing regression was 2.4 mmol/L. However, in-trial LDL cholesterol was greater in other trials in which substantial regression occurred, e.g. the colestipol-niacin group in FATS (3.3 mmol/L), MAAS (3.0 mmol/L) [17], SCRIP (3.12 mmol/L) [19] and the diet-cholestyramine group in STARS (3.37 mmol/L). In 8 trials in which regression was substantial, mean in-trial LDL cholesterol level was 2.9 mmol/L.

In 6 trials in which little or no regression was observed, mean in-trial LDL cholesterol was higher, 3.6 mmol/L. But among these were two (POSCH [12] and HARP [20]) in which LDL cholesterol averaged 2.7 and 2.23 mmol/L, respectively. Regression of angiographic outcome on LDL cholesterol suggests that over a wide range, the lower the LDL cholesterol the better. The crude results of regression trials are also compatible with the view that the extent of lipid lowering is important. Clarification will require careful meta-analyses that take into account the variety of angiographic endpoints and also the important effect of baseline severity of disease on outcome. Pending such data, the extent of lipid lowering should be chosen in the light of overall risk factor status, as in current guidelines.

Associations with Nutrient Intake

Angiographic trials have provided an opportunity to examine the relation between nutrient intake and progression. In the pioneering uncontrolled Leiden trial of a vegetarian high-polyunsaturate diet, progression was directly related to the serum cholesterol:HDL-cholesterol ratio [35]. Analysis of nutritional data from the placebo group of CLAS [36] showed that subjects who developed new lesions had higher intakes of fat, saturated fat, monounsaturated fat, and polyunsaturated fat. In LIFESTYLE [14], interventions included a vegetarian low fat diet and weight loss; the level of compliance correlated with a favorable angiographic outcome. In STARS [10], one group received an isocaloric diet as the single intervention while controls received usual care. The combined diet and usual care groups provided a wide range of nutrient intakes, assessed several times during the trial. STARS thus afforded a unique opportunity to study associations between nutrient intake and progression/regression (Table 3) [37,38]. On univariate analysis, significant and substantial proportions of the variance in angiographic course were explained by intakes of energy, fat, and saturated fat; of the latter, myristic, palmitic, and stearic acids were strongly related to progression. Dietary cholesterol was directly, near-significantly, related.

Table 3. Relationships between nutrient intake and progression of coronary artery disease [37,38]. STARS.

	% Variance Explained	Regression	p
Univariate			
Energy, kcal/d	21.7	-0.001	0.001
Fat, g/d	29.7	-0.010	< 0.001
Saturated Fat, g/d	19.5	-0.010	0.001
Monounsaturated Fat, g/d	11.4	-0.010	0.016
Polyunsaturated Fat, g/d	0.6	-0.006	0.592
Cholesterol, mg/d	7.3	-0.001	0.058
Fiber, g/d	0.7	-0.003	0.561
C14:0	15.5	-0.007	0.003
C16:0	20.8	-0.002	< 0.001
C18:0	23.8	-0.005	< 0.001
Total Trans	19.7	-0.010	< 0.001
Multivariate			
C16:0*	13.2	-0.002	0.026
C18:0*	17.0	-0.005	0.009
Total Trans*	16.6	-0.008	0.013

*significant associations largely explained by intakes of dairy fats and lamb.

Transunsaturated fatty acid intake was positively associated with progression. On multivariate analysis, intakes of palmitate, stearate and trans acids retained significance, but because of strong intercorrelations their independent contributions could not be determined. As in CLAS, associations between mono- and polyunsaturated fatty acid intakes and progression were positive; i.e. no 'protective' effect was detected. Since the main sources of monounsaturates in the STARS population were dairy fats and meat fat, the associations may have been confounded by intakes of saturated fatty acids from these foods.

Lipid Lowering and Progression in Women and Men

Women participated in six angiographic trials of lipid lowering. A significant treatment effect was observed in women, but not in men, with familial hypercholesterolemia in SCOR [9]. In LIFESTYLE [14] all five female participants showed net regression. Less progression occurred in treated women in MARS [15] and SCRIP [19] than in treated men. Reduction in minimum lumen diameter was the same in women in CCAIT as in all participants [16]. Only in FHRS, which did not have a usual care group, did women fare less well than men [25].

Is a Favorable Angiographic Outcome Dependent on Serum Cholesterol at Entry?

This question was brought to attention by HARP [20] in which entry was limited to subjects with entry serum cholesterol level < 6.5 mmol/L; despite successful cholesterol lowering, no significant angiographic benefit was seen. In several other trials with wider entry criteria, results have been examined in groups stratified by serum cholesterol at entry; in CLAS [7] and MARS [15] there were favorable treatment effects on coronary arteries both when entry cholesterol level was < 6.22 mmol/L and > 6.22 mmol/L; this was also the case in the carotid arteries in ACAPS [31] when LDL cholesterol was < 4.1 mmol/L and > 4.1 mmol/L at entry. Strikingly, there was a more favorable treatment effect in FATS [39] when entry LDL cholesterol was < 4.1 mmol/L than > 4.1 mmol/L. Findings were ambiguous in CCAIT [16]; there was no significant treatment effect when entry levels were < 6.4 mmol/L, however, the graded therapy protocol led to use of a lower dose of lovastatin in this subset. It should be noted that in HARP [20] the controls also received treatment; a diet was prescribed, and 10 of 39 subjects received lipid-lowering drugs. This would attenuate the power to detect a treatment effect. Minimum diameter of all lesions decreased less in the intervention group than in controls, though nonsignificantly.

An analysis of 8 trials has suggested that angiographic improvement is greatest when pre-treatment LDL cholesterol levels are high [54]. Hence it seems that angiographic benefit occurs over a wide range of pretreatment cholesterol levels, but that there may be diminishing returns at low levels; this is compatible with the positive log-linear epidemiological relationship between plasma cholesterol and the incidence of coronary heart disease.

The Relation Between Angiographic Change and Clinical Events: Its Significance for Prevention

The Acute Occlusive Event

Plaque fissuring as a cause of occlusive coronary thrombosis was reported in 1967 [40]. That fissuring of the fibrous cap, followed by thrombosis, underlies the great majority of Q-wave myocardial infarcts, sudden ischemic cardiac deaths and unstable angina, as well as silent rapid plaque growth, has become evident through careful quantitative studies by

Davies et al. [41-43] and by Fuster et al. [44].

THE CONCEPT OF THE INFARCTOGENIC PLAQUE

Growing insight into the mechanisms and causes of this acute process has been gained. The morphology of vulnerable plaques has been clarified. Circumferential stress, the immediate cause of fissuring, has been found by computer modeling to be greatest in the thin fibrous caps of lipid-rich plaques [42]. Thinness of the cap profoundly increases circumferential stress; severity of stenosis diminishes it [45]; in plaques causing < 75% stenoses, the presence of a lipid pool profoundly increases stress. In aortic plaques the presence of a lipid pool comprising > 40% of cross-sectional area is critical to fissuring and thrombosis [43].

In myocardial infarction patients who had fortuitously undergone coronary angiography months previously, small- to moderate-sized plaques are likeliest to lead to infarction, e.g. [46]. Thus infarct-related lesions are often hemodynamically insignificant even shortly before major clinical events. Such plaques are far more numerous than those producing > 70% stenoses.

Interacting with these physical factors are potent biological ones. There is a 5-fold increase in the macrophage content of fibrous caps of fissured plaques compared with unfissured ones [43]; but smooth muscle cell content is much diminished. Growing evidence indicates that the presence of macrophages and T-lymphocytes is important in rendering the cap vulnerable to physical stresses, and Libby [47] proposes a role for chronic inflammation. The cytokine IFN-γ released by T-lymphocytes inhibits interstitial collagen synthesis by smooth muscle, and macrophage foam cells from experimental atherosclerotic plaques release stromelysin and interstitial collagenase, proteases that can break down various components of the extracellular matrix of the arterial wall. Libby found excess matrix-degrading activity in the vulnerable shoulder region of human plaques.

LIPID LOWERING-INDUCED REGRESSION AND THE INFARCTOGENIC PLAQUE

Many processes have been invoked to explain the link between widened arterial lumen and reduced coronary event rate. That true regression of lesions, due to depletion of the lipid pool, is one such process is reasonably certain, by analogy with changes seen in animal studies of regression [4,5]; prevention of new lesions and arrest of progression in human trials have their counterpart in the prevention of atherosclerosis by early cholesterol lowering in genetically-hyperlipidemic rabbits [48]. Speculative mechanisms include restored endothelium-dependent vasodilatation, lysis of thrombi, and vascular remodeling; that reduced IMT has regularly been observed in carotid arteries [29-32], however, suggests that these are not necessary elements. Plaque "stabilization" is commonly invoked to account for reduced event rates; but apart from an insightful discussion by Brown et al. [49], to whom this account owes much, few have attempted to define stabilization.

In their study of plaque regression in primates, Small et al. [50] examined the time course of the processes involved. After 6 months of lipid lowering, when intimal thickness was only slightly reduced, there was striking depletion of macrophage-derived foam cells.

Cholesteryl ester content had begun to diminish. In man, foam cell depletion may be one of the processes that reduce coronary events during lipid lowering. Diminished LDL and IDL influx [51] slowly deplete the lipid pool, also lessening stress on the plaque cap; the reduced lipid content seen in animal models [4,5,50] is evident angiographically as lumen widening or decreased IMT.

Implications for Prevention

Preventive strategy should take these new insights into account. The concept of targeted vigorous lipid lowering is established [52], but such efforts need increasingly to be focused on the presence of infarctogenic plaques. In cardiological practice, a change of emphasis is required: hemodynamically-unimportant lesions seen angiographically are highly significant in the context of prevention by lipid lowering. In this sense, overt cardiovascular disease, with its attendant 6-7-fold increase in risk of recurrent coronary events, is best regarded as a marker for the presence of further infarctogenic plaques.

In the asymptomatic subject the decision to treat conservatively or intensively is more difficult, since noninvasive procedures for imaging coronary arteries, e.g. by ultrafast tomographic scanning for detecting coronary calcification, have yet to be widely introduced and may be prohibitively expensive. Current practice, of multifactorial risk assessment to identify the hyperlipidemic patient who requires vigorous and often pharmacological treatment, may well be effective through being an indirect means of detecting patients likely to have infarctogenic plaques. Until coronary imaging becomes more accessible, risk assessment is best reinforced by carotid ultrasonography [53], the better to target the patient in need of vigorous preventive measures. These trends will deemphasize the distinction between primary and secondary prevention, may widen the range of patients for whom intensive lipid lowering is indicated, and will improve targeting of such therapy.

References

1. Ost RC, Stenson S. Regression of peripheral atherosclerosis during therapy with high doses of nicotinic acid. Scand J Clin Lab Invest 1967;99:241-45.
2. Barndt R, Blankenhorn DH, Crawford DW. Regression and progression of early femoral atherosclerosis in treated hyperlipoproteinemic patients. Ann Intern Med 1977;86:139-46.
3. Duffield RGM, Lewis B, Miller NE, Jamieson CW, Brunt JNH, Colchester ACF. Treatment of hyperlipidaemia retards progression of symptomatic femoral atherosclerosis. Lancet 1983;ii:639-42.
4. Armstrong ML, Megan MB. Lipid depletion in atheromatous coronary arteries in monkeys after atherogenic and regression diets. Circ Res 1972;30:675-80.
5. Wissler RW, Vesselinovitch D. Can atherosclerotic plaques regress? Anatomic and biochemical evidence from animal models. Am J Cardiol 1990;65:33-40.
6. Brensike JF, Levy RI, Kelsey SF, et al. Effects of therapy with cholestyramine onprogression of coronary arteriosclerosis: Results of the NHLBI Type II Coronary Intervention Study. Circulation 1994;69:313-24.
7. Blankenhorn DH, Nessim SA, Johnson RL, Sanmarco ME, Azen SP, Cashin-Hemphill L.

Beneficial effects of combined colestipol-niacin therapy on coronary atherosclerosis and coronary venous bypass grafts. JAMA 1987;257:3233-40.

8. Brown G, Albers JJ, Fisher LD, et al. Regression of coronary artery disease as a result of intensive lipid-lowering therapy in men with high levels of apolipoproteinB. N Engl J Med 1990;323:1289-98.
9. Kane JP, Malloy MJ, Ports TA, Phillips NR, Diehl JC, Havel RJ. Regression of coronary atherosclerosis during treatment of familial hypercholesterolemia with combined drug regimes. JAMA 1990;264:3007-12.
10. Watts GF, Lewis B, Brunt JNH, et al. Effects on coronary artery disease of lipid-lowering diet, or diet plus cholestyramine, in the St. Thomas' Atherosclerosis Regression Study (STARS). Lancet 1992;339:563-69.
11. Cashin-Hemphill L, Mack WJ, Pogoda JM, Sanmarco ME, Azen SP, Blankenhorn DH. Beneficial effects of colestipol-niacin on coronary atherosclerosis; a 4-year follow-up. JAMA 1990;264:3013-17.
12. Buchwald H, Varco RL, Matts JP, et al. Effect of partial ileal bypass surgery on mortality and morbidity from coronary heart disease in patients with hypercholesterolemia. N Engl J Med 1990;323:946-55.
13. Schuler G, Hambrecht R, Schlierf G, et al. Regular physical exercise and low fat diet. Effects on progression of coronary artery disease. Circulation 1992;86:1-11.
14. Ornish D, Brown SE, Scherwitz LW, et al. Can lifestyle changes reverse coronary heart disease: The Lifestyle Heart Trial. Lancet 1990;336:129-33.
15. Blankenhorn DH, Azen SP, Kramsch DM, et al. Coronary angiographic changes with lovastatin therapy. Ann Intern Med 1993;119:969-76.
16. Waters D, Higginson L, Gladstone P, et al. Effects of monotherapy with an HMG-CoA reductase inhibitor on the progression of coronary atherosclerosis as assessed by serial quantitative arteriography. Circulation 1994;89:959-68.
17. MAAS Investigators. Effect of simvastatin on coronary atheroma: The Multicentre Anti-Atheroma Study (MAAS). Lancet 1994;344:633-38.
18. Jukema JW, Bruschke JVD, van Boven AJ, et al. Effects of lipid lowering by pravastatin on progression and regression of coronary artery disease in symptomatic men with normal to moderately elevated serum cholesterol levels. Regression Growth Evaluation Statin Study (REGRESS). Circulation 1995;91:2528-40.
19. Haskell WL, Alderman EL, Fair JM, et al. Effects of intensive multiple risk factor reduction on coronary atherosclerosis and clinical cardiac events in men and women with coronary artery disease. Circulation 1994;89:975-90.
20. Sacks FM, Pasternak RC, Gibson CM, et al. Effect on coronary atherosclerosis of decrease in plasma cholesterol concentrations in normocholesterolaemic patients. Lancet 1994;344:1182-86.
21. Nikkila EA, et al. Prevention of progression of coronary atherosclerosis by treatment of hyperlipidaemia. A seven year prospective angiographic study. Brit Med J 1984;289:220-23.
22. Hahmann HW, Bunte T, Hellwig L, et al. Progression and regression of minor coronary arterial narrowings by quantitative angiography after fenofibrate therapy. Am J Cardiol 1991;67:957-61.
23. Tatami R, Inoue N, Otih H, et al. Regression of coronary atherosclerosis by combined LDL apheresis and lipid-lowering drug therapy in familial hypercholesterolemia: A multicentre study. Atherosclerosis 1992;95:1-13.
24. Schuff-Werner P, Gohlke H, Bartmann U, et al. The HELP-LDL-apheresis multicentre study.

Europ J Clin Invest 1994;24:724-32.
25. Thompson GR, Maher VMG, Matthews S, et al. Familial Hypercholesterolaemia Regression Study: A randomized trial of LDL apheresis. Lancet 1995;345:811-16.
26. Olsson AG, Ruhn G, Erikson U. The effect of serum lipid regulation on the development of femoral atherosclerosis in hyperlipidaemia. A nonrandomized controlled study. J Intern Med 1990;227:381-90.
27. Blankenhorn DH, Azen SP, Crawford DW, et al. Effects of colestipol-niacin therapy on human femoral atherosclerosis. Circulation 1990;83:438-47.
28. Walldius G, Erikson U, Olsson AG, et al. The effect of probucol on femoral atherosclerosis: The Probucol Quantitative Regression Swedish Trial. Prev Cardiol 1994;74:875-83.
29. Salonen R, Nyyssonen K, Porkkala E, et al. Kuopio Atherosclerosis Prevention Study (KAPS): A population-based primary prevention trial of the effect of LDL lowering on atherosclerosis progression on carotid and femoral arteries. Circulation 1995; in press.
30. Blankenhorn DH, Selzer RH, Crawford DW, et al. Beneficial effects of colestipol-niacin therapy on the common carotid artery: Two- and four-year reduction of intima-media thickness measured by ultrasound. Circulation 1993;88:20-28.
31. Furberg CD, Adams HP, Applegate WB, et al. Effect of lovastatin on early carotid atherosclerosis and cardiovascular events. Circulation 1994;90:1679-87.
32. Crouse JR III, Byington RP, Bond MG, et al. Pravastatin, Lipids, and Atherosclerosis in the Carotid Arteries (PLAC II). Am J Cardiol 1995;75:455-59.
33. Cashin-Hemphill L, Mack W, LaBree L, et al. Coronary progression predicts future cardiac events. Circulation 1993;88(I):I-363.
34. Watts GF, Mandalia S, Brunt JNH, Slavin B, Coltart DJ, Lewis B. Independent associations between plasma lipoprotein subfraction levels and the course of coronary artery disease in the St. Thomas' Atherosclerosis Regression Study (STARS). Metabolism 1993;42:1461-67.
35. Arntzenius AC, Kromhout D, Bart JD, et al. Diet, lipoproteins, and the progression of coronary atherosclerosis. N Engl J Med 1985;312:805-11.
36. Blankenhorn DH, Johnson RL, Mack WJ, et al. The influence of diet on the appearance of new lesions in human coronary arteries. JAMA 1990;263:1646-52.
37. Watts GF, Jackson P, Mandalia S, et al. Nutrient intake and progression of coronary artery disease. Am J Cardiol 1994;73:328-32.
38. Watts GF, Lewis B, Jackson P, Lewis ES, Burke V. Nutritional determinants of atherosclerosis progression in man: the STARS trial. In: Woodford FP, Davignon J, Sniderman A, editors. Atherosclerosis X. Amsterdam: Elsevier Science, 1995:292-97.
39. Stewart BF, Brown BG, Zhao X-Q, et al. Benefits of lipid-lowering therapy in men with elevated apolipoprotein B are not confined to those with very high LDL cholesterol. JACC 1994;23:899-906.
40. Constantinides P. Plaque fissuring in human coronary thrombosis. J Atheroscler Res 1966;6:1-17.
41. Davies M, Thomas AC. Plaque fissuring - the cause of acute myocardial infarction, sudden death and crescendo angina. Br Heart J 1985;53:363-73.
42. Richardson PD, Davis MJ, Born GVR. Influence of plaque configuration and stress distribution on fissuring of atherosclerotic plaques. Lancet 1989;ii:941-44.
43. Davis MJ, Richardson PD, Woolf N, Katz DR, Mann J. Risk of thrombosis in human atherosclerotic plaques: Role of extracellular lipid, macrophage, and smooth muscle content. Br Heart J 1993;69:377-81.
44. Fuster V, Badimon JJ, Badimon L. Clinical-pathological correlations of coronary disease

progression and regression. Circulation 1992;86(III):III-1-III-2.
45. Loree HM, Kamm RD, Stringfellow RG, Lee RT. Effects of fibrous cap thickness on peak circumferential stress in atherosclerotic vessels. Circ Res 1992;71:850-58.
46. Ambrose JA, Tannenbaum MA, Alexopoulos D, et al. Angiographic progression of coronary artery disease and the development of myocardial infarction. JACC 1988;12:56-62.
47. Libby P. Molecular bases of the acute coronary syndromes. Circulation 1995;91:2844-50.
48. La Ville AE, Seddon AM, Shaikh M, Rowles PM, Woolf N, Lewis B. Primary prevention of atherosclerosis by lovastatin in a genetically hyperlipidaemic rabbit strain. Atherosclerosis 1989;78:205-10.
49. Brown BG, Zhao X-Q, Sacco DE, Albers JJ. Lipid lowering and plaque regression. Circulation 1993;87:1781-91.
50. Small DM, Bond MG, Waugh D, Prack M, Sawyer JK. Physicochemical and histological changes in the arterial wall of nonhuman primates during progression and regression of atherosclerosis. J Clin Invest 1984;73:1590-1605.
51. Nordestgaard BG, Tybjaerg-Hansen A, Lewis B. Influx in vivo of low density, intermediate density, and very low density lipoproteins into aortic intimas of genetically hyperlipidemic rabbits. Arteriosclr Thromb 1992;12:6-18.
52. Prevention of coronary heart disease - scientific background and new clinical guidelines. Nutr Metab Cardiovasc Dis 1992;2:113-56.
53. Salonen JT, Salonen R. Ultrasonographically assessed carotid morphology and the risk of coronary heart disease. Arterioscler Thromb 1991;11:1245-49.
54. Sacks FM, Gibson M, Rosner B, et al. The influence of pretreatment LDL cholesterol concentrations on the effect of hypocholesterolemic therapy on coronary atherosclerosis in angiographic trials. Am J Cardiol 1995;76:78c-85c.

CLINICAL CONSEQUENCES OF LOWERING CHOLESTEROL

M.R. Law
Department of Environmental and Preventive Medicine, Wolfson Institute of Preventive Medicine, The Medical College of St Bartholomew's Hospital, Charterhouse Square, London EC1M 6BQ, United Kingdom

Introduction

There is much published data on serum cholesterol and ischemic heart disease (IHD), and no doubt that a causal relationship exists between the two. The need has been to determine the size and speed of reversal of the relationship according to age. In doing so, both observational data (cohort studies) and intervention data (randomized controlled studies) are necessary [1,2]. The two are complementary, each has specific advantages that the other lacks. Table 1 summarizes these.

Table 1. Relative advantages of cohort studies and randomized trials in assessing the relation between serum cholesterol and ischemic heart disease (IHD).

Objective	Advantage	Reason/Comment
Statistical power	Cohort studies	18,000 IHD events (cohort studies) versus 4,000 (trials)
Dose-response effect of cholesterol on IHD	Cohort studies	3.0 mmol/l cholesterol difference (10th-90th centile in cohort studies) versus 0.6 mmol/l (average reduction in trials)
Wide age range	Cohort studies	IHD events at age 35-85 versus 55-65
Long-term effects of cholesterol differences	Cohort studies	Decades of "exposure" (cohort studies) versus 5 years (trials)
Short-term effects of cholesterol differences	Randomized trials	Only an intervention study can show this
Avoid bias	Randomized trials	Not a major advantage. Confounding by other IHD risk factors and underestimation biases in cohort studies can be allowed for

A. M. Gotto, Jr. et al. (eds.), Drugs Affecting Lipid Metabolism, 137–143.

The cohort studies recruited large cohorts (groups) of men, divided them into subgroups (usually quintile groups or fifths) according to ranked cholesterol measurements, and measured the dose-response relationship between cholesterol and subsequent IHD mortality rates across the subgroups. The cholesterol differences between individuals (predominantly genetically determined) will have been present for many years before the start of the study, so cohort studies estimate the long-term effect of a difference in serum cholesterol on risk of IHD. In the randomized trials the duration of the cholesterol reduction was short (five years on average, deaths occurring on average only two-to-three years from the start of treatment); the trials estimate the extent to which the maximum benefit, as estimated from the cohort studies, can be attained in the short term. The cohort studies have greater statistical power, since they recorded many more IHD events than the trials, and were able to examine larger differences in serum cholesterol between individuals. They were also able to estimate the association of cholesterol with IHD over a wide age range, whereas in the trials almost all the IHD events occurred in the ten-year age range, 55-64 years.

Cholesterol And IHD

Most of the studies of cholesterol and IHD recruited men, for reasons of economy as IHD is more common in men. These data are summarized below. The limited data for women indicate a similar effect as in men [2].

COHORT STUDIES

The nature of the association between cholesterol and IHD. The incidence of IHD, plotted on a logarithmic scale according to quintile groups (fifths) of the ranked serum cholesterol concentration in the ten largest cohort studies of serum cholesterol and IHD [2], shows a remarkable consistency in the pattern of results. There is no threshold below which a further decrease in serum cholesterol is not associated with a further decrease in risk of IHD. The two largest studies establish this beyond doubt in that the 95% confidence limits of the risk estimates in each quintile group do not overlap; the other studies are entirely consistent with this relationship. In the ten studies the relationship was described by a straight line linking the proportional change in ischemic heart disease with given absolute differences in serum cholesterol. In the largest study (MRFIT Screenees) the fit of this model was almost perfect ($r = 0.997$). Thus a constant absolute difference in serum cholesterol concentration of, say, 0.6 mmol/l, from any point on the cholesterol distribution is associated with a constant percentage difference in the incidence of IHD.

Underestimation of the size of the effect. Cohort studies underestimate the size of the dose-response relationship between serum cholesterol and IHD [1]. The major source of underestimation is regression dilution bias, which affects all observational studies in which the explanatory (horizontal axis) variable is, like serum cholesterol, subject to random fluctuation within an individual over time. Since the same cholesterol measurements were used to divide the cohort into subgroups and to calculate the mean cholesterol concentration of each subgroup, the subgroups with higher cholesterol concentrations will include a disproportionate number of men selected because the single measurement was, by chance, higher than their long-term average value. The long-term mean cholesterol concentration of these subgroups will therefore be overestimated. Similarly, the cholesterol concentration of the groups with lower cholesterol will be underestimated. This tends to link given differences in IHD mortality with a wider range of serum cholesterol levels than is in fact the case, thereby underestimating the "dose-response." A second source of underestimation arises because differences in total cholesterol between individuals in cohort studies include not only differences in low density lipoprotein (LDL) cholesterol but differences in other subfractions of total cholesterol. These observational differences, however, are to be linked to the effect of interventions which, though they were measured as a reduction in total cholesterol, in fact lowered LDL cholesterol almost exclusively. Correction for the two sources of underestimation makes the association in cohort studies about half as strong again [1].

The size of the effect. Table 2, using data from the ten cohort studies, shows the estimates of the percentage decrease in the risk of IHD according to the extent of the decrease in serum cholesterol concentration and age at death [2]. With a cholesterol reduction of 0.6 mmol/l (10%), which can realistically be attained by a moderate change in diet, the decrease in IHD is about 50% at age 40, 40% at 50, 30% at 60, and 20% at 70-80. While the proportional change in risk of IHD decreases with increasing age, the absolute change will increase because IHD becomes so much more common with age.

Table 2. Estimates (from ten cohort studies) of the percentage decrease in risk of IHD with serum cholesterol reduction, according to age.

Age (years)	Approximate Percentage Decrease in Risk for a Serum Cholesterol Reduction (mmol/l) of:			
	0.3	0.6	1.2	1.8
40	32%	54%	79%	90%
50	22%	39%	63%	77%
60	15%	27%	47%	61%
70	11%	20%	36%	49%
80	10%	19%	34%	47%

RANDOMIZED TRIALS

Data has been analyzed from 28 randomized controlled trials of serum cholesterol reduction and IHD [2]. Nearly all the IHD events in these trials occurred in the age range 55-64 (average 60) years, and the mean serum cholesterol reduction was about 0.6 mmol/l (10%). Figure 1 shows the overall reduction in incidence of IHD in all the trials combined for a 0.6 mmol/l reduction in serum cholesterol according to time since entry into the trial. In the first two years there was almost no effect of serum cholesterol reduction. From 2-to-5 years the average reduction in IHD was 22%, and after five years the reduction was 25%. This estimate of 25% is close to the estimate of 27% from the cohort studies (Table 2) for the long-term association at the same age (60) and same cholesterol difference (0.6 mmol/l). Figure 1 summarizes these results.

The HMG-CoA reductase inhibitor ("statin") class of drugs can lower total and LDL cholesterol by about 1.8 mmol/l. Table 2 shows that these drugs would be expected to lower IHD mortality in the long term by an estimated 61% at age 60 (given that a reduction of 0.6 mmol/l lowers risk by 27%, or to 73% (100% - 27% = 73%), a reduction three times as great will reduce risk to 0.73^3, or 39%, a reduction of 61%). In the recently published Scandinavian Simvastatin Survival Study (4S) trial the mean serum cholesterol reduction was 1.8 mmol/l [3]. The reduction in IHD mortality after two years was close to this estimate of 61% from the cohort studies (Table 2) for the long-term association at the same age (60) and same cholesterol difference (1.8 mmol/l).

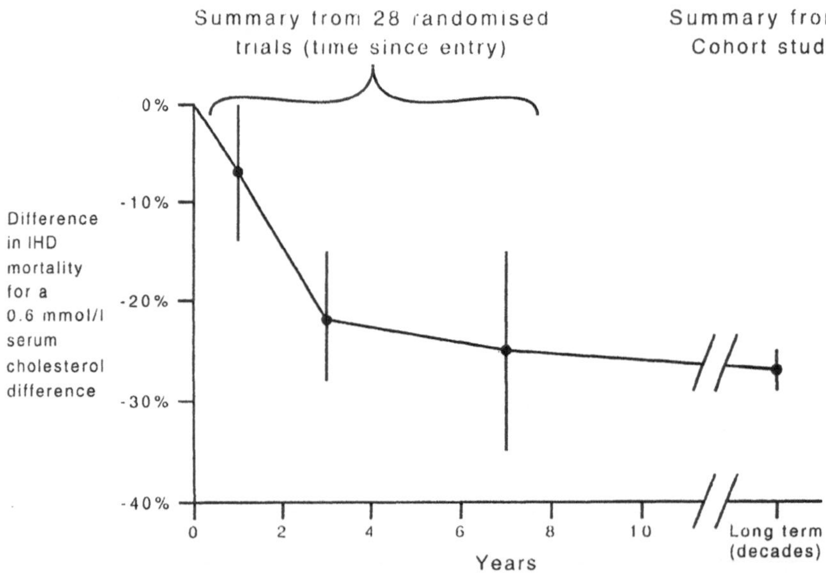

Figure 1. Decrease in the incidence of IHD per 0.6 mmol/l decrease in serum cholesterol in the randomized trials according to time since entry, and in the cohort studies (estimating the long-term difference). All data apply to the age group 55-64 years [2].

CONCLUSIONS ON IHD

The randomized trials show that the maximal reduction in IHD following a given cholesterol reduction is attained rapidly. The effect is virtually fully reversed after 5 years, and the greater part of the effect is reversed after 2 years. The effect of serum cholesterol reduction is large and important. While the change in serum cholesterol that can easily be attained by an individual trying to alter his or her diet apart from his family, friends, and workmates is relatively small (5%), a serum cholesterol reduction of 0.6 mmol/l (10%) by dietary change is realistic on a population basis. It has been attained for example over periods of ten years or so in communities in the United States and in Finland [4]. This cholesterol reduction would lower IHD mortality by about 30% at age 60. The evidence on the lack of a threshold is important in dispelling the notion that the major application of cholesterol lowering treatments is to reduce comparatively high cholesterol levels down to the average levels in the population. The average serum cholesterol levels in Western populations, about 6 mmol/l, are high compared to typical levels of about 3.5 mmol/l in hunter-gatherer societies (which represent the evolutionary norm). Everybody in a Western society would reduce their risk of IHD by reducing their existing serum cholesterol level. The "statin" group of cholesterol lowering drugs, in reducing total and LDL cholesterol by about 1.8 mmol/l, would reduce heart disease mortality by about half even in old age, and by well over half at ages of 60 and under, as shown in Table 2. These drugs are appropriate for all patients at high overall risk of myocardial infarction even if the serum cholesterol level is "average."

Possible Hazards Of Cholesterol Reduction

COHORT STUDIES

In cohort studies the cholesterol measurement on entry can be lowered by many diseases in their preclinical or early clinical stages, and by many causes of disease, such as alcoholism, smoking, and infection. A British survey showed that nonspecified intercurrent illness lowered serum cholesterol by 0.5 mmol/l (8%) on average. Associations of low cholesterol with early disease, or with causes of disease, at the outset of a cohort study will produce subsequent spurious associations between low cholesterol and mortality.

This effect can be minimized by dividing the cohort studies into two groups, one in which the men were recruited by virtue of their employment status, and the other based on recruitment from community sources (population registers, community groups, etc). The cohort studies of employed individuals, which will tend to include only individuals who are healthy on entry, show no relationship (relative risk 1.00) between low serum cholesterol and mortality from causes other than IHD [5]. Excess mortality was present only in the community cohorts, which necessarily included some individuals with disease on entry. Analysis of mortality data across communities with different cholesterol levels supported the data from the employed cohorts in showing no overall association with non-IHD mortality [5].

RANDOMIZED TRIALS

Analysis of cause-specific mortality data in all the randomized trials combined showed no statistically significant excess mortality from any specific cause except one, deaths due to gallstones in trials using the drug clofibrate (which is known to cause gallstones) [5].

There has been particular concern relating to excess mortality from accidents and suicide, because of a cross-sectional association in several studies with low serum cholesterol and depression. The evidence indicates that this association arises not because low serum cholesterol causes depression, but because depressed people eat less on average and so have lower serum cholesterol [5]. Effective treatment of depression leads to an increase in serum cholesterol concentration. Two large trials of "statin" drugs have shown that lowering cholesterol does not lead to depression or other disturbances of mood. Two of the older trials gave rise to concern despite the results not being statistically significant (11 versus 4 and 9 versus 5 deaths from accidents and suicide in the treated versus control groups), but the excess was concentrated in patients who did not take the cholesterol lowering drugs, so cholesterol reduction cannot have caused it. Some 34,000 patient years of observation has now accrued in trials of statin drugs, and the absence of any excess noncardiac mortality in treated patients is reassuring because of the large reduction in cholesterol that these drugs produce.

Conclusions

A reduction of 0.6 mmol/l (10%) in average serum LDL and total cholesterol levels is readily achievable by changes in dietary practice among communities, if groups act in concert to reduce their saturated fat intake, and substitute mono- and polyunsaturated fats and complex carbohydrates (cereals, fruit, and vegetables). Reductions of about 10% have been achieved in a number of communities [4]. The consequent reduction in IHD of 30% in middle-aged people and 20% in older people represents one of the largest and most readily achieved public health targets of the Western world. Larger reductions attainable by cholesterol lowering drugs would reduce IHD mortality rates by over half, and there is no evidence that such reduction will cause any material adverse effects. Use of cholesterol lowering drugs is of major importance in patients at high risk of IHD death.

References

1. Law MR, Wald NJ, Wu T, Hackshaw, Bailey A. Systematic underestimation of association between serum cholesterol concentration and ischemic heart disease in observational studies: Data from the BUPA study. BMJ 1994;308:363-66.
2. Law MR, Wald NJ, Thompson SG. Serum cholesterol reduction and health: By how much and how quickly is the risk of ischemic heart disease lowered? BMJ 1994;308:367-72.
3. Scandinavian Simvastatin Survival Study Group. Randomized trial of cholesterol lowering in 4444 patients with coronary heart disease: The Scandinavian Simvastatin Survival Study (4S). Lancet 1994; 344:1383-89.

4. Law MR, Wald NJ. An ecological study of serum cholesterol and ischemic heart disease between 1950 and 1990. Eur J Clin Nutrition 1994; 48:305-25.
5. Law MR, Thompson SG, Wald NJ. Serum cholesterol reduction and health: assessing possible hazards. BMJ 1994;308:373-79.

DEFINING THE CLINICAL BENEFIT OF CHOLESTEROL LOWERING

Antonio M. Gotto, Jr.
Department of Medicine, Baylor College of Medicine, and Internal Medicine Service, The Methodist Hospital, 6550 Fannin, Houston, Texas 77030, USA

The evidence supporting the clinical benefit of cholesterol lowering has grown extensively within the last few years. Primary- and secondary-prevention clinical trials have demonstrated that reducing plasma cholesterol can lead to significant decreases not only in atherosclerotic coronary heart disease (CHD) morbidity and mortality rates, but also in all-cause mortality rate [1-5]. A meta-analysis by Law et al. [6] of 28 randomized, controlled lipid-lowering trials using a variety of interventions showed that, in men aged 55 to 64, a 23 mg/dL (about 10%) reduction in total cholesterol was associated with a 22% reduction in ischemic heart disease events within 2 to 5 years after initiating therapy, and a 25% reduction thereafter. Data from 10 prospective cohort studies showed a 23 mg/dL reduction in total cholesterol in men to reduce ischemic heart disease events by about 50% at age 40, 40% at age 50, 30% at age 60, and 20% at age 70. Data for women were limited but indicated a similar effect [6].

In another analysis of data from the observational and interventional studies [7], Law et al. found no evidence that low or reduced plasma cholesterol increases the mortality rate from any cause other than hemorrhagic stroke, a risk affecting only people with very low cholesterol concentrations (about 6% of people in Western populations). Yet even in this subgroup, the heart disease benefits of cholesterol lowering outweighed any increased risk.

The Scandinavian Simvastatin Survival Study (4S), a randomized trial in which the only primary endpoint was total mortality rate, showed that lipid lowering was associated with a significant reduction in this endpoint [2]. Over a median 5.4-year follow-up, 4,444 men and women with a history of myocardial infarction or angina pectoris and total cholesterol of 212 to 310 mg/dL were treated with either 20 mg/d of the 3-hydroxy-3-methylglutaryl coenzyme A (HMG-CoA) reductase inhibitor simvastatin or placebo. Simvastatin dosage was titrated over the course of the study to reduce total cholesterol to between 116 and 201 mg/dL; thus, 37% of patients in the simvastatin group received 40 mg/d and 2 patients received only 10 mg/d. A 25% reduction in total cholesterol and a 35% reduction in low-density lipoprotein (LDL) cholesterol in the simvastatin group coincided with a 30% reduction in risk for dying from any cause ($p = 0.0003$). Subanalysis of the causes of death showed that simvastatin treatment was not associated with increased deaths from non-CHD causes (67 in the placebo versus 71 in the simvastatin group), thus

A. M. Gotto, Jr. et al. (eds.), Drugs Affecting Lipid Metabolism, 145–149.

establishing that the primary effect of simvastatin therapy on mortality was in reducing CHD deaths (189 coronary deaths in the placebo versus 111 in the simvastatin group, a 42% risk reduction). Simvastatin therapy was also associated with a 34% reduction in the risk for having one or more major coronary events ($p < 0.00001$) and a 37% reduction in the risk for undergoing revascularization procedures [2]. CHD benefit was found across all quartiles of baseline total, LDL, and high-density lipoprotein (HDL) cholesterol, with similar benefit in each quartile [3].

A prospectively planned pooled analysis of four regression trials using the HMG-CoA reductase inhibitor pravastatin further illustrates the benefit of lowering cholesterol [4]. Data from the Pravastatin Limitation of Atherosclerosis in the Coronary Arteries (PLAC I) trial, the Pravastatin, Lipid, and Atherosclerosis in the Carotid Arteries (PLAC II) trial, the Kuopio Atherosclerosis Prevention Study (KAPS), and the Regression Growth Evaluation Statin Study (REGRESS) were combined. All were randomized, placebo-controlled trials. In PLAC I, REGRESS, and KAPS, drug recipients were administered 40 mg pravastatin once daily for 2 to 3 years. In PLAC II, the pravastatin dosage was titrated between 20 and 40 mg/d in order to achieve an LDL cholesterol level of at least 110 mg/dL. Change in vessel stenosis was monitored by angiography of the coronary arteries in PLAC I and REGRESS and by ultrasonography of the carotid arteries in PLAC II and KAPS. Subjects in PLAC I, PLAC II, and REGRESS had a history of CHD, whereas the subjects in KAPS were drawn from the general population without regard to their disease status. In total, data from 1,891 men and women were analyzed. The results of this meta-analysis showed a 62% decrease in risk for a coronary event with cholesterol lowering ($p = 0.001$). The same analysis reported a 53% reduction in the combined endpoint of nonfatal myocardial infarction or all-cause mortality rate ($p = 0.003$) and a 51% reduction in the combined endpoint of nonfatal myocardial infarction or CHD death ($p = 0.006$).

The biophysical antecedent to most coronary events is believed to be the rupture of the atherosclerotic plaque, which initiates a thrombogenic chain of events that leads to arterial occlusion. Lipid-lowering therapy is thought to mediate benefit by stabilizing those atherosclerotic lesions at high risk for rupture. Such plaques are called culprit lesions. The characteristics of the culprit lesion include a soft, lipid-rich core and a weak fibrous cap with a high macrophage content and few smooth muscle cells. The precursor of the atherosclerotic plaque is the fatty streak, which arises from the subintimal aggregation of foam cells, which are macrophages that are rich in lipid content. The cytotoxic products of lipoprotein oxidation, especially oxidized LDL, may aggravate injury to the vascular endothelium and are particularly susceptible to macrophage uptake. Ideally, fibrous tissue and smooth muscle cells develop over the lesion to separate its thrombogenic contents from the plasma compartment of the vessel. However, the high degree of macrophage activity facilitates an inflammatory response that reduces the mechanical strength of the fibrous cap by both inhibiting smooth muscle cell proliferation and degrading existing connective tissues [8]. Intimal rupture that extends from the lumen into the lipid-rich core of the vulnerable lesion is found in 80% to 90% of cases of infarction [9].

High-risk lesions also tend to be only mildly to moderately stenotic (less than 70% blockage). Lesions that contribute greater than 70% stenosis are less common than the moderately stenotic class, and it has been suggested that vessels affected by severe stenosis are more likely to have developed collateral systems that circumvent the blockage. These vessels are more likely to occlude silently than to initiate an ischemic event [10].

Lipid-lowering therapy may stabilize lesions by normalizing endothelial function. Atherosclerotic disease has been implicated in dysfunctional endothelial response to, and release of, the powerful vasodilator endothelium-derived relaxing factor (EDRF), which is nitric oxide or one of its analogues [9]. Interference with the action of EDRF would account for the paradoxical vasoconstriction seen in patients with CHD upon exercise; vasoconstriction reduces the vessel's ability to respond to stress and increases the risk for plaque rupture. A study by Egashira et al. [11] showed that lipid regulation improved blood flow and vasodilatory response to acetylcholine in hypercholesterolemic patients. Nine patients with hypercholesterolemia and a history of angina pectoris, but not of myocardial infarction, were initially given 10 mg/d of pravastatin, which was titrated to 20 mg/d after 2 weeks if total cholesterol did not fall below 200 mg/dL. After 6 to 9 months of pravastatin treatment, total cholesterol fell by 31%, acetylcholine-induced vasoconstriction was reduced ($p < 0.05$), and acetylcholine-induced perfusion was increased ($p < 0.001$). This evidence supports the hypothesis that cholesterol-lowering therapy helps restore endothelium-dependent vasomotor function. Other mechanisms that have been postulated to underlie the beneficial effects of lipid regulation on lesion susceptibility are improvement in vascular reactivity, depletion of the lesion's lipid core by reverse cholesterol transport, alleviation of the inflammatory response described above, and reduction of thrombogenicity.

Kobashigawa et al. [12] found that pravastatin treatment in heart transplant recipients improved not only cholesterol levels, but also the overall survival rate 1 year after the transplantation. Ninety-seven hypercholesterolemic male and female transplant patients were given either 40 mg pravastatin or placebo per day, in addition to their immunosuppressive therapy. After 1 year of therapy, the patients receiving pravastatin had a lower mean total cholesterol concentration (193 mg/dL versus 248 mg/dL), fewer cases of cardiac rejection accompanied by hemodynamic compromise (3 versus 14, $p = 0.005$), better survival (94% versus 78%, $p = 0.025$), and a lower incidence of coronary vasculopathy as determined by angiography or autopsy (3 versus 10 patients, $p = 0.049$). Heart transplantation is usually accompanied by hypercholesterolemia and accelerated development of atherosclerosis, placing graft recipients at particularly high risk for CHD events. Although the risk for myopathy sometimes seen with statin therapy increases with the concomitant use of cyclosporine, this study reported no incidence of such side effects.

Since the time of the twelfth Drugs Affecting Lipid Metabolism conference, the results of the West of Scotland Coronary Prevention Study (WOSCOPS) have become available [5], adding to the body of knowledge of the benefit of aggressive lipid regulation. In this trial, 6,595 men, 45 to 64 years old, with no history of myocardial infarction were randomized to receive 40 mg/d of pravastatin or placebo. Pravastatin therapy led to a 20% reduction in total plasma cholesterol and a 26% reduction in LDL cholesterol. This study also reported significant reductions in clinical events. There was a 31% reduction in the risk for nonfatal myocardial infarction or CHD death ($p < 0.001$) and a 33% reduction in definite plus suspected deaths from myocardial infarction ($p = 0.033$). The all-cause mortality rate was reduced by 22% ($p = 0.051$). Taken in conjunction with the results of 4S, this finding should assuage doubts about the safety of lipid lowering as an appropriate strategy for managing CHD risk whether in primary or secondary prevention.

Approximately 95% of the WOSCOPS population was ostensibly free of CHD (5% had evidence of angina pectoris). The guidelines of the Second Adult Treatment Panel (ATP II) of the U.S. National Cholesterol Education Program recommend that drug therapy be considered in patients free of CHD when LDL cholesterol is 190 mg/dL or higher and fewer than two other risk factors are present, or 160 mg/dL or higher and two or more other risk factors are present [13]. In many of the earlier clinical trials, the mean baseline LDL cholesterol level tended to be 200 mg/dL or higher. The mean baseline LDL cholesterol in the WOSCOPS population was 192 mg/dL. The clinical benefits seen in WOSCOPS suggest that the ATP II intervention levels for primary prevention may be too conservative and that drug therapy may be beneficial at lower baseline levels of LDL cholesterol. For example, it may be effective to consider drug therapy in asymptomatic patients with fewer than two other risk factors when dietary and other lifestyle interventions fail to lower LDL cholesterol below 160 mg/dL. In patients with two or more other risk factors, drug therapy could possibly be considered at 130 mg/dL.

Refining the existing treatment guidelines for dyslipidemia represents a future direction of atherosclerosis research, as does deciphering the complex mechanisms underlying both atherogenesis and the benefit of lipid lowering. The preponderance of clinical evidence supports the current strategy of managing CHD risk by managing dyslipidemia; significant clinical benefit can be achieved with aggressive lowering of cholesterol.

References

1. Levine GN, Keaney JF Jr, Vita JA. Cholesterol reduction in cardiovascular disease: Clinical benefits and possible mechanisms. N Engl J Med 1995;332(8):512-21.
2. The Scandinavian Simvastatin Survival Study Group. Randomised trial of cholesterol lowering in 4444 patients with coronary heart disease: The Scandinavian Simvastatin Survival Study (4S). Lancet 1994;344:1383-89.
3. Scandinavian Simvastatin Survival Study Group. Baseline serum cholesterol and treatment effect in the Scandinavian Simvastatin Survival Study (4S). Lancet 1995;345:1274-75.
4. Byington RP, Jukema JW, Salonen JT, et al. Reduction in cardiovascular events during pravastatin therapy. Pooled analysis of clinical events of the Pravastatin Atherosclerosis Intervention Program. Circulation 1995;92:2419-25.
5. Shepherd J, Cobbe SM, Ford I, et al., for the West of Scotland Coronary Prevention Study Group. Prevention of coronary heart disease with pravastatin in men with hypercholesterolemia. N Engl J Med 1995;333(20):1301-307.
6. Law MR, Wald NJ, Thompson SG. By how much and how quickly does reduction in serum cholesterol concentration lower risk of ischaemic heart disease? BMJ 1994;308:367-72.
7. Law MR, Thompson SG, Wald NJ. Assessing possible hazards of reducing serum cholesterol. BMJ 1994;308:373-79.
8. Libby P. Molecular bases of the acute coronary syndromes. Circulation 1995;91(11):2844-50.

9. Brown BG. Lipid-lowering therapy for the stabilization of the vulnerable atherosclerotic plaque. Current Opinion in Lipidology 1993;4:305-309.
10. Falk E. Why do plaques rupture? Circulation 1992;86(III):III-30-III-42.
11. Egashira K, Hirooka Y, Kai H, et al. Reduction in serum cholesterol with pravastatin improves endothelium-dependent coronary vasomotion in patients with hypercholesterolemia. Circulation 1994;89(6):2519-24.
12. Kobashigawa JA, Katznelson S, Laks H, et al. Effect of pravastatin on outcomes after cardiac transplantation. N Engl J Med 1995;333:621-27.
13. Expert Panel on Detection, Evaluation, and Treatment of High Blood Cholesterol in Adults. Summary of the second report of the National Cholesterol Education Program (NCEP) Expert Panel on Detection, Evaluation, and Treatment of High Blood Cholesterol in Adults (Adult Treatment Panel II). JAMA 1993;269:3015-23.

EXTENDING THE BENEFIT OF LIPID LOWERING: A LOOK AHEAD

James Shepherd
Institute of Biochemistry, Royal Infirmary, Glasgow G4 0SF, United Kingdom for the West of Scotland Coronary Prevention Study Group

The statins, following their introduction into clinical practice almost a decade ago, have captured and expanded the cholesterol lowering drug market. They act primarily by inhibiting hepatic 3-hydroxy-3-methylglutaryl coenzyme A reductase (HMG-CoA reductase), the rate limiting enzyme in the important metabolic cascade leading to cholesterol biosynthesis [1]. In consequence, the availability of cholesterol within hepatocytes is limited and low density lipoprotein (LDL) receptors on their membranes upregulated. This leads to accelerated plasma clearance not only of LDL but also of its precursors, very low density and intermediate density lipoproteins (VLDL and IDL). Circulating LDL levels therefore fall, partly because of an increase in catabolism and also because LDL precursor availability is curtailed. Since HMG-CoA reductase is responsible for the production of mevalonate, and therefore operates at an early stage in the cholesterol synthetic pathway, there is no build up of later intermediary metabolites en route to cholesterol which led to the disastrous failure of triparanol [2].

The runaway clinical success of the statins springs from their apparently exemplary hypolipidemic actions. Total plasma cholesterol falls by 15-30% and LDL cholesterol by 20-40%, while high density lipoprotein (HDL) cholesterol rises by 5-10% in response to regular treatment [3]. As a bonus, there is a welcome though less spectacular reduction of 10-20% in plasma triglyceride. Considerable aggregate clinical benefits accrue from these changes. The best examples to date come from a series of projects designed to examine the value of statin mediated lipid reduction in individuals with pre-existent vascular disease. The Scandinavian Simvastatin Survival Study (4S) followed the impact of therapy in 4,444 individuals with previous myocardial infarction or stable angina pectoris and showed that simvastatin treatment reduced overall deaths by 30% by targeting coronary morbidity and mortality. Nonfatal and fatal myocardial infarctions were reduced by 37% and 42% respectively [4].

Other studies, though smaller, also showed impressive reductions in cardiovascular events in response to statin therapy. One of the earliest of these, PLAC-II [5] used monotherapy with pravastatin, again in patients with coronary artery disease, adopting ultrasound assessment of progression of early carotid atherosclerosis as the primary outcome variable. Despite its small size and relatively short followup, the study recorded

A. M. Gotto, Jr. et al. (eds.), Drugs Affecting Lipid Metabolism, 151–155.

a significant reduction in vascular event rates and a slowing in the progression of early carotid atherosclerosis in the group of individuals prescribed active lipid lowering therapy [6]. A similarly designed project using another statin, lovastatin, produced equally gratifying results [7]; and when these and other statin-related trials of secondary coronary prevention are viewed in aggregate, there can no longer be any doubt about the benefit and safety of treating hypercholesterolemia in patients who have had a myocardial infarction [8,9].

But what is the role of cholesterol reduction in the primary prevention of coronary disease? Three major trials have already reported on this question, prior to the statin era. The first, the World Health Organization (WHO) clofibrate trial, [10,11] demonstrated a reduction in the rate of nonfatal myocardial infarction in the drug-treated group but also indicated that clofibrate therapy was associated with a rise in total mortality. This finding raised doubts over the benefits of widespread use of lipid lowering agents. The publication of the Lipid Research Clinics Coronary Primary Prevention Trial (LRC-CPPT) in 1984 [12-14] and the Helsinki Heart Study (HHS) in 1987 [15,16] reversed this attitude to some extent, but many still remain skeptical because of the inability of these later trials to show a significant effect on coronary or total mortality. In the LRC-CPPT, an 11% decrease in levels of LDL cholesterol was associated with a significant decrease (of 19%) in cardiac events (fatal plus nonfatal myocardial infarction). The performance of this study was less than predicted due to compliance problems. In HHS, the drug used (gemfibrozil) was less potent but was palatable and compliance among subjects at trial visits was high. The drug reduced LDL cholesterol and triglyceride levels by 8% and 35%, respectively, and increased levels of HDL cholesterol by about 10%. These lipid changes were associated with a significant reduction (34%) in the incidence of CHD as measured by the combined fatal plus nonfatal myocardial infarction endpoint.

Neither the LRC-CPPT nor HHS had the statistical power to address the question of the benefits of lipid lowering agents in preventing coronary death. To do this, it is necessary (a) to study a population with a higher event rate; (b) to increase the sample size; and/or (c) to use a more effective lipid lowering agent. The West of Scotland Coronary Prevention Study (WOSCOPS), using pravastatin, attempts to address each of these issues [17]. The trial compares the effects of pravastatin (40 mg taken at night) versus placebo in men aged 45-64 years. The 6,595 recruits for this study were identified by population screening. The men who met the inclusion criteria were screened for CHD risk factors and were invited for a second visit if their total cholesterol levels were ≥ 251 mg/dL (6.5 mmol/L) as measured by a Reflotron® bench-top analyzer (Boehringer Mannheim, Lewes, Kent). Subjects fasted during the second visit, which took place after a minimum of 4 weeks on a standard cholesterol lowering diet. A full lipoprotein profile was obtained on this visit (plasma, LDL, HDL, VLDL, cholesterol, and plasma triglyceride). Progress to the third visit, on which a fasting lipoprotein profile was also obtained after a further 4 weeks of diet, required a fasting LDL cholesterol level ≥ 155 mg/dL (4.0 mmol/L) at visit 2. Invitation to the randomization visit (visit 4) required fasting LDL cholesterol to be ≥ 155 mg/dL (4.0 mmol/L) at visits 2 and 3, at least one of them to be ≥ 174 mg/dL (4.5 mmol/l), and at least one of them to be ≤ 232 mg/dL (6.0 mmol/L). Subjects were required to be free of significant evidence of CHD, although subjects with angina, identified as those with a positive Rose questionnaire at baseline, who had not been hospitalized in the previous 12 months, were eligible for entry. Further details of inclusion and exclusion criteria are given in the study design paper [17].

The study is designed to have adequate power to address the endpoint of CHD death plus nonfatal myocardial infarction. In addition, the incidence of important events (CHD death only [whether preceded by a nonfatal myocardial infarction or not] and nonfatal myocardial infarction only) will be reported as indicated in the study design paper. In addition, a report on all-cause mortality will be provided. Although not originally specified, results for all cardiovascular deaths will be published to permit comparison with other studies.

Based on the log rank test with a two-sided significance level of 0.05, a comparison between pravastatin and placebo groups has 99% power for attaining the combined endpoint (fatal coronary events plus nonfatal myocardial infarction) and 66% power for attaining the single endpoint of fatal coronary events. If the reduction in events due to treatment is 35%, then the power for fatal coronary events is 80%. This study does not have adequate power to address the endpoint of total mortality.

The WOSCOPS trial has achieved its basic aim to recruit a cohort of more than 6,000 men aged 45-64 years with elevated levels of LDL cholesterol (mean level of approximately 193 mg/dL [5 mmol/L]). The randomized participants possess other risk factors for CHD (44% are current smokers, 15.8% are hypertensive, 5.2% have positive Rose questionnaires for angina, 1.2% are diabetic). More than 30,000 patient years of followup had accrued by the final followup examination, which occurred in May 1995.

At this evaluation, subjects had a final study ECG recorded in addition to the completion of routine case report forms. The actual date of attendance was taken as the censoring date for each individual's followup evaluation. Subjects not attending the final visit within the visit window were allocated the final day of their visit window as their followup censoring date and their status at that time were obtained by personal contact, contact with general practitioners, and by reference to national registries of deaths and hospitalizations. The results of the study will be reported in November 1995 at the American Heart Association meeting in Anaheim and published in tandem in the medical literature. At the same time, each subject and his general practitioner will be unblinded to the subject's trial medication and will receive a summary of the lipid results before and during the trial so that appropriate ongoing treatment can be assessed.

The characteristics summarized in this paper indicate that WOSCOPS, both individually and in combination with other ongoing trails involving statins, will make a significant contribution to the debate on the appropriate policy for the use of cholesterol lowering agents in the prevention of CHD.

References

1. Grundy SM. HMGCoA reductase inhibitors for treatment of hypercholesterolemia. New Engl J Med 1988;319:23-33.
2. Avigan J, Steinberg D, Vroman HE, et al. Studies of cholesterol biosynthesis I. The

identification of desmosterol in serum and tissues of animals and man treated with MEK-29. J Biol Chem 1960;253:3123-26.
3. Feussner G. HMGCoA reductase inhibitors. Current Opinion in Lipidology 1994;5: 59-68.
4. Scandinavian Simvastatin Survival Study Group. Randomised trial of cholesterol lowering in 4444 patients with coronary heart disease: The Scandinavian Simvastatin Survival Study (4S). Lancet 1994;344:1383-89.
5. Crouse JR, Byington RP, Bond MG, et al. Pravastatin, Lipids and Atherosclerosis in the Carotid Arteries: Design features of a clinical trial with carotid atherosclerosis outcome. Controlled Clinical Trials 1992;13:495-506.
6. Crouse JR, Byington RP, Bond MG, et al. Pravastatin, Lipids and Atherosclerosis in the Carotid Arteries (PLAC-II). Am J Cardiol 1995;75:455-59.
7. Furberg CD, Adams HP, Applegate WB, et al. Effect of lovastatin on early carotid atherosclerosis and cardiovascular events. Circulation 1994;90:1679-87.
8. Furberg CD, Byington RP, Crouse JR, Espeland MA. Pravastatin, lipids and major coronary events. Am J Cardiol 1994;73:1133-34.
9. Rossouw JE, Lewis B, Rifkind BM. The value of lowering cholesterol after myocardial infarction. New Engl J Med 1990;323:1112-19.
10. Committee of Principal Investigators. WHO Clofibrate Trial. A cooperative trial on the primary prevention of ischaemic heart disease using clofibrate, report. Br Heart J 1978;40:1069-1118.
11. Committee of Principal Investigators. WHO Clofibrate Trial. Cooperative trial on primary prevention of ischaemic heart disease using clofibrate to lower serum cholesterol: Mortality followup report. Lancet 1980;2:379-85.
12. The Lipid Research Clinics Program. The Coronary Primary Prevention Trial: Design and implementation. J Chron Dis 1979;32:609-31.
13. The Lipid Research Clinics Program. The Lipid Research Clinics Coronary Primary Prevention Trial results, I. Reduction in incidence of coronary heart disease. JAMA 1984;251-364.
14. Lipid Research Clinics Program. The Lipid Research Clinics Coronary Primary Prevention Trial results, II. The relationship of reduction in incidence of coronary heart disease to cholesterol lowering. JAMA 1984;251:365-374.
15. Mäntärri O, Elo O, Frick MH, et al. The Helsinki Heart Study: Basic design and randomisation procedure. Eur Heart J 1987;8:(I):1-29.
16. Frick MH, Elo O, Haapa K, et al. The Helsinki Heart Study: Primary prevention trial with gemfibrozil in middle-aged men with dyslipidemia: Safety of treatment, changes in risk factors, and incidence of coronary heart disease. New Engl J Med 1987;317:1237-45.
17. The West of Scotland Coronary Prevention Study Group. A coronary primary prevention study of Scottish men aged 45-64 years. Trial design. J Clin Epidemiol 1992;45:849-60.

Appendix

THE WEST OF SCOTLAND CORONARY PREVENTION STUDY GROUP

Prof. James Shepherd (Chairman, Co-Principal Investigator)
University of Glasgow, Institute of Biochemistry
Glasgow Royal Infirmary

Prof. Stuart M Cobbe	(Chairman Cardiovascular Endpoints Committee, Co-Principal Investigator), University of Glasgow Department of Medical Cardiology, Glasgow Royal Infirmary
Prof. A Ross Lorimer	(Chairman, Adverse Events Committee) Department of Medical Cardiology, Glasgow Royal Infirmary
Prof. James McKillop	(General Medicine and Cardiology Liaison) University of Glasgow, Department of Medicine Glasgow Royal Infirmary
Prof. Ian Ford	(Trial Statistician, Director of Data Centre) Department of Statistics, University of Glasgow
Prof. Chris Packard	(Study Director, Laboratory Coordinator) Institute of Biochemistry, Glasgow Royal Infirmary
Prof. Peter Macfarlane	(ECG Laboratory Coordinator) University of Glasgow, Department of Medical Cardiology Glasgow Royal Infirmary
Dr. Chris Isles	(Dumfries and Galloway Coordinator) Department of Medicine Dumfries & Galloway District General Hospital

HIGH RISK STRATEGIES FOR HEART DISEASE PREVENTION

James Shepherd
Institute of Biochemistry, Royal Infirmary, Glasgow G4 0SF, United Kingdom

Coronary heart disease (CHD) is so prevalent in industrialized countries that the interventive cardiologist cannot be expected to do more than blunt the impact of its worst excesses. The underlying problem, atherosclerosis, is advanced by the time symptoms have occurred and we are therefore inevitably faced with palliation rather than cure. For one quarter of myocardial infarct sufferers the best technology in the world cannot even offer a glimmer of hope. They die outside of hospital before therapy can be given. And, according to the British Regional Heart Study, for every 40-59-year-old male who dies, there are approximately 50 others with detectable underlying disease who are at risk of being the next victim. No health care facilities, however elaborate or extensive, could possibly hope to make a significant impact on a problem of this size. It is therefore not surprising that implementation of appropriate preventive programs [1-4] is recognized by clinician and politician alike as the only practicable means of reducing the medical and economic burden that CHD places on society. Opinion has been moving in this direction for some time but implementation of such a program is still a controversial issue. That said, national experience in the USA, Australia, and Israel suggests that worthwhile and significant reductions in coronary heart mortality are to be expected as population awareness of the risks of smoking and the benefits of a healthier lifestyle increases. The revelations from the North Karelia district of Finland are particularly enlightening [5]. There, a ten-year community-based program achieved significant reductions in cigarette smoking (25%), serum cholesterol (3%), and blood pressure (systolic reduction, 3%; diastolic, 1%) in men and was associated with a 24% decline in male ischemic heart disease mortality at a time when the fall in those parts of the country which had not been subjected to intervention was only 12%. It seems then that activities of this kind offer substantial benefit to the population in terms of reduced cardiovascular morbidity and mortality but their implementation raises the question of the merit of offering blanket advice to the population at large (the population approach) or focusing selectively on individuals at particular risk (the high risk approach). Most doctors would agree that these two strategies are complementary and work well when applied together. The prevalence of life threatening coronary risk factors in the US population is high. About 10% of apparently healthy middle-aged individuals are hypertensive, 25-45% smoke (depending on state and social class), and up to 50% have higher than desirable blood cholesterol levels (> 5.2 mmol/l). The only way to address successfully a problem of this

A. M. Gotto, Jr. et al. (eds.), Drugs Affecting Lipid Metabolism, 157–159.

magnitude is through the family practitioner. Primary health care services are uniquely placed to implement preventive medicine for both individuals and populations.

That being so, why have we been so unsuccessful in integrating CHD prevention programs into clinical practice? Lack of availability of advice in the form of recommendations or guidelines is certainly not to blame. Coronary heart disease prevention has been the subject of intense scrutiny for the last three decades and a wide variety of pronouncements have emerged at national and international level aimed at helping medical practitioners to apply appropriate preventive measures. Despite the remarkable coherence of these recommendations, extremist views for and against taking action have sparked the greatest amount of media publicity and have led many practitioners to the belief that while such bickering continues, inaction is the most appropriate policy. In an attempt to dispel this inertia, at least in Europe, a Task Force representing the European Society of Cardiology, the European Atherosclerosis Society, and the European Society of Hypertension has reviewed the available evidence and drawn the key elements from the recommendations of each Society in order to produce a common, agreed-upon policy on CHD prevention. This policy is intended to complement guidelines published earlier by the Societies [6-8] and the interested physician is referred to the latter for more detailed management information.

The central tenet of the joint guidelines is based on the concept of the total burden of risk exposure faced by the individual. This approach, in line with other guidelines, acknowledges first that CHD is multifactorial and secondly that we as physicians need to deal with patients rather than isolated risk factors.

In a world of dwindling resources, there is a clear appreciation that we need to set priorities for prevention. Highest among these are patients with established CHD. They constitute a discrete and readily identifiable population who are at very high risk for major CHD events and who therefore account for a disproportionately large amount of coronary disease. Focusing treatment on these patients is therefore relatively easy, highly beneficial to these individuals, and provides a good outcome dividend in proportion to the resources invested.

It is important to note that although intensive treatment of patients with dramatically elevated levels of one risk factor is beneficial to individuals, these patients represent only a small fraction of the total population. Contrary to popular belief, the majority of those who develop CHD have cholesterol levels close to the mean value for the population. Consequently, in order to make an impact on the burden of CHD, we must combine identification and treatment of high risk individuals with mass strategies aimed at the much larger number of people whose aggregate risk is high despite the lack of prominence of any one risk factor. The perception of a mass strategy to lower cholesterol as costly and of limited effectiveness is inaccurate. The benefits of such a strategy compare favorably with other well-established public health measures.

References

1. Shaper AG, Pocock SJ, Walker M, Cohen NM, Wale CJ, Thomson AG. British Regional Heart Study: Cardiovascular risk factors in middle-aged men in 24 towns. Brit Med J

1982;283:179-186.

2. The Expert Panel: Report of the National Cholesterol Education Program expert panel on detection, evaluation and treatment of high blood cholesterol in adults. Arch Intern Med 1988;148:36-69.
3. Smith SC, Blair SN, Criqui MH, et al. Preventing heart attack and death in patients with coronary disease. Circulation 1995;92:2-4.
4. Pyorala K, de Backer G, Poole-Wilson P, Wood D. Prevention of coronary heart disease in clinical practice. Recommendations of the task force of the European Society of Cardiology, European Atherosclerosis Society and European Society of Hypertension. Eur Heart J 1994;15:1300-31 and Atherosclerosis 1994;110:121-61.
5. Salonen JT, Puska P, Mustaniemi H. Changes in morbidity and mortality during comprehensive community program to control cardiovascular disease during 1972-7 in North Karelia. Brit Med J 19"9;2:1178-83.
6. Prevention of coronary heart disease: Scientific background and new clinical guidelines. Recommendation of the European Atherosclerosis Society. Nutr Metab Cardiovasc Dis 1992,2:113-56.
7. Study Group of the European Atherosclerosis Society. Strategies for the prevention of coronary heart disease. Eur Heart J 1987;8:77-88.
8. Guidelines Subcommittee. 1993 guidelines for the management of mild hypertension. J Hypertens 1993;11:905-18.

THE ROLE OF RISK FACTORS IN THE RAPID DEVELOPMENT OF SEVERE CORONARY ARTERY ATHEROSCLEROSIS IN YOUNG PEOPLE

Robert W. Wissler, Laura Hiltscher, Matthew Wahden, and the PDAY Group
Department of Pathology and the PDAY Administration, University of Chicago Medical Center, 5841 South Maryland Avenue, Chicago, Illinois 60637, USA

Introduction

This report is concerned with the unexpected results of a study of the coronary arteries and the aortas from approximately 1,000 cases of sudden death victims between the ages of 15 and 35. These cases are a part of the research program entitled the Pathobiological Determinants of Atherosclerosis in Youth (PDAY) which now includes more than 3,000 cases. This selected group of 1,000 cases consists of the only PDAY autopsies which have available gross close-up photographs of the aortic standard sampling areas (#'s 01, 16, and 18) in which the unstained lesions in each of these areas had been classified by color-coded strips grossly and depicted in a close-up macrolens photograph. Sections prepared through the center of these samples and stained with Oil Red O (ORO) and counterstained with hematoxylin make it possible to obtain valid gross/microscopic comparisons.

We have discovered that there are many more advanced, so called "fibrous," plaques with microscopic necrotic lipid-filled centers and fibrous caps in the proximal left anterior descending (LAD, #45) artery samples than in the standardized lower abdominal aorta samples (#16) from these same cases. Our study reveals that the advanced fibrous plaques in the coronary arteries and aorta can rather easily be divided between plaques with a relatively large necrotic center and a thin fibrous cap, and plaques with relatively small necrotic centers and a thick fibrous cap. In addition, they can be divided into relatively large space-occupying plaques producing from 25 to 50 percent stenosis of the lumen of the LAD coronary artery and smaller advanced plaques with all of the characteristics of fibrous plaques but occupying less than a quarter of the original coronary artery lumenal area.

Investigation of the risk factors which were determined postmortem correlated with the development of the advanced proximal LAD coronary plaques indicated that approximately 70 percent of these individuals presented evidence of smoking as ascertained by serum thiocyanate determinations and that the next most common risk factors correlated with these fibrous plaques were the elevated serum lipid (cholesterol) values, or the combination of elevated lipid values and thiocyanate values.

On the other hand, even though race, obesity, glycosylated hemoglobin, and elevated

A. M. Gotto, Jr. et al. (eds.), Drugs Affecting Lipid Metabolism, 161–168.

hypertension indices were correlated with an increase in the extent of sudanophilia and often with raised coronary lesions by gross evaluation in previous PDAY studies, these risk factors did not correlate in any meaningful way with the advanced fibrous plaques with necrotic cores and fibrous caps as determined by microscopic evaluation.

Discussion

Table 1 indicates the overall distribution among the various lesion types in the ORO microscopic sections of the proximal LAD coronary artery (sample #45) and the lower abdominal aortic lesions (sample #16).

Table 1. The analysis of the microscopic lesion classification in the more than 800 cases in which risk factor data and useable slides were available.

Sample Location	No Micro Lesion	Micro Fatty Streaks	Fatty Plaques	Fibrous Plaques
Lower Abdominal Aorta #16	250	53	479	38
Proximal LAD #45	388	47	337	102

Note that there are three paradoxical results reflected in this table. They are as follows:

- There are many more samples with no microscopic evidence of lipid-containing atheromatous change in the LAD coronary artery sections than in the lower abdominal aorta.
- There are many more so-called fatty plaques (intermediate raised lesions) in the lower abdominal aorta than in the proximal LAD coronary artery sections.
- There are almost 2-1/2 times as many fibrous plaques (advanced raised lesions with a necrotic core and a fibrous cap) in the LAD coronary artery sections than in the lower abdominal aortic sections, both taken through the areas of greatest prevalence of atherosclerotic plaque progression [1,2].

The latter of these three unexpected results is especially surprising in view of the commonly held dictum that the lower abdominal aorta is the predominant site of the progression of the atheromatous process in young individuals, a decade or so prior to the progression of the disease in the proximal LAD. But one has to keep in mind that these microscopic sections were evaluated and classified as fibrous plaques only if there were definite core areas which were very lipid-rich and acellular (necrotic), which is one of the hallmarks of severity that determines whether a lesion can be classified as a type IV and/or type V [3]. This is not necessarily the case with the gross evaluations which have been used for many previous studies.

A more definitive study of the fibrous plaques in the 102 cases in which the microscopic slides of the pressure perfusion fixed proximal LAD coronary arteries showed advanced lesions revealed that 24 of these were severe enough to fill in from 25 to 50 percent of the lumenal area, whereas 78 advanced lesions, which were typical in that they had a definite necrotic center and a fibrous cap, were much less massive. On cross-section, these fibrous plaques filled in less than 25 percent of the lumenal area.

There was a rather easily ascertained division in almost all instances of the ratio between the fibrous components of the lesion and the necrotic core. As is shown in Table 2, 8 of the large advanced lesions had a relatively thick fibrous cap and a relatively smaller acellular lipid-rich core, whereas 16 lesions were large in volume but had much thinner fibrous caps so that the grossly soft grumous center was very close to the lumen.

Table 2. Large and small coronary fibrous plaques with enumeration of thin and thick fibrous caps.

Plaque Size	Total	# with Thin Fibrous Caps	# with Thick Fibrous Caps
Large LAD Plaques	24	16	8
Small LAD Plaques	78	34	44
Total	102	50	52

Table 2 also shows that this same division into two general types of lesions applies to the smaller, less stenosing, advanced plaques. As Fuster et al. have emphasized, these plaques with thin fibrous caps and relatively large lipid-rich cores are unstable and the most dangerous to the patient since they are probably much more likely to develop a break in their fibrous cap [4,5]. This fracture or rupture may greatly enhance the condition leading to immediate thrombosis even when the plaques are relatively small and virtually undetectable by any existing methods of predicting coronary disease on the basis of imaging in the living subject. This of course is especially true of the smaller, less voluminous plaques with thin fibrous caps and relatively large necrotic centers of the type illustrated in Figure 1.

When we studied the relationship of risk factors to these advanced plaques, it became evident that the great majority of the 102 cases in which fibrous plaques were present had strong evidence of the use of tobacco [6,7]. This was reflected in elevated thiocyanate tests, a chemical analysis of serum or urine which is frequently used clinically to detect a history of recent smoking. This correlation of risk factors also revealed that the presence of hyperlipidemia and/or the combination of hyperlipidemia and smoking carried a positive correlation with these advanced lesions [7,8].

On the other hand the relatively large coronary artery plaques with a thick fibrous cap may not be nearly as likely to lead to life-threatening clinical events as their size might suggest. They may be regarded as stable plaques.

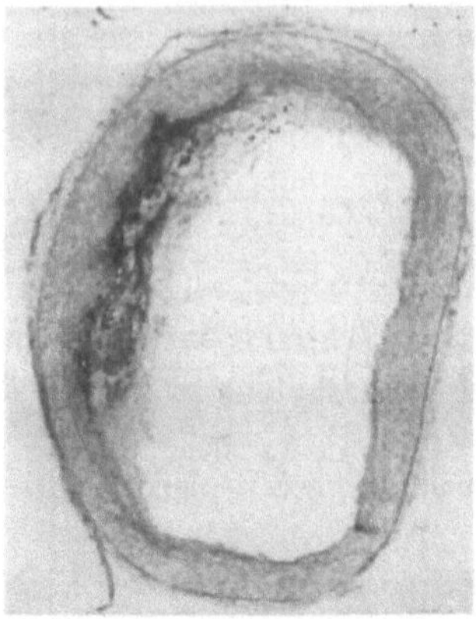

Figure 1. This plaque, which probably would not be visualized by angiography, is from a 22-year-old black male and shows a very thin fibrous cap and a relatively large acellular center which stains intensively for both lipid and calcium.

A further refinement of these correlative studies was undertaken. Table 3 summarizes the results of this further analysis of the four types of advanced plaques and the mean quantitative risk factor values for hyperlipidemia and thiocyanate levels.

It should be noted that two important trends are apparent in this tabulation.

- The large fibrous plaques, with their thin fibrous caps, perhaps potentially the most clinically important lesion type, are definitely associated rather conspicuously with elevated serum thiocyanate levels and elevated serum cholesterol levels.
- The smaller fibrous plaques with relatively thick fibrous caps also seem to be associated with an elevated serum thiocyanate level combined with a somewhat elevated serum cholesterol.

Both of these observations are noteworthy and need further study and documentation.

The other risk factors which were quantitatively measured in the majority of these cases reveal no correlation with the occurrence of fibrous plaques in the proximal LAD coronary artery even though they were often related to the extent of the aortic and coronary artery lesions [9,10,11,12]. These include measures of obesity, glycosylated hemoglobin as an indicator of high risk of diabetes, and indices of hypertension.

This is probably the first time that these advanced plaques have been carefully evaluated microscopically to ascertain the relative proportions of fibrous cap and necrotic core. Since these sections indicate a wide diversity in the prominence of the fibrous cap it is not surprising that the results are not similar to those obtained by visual gross grading which is primarily aimed at judging extent of disease and only secondarily focused on severity of the disease, and then mostly relying on the thickness of the fibrous cap for making a decision. The evaluation which is reported here included all lesions with a definite lipid-rich, acellular core.

Table 3. Risk factor mean values as related to the four main types of fibrous plaques in 102 proximal lad coronary artery samples.

Type of Lesion	Average Age	Mean Serum Values	
		Thiocyanate (μM/l)	Cholesterol (mg/100 ml)
Large fibrous plaque with thin fibrous cap and large necrotic core.	29.6	124.3	248.1
Large fibrous plaque with thick fibrous cap and relatively small necrotic core.	29.2	93.3	202.7
Smaller fibrous plaque with thin fibrous cap and large necrotic core.	27.8	88.4	187.4
Smaller fibrous plaque with thick fibrous cap and relatively small necrotic center.	29.7	131.7	221.6

These advanced coronary artery fibrous plaques were found predominantly in males and, while all of the subjects were less than 35 years of age, there was also a definite predominance of these advanced plaques in individuals in the two higher five-year age groups, i.e. 25-29 and 30-34. On the other hand, no relationship could be found between the presence of these advanced lesions and the two racial groups which are almost equally represented in the PDAY study. They were also almost equally represented in these four groups of advanced lesions, i.e. the larger versus the smaller, and the more fibrous versus the less fibrous plaques.

One of the more hopeful aspects of the results of this study of advanced coronary plaques in young people is based on the observations we have recorded and reported in our many years of study of regression of arterial plaques in rhesus monkeys with advanced experimental atherosclerosis in their coronary arteries as well as their aortas.

These results, which have been summarized in relevant publications [13,14] indicate very strongly that lipid is relatively easily removed from fibrous plaques even from those with large lipid-rich acellular cores. This would suggest that clinically the most "dangerous" advanced plaques would be the most amenable to lipid lowering therapeutic intervention since the collagen and elastin are reduced much more slowly [15,16]. Under these circumstances the plaques can be greatly reduced in size in one of the experimental models which most closely resembles the advanced human disease in lesion components and in the variety of patterns in which the atherosclerotic plaques appear.

The major problem at present is in identifying small but dangerous plaques with thin fibrous caps, like the one printed in Figure 1. We definitely need ways of identifying the relative size of components in relatively small lesions which generally would not be detected in contrast media angiography of coronary arteries. A major advance in technology is needed in order to identify these lesions as well as the relative size of their components.

Acknowledgements

This work was partially supported by HL 33740 and HL 45715 from the NIH Heart, Lung and Blood Institute. Special thanks and recognition are due to Gertrud Friedman, Blanche Berger, Taryn McFadden, and Ashish Mahajan. See acknowledgements of the PDAY scientific group as Appendix following references.

References

1. Cornhill JF, Herderick EE, and the Pathobiological Determinants of Atherosclerosis in Youth (PDAY) Research Group. Arterial disease in young people. In: Blankenhorn DH, editor. Atherogenesis and regression. Part I. Development of atherosclerosis. New York: Cahners Healthcare Communications, 1993:4-10.
2. Svindland A. The localization of sudanophilic and fibrous plaques in the main left coronary bifurcation. Atherosclerosis 1983;48:139-145.
3. Stary HC, Chandler AB, Dinsmore RE, et al. Definitions of advanced types of atherosclerotic lesions and a histological classification of atherosclerosis. Arterioscler Thromb Vasc Biol 1995;15:1512-31.
4. Fuster V, Badimon L, Badimon JJ, Chesebro JH. The pathogenesis of coronary artery disease and the acute coronary syndromes (first of two parts). N Engl J Med 1992;326:242-50.
5. Fuster V, Badimon L, Badimon JJ, Chesebro JH. The pathogenesis of coronary artery disease and the acute coronary syndromes (second of two parts). N Engl J Med 1992;326:310-18.
6. Wissler RW, Hiltscher L, Oinuma T and the PDAY Research Group. Pathogenesis of atherosclerosis--the lesions of atherosclerosis in the young: From fatty streaks to intermediate lesions. In: Fuster V, Ross R, Topol E, editors. Atherosclerosis and coronary artery disease. New York: Raven Press, 1996:475-79, & colorplates 12-16.
7. Wissler RW, Hiltscher L, Wahden M. Early evolution of coronary artery lesions in young people: From fatty streak to fibrous plaque - implications for imaging. In: Fuster V, editor. Syndrome of atherosclerosis: Correlations of clinical imaging and pathology. New York: Futura Publishing Company, 1996:65-80.
8. PDAY Research Group. Relationship of atherosclerosis in young men to serum lipoprotein cholesterol concentrations and smoking: A preliminary report from the Pathobiological Determinants of Atherosclerosis in Youth (PDAY) Research Group. JAMA 1990;264:3018-3024.
9. Strong JP, Oalmann MC, Malcom GT, and the Pathobiological Determinants of Atherosclerosis in Youth (PDAY) Research Group. Atherosclerosis in youth: Relationship of risk factors to arterial lesions. In: Lauer RM, Luepker RV, Filer LJ Jr, editors. Monograph

on prevention of atherosclerosis and hypertension beginning in youth. Malvern, PA: Lea and Febiger, 1994:13-20.

10. McGill HC Jr, McMahan A, Malcom GT, Oalmann MC, Strong JP and the Pathobiological Determinants of Atherosclerosis in Youth (PDAY) Research Group. Relation of glycohemoglobin and adiposity to atherosclerosis in youth. Arterioscler Thromb Vasc Biol 1995;15:431-40.
11. Strong JP, for the Pathobiological Determinants of Atherosclerosis in Youth (PDAY) Research Group. Natural history and risk factors for early human atherogenesis. Clin Chem 1995;42:134-38.
12. McGill HC, Strong JP, Tracy RE, McMahan A, Oalmann MC, and the Pathobiological Determinants of Atherosclerosis in Youth (PDAY) Research Group. Relation of a postmortem renal index of hypertension to atherosclerosis in youth. Arterioscler Thromb Vasc Biol 1995; in press.
13. Wissler RW, Vesselinovitch D. Interaction of therapeutic diets and cholesterol-lowering drugs in regression studies in animals. In: Malinow MR, Blaton VH, editors. Regression of atherosclerotic lesions. New York: Plenum Press, 1984: 21-41.
14. Wissler RW, Vesselinovitch D. The time course of atherosclerotic lesion regression in macaque monkeys. In: Descovitch CG, Gaddi A, Magri GL, Lenzi S, editors. Atherosclerosis and cardiovascular disease. 7th Intl. Meeting. Dordrecht, The Netherlands: Kluwer Academic Publishers, 1990:391-400.
15. Vesselinovitch D, Wissler RW, Hughes R, Borensztajn J. Reversal of advanced atherosclerosis in rhesus monkeys. I. Light microscopic studies. Atherosclerosis 1976;23: 155-76.
16. Armstrong ML. Connective tissue changes in regression. In: Schettler G, Goto Y, Hata Y, Klose G, editors. Atherosclerosis IV. Berlin: Springer Verlag, 1977:405-413.

Appendix

PATHOBIOLOGICAL DETERMINANTS OF ATHEROSCLEROSIS IN YOUTH (PDAY) RESEARCH GROUP

Directors. Program Director; R.W. Wissler, Ph.D.,M.D., University of Chicago. Associate Directors: A.L. Robertson, Jr.,M.D., Ph.D., University of Illinois (1987-1992); J.P. Strong, M.D., Louisiana State University (1992-present)

Steering Committee. J.F. Cornhill, Ph.D., Ohio State University; H.C. McGill, Jr., M.D., Southwest Foundation for Biomedical Research; C.A. McMahan, Ph.D., University of Texas Health Science Center (San Antonio); Abel Robertson,Jr.,M.D.,Ph.D., University of Illinois; J.P. Strong, M.D., Louisiana State University Medical Center; R.W. Wissler, Ph.D., M.D., University of Chicago

Standard Operating Protocol and Manual of Procedures Committee Chairman. M.C. Oalmann, Ph.D., Louisiana State University Medical Center

Participating Centers. University of Alabama (Birmingham), Department of Medicine - Principal Investigator (P.I.): S. Gay, M.D., Coinvestigators: R.E. Gay, M.D., C.-Q. Huang, M.D. (HL-33733); Department of Biochemistry - P.I.: E.J. Miller, Ph.D.; Coinvestigators: D.K. Furuto, Ph.D., M.S. Vail, A.J. Narkates (HL-33728)

Albany Medical College (Albany, NY) - P.I.: A. Daoud, M.D., Coinvestigators: A.. Frank, Ph.D., M.A. Hyer, E.C. McGovern (HL-33765)

Baylor College of Medicine (Houston) - P.I.: L.C. Smith, Ph.D., Coinvestigator - F. M. Strickland, Ph.D. (HL-33750)

University of Chicago (Chicago) - P.I.: R.W. Wissler, Ph.D., M.D., Coinvestigators: D. Vesselinovitch, M.S., D.V.M., A. Komatsu, M.D., Ph.D., Y. Kusumi, M.D., G.M. Culen, D.P.M., A. Chien, B.A., A. Demopoulos, B.A., G. Friedman, B.A., R.T. Bridenstein, M.S., R. H. Kirschner, M.D., M. Bekermeier, ASCP, B. Berger, ASCP, L. Hiltscher, ASCP (HL-33740)

University of Illinois (Chicago) - P.I.: A.L. Robertson, Jr.,M.D.,Ph.D., Coinvestigators: E.R. Donoghue, M.D., R.J. Buschmann, Ph.D., Y. Katsura, M.D., T. Lyong An, M.D., E. Choi, M.D., N. Jones, M.D., M.S. Kaleikar, M.D., Y. Konakei, M.D. B. Lifschultz, M.D., V.R. Gumidyala, M.D., R.H. Harper, B.S., F. Nerns, H.T.L.(ASCP) (HL-33758)

Louisiana State University Med Ctr (New Orleans) - P.I.: J.P. Strong, M.D., Coinvestigators: G.T. Malcom, Ph.D., W.P. Newman III, M.D., M.C. Oalmann, Ph.D., P.S. Roheim, M.D., A.K. Bhattacharyya, Ph.D., M.A. Guzman, Ph.D., A.A. Hatem, M.D., C.A. Hornick, Ph.D., C.D. Restrepo, M.D., R.E. Tracy, M.D.,Ph,D., C.C. Breaux, M.S., S.E. Hubbard, C.S. Zsembik, D.G. Gibbs, D.A. Troxclair (HL-33746)

University of Maryland (Baltimore) - P.I.: W. Mergner, M.D.,Ph.D., Coinvestigators: J.H. Resau, Ph.D., R.D. Vigorito, M.S.,P.A., Q.-C. Yu, M.D., J. Smialek, M.D. (HL-33752)

Medical College of Georgia (Augusta) - Co-P.I: A.B. Chandler, M.D., R.N. Rao, M.D., Coinvestigators: D.G. Falls, M.D., R. G. Gerrity, Ph.D., B.O. Spurlock, B.A., Associate Investigators: K.B. Sharma, M.D., J.S. Sexton, M.D., Research Assistants: K.K. Smith, HT (ASCP), G.W. Forbes (HL-33772)

University of Nebraska Med Ctr (Omaha) - P.I.: B.M. McManus, M.D.,Ph.D., Coinvestigators: J.W. Jones, M.D., T.J. Kendall, M.S., J.A. Remmenga, B.S., W.C. Rogier, B.S. (HL-33778)

Ohio State University (Columbus) - P.I.: J.F. Cornhill, Ph.D., Coinvestigators: W.R. Adrion, M.D., P.M. Fardel, M.D., B. Gara, M.S., E. Herderick, J. Meimer, M.S., L.R. Tate, M.D. (HL-33760)

Southwest Foundation for Biomedical Research (San Antonio) - P.I.: J.E. Hixson, Ph.D., P.K. Powers (HL-39913)

University of Texas Health Science Ctr (San Antonio) - P.I.: C.A. McMahan, Ph,D., Coinvestigators: H.C. McGill, Jr.,M.D., Y. Marinez, M.A., T.J. Prihoda, Ph.D., H.S. Wigodsky, M.D., Ph.D. (HL-33749)

Vanderbilt University (Nashville) - P.I.: R. Virmani, M.D., Coinvestigators: J.B. Atkinson, M.D., Ph.D., C.W. Harlan, M.D. (HL-33770)

West Virginia University (Morgantown) - P.I.: S.N. Jagannathan, Ph.D., Coinvestigators: B. Caterson, Ph.D., J.L. Frost, M.D., K. Murali, K. Rao, M.D., S. Jagannathan, P. Johnson, N.F. Rodman, M.D. (HL-33748)

SIMVASTATIN-INDUCED REDUCTION IN RISK OF MAJOR CORONARY EVENTS IS RELATED MAINLY TO REDUCTION IN LDL CHOLESTEROL BUT ALSO TO INCREASE IN HDL CHOLESTEROL

Anders G. Olsson for the 4S Group
Department of Internal Medicine, University Hospital, S-581 85 Linköping, Sweden

Introduction

Efforts to reduce coronary heart disease (CHD) risk in patients who already have the disease is called secondary prevention. For this purpose plasma lipid lowering drugs have been tried since the 1970s with varying results. In the Newcastle [1] and Scottish [2] studies, benefit was noted in the subgroup of patients with angina pectoris. In the Coronary Drug Project (CDP), five treatment principles were used: estrogen in two doses, dextrothyroxin, clofibrate, and nicotinic acid [3]. Dextrothyroxin and the two doses of estrogen had to be stopped prematurely because of serious side effects. There was no evidence of the efficacy of clofibrate [4]. The five-year incidence of definite, nonfatal myocardial infarction on nicotinic acid in CDP was 8.9% in the nicotinic acid group and 12.2% in the placebo group, a significant difference. No effect was seen on total mortality, the primary endpoint in CDP. In a 15-year follow-up of CDP, it was shown that total mortality in the nicotinic acid group was 52.0% versus 58.2% in the placebo group, an 11% and highly significantly lower rate [5]. The open Stockholm Ischaemic Heart Disease Secondary Prevention Study using a combined treatment with clofibrate and nicotinic acid showed a 26% lower total mortality in the treatment group compared to placebo (61 versus 82 cases, $p < 0.05$) [6]. Therefore, even if several studies have indicated beneficial effects of lipid lowering in secondary prevention, no study fulfilling present-day requirements for an intervention study so far has proven that these effects are real.

The introduction of the 3-hydroxy-3-methylglutaryl coenzyme A (HMG-CoA) reductase inhibitors in the treatment of hyperlipidemia led to improved possibilities in the prevention of CHD through lipid lowering.

The Scandinavian Simvastatin Survival Study (4S) [7,8] is the first study using this new therapy. Primary endpoint was total mortality.

Patients and Methods

4S is a double-blind, randomized, placebo-controlled study of simvastatin in patients with

A. M. Gotto, Jr. et al. (eds.), Drugs Affecting Lipid Metabolism, 169–174.

CHD either as myocardial infarction or angina pectoris. It comprised 4,444 male and female patients, 2,221 in the placebo and 2,223 in the actively treated group, aged between 35 and 70 years, with serum cholesterol between 5.5 and 8.0 mmol/l (213 and 310 mg/dl) and serum triglycerides below 2.5 mmol/l (221 mg/dl). All participants received dietary advice. Treatment goal regarding cholesterol was between 3.0 and 5.2 mmol/l (115 and 200 mg/dl). This was obtained through a dosage titration procedure. Starting dose of simvastatin was 20 mg daily. If the patients did not reach the upper target cholesterol of 5.2 mmo/l during the first 18 weeks of treatment, dosage was increased to 40 mg daily. Thirty-seven percent of the patients in the simvastatin group increased the dose to 40 mg. A similar dummy procedure was performed in the placebo group to ensure double blindness.

A total number of 440 deaths was considered necessary to determine efficacy and was used as breaking point for the study. This occurred after a median duration of 5.4 years of study.

Effects on Serum Lipids and Lipoproteins

The mean basal cholesterol concentration of 6.4 mmol/L (260 mg/dl) decreased to 4.7 mmol/l (182 mg/dl) at 12 months in those who received 20 mg and to 5.1 mmol/l (197 mg/dl) in those who received 40 mg simvastatin daily. Initial low density lipoprotein (LDL) was 4.7 (182 mg/dl) in 20 mg patients and 5.1 mmol/l (197 mg/dl) in 40 mg patients and their levels on treatment were 2.9 (112) and 3.3 (128) mmol/l (mg/dl), respectively. Simvastatin treatment decreased cholesterol by 25% and LDL cholesterol by 35% (Figure 1). Plasma triglycerides decreased by 10% and high density lipoprotein (HDL) cholesterol increased by 8%. These effects were maintained through the study for all lipids and lipoproteins. A slight increase in total and LDL cholesterol may be due to a number of patients, who left blood samples for lipid determination but did not take the drug during the later part of the study ("intention to treat" principle).

Effects on Clinical Endpoints and Tolerance

The study demonstrated that treatment with simvastatin for 5.4 years decreased total mortality from 256 (11.5%) in the placebo group to 182 (8.2%) or by 30% ($p < 0.0003$) (Figure 2). This was due to a reduction in CHD mortality from 189 in the placebo group to 111 or by 42% ($p < 0.00001$). The risk of major coronary events, i.e. fatal and nonfatal myocardial infarctions, decreased by 34%. The need for coronary artery bypass grafting and percutaneous transluminal coronary angioplasty decreased in the simvastatin group to 252 from 383 in the placebo treated group, a 37% reduction in the risk. In a post hoc analysis it was furthermore shown that the number of patients with nonfatal cerebrovascular events decreased from 98 to 70 by the treatment ($p = 0.024$). In women the effect on major coronary events was similar to that in men. Age did not influence outcome in any significant way; simvastatin was effective in all ages included in 4S.

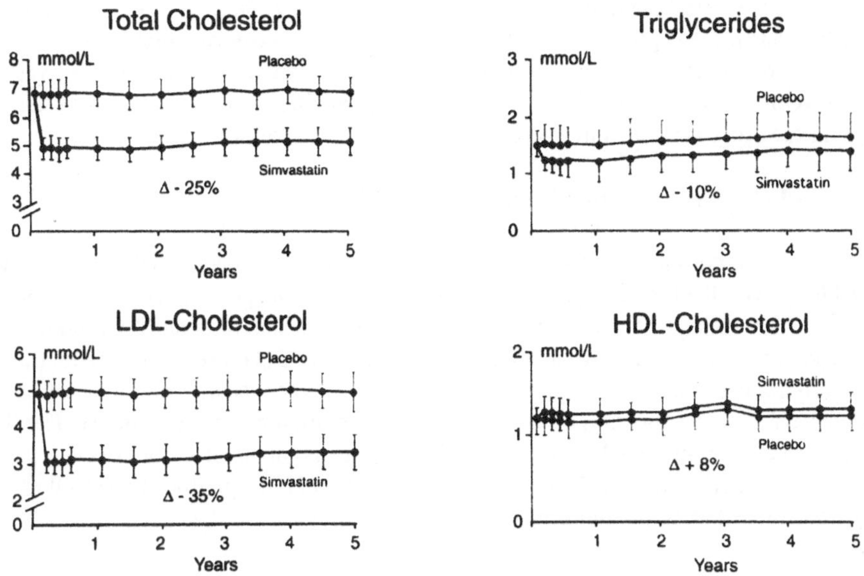

Figure 1. Serum lipid and lipoprotein concentrations in simvastatin and placebo groups during the study.

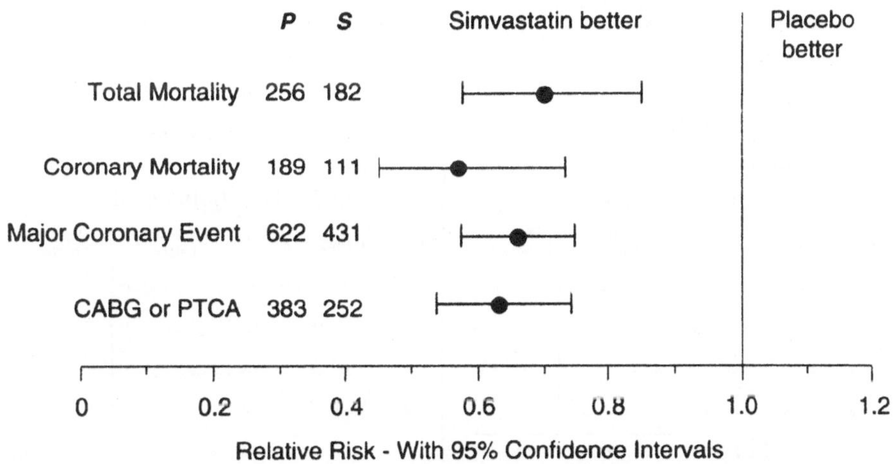

Figure 2. Relative risks with 95% confidence intervals for different clinical endpoints in 4S. P and S indicate number of cases in placebo and simvastatin groups, respectively. Risk reduction = (1-relative risk) x 100%. CABG = coronary artery bypass grafting, PTCA = percutaneous transluminal coronary angioplasty.

Simvastatin was well tolerated. The overall frequency of adverse events was similar in simvastatin and placebo groups. No differences were noted in cancer, suicide, or traumatic deaths. No differences were seen in nonfatal cancers. One woman on 20 mg simvastatin daily developed myalgia and high creatine kinase activities but symptoms vanished on stopping the drug. Increased liver enzyme activities were rare on drug treatment.

Effects in Relation to Baseline Lipids

The risk of major coronary events (coronary death and nonfatal myocardial infarction) was related to baseline lipid and lipoprotein concentrations [9]. The percentage of patients with major coronary events tended to increase with increasing baseline total and LDL cholesterol levels and to decrease with increasing HDL cholesterol levels (Figure 3). The reductions in relative risk was similar in each quartile for each lipid. There was no significant difference in relative risk between quartiles for any of the lipids and lipoproteins determined. The 95% confidence intervals, given in Figure 3, show that the effects on major coronary events were significant even in the lowest LDL quartile and the highest HDL quartile. The absolute risk reductions tended to be greater with higher baseline lipids.

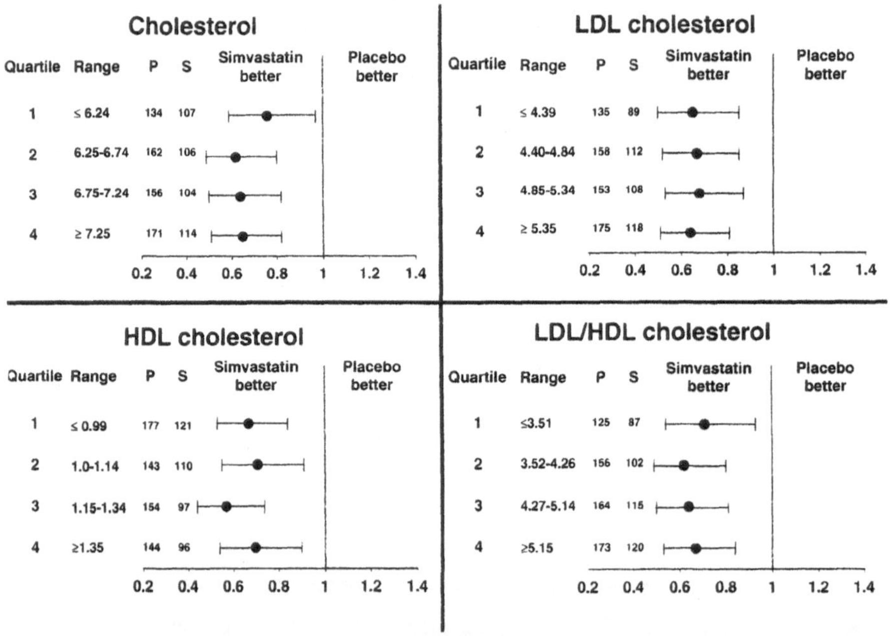

Figure 3. Relative risk with 95% confidence intervals for baseline quartiles of serum lipids and lipoproteins. P and S indicate number of cases in placebo and simvastatin groups, respectively. Risk reduction = (1-relative risk) x 100%.

Effects in Relation to Change in Lipids and on Treatment Levels

The relations between change in lipids and lipoproteins and lipid levels achieved during treatment and clinical outcome measures are currently under investigation. Percentage change of lipid values during the study in the simvastatin group was calculated as area under the curve and related to the rate of major coronary events in a Cox proportional hazards model. Changes of total cholesterol, LDL cholesterol, and the ratio LDL/HDL cholesterol were all highly statistically significantly related to risk. Choosing one lipid measure as a primary explanatory variable, the independent contribution to the relationship with events of each of the other lipid changes was assessed. All explanatory power shared between the primary and secondary lipid variable was allocated to the primary variable. In almost all combinations of two variables, the secondary explanatory variable gave statistically significant additional information on risk.

Comment

4S demonstrates that simvastatin treatment in secondary prevention is effective in decreasing total mortality. This effect is mediated through decreased coronary mortality. The treatment also diminishes dramatically nonfatal coronary manifestations. The treatment is safe and no suspicions of untoward effects, induced by the pronounced cholesterol lowering, on noncardiovascular disease or mortality are raised. The fact that all included patients benefitted from treatment regardless of initial cholesterol levels implies that whenever a patients has coronary heart disease his or her LDL cholesterol is too high for that person´s coronary arterial wall. The fact that changes in total and LDL cholesterol during treatment was highly statistically significantly related to risk indicates that a maximum change of the lipid levels should be the goal. The finding of independent contribution to risk reduction from both changes in LDL cholesterol and HDL cholesterol suggests that the effect of simvastatin on outcome involves a broader lipoprotein spectrum than just LDL cholesterol.

References

1. Group of physicians of the Newcastle upon Tyne region. Trial of clofibrate in the treatment of ischaemic heart disease. Brit Med J 1971;4:767-74.
2. Research Committee of the Scottish Society of Physicians. Ischaemic heart disease: A secondary prevention trial using clofibrate. Brit Med J 1971;4:775-84.
3. Coronary Drug Project Research Group. The Coronary Drug Project: Design, methods and baseline results. Circulation 1973;47(1):I1-I50.
4. Coronary Drug Project Research Group. Clofibrate and niacin in coronary heart disease. JAMA 1975;231:360-81.
5. Canner PL, Berge KK, Wenger NK, et al. Fifteen year mortality in Coronary Drug Project patients: Long-term benefit with niacin. J Am Coll Cardiolog 1986;8:1245-55.
6. Carlson L, Rosenhamer G. Reduction of mortality in the Stockholm Ischaemic Heart Disease Secondary Prevention Study by combined treatment with clofibrate and nicotinic acid. Acta Med Scand 1988;223:405-18.

7. The Scandinavian Simvastatin Survival Study Group. Design and baseline results of the Scandinavian Simvastatin Survival Study of patients with stable angina and/or previous myocardial infarction. Am J Cardiol 1993;71:393-400.
8. The Scandinavian Simvastatin Survival Study Group. Randomized trial of cholesterol lowering in 4444 patients with coronary heart disease: The Scandinavian Simvastatin Survival Study (4S). Lancet 1994;344:1383-89.
9. The Scandinavian Simvastatin Survival Study Group. Baseline serum cholesterol and treatment effect in the Scandinavian Simvastatin Survival Study (4S). Lancet 1995; 345:1274-75.

OBJECTIVES OF THE AGENCY FOR HEALTH CARE POLICY AND RESEARCH AND CLINICAL TRIALS

Lynn A. Bosco
Agency for Health Care Policy and Research, Center for Outcomes and Effectiveness Research, 2101 E. Jefferson Street, Suite 605, Rockville, Maryland 20852, USA

Introduction

The Agency for Health Care Policy and Research (AHCPR) was established December 19, 1989 by Title IX of the Omnibus Budget Reconciliation Act of 1989. The Agency replaced the National Center for Health Services Research and Health Care Technology Assessment. According to the authorizing legislation [1]:

> The purpose of the Agency is to enhance the quality, appropriateness, and effectiveness of health care services and access to such services, through the establishment of a broad base of scientific research and through the promotion of improvements in clinical practice and in the organization, financing, and delivery of health care services.

The legislation further states that the general authorities and duties of the agency require that:

> The Administrator shall conduct and support research, demonstration projects, evaluations, training, guideline development, and dissemination of information on health care services and on systems for the delivery of such services, including activities with respect to:
> (1) the effectiveness, efficiency, and quality of health care services;
> (2) the outcomes of health care services and procedures;
> (3) clinical practice, including primary care and practice-oriented research;
> (4) health care technologies, facilities, and equipment;
> (5) health care costs, productivity, and market forces;
> (6) health promotion and disease prevention;
> (7) health statistics and epidemiology; and

A. M. Gotto, Jr. et al. (eds.), Drugs Affecting Lipid Metabolism, 175–180.

(8) medical liability

AHCPR is a component of the US Department of Health and Human Services (HHS). The Department consists of health agencies with a broad variety of responsibilities, including regulatory, direct health care delivery, reimbursement, and intra- and extra-mural research.

The National Institutes of Health is the primary funding agency for biomedical research, while AHCPR funds health services, medical effectiveness and outcomes research. Biomedical research seeks to answer questions about the physical determinants of causality and prevention of diseases. Health services research addresses the social, financial, organizational and cultural facets of health and health care. Outcomes research addresses issues of clinical practice.

The Medical Treatment Effectiveness Program

The Center for Outcomes and Effectiveness Research is the principal component within AHCPR responsible for research within the Medical Treatment Effectiveness Program (MEDTEP). In addition to clinically oriented effectiveness and outcomes studies, MEDTEP also includes three other integrated programs: (1) data development; (2) the guidelines development program; and (3) dissemination. AHCPR's effectiveness and outcomes research focuses on the question of what works and what does not in the routine practice of medicine. Most of this research is disease or condition specific. Further defining characteristics include high prevalence, significant resource utilization, and serious morbidity or death. AHCPR guidelines and outcomes research focus on the same set of priorities: the determination of the most appropriate and cost effective treatment of common and costly diseases.

A distinction is made in MEDTEP between the terms "efficacy" and "effectiveness." Efficacy is defined as evidence gathered under controlled circumstances with select populations. A study of efficacy will most often be done as a randomized, controlled clinical trial. Frequently patients will be volunteers, selected because of the absence of significant comorbidity and the high probability that they will actually complete the study. Children, the very elderly, and women who could become pregnant, are likely to be excluded. In efficacy studies, patients are monitored more closely than they would be in routine medical practice thus changing the dynamics of treatment. Incentives are provided for compliance with the requirements of the study and treatment follows a defined protocol that allows for minimal deviation.

Effectiveness studies differ from efficacy studies because a variety of methods for collecting data are acceptable and the population selection criteria is usually less stringent. An effectiveness study may also be a randomized trial but monitoring is equivalent to that which one would experience in the routine practice of medicine. Any person with the disease under study is a potential candidate for inclusion and exclusions are kept to a minimum. These studies will also gather information on the impact of variation in provider and patient behavior on the outcomes of treatment.

Efficacy studies determine whether an intervention can reach a previously determined endpoint safely, while minimizing patient and provider variations related to the treatment. Effectiveness studies allow for greater generalizability to larger populations.

AHCPR studies effectiveness in terms of a broad range of treatment outcomes. In addition to the traditional measures of mortality and hospitalization, outcomes studies include patient factors, such as satisfaction with care, quality of life, and functional status. All outcomes must be measures of patient impact rather than process.

Much of AHCPR MEDTEP research has focused on unregulated aspects of medical care, particularly surgical procedures (e.g. cholecystectomy and prostatectomy) and diagnostic procedures (e.g. diagnosis of cholecystitis) where even efficacy studies were unavailable or inconclusive. The largest program thus far has been the Patient Outcomes Research Teams (PORT and PORT II). This extramural research program began in 1989 and is ongoing [2].

The Outcomes of Pharmaceutical Therapy Program

The Outcomes of Pharmaceutical Therapy Program became a part of MEDTEP in 1990. This extramural research program sought to sponsor research that would move beyond the Food and Drug Administration (FDA) required safety and efficacy data, since the FDA's regulations do not contain a requirement for studies of comparative effectiveness between alternative therapies (e.g. drug versus surgery or drug versus drug), or studies of cost effectiveness. Most of the MEDTEP pharmaceutical studies funded to date address questions pertinent to the FDA defined postmarketing or phase IV period of drug development, including both the studies of pharmacoepidemiology and pharmacoeconomics. Pharmacoeconomics has become the most prominent of these two areas of research. Recently AHCPR identified pharmacoeconomic research as a top priority through the release of a request to the academic community for grant application focused in this field.

Pharmacoeconomics

FDA has been particularly interested in pharmacoeconomics lately because of the desire on the part of the pharmaceutical industry to conduct cost-effectiveness studies and use the results of these studies for promotional purposes. Pharmaceutical firms perceive a need to demonstrate cost effectiveness so that insurers place them on formularies, bulk purchasers include them, and pharmacy and therapeutics committees approve them. Most of the time comparative data on both cost and effectiveness has been unavailable, since drugs are approved with only efficacy data. Unlike countries such as Australia, no comparative cost effectiveness data is required for marketing in the United States. The current FDA policy on pharmacoeconomic claims is as follows [3]:

> FDA currently reviews all drug promotions to assure that claims are not false or misleading. Comparative economic claims must be substantiated by "adequate and well-controlled" studies that support the comparative effectiveness portion of the economic claim. (For comparisons of

treatments with small differences in effectiveness, randomization of treatment groups is considered necessary.) The methods of collection and analysis of cost data must be fully transparent and disclosed.

Managed care organizations and hospitals have also attempted to perform pharmacoeconomic analyses to support reimbursement and formulary decisions. Unfortunately, because many studies are performed and published by organizations with a financial interest in the study outcome, the objectivity of this kind of research may be jeopardized by an apparent conflict of interest.

Concerns about the adequacy of pharmacoeconomic studies have generated a call for standardized principles of pharmacoeconomics and numerous guidelines and checklists have actually been published [4]. To summarize what has been written to date, these guidelines recommend that a pharmacoeconomic study always include the following appropriately completed steps: 1) the question is stated; 2) the perspective (e.g. patient, institution) is identified; 3) the study design is well described and answers the question from the appropriate perspective; 4) all alternative treatments are considered; 5) future costs are discounted; 6) all costs and outcomes are identified and correctly valued; 7) a sensitivity analysis is included; 8) all possible conclusions and limitations are explored; and 9) study sponsorship is identified.

Adherence to these principles appears to be incomplete. A critical appraisal of seven studies on cholesterol-lowering agents published in the journal *Pharamcoeconomics* [5] found that none of the studies reviewed completely followed these principles. Most commonly studies failed to included all alternative treatments in the analysis or to use credible values for the study variables.

Primary data collection of costs and outcomes in the same population in a study, such as a randomized trial, assures that data collected validly represents costs and outcomes. Unfortunately, data collected from a trial may not generalize to the routine practice of medicine unless the trial has an adequate sample size and closely mimics routine clinical practice. Since these trials are only rarely done and even more rarely do they include an economic component, researchers must seek out additional sources of data.

Drug Cost Data

Unfortunately for the pharmacoeconomist, there is no perfect source of drug cost data. Below is a list of data sources and associated problems.

For pricing individual prescription drugs, the most commonly recommended source, and probably the only one that is easily accessible, is the published "average wholesale price" (AWP). This is published annually with periodic updates. A number of companies provide this information inexpensively and use is usually not restricted by copyright. The publishers obtain the prices directly from the manufacturer. For a somewhat steeper price one can get the information on CD-ROM or through an online service. A dispensing fee is nearly always added to the AWP. Controversy exists as to whether AWP truly represents pharmaceutical costs because of the variability between mark-ups and the unmeasured impact of discounts to large purchasers.

Other commercial sources collect prescription drug cost data at all levels within the market. These data are usually collected directly through a computerized system of a sample of the market of interest and are usually robust enough to provide a national projection. These data can even provide patient level pharmacy cost data for individual drugs and even specific dosages. A number of companies provide this kind of data. which is copyrighted and must be purchased. Most of these companies will provide a limited amount of data free to academic researchers, otherwise the data are considerably more costly than the AWP.

The government collects information on drug costs through three surveys. AHCPR collects patient-based cost data with the National Medical Expenditure Survey (NMES) which is undertaken only every ten years. In 1987 it included 14,000 families, who responded to questionnaires and kept diaries of medical expenditures for one year. At least one validation study of this database suggested that both cost and utilization are underreported. Diagnostic information may be linked to utilization but for individual drugs, sample size may be inadequate to answer many research questions.

The Health Care Financing Administration (HCFA) collects data on an annual basis, of national medical expenditures, including drug costs. These data are most useful for aggregate analyses rather than studies of individual drugs.

The Bureau of Labor statistics annually collects data on expenditures on a "market basket" or representative sample of pharmaceuticals. A producer and consumer price index are calculated. These indices are mostly designed to measure inflation and are used within the context of a price index for all commodities and one that measures medical care. Lately these indices have been criticized as overstating increases. Although these indices can be broken out into broad indication classes, they may have minimal usefulness for individual products. New products are underrepresented in the sample because they are not included until their second year on the market.

Medicaid billing data that are compiled for the Health Care Financing Administration (HCFA) also include cost, utilization, and diagnostic information. However, the population covered by Medicaid and the health care they receive is very different from the general population. These data are usually purchased through HCFA contractors.

In addition to HCFA, AHCPR, commercial firms, and the Bureau of Labor Statistics, the National Center for Health Statistics, National Ambulatory Medical Care Survey collects drug utilization data but no costs. Other sources of data include local billing data for large organizations, such as multi-state HMOs.

Conclusions

Because of the perceived need to reduce the cost of medical care, tools are being developed to compare the value of prescription drugs. Very little work has been done to validate available cost data or to link drug utilization, cost, and outcomes. It is also the rare study that links actual costs to outcomes in a population large and representative enough to permit generalization of study findings. Ultimately, if the data used misrepresent the true costs and outcomes of treatment, patients may be deprived of appropriate therapy and may not experience optimal outcomes. The extent to which pharmacoeconomic studies are used to make resource allocation decisions is unknown. Institutional pharmacy and therapeutic committees have for many years made formulary decisions using published efficacy information. They have also used acquisition costs to assist in decisions where there was no discernible difference in reported efficacy for competing alternatives. It is not completely clear how newly developed tools to combine cost and outcomes are being used.

This lack of information points to the need for research not biased by economic self-interest or even the appearance of a conflict of interest. The AHCPR Outcomes of Pharmaceutical Therapy Program welcomes such pharmacoeconomic study proposals through its investigator-initiated grant program and through the occasional release of Request for Applications (RFA). However, current uncertainties regarding grant sponsored health services and outcomes research suggest the need to develop alternative and innovative sources of funding to encourage and facilitate optimal use of resources.

Acknowledgement

I would like to acknowledge the assistance of Richard Greene, MD, PhD and Claire Maklan, PhD.

Disclaimer

The opinions expressed here are solely those of the author and do not represent the policy of the Agency for Health Care Policy and Research.

References

1. Omnibus Budget Reconciliation Act of 1989. US Congress, 1989. Washington DC
2. Medical Treatment Effectiveness Research: PORT-II. NIH Guide to Grants and Contracts Vol. 23, No. 18, May 13, 1994.
3. Personal Communication, Laurie B. Burke, Food and Drug Administration
4. Sanchez, L.A. Evaluating the Quality of Published Pharmacoeconomic Evaluations. Hospital Pharmacy 1995;30:146-152.

THE ROLE OF HMG-CoA REDUCTASE INHIBITORS IN HOMOZYGOUS FAMILIAL HYPERCHOLESTEROLEMIA

A. David Marais, Jean C. Firth, Rossitza P. Naoumova*, and Gilbert R. Thompson*
*Department of Medicine, University of Cape Town Medical School, Observatory 7925, Cape Town, South Africa and *MRC Lipoprotein Team, Clinical Sciences Centre, Royal Postgraduate Medical School, Hammersmith Hospital, Du Cane Road, London W12 ONN, United Kingdom*

Introduction

The past two decades have been remarkable for the unravelling and manipulation of sterol and lipoprotein metabolism but have also seen some paradigm shifts as insight has improved. This is true also for the understanding of familial hypercholesterolemia (FH) and its treatment with hydroxymethylglutaryl coenzyme A reductase inhibitors.

Several metabolic errors give rise to excesses of plasma sterols. FH is an autosomal dominant disorder in which defective low density lipoprotein (LDL) receptors cause an increase in plasma LDL concentration [1]. The gene prevalence is about 1 in 500 of the population, so that the homozygous state is rarely encountered. In South Africa, a "founder effect" has resulted in an higher prevalence of FH in Afrikaners [2,3], as well as in other sectors of the population [4]. We therefore have an almost unique opportunity to study this disorder and its treatment.

Heterozygous FH is characterized by a plasma total cholesterol concentration greater than 7.8 mM/L (300 mg/dL), tendon xanthomata, and premature ischemic heart disease. The impact of homozygous FH is much more severe. The homozygote typically develops tendinous and cutaneous lipid deposits before the age of 10 years, and ischemic heart disease commonly sets in before the third decade beyond which survival is extremely unlikely without intervention. The plasma cholesterol concentration is usually in excess of 16 mM/L (600 mg/dL). Homozygous FH is diagnosed by the clinical setting as well as either a demonstration of low LDL receptor binding activity in cultured skin fibroblasts, or the presence of LDL receptor mutations. Genotyping and LDL binding studies yield information about the cell biology of the LDL receptor [5]. There are five classes of mutations in the LDL receptor and these influence the high affinity binding of LDL in the maximally upregulated state: from "receptor-negative" to "receptor-defective."

The management of homozygous FH is outlined in Table 1. Attitudes have changed from nihilism to aggressive and successful intervention by plasmapheresis to a guarded

A. M. Gotto, Jr. et al. (eds.), Drugs Affecting Lipid Metabolism, 181–186.

optimism that gene therapy could cure the disorder. Aggressive surgery such as porto-systemic shunting and liver transplant are not without their own risks.

Table 1. Management of homozygous familial hypercholesterolemia (HoFH). The treatment of choice is plasmapheresis while auxiliary treatment with HMG-Co reductase inhibitors may now be accepted if proven to reduce plasma cholesterol rebound in the individual. While portacaval shunt is no longer advised, liver transplantation should be considered if cardiac transplantation is indicated.

Management of HoFH	
Approach	Comments
Health Lifestyle	Very low fat diet, habits
Plasmapheresis	Plasma exchange Dextran sulphate adsorption Extracorporeal precipitation Double filtration Immuno-affinity
Surgery	Porto-systemic shunting Coronary bypass grafts Liver transplantation Aortic valve replacement
Drug Therapy	Niacin Bile salt sequestrants HMG-CoA reductase inhibitors
Gene Therapy	Still Experimental

In the interim, plasmapheresis to repetitively remove cholesterol is the treatment of choice. We still use plasma exchange [6] but more recent developments [7] include double filtration, dextran sulphate adsorption, and immuno-affinity column perfusion, as well as extracorporeal lipoprotein precipitation. Although plasmapheresis is effective in improving clinical manifestations [8], aortic stenosis gradients [9], and survival [10], it is not always met with complete success. Typically, in our center where we exchange about 1.5 times the plasma volume, the postplasmapheresis LDL cholesterol concentration is about 3 mM/L (115 mg/dL) and rises during a fortnight to about 12 mM/L (450mg/dL). Unless plasmapheresis can be done at shorter intervals, additional measures should be sought to improve cholesterol control and curb atherosclerosis.

Drug therapy aimed at modifying the lipoprotein abnormality in homozygous FH has been disappointing. Consideration of the classical lipoprotein pathway indicates that drugs are unlikely to dramatically modify LDL concentration. A constant secretion of VLDL from the liver occurs into plasma before it is converted through intermediate density lipoproteins to LDL. A reduction of LDL receptor activity reduces the uptake of intermediate density lipoproteins and favors their conversion to LDL, the concentration of which is also increased by diminished clearance. Both HMG-CoA reductase inhibitors and bile acid sequestrants are thought to act by depleting the intrahepatic cholesterol so that there is upregulation of the LDL receptor. In heterozygous FH, the diminished *de novo* synthesis due to HMG-CoA reductase inhibitors results in upregulation of normal and abnormal LDL receptor alleles and thus the LDL concentration will diminish. In the homozygote both LDL receptor alleles represent nonfunctional receptors so that it is reasonable to assume that HMG-CoA reductase inhibitors will not be effective. For similar reasons, bile acid sequestrants are also not expected to be effective in homozygous FH. The use of probucol has been associated with improvement of xanthomata [11], presumably due to different properties of LDL. Niacin is also relatively ineffective and frequently is poorly tolerated.

We were interested in testing the HMG-CoA reductase inhibitors as auxiliary therapy to plasma exchange for homozygous FH. FH homozygotes with residual LDL receptor activity may have some benefit, as suggested by a study of simvastatin in Cape Town [9], but other mechanisms of action could also apply, especially at more powerful inhibition of *de novo* cholesterol synthesis. There have been reports in animal [12] and human [13] studies that VLDL secretion or composition was altered. Recently, a receptor-negative FH homozygote [14] was described as having a surprising response to an HMG-Co A reductase inhibitor.

Discusssion

We explored the safety and efficacy of simvastatin and more recently, atorvastatin, in homozygous FH. Both are efficient inhibitors of HMG-CoA reductase but atorvastatin has had maximal effects on LDL cholesterol concentration [15]. Although some patients were studied on both drugs, data in one subject receiving auxiliary atorvastatin is illuminating. The study on simvastatin has been published in detail [9] but some important features will be reviewed and contrasted with the atorvastatin study.

The simvastatin study compared the LDL cholesterol concentrations in 6 homozygous FH subjects with a range of residual LDL receptor binding capacities in maximally upregulated cultured skin fibroblasts. These defects ranged from receptor-negative, through low defective receptor status (5-20%), to high defective status (20-30%). The study commenced with 10 mg at night for 6 exchanges, increased to 20 mg at night for the same period, and then the subjects remained on 40 mg for 12 exchanges. One boy, CI, whose mass was half that of the others, was limited to 20 mg at night. LDL cholesterol, calculated by the Friedewald formula [16], was used to assess responses. There seemed to be little impact until the maximum recommended dose of simvastatin was used. There was an improvement in the group's LDL cholesterol concentration before plasma exchange. The average of 18% decrease was significant but reflected quite a range of response. One individual (VDP) decreased his LDL cholesterol concentration by 30% and reacted unexpectedly well in relation to his maximal LDL receptor activity which was "low defective." He may represent an unusual sensitivity. The remainder of the subjects responded in accordance with their LDL receptor binding capacities. The receptor-negative subject appeared insensitive to simvastatin: his LDL cholesterol concentration decreased by 3%, while the subject with the highest LDL binding capacity responded with a 27% decrease which could be regarded as therapeutically useful.

Subject CI from this study, after due wash-out from the simvastatin, has been tested with atorvastatin as auxiliary treatment. The subject again took the drug at night, but the adult dose of 80 mg was taken as he had grown. Three pre-exchange LDL cholesterol concentrations were compared with three values measured after the subject had been on atorvastatin for 4 weeks. There were no adverse effects. The plasma LDL cholesterol concentrations are compared in Figure 1. There was a gratifying reduction of 19% which can be regarded as therapeutically useful. The mechanism(s) of action cannot involve the LDL receptor.

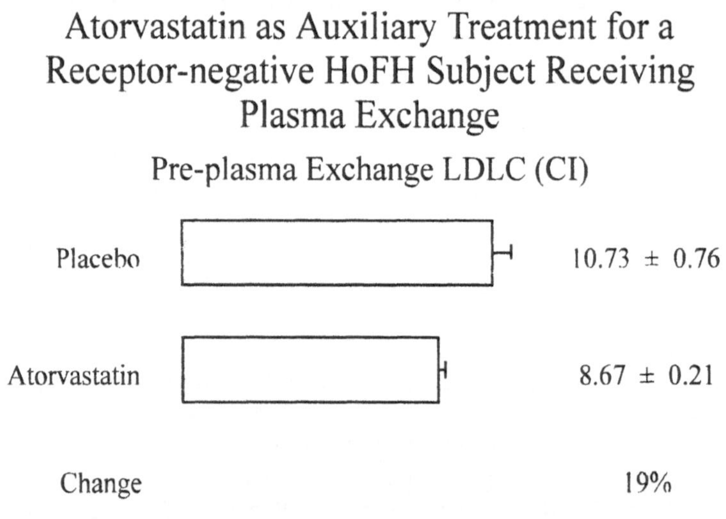

Figure 1. LDL cholesterol response in receptor-negative homozygous FH subject receiving 80 mg of atorvastatin daily. The average and standard deviations of 3 measurements on placebo and the drug are indicated.

We have previously studied plasma mevalonic acid concentration in heterozygous FH subjects on various HMG-CoA reductase inhibitors [17] and found atorvastatin the most powerful: it depressed the early morning fasted-state plasma mevalonic acid concentration by 62%. The average fasted plasma mevalonic acid concentration measured [18] in CI conformed to usual range observed in normal subjects, and decreased by 41% from 4.90 to 2.87 ng/ml. From this result it is inferred that cholesterol synthesis was significantly suppressed by the drug, but it is not clear whether this individual's response is less than expected.

The observed responses to simvastatin and atorvastatin could possibly be explained by their impact on *de novo* synthesis of cholesterol. The overall cholesterol balance of cholesterol in the liver is complex. Fluxes occurring into a cholesterol pool include LDL cholesterol (receptor and/or nonreceptor mediated uptake), *de novo* synthesis, as well as hydrolysis of cholesterol esters. Fluxes out of this pool include bile acid synthesis, direct secretion into bile, and secretion in lipoproteins. It is suggested that, in homozygous FH, LDL receptors are not maximally upregulated even in the face of a marked reduction in the plasma concentration by plasma exchange. Presumably the high concentrations of plasma LDL for even few days before the ensuing plasmapheresis permit cholesterol accumulation in the liver. This may influence lipoprotein production in such a way that more cholesterol is secreted in VLDL or in smaller cholesterol-rich lipoprotein species. Incomplete diurnal suppression of *de novo* synthesis may not deplete cholesterol ester pools but would still result in upregulation of LDL receptors. Atorvastatin, probably by a nearly complete suppression of *de novo* cholesterol synthesis, will additionally influence lipoprotein production because cholesterol ester pools are depleted.

It is tempting to speculate that *de novo* synthesized cholesterol modulates the assembly and/or secretion rates [12] of usual lipoprotein particles or alters their composition and/or metabolism [19]. One subject in our simvastatin study represents an unusual sensitivity to HMG-CoA reductase inhibitors, resembling the unusual reported case [14]. Both cases may have unusually high requirements for *de novo* synthesized cholesterol so that lipoprotein secretion may be profoundly affected by HMG-CoA reductase inhibitors.

In conclusion, HMG-Co A reductase inhibitors may not only influence plasma LDL concentration by modulating LDL receptor activity, but may also influence lipoprotein secretion. Though previously believed to be ineffectual in homozygous FH, these drugs may play a role in their management, as auxiliary agents for plasmapheresis. There may be some unusually sensitive subjects who can currently only be identified by trial. Atorvastatin seems to have a greater efficacy than other currently available HMG-Co A reductase inhibitors and this could be due to a longer period of action.

References

1. Brown MS, Goldstein JL. A receptor-mediated pathway for cholesterol homeostasis. Science 1986;232:34-47.
2. Seftel HC, Baker SG, Sandler MP, et al. A host of hypercholesterolemic homozygotes in South Africa. Br Med J 1980:281:633-36.
3. Gevers W. Three mutations that cause familial hypercholesterolemia in Afrikaners identified - a milestone in South African medicine. S Afr Med J 1989;76:393-94.

4. Rubinsztein DC, van der Westhuyzen DR, Coetzee GA. Monogenic primary hypercholesterolemia in South Africa. S Afr Med J 1994;84:339-44.
5. Hobbs HH, Russell DW, Brown MS, Goldstein JL. The LDL receptor locus in familial hypercholesterolemia: Mutational analysis of a membrane protein. Ann Rev Genet, 1990;24:133-70.
6. Marais AD, Wood L, Firth JC, Hall JM, Jacobs P. Plasma exchange for homozygous familial hypercholesterolemia: The Cape Town experience. Transfus Sci 1993; 14:239-47.
7. Kitano Y, Thompson GR. Role of LDL apheresis in the management of hypercholesterolemia. Transfus Sci 1993;14:269-80.
8. Thompson GR, Myant NB, Kilpatrick D, Oakley CM, Raphael MJ, Steiner RE. Assessment of long-term plasma exchange for familial hypercholesterolemia. Br Heart J 1980;43:680-88.
9. Keller C, Schmitz H, Theisen K, Zollner N. Regression of valvular aortic stenosis due to homozygous familial hypercholesterolemia following plasmapheresis. Klin Wochenschr 1986;64:338-41.
10. Thompson GR, Miller JP, Breslow JL. Improved survival of patients with homozygous familial hypercholesterolemia treated by plasma exchange. Br Med J 1985;291:1671-73.
11. Yamamoto A, Matsuzawa Y, Yokoyama S, Funahashi T, Yamamura T, Kishino B. Effects of probucol on xanthoma regression in familial hypercholesterolemia. Am J Cardiol 1986;57:29H-35H.
12. Khan B, Wilcox HG, Heimberg M. Cholesterol is required for secretion of very-low density lipoprotein by rat liver. Biochem J 1989;259:807-16.
13. Uauy R, Vega GL, Grundy SM, Bilheimer DM. Lovastatin therapy in receptor-negative homozygous familial hypercholesterolemia: Lack of effect on low-density lipoprotein concentrations or turnover. J Pediatr 1988;113:387-92.
14. Feher MD, Webb JC, Patel DD, et al. Cholesterol-lowering drug therapy in a patient with receptor-negative homozygous familial hypercholesterolemia. Atherosclerosis 1993;103:171-80.
15. Nawrocki JW, Weiss SR, Davidson MH, et al. Reduction of LDL cholesterol by 25% to 60% in patients with primary hypercholesterolemia by atorvastatin, a new HMG-CoA reductase inhibitor. Arterioscler Thromb 1995;15:678-82.
16. Friedewald WT, Levy RI, Frederickson DS. Estimation of the concentration of low density lipoprotein cholesterol in plasma, without use of the ultracentrifuge. Clin Chem 1972;18:499-502.
17. Naoumova RP, Marais AD, Firth JC, Rendell NB, Taylor GW, Thompson GR. Plasma mevalonic acid, an index of cholesterol synthesis in vivo and responsiveness to HMG-CoA reductase inhibitors in familial hypercholesterolemia. Atherosclerosis 1996;119:203-13.
18. Scoppola A, Maher VMG, Thompson GR, Rendell NB, Taylor GW. Quantitation of plasma mevalonic acid using gas chromatography-electron capture mass spectrometry. J Lipid Res 1991;32:1057-60.
19. Watts GF, Naoumova R, Cummings MH, et al. Direct correlation between cholesterol synthesis and hepatic secretion of apoliopoprotein B-100 in normolipidaemic subjects. Metabolism 1995;44:1052-57.

EMERGING EVIDENCE FOR TRIGLYCERIDE AS A RISK FACTOR FOR CORONARY ARTERY DISEASE: A REVIEW OF THE EPIDEMIOLOGIC DATA

Melissa A. Austin and John E. Hokanson*
*Department of Epidemiology, School of Public Health and Community Medicine, Box 357236 and *Division of Metabolism, Endocrinology and Nutrition, Department of Medicine, School of Medicine, Box 356426, University of Washington, Seattle, Washington 98195, USA*

Introduction

Plasma triglyceride has long been implicated as a risk factor for coronary heart disease. The first case-control study by Albrink and Man in 1957 [1] showed that fasting triglyceride levels were increased among coronary heart disease (CHD) cases compared to control subjects. Similarly, the earliest prospective study of triglyceride and ischemic heart disease (IHD) demonstrated increased incidence of IHD among men in the cohort with elevated triglyceride levels at baseline, compared with men with lower levels [2]. However, even in this early study, the authors speculated that the triglyceride association may not have been independent of other plasma lipid levels.

In the decades following these studies, an extensive literature developed examining the role of triglyceride as a risk factor for cardiovascular disease. In a review of these studies, Austin noted that most studies showed a relationship between triglyceride and CHD [3]. However, a number of studies found that this association did not remain statistically significant after controlling for other lipid risk factors, especially high-density lipoprotein (HDL) cholesterol. In reviewing this and other evidence, the National Institutes of Health Consensus Development Panel on Triglyceride, High Density Lipoprotein, and Coronary Heart Disease concluded that, "For triglyceride, the data are mixed, although strong associations are found in some studies, the evidence for a causal relationship [with CHD] is still incomplete" [4]. Similarly, recent data from the Lipid Research Clinics (LRC) follow-up study demonstrated that triglyceride was related to 12-year CHD mortality in both men and women [5], but this relationship was no longer statistically significant after adjustment for covariates. Thus, the role of triglyceride as a risk factor for CHD remains to be fully elucidated.

This chapter will focus on the relationship between triglyceride and cardiovascular disease. First, the semiquantitative techniques of meta-analysis will be applied to population-based, prospective studies of triglyceride and cardiovascular disease (CVD) to estimate of

A. M. Gotto, Jr. et al. (eds.), Drugs Affecting Lipid Metabolism, 187–194.

the strength of this association in the general population, and to evaluate the effect of other risk factors, especially HDL cholesterol [6,7]. Second, the familial forms of hypertriglyceridemia will be reviewed, and ongoing studies of these disorders will be described.

Meta-analysis of Triglyceride and Cardiovascular Disease

Published studies from the literature were selected for the meta-analysis based on several criteria [6]. First, only studies using a prospective study design were selected, insuring that elevations in plasma triglyceride preceded the onset of disease. Second, only studies using population-based samples of study subjects were selected, so that relative risk estimates are as applicable as possible to the general population. Because the results from the LRC follow-up study [5] were based on a sample enriched with hyperlipidemic subjects, the relative risks for this analysis were adjusted for ascertainment (hyperlipidemic versus random sample) based on results kindly provided by Dr. M.H. Criqui (personal communication). To exclude the possibility of postprandial effects, only studies evaluating fasting triglyceride levels were included. Each study cohort was included only once in the analysis, using the publication reporting the longest follow-time. Both fatal and nonfatal cardiovascular endpoints were included, although most studies focused on myocardial infarction or CHD death. Finally, only Caucasian study subjects were included in the analysis, since little data is currently available on other ethnic groups.

A total of seventeen studies conforming to these selection criteria were identified [2,5,8-24], including sixteen studies representing 2,445 events among 46,413 men followed for an average of 8.4 years, and five studies representing 439 events among 10,864 women followed for an average 11.4 years. Study subjects ranged in age from 15 to 81 years old in all the studies. Among men, six studies were from the USA, six from Scandinavian countries, and one each from France, Germany, Italy, and the United Kingdom. Among women, three studies were from the USA and two from Scandinavia.

The meta-analysis was performed separately for men and women using the techniques described by Greenland [7]. Briefly, relative risk (RR) estimates are determined for each individual study by calculating β, the estimated slope from logistic regression analysis, standardized to a 1 mmol/L increase in triglyceride. To determine the statistical significance of the association and to calculate confidence intervals (CI), the variance of β is next computed. The β value for each study is then weighted by the inverse of the variance, reflecting both the sample size of size and follow-up time of study. Finally, the weighted β values are averaged and converted to the summary RR value, so that the larger the study and the longer the follow-up time, the greater its contribution to the summary RR. These procedures result in the <u>univariate summary RR</u> for the association between triglyceride and CVD. To determine the effect of covariates on this estimate, the same procedures were used to estimate the <u>multivariate summary RR</u> using the six studies that included HDL cholesterol as a covariate [5,8,16,20,22,23]. Of these studies, four also included adjustment for age, four for total cholesterol, two for LDL cholesterol, four for smoking, six for body mass index, and five for blood pressure. To maximize the potential effects on the multivariate summary RR, all these covariate adjustments were included in the analysis.

As shown in Figure 1, univariate RR estimates for cardiovascular disease associated with a 1 mmol/L increase in triglyceride ranged from 1.07 to 1.98 for men with a summary RR of 1.32 (95% CI 1.26-1.39). This indicates a 32% increase in disease risk associated with triglyceride. Among the five prospective studies in women, individual RR estimates for triglyceride ranged from 1.69 to 2.05 (Figure 1), all of which were statistically significant. The summary univariate RR was higher for women than men, 1.76 (95% CI 1.50-2.07), although the confidence interval is somewhat wider due to the smaller sample size (approximately 10,800 women). Thus, a 1 mmol/L increase in triglyceride was associated with a 76% increase in risk of incident cardiovascular disease in women. Because only population-based studies were included, the summary relative risk estimates derived from this analysis provide the best available overall estimates for relationship between triglyceride and CVD.

It has long been noted that triglyceride is a more potent risk factor in Scandinavian countries than in other countries [3], and meta-analysis allows a quantitative comparison of RR risk values in different geographic locations. Among men, RR values were 1.49, 1.25, and 1.34 for studies conducted in Scandinavia, other countries in Europe, and the USA, respectively (all $p < 0.05$). Among studies in women, RR values were also higher in Scandinavian countries than in the USA, 2.02 and 1.71, respectively. Thus, in both men and women, univariate RRs are indeed higher for studies conducted in Scandinavian countries compared to studies conducted elsewhere.

As expected, multivariate RR estimates with adjustment for HDL cholesterol were attenuated. For men, the multivariate RRs for triglyceride ranged from 0.98 to 1.39 with the summary RR of 1.14 being statistically significant (95% confidence interval 1.05-1.28). In women, the summary multivariate RR was higher than for men, with a value of 1.37 (95% CI 1.13-1.66). Thus, even after adjustment for HDL cholesterol, a statistically significant increase in risk of incident cardiovascular disease was associated with triglyceride for both men and women. Importantly, studies conducted in Scandinavia, in which univariate RRs are highest, are not included in these multivariate RRs since HDL cholesterol adjustments were not reported. Thus, the multivariate RRs reported here for triglyceride are likely to be conservative. Furthermore, when an external adjustment procedure is used to evaluate the confounding effect of HDL cholesterol among those not reporting adjustment for this variable [7], the multivariate summary RR was 1.22 (95% CI 1.15-1.29) for men and 1.44 (95% CI 1.23-169) in women (Figure 2).

To summarize, based on all the available data from population-based, prospective studies, meta-analysis shows that increases in plasma triglyceride are associated with a significant increase in risk of incident cardiovascular disease among both men and women. In men, an increase of 1 mmol/L was associated with a 32% increase in risk of disease. A higher, 76% increased risk, was found in women. Based on data from studies that reported adjustment for HDL cholesterol and other risk factors, multivariate RR estimates were attenuated, but were still statistically significant, representing a 14% increase in risk for men and a 37% increase in risk for women. Importantly, because only population-based studies

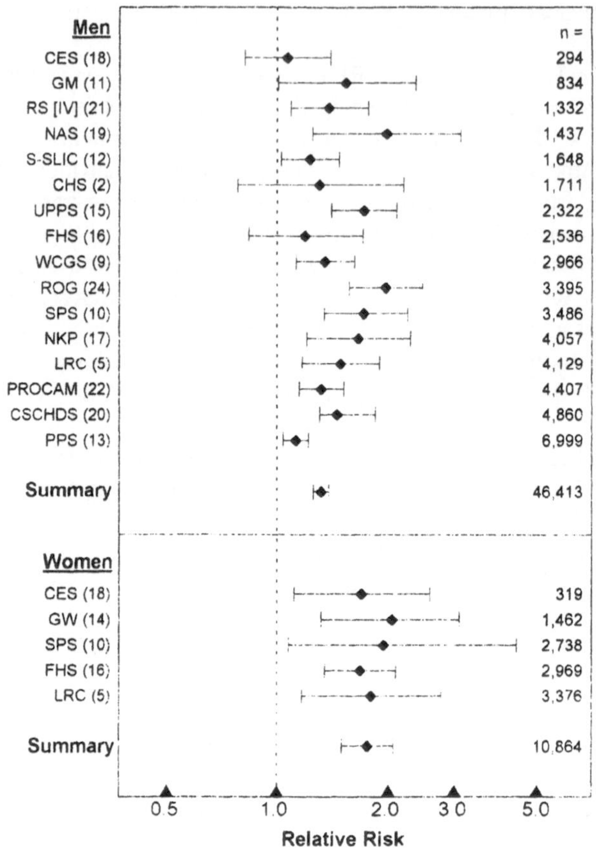

Figure 1. Univariate relative risk estimates and 95% confidence intervals for the association between incident cardiovascular disease and a 1 mmol/L increase in triglyceride, by gender. Relative risk values are given on the X-axis on a natural logarithm scale. The Y-axis lists each study included in the meta-analysis and reference numbers, ordered by sample size, and the summary relative risk. A relative risk of 1.0 (vertical dotted line) represents no association, and confidence intervals that do not cover 1.0 indicate relative risks that are statistically significant at the p = 0.05 level. Study abbreviations: CHS, Cardiovascular Health Center [2]; WCGS, Western Collaborative Health Study [8,9]; SPS, Stockholm Prospective Study [10]; GM, Men Born in 1913 Study [11]; S-SLIC, Suomi-Salama Life Insurance Cohort [12]; PPS, Paris Prospective Study [13]; WG, Study of Women in Gothenburg [14]; UPPS, Uppsala Primary Preventive Study [15]; FHS, Framingham Heart Study [16]; NKP, North Karelia Project [17]; CES, Cardiovascular Epidemiology Study [18]; NAS, Normative Aging Study [19]; CSCHDS, Caerphilly and Speedwell Collaborative Heart Disease Studies [20]; RS(IV), Reykjavik Study, Stage IV [21]; PROCAM, Prospective Cardiovascular Munster Study [22]; ROG, Rome Occupational Groups [23,24]; LRC, Lipid Research Clinics Follow-up Study [5]. Figure adapted from reference [6].

were included in the analysis, these results provide the best available estimates of triglyceride risk in the general population. Therefore, triglyceride is a risk factor for cardiovascular disease, independent of HDL cholesterol.

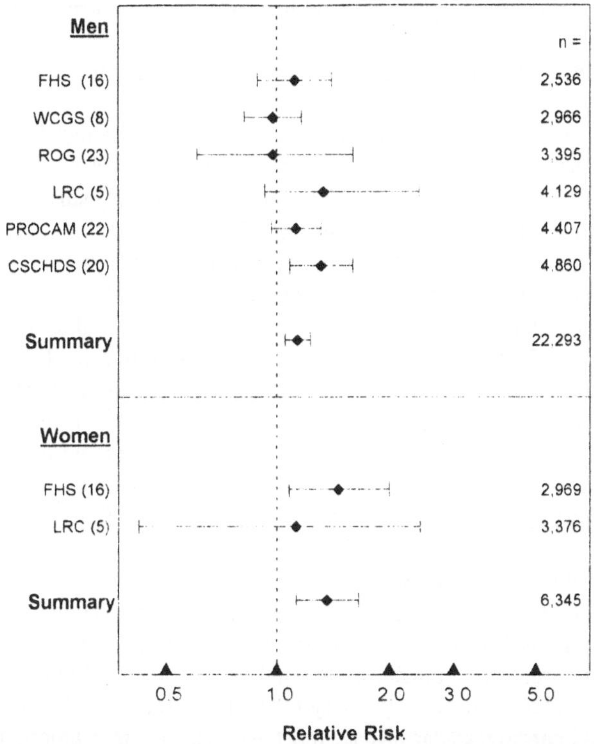

Figure 2. Multivariate-adjusted relative risk estimates and 95% confidence intervals for the association between incident cardiovascular disease and a 1 mmol/L increase in triglyceride, by gender, for those studies that adjusted for HDL cholesterol. Relative risk values are given on the X-axis on a natural logarithm scale. The Y-axis lists each study included in the meta-analysis and reference numbers, ordered by sample size, and the summary relative risk. Note that a relative risk of 1.0 (vertical dotted line) represents no association, and confidence intervals that do not cover 1.0 indicate relative risks that are statistically significant at the $p = 0.05$ level. See Figure 1 for study abbreviations. Figure adapted from reference [6].

However, as demonstrated by the attenuated multivariate RR estimates, a major proportion of the risk of CVD attributable to triglyceride is accounted for by HDL cholesterol, body mass index, blood pressure, and possibly other risk factors. Austin et al.

[25] have proposed an "Atherogenic Lipoprotein Phenotype" characterized by small, dense LDL, increased triglyceride, and lower HDL cholesterol. The insulin resistance syndrome [26] is characterized by a similar constellation of abnormal lipids, glucose intolerance, and hypertension, as well as insulin resistance itself. These complex metabolic syndromes that include plasma triglyceride suggest that the search for "independent" risk factors may mask the multifactorial nature of the pathophysiology involved. Rather, it may be useful to combine these correlated risk factors into a small number of composite variables using multivariate factor analysis [27] to elucidate the underlying disease mechanisms.

Familial Forms of Hypertriglyceridemia and Coronary Heart Disease

The two familial forms of hypertriglyceridemia, familial "monogenic" hypertriglyceridemia (FHTG) and familial combined hyperlipidemia (FCHL) were first characterized by Goldstein and colleagues based on families of myocardial infarction (MI) survivors [28]. FHTG is characterized by familial aggregation of elevated plasma triglyceride levels in relatives, but with normal plasma cholesterol values. In contrast, relatives in families with FCHL have elevated triglyceride, elevated cholesterol or both, and these lipid phenotypes can vary over time. These two familial disorders were the most common in families of the MI survivors, with a prevalence of 16% and 32%, respectively. Importantly, both disorders were associated with increased risk of coronary heart disease in relatives of the probands.

Brunzell and colleagues further characterized these disorders based on families with familial aggregation of hypertriglyceridemia, regardless of CVD status [29]. In contrast to the Goldstein studies, only FCHL hyperlipidemic relatives were at increased risk. On the basis of these findings, FCHL is thought to be associated with familial risk of CHD, while FHTG is not.

However, this conclusion remains to be confirmed prospectively, and the underlying genetic basis of these disorders is not yet understood. The "Genetic Epidemiology of Triglyceride" (GET Study), is currently in progress to follow-up these families after more than 20 years to address these questions. A total of 108 extended kindreds from both sets of families are included, with three primary goals. First, the study will determine whether total mortality and cardiovascular disease mortality are increased among relatives in these two types of families, as well as evaluating the relationship between of triglyceride levels at baseline in relation to subsequent mortality. Second, the genetic epidemiology of a variety of lipoprotein-related risk factors are being evaluated based on new blood samples from surviving family members. Since FCHL and FHTG may be heterogeneous, these analyses may lead to refinement of the lipoprotein phenotypes that characterize these disorders. Finally, a repository of DNA is being developed for studies to determine the genetic basis of these common triglyceride-related familial disorders.

Summary and Conclusions

In conclusion, meta-analysis of data from population-based prospective studies demonstrates that increased plasma triglyceride is associated with a 32% increase in risk of cardiovascular disease in men and a 76% increase in risk among women. After adjustment for HDL cholesterol and other risk factors, these risks were reduced to 14% in men and 37% increase in women, but remained statistically significant. These results, based on more than 46,000 men and 10,800 women, show that plasma triglyceride is an independent risk factor for cardiovascular disease. However, few of studies have included women and non-Caucasian ethnic groups and more data is urgently needed in these populations. Furthermore, better understanding of the familial forms of hypertriglyceridemia will be important in determining how triglyceride may be involved in genetic susceptibility to CHD.

Acknowledgements

This work was supported by NIH Program Project Grant HL30086 and by NIH R01 Grant HL45913, and was performed during Dr. Austin's tenure as an Established Investigator of the American Heart Association.

References

1. Albrink MJ, Man EB. Serum triglycerides in coronary artery disease. Arch Intern Med 1959;103:4-8.
2. Brown DF, Kinch SH, Doyle JT. Serum triglycerides in health and in ischemic heart disease. N Engl J Med 1965; 273:947-52.
3. Austin MA. Plasma triglyceride and coronary heart disease. Arterioscler Thromb 1991;11:2-14.
4. NIH Consensus Development Panel on Triglyceride, High Density Lipoprotein, and Coronary Heart Disease. Triglyceride, high density lipoprotein, and coronary heart disease. JAMA 1993;269:505-10.
5. Criqui MH, Heiss G, Cohn R, et al. Plasma triglyceride level and mortality from coronary heart disease. N Engl J Med 1993;328:1220-25.
6. Hokanson JE, Austin MA. Plasma triglyceride is a risk factor for cardiovascular disease independent of high-density lipoprotein cholesterol. A meta-analysis of population-based prospective studies. J Cardiovasc Risk, in press.
7. Greenland S. Quantitative methods in the review of epidemiologic literature. Epidemiol Rev 1987;9:1-30.
8. Hulley SB, Rosenman RH, Bawol RD, Brand RJ. Epidemiology as a guide to clinical decisions. The association between triglyceride and coronary heart disease. N Engl J Med 1980;302:1383-89.
9. Rosenman RH, Brand RJ, Jenkins CD, Friedman M, Straus R, Wurm M. Coronary heart disease in the Western Collaborative Group Study. Final follow-up experience of 8 1/2 years. JAMA 1975;233:872-77.
10. Bottinger LE, Carlson LA. Risk factors for death for males and females. A study of death pattern in the Stockholm Prospective Study. Acta Med Scand 1982;211:437-42.
11. Wilhelmsen L, Wedel H, Tibblin G. Multivariate analysis of risk factors for coronary heart disease. Circulation 1973;XLVIII:950-58.
12. Pelkonen R, Nikkilä EA, Koskinen S, Penttinen K, Sarna S. Association of serum lipids and obesity with cardiovascular mortality. BMJ 1977;2:1185-87.

13. Cambien F, Jacqueson A, Richard JL, Warnet JM, Ducimetiere P, Claude JR. Is the level of serum triglyceride a significant predictor of coronary death in "normocholesterolemic" subjects? The Paris Prospective Study. Am J Epidemiol 1986;124:624-32.
14. Bengtsson C, Bjorkelund C, Lapidus L, Lissner L. Association of serum lipid concentrations and obesity with mortality in women: 20 year follow-up of participants in prospective population study in Gothenburg, Sweden. BMJ 1993; 307:1385-88.
15. Åberg H, Lithell H, Selinus I, Hedstrand H. Serum triglycerides are a risk factor for myocardial infarction but not for angina pectoris. Results from a 10-year follow-up of Uppsala Primary Preventive Study. Atherosclerosis 1985;54:89-97.
16. Wilson P, Larson G, Castelli W. Triglycerides, HDL-cholesterol and coronary artery disease: A Framingham update on the interactions. Can J Cardiol 1994;10(lB):5B-9B.
17. Salonen JT, Puska P. Relation of serum cholesterol and triglycerides to the risk of acute myocardial infarction, cerebral stroke and death in eastern Finnish male population. In J Epidemiol 1983;12:26-31.
18. Heyden S, Heiss G, Hames CG, Bartel AG. Fasting triglycerides as predictors of total and CHD mortality in Evans County, Georgia. J Chron Dis 1980;33:275-82.
19. Glynn RJ, Rosner B, Silbert JE. Changes in cholesterol and triglyceride as predictors of ischemic heart disease. Circulation 1982;66:724-31.
20. Bainton D, Miller NE, Bolton CH, et al. Plasma triglyceride and high density lipoproteins cholesterol as predictors of ischaemic heart disease in British men. The Caerphilly and Speedwell Collaborative Heart Disease Studies. Br Heart J 1992; 68:60-66.
21. Sigurdsson G, Baldursdottir, Sigvaldason H, Agnarsson U, Thorgeirsson G, Sigfusson N. Predictive value of apolipoproteins in a prospective survey of coronary artery disease in men. Am J Cardiol 1992;69:1251-54.
22. Assmann G, Schulte H. Relation of high-density lipoprotein cholesterol and triglyceride to incidence of atherosclerotic coronary artery disease (the PROCAM experience). Am J Cardiol 1992;70:733-27.
23. Menotti A, Spagnolo A, Scanga M, Dima F. Multivariate prediction of coronary disease deaths in a 10 year follow-up of an Italian occupational male cohort. Acta Cardiologica 1992;XLVII:311-20.
24. Menotti A, Scanga M, Morisi G. Serum triglycerides in the prediction of coronary artery disease (an Italian experience). Am J Cardiol 1994;73:29-32.
25. Austin MA, King M-C, Vranizan KM, Krauss RM. Atherogenic lipoprotein phenotype. A proposed genetic marker for coronary heart disease risk. Circulation 1990;82:495-506.
26. Reaven G. Role of insulin resistance in human disease. Diabetes 1988;37:1595-1607.
27. Edwards KL, Austin MA, Newman B, Mayer E, Krauss RM, Selby JV. Multivariate analysis of the insulin resistance syndrome. Arterioscler Thromb 1994;14:1940-45.
28. Goldstein JL, Schrott HG, Hazzard WR, Bierman EL, Motulsky AG. Hyperlipidemia in coronary heart disease. II. Genetic analysis in 176 families and delineation of a new inherited disorder, combined hyperlipidemia. J Clin Invest 1973;52:1544-68.
29. Brunzell JD, Schrott HG, Motulsky AG, Bierman EL. Myocardial infarction in the familial forms of hypertriglyceridemia. Metabolism 1976;25:313-20.

TRIGLYCERIDES ARE INDEPENDENTLY PREDICTIVE OF THE EXTENT OF CORONARY ATHEROSCLEROSIS

Heinz Drexel[1], Jörg Muntwyler[1], Jan Beran[3], Hansruedi Schmid[2], Theo Gasser[3], and Franz W. Amann[1]
[1]The Division of Cardiology, Department of Medicine, and [2]the Institute of Clinical Chemistry, University Hospital Zurich, and [3]the Department of Biostatistics, Institute of Social and Preventive Medicine, University of Zurich, Zurich, Switzerland

Introduction

The plasma concentrations of cholesterol and of its main component, low density lipoprotein (LDL)-cholesterol, are established risk factors for the incidence of atherosclerotic vascular complications [1]. Epidemiologic studies also have consistently demonstrated that plasma concentrations of high density lipoprotein (HDL)-cholesterol levels are inversely correlated with the incidence of coronary artery disease [2,3].

A long standing debate is to what extent triglycerides contribute to the risk of atherosclerosis. In cross-sectional studies triglycerides show a univariate association with clinical events from coronary artery disease, and this association persists after taking cholesterol or LDL-cholesterol into account [4]. However, in prospective studies controlling also for HDL-cholesterol concentration, triglycerides are eliminated as an independent risk factor in most studies [4].

Clinical events (and mortality) may be suboptimal endpoints to assess atherogenicity because they represent the last step in a cascade of events triggered by atherogenic and thrombogenic factors; thrombogenic factors ultimately determine whether or not infarction occurs [5,6]. Therefore, the incidence of myocardial infarctions is related to both thrombogenicity and atherosclerosis. Angiography preferentially assesses atherosclerosis. The status of triglycerides as an atherogenic risk factor independent from LDL-cholesterol and HDL-cholesterol has not been assessed by angiography. We therefore studied the relations of LDL-cholesterol, HDL_2-cholesterol, HDL_3-cholesterol, and triglycerides to the extent of coronary atherosclerosis in 500 angiographied patients.

A. M. Gotto, Jr. et al. (eds.), Drugs Affecting Lipid Metabolism, 195–201.

Methods

PATIENT SELECTION

The study group comprised consecutive patients undergoing elective coronary angiography for evaluation of established or suspected coronary artery disease (CAD). Details are given elsewhere [7]. Five hundred patients (418 men and 82 women) were enrolled in the study.

CORONARY ANGIOGRAPHY

Selective coronary angiograms were obtained using the Judkins or Sones technique. For quantitative evaluation of atherosclerosis, the coronary circulation was divided into 12 segments [7]. CAD was determined by extent, which was defined as the number of ≥ 50% stenoses. A total of 1,006 significant lesions were documented. In 105 patients no significant stenoses were found. This proportion of patients without angiographic lesions (75 out of 444 or 17%) compares well with a large angiographic study on lipids [8].

LIPID AND LIPOPROTEIN MEASUREMENTS

After a supervised overnight fast of 12 to 13 hours and after complete abstinence from ethanol for at least 24 hours, venous blood was collected from an antecubital vein. HDL-, HDL_2-, and HDL_3-cholesterol were determined using a stepwise precipitation procedure with dextran sulfate [9]. Non-HDL-cholesterol was found by subtracting HDL-cholesterol from total plasma cholesterol. LDL-cholesterol and very low density lipoprotein (VLDL)-cholesterol were calculated using Friedewald's formula [10]. Further details have been described previously [7,11].

STATISTICS

The extent of coronary atherosclerosis varied between 0 and 10 lesions. To obtain statistically sensible results, we distinguished the following four categories: category 1, no lesions; category 2, 1 to 3 lesions; category 3, 4 to 6 lesions; and category 4, 7 to 10 lesions, respectively. By stepwise ordinal polychotomous regression analysis, extent of disease was investigated for associations with the factors total cholesterol, LDL-cholesterol, HDL_2-cholesterol, HDL_3-cholesterol, VLDL-cholesterol, non-HDL-cholesterol, triglycerides, apolipoprotein B, age, and gender [12]. The limits (p values) for entering or removing a factor were set to 0.1 and 0.15, respectively. The term HDL-cholesterol was not included into stepwise regression models because HDL-cholesterol represents the exact sum of HDL_2-cholesterol and HDL_3-cholesterol and therefore contains all the variability of the two subfractions.

Results

From the 500 patients enrolled in the study, 56 were excluded from analysis because they were taking lipid lowering drugs. From the remaining 444 subjects, 339 had one or more significant (≥ 50%) coronary lesions (CAD+); 105 were free of such lesions (CAD-). Table 1 lists the demographic characteristics of these two patient groups. As expected, the proportion of smokers was higher in CAD+ patients than in CAD- patients. By contrast, there were no significant differences with respect to age, body mass index, systolic or diastolic blood pressure, or alcohol intake.

Table 1. Demographic characteristics of patients with (CAD+) and without (CAD-) significant coronary lesions*.

Characteristic	CAD+	CAD-
No. of Patients	339	105
Age (yrs)	58 ± 0.5	58 ± 1.0
Sex Distribution (M/F)	302/37	66/39
BMI ($kg.m^{-2}$)	25.9 ± 0.2	25.3 ± 0.3
Systolic Blood Pressure (mm Hg)	129 ± 1	133 ± 2
Diastolic Blood Pressure (mm Hg)	80 ± 1	83 ± 1
Smokers (%)	70	51
Ethanol Intake ≥ 5g/day (%)	56	54

* (mean ± SEM unless stated)

The results of the stepwise polychotomous logistic regression demonstrate a significant independent association with disease extent for all three cholesterol subfractions, LDL-, HDL_2-, and HDL_3-cholesterol, as well as for age and gender (Table 2). However, the stepwise procedure also included triglycerides and apolipoprotein B. The contribution to the model was highly significant for triglycerides ($p = 0.005$) but not for apolipoprotein B ($p = 0.078$). An increase in age by 10 years increased the risk for falling into a higher category of CAD extent by an approximate factor of 1.6 (95% confidence interval 1.34-2.01), provided that all other factors were kept constant. The same increase was obtained by increasing LDL-cholesterol by about 36 mg/dL, or by increasing plasma triglycerides by about 88 mg/dL. The amounts of HDL_2-cholesterol and HDL_3-cholesterol by which this increase would be compensated, were -8 mg/dL and -18 mg/dL, respectively. Average for total HDL-cholesterol was -12 mg/dL.

Table 2. Relation of risk factors to the extent of coronary atherosclerosis.

Factor	β_i*	SD	β_i/SD#
LDL-Cholesterol	0.5371	0.192	2.79
HDL_2-Cholesterol	-2.432	-0.958	2.54
HDL_3-Cholesterol	-1.067	0.506	-2.11
Triglycerides	0.4899	0.176	2.79
Age	0.0493	0.010	4.76
Gender§	-1.124	0.284	-3.96
Apo B	1.190	0.675	1.76

* a positive coefficient indicates that the corresponding factor tends to increase the number of lesions, a negative factor indicates that the factor tends to decrease the number of lesions.
§ (male=0, female=1)
# This column measures how strongly significant the corresponding effect is (if the term is ≥ 1.96 in absolute value, the effect is significant at the 5%-level).

This formula can be adopted to estimate the potential vascular benefit of lipid lowering drugs. For example, a typical response to gemfibrozil, i.e. a reduction of triglycerides from 360 to 260 mg/dL, reduction of LDL-cholesterol from 160 to 150, and an increase of HDL-cholesterol from 30 to 35 mg/dL, respectively, indicates 3-, 10-, and 5-year equivalents, i.e. a total of 18-year equivalents of potential vascular benefit. Likewise, changes induced by pravastatin (a decrease of LDL-cholesterol from 200 to 140 and of triglycerides from 160 to 150, and an increase of HDL-cholesterol from 50 to 55 mg/dL, respectively) indicates 15+1+5, i.e. 21-year equivalents of potential vascular benefit.

Discussion

Extent is a sensitive marker of coronary atherosclerosis because every stenosis represents a separate endpoint. This study documented 1,006 endpoints, four-to-eight times more than reported from large prospective studies [13]. Three fractions of blood cholesterol (LDL-cholesterol, HDL_2-cholesterol, and HDL_3-cholesterol) were strongly and independently related to the angiographic extent of coronary atherosclerosis.

Our finding of a strong independent predictive power of LDL-cholesterol, HDL_2-, and HDL_3-cholesterol, respectively, for the extent of coronary atherosclerosis has been discussed in detail [11,14,15].

Apart from age, gender, and the three cholesterol subfractions, triglycerides emerged as a significant and independent predictor for the extent of coronary atherosclerosis. It fits well into this notion that hypertriglyceridemia is frequently encountered in diabetic patients [4] in whom extent of coronary atherosclerosis is greater than in nondiabetics and related to triglyceride levels [16]. However, a very sensitive tool is required to prove this association of triglycerides with disease extent also for nondiabetics who have a lower prevalence of hypertriglyceridemia. From the three published angiographic studies where triglyceride levels were adjusted for HDL-cholesterol, the triglyceride association with disease extent remained significant in two [17,18] but did not in one [19]. However, none of them studied HDL subfraction cholesterol together with triglycerides.

Because of the correlation between HDL-cholesterol and triglycerides, in most studies, triglycerides are eliminated as an independent risk factor when HDL-cholesterol is included in multiple logistic models [4]. A widely held view therefore is that high triglycerides are not directly atherogenic but act via decreased HDL levels. In contrast, our data point to a role for triglycerides to increase disease extent independently from HDL and LDL. The theoretical possibility that triglycerides are only an indicator of the atherogenicity residing in the cholesterol of triglyceride-rich particles can be excluded because VLDL-cholesterol was not a significant variable in the statistical model.

One mechanism to explain an intrinsic atherogenicity of triglycerides is that high plasma triglyceride levels drive core lipid exchange between lipoproteins. Triglycerides are thereby transferred from triglyceride-rich lipoproteins to LDL in exchange with cholesteryl esters [20]. Subsequently, the triglyceride of LDL is hydrolyzed by lipoprotein lipase and/or hepatic lipase, which reduces size and increases density of these LDL. Small, dense LDL are the hallmark of the LDL subclass pattern B also known as the "atherogenic lipoprotein phenotype" [21]. This is present in about 30% of the population [4] and confers a high risk for myocardial infarction [22]. In this context, triglycerides can be viewed as molecules that toxify LDL. This interpretation is consistent with the data from the PROCAM study [23] where, among individuals with a LDL/HDL cholesterol ratio > 5.0, hypertriglyceridemia proved a powerful additional risk factor for atherosclerotic events.

The design of our study with its high number of endpoints also enabled us to compare reliably the power of the risk factors age, LDL-cholesterol, triglycerides, and of the protective factors HDL_2-cholesterol and HDL_3-cholesterol. Ten years of age had the same effect on CAD extent as an increase of 36 mg/dL in LDL-cholesterol or of 88 mg/dL in triglycerides and equalled the protective effect of 8 mg/dL of HDL_2-cholesterol or of 18 mg/dL of HDL_3 cholesterol. No such data on the relative power of these risk factors have been reported so far except that one study compared the effect of LDL-cholesterol and HDL-cholesterol (without subfraction analysis) on total cardiovascular mortality: An increase in LDL-cholesterol of 30 mg/dl was found equivalent to a decrease in HDL-cholesterol of 10 mg/dl in men [24]. These numbers compare well to our risk ratios. We used 12 mg/dL for total HDL-cholesterol as the equivalent. If the above formula is adopted to typical lipid effects induced by fibrates or inhibitors of HMG-CoA reductase, it is evident that both classes of compounds provide a similar potential vascular benefit, 18- and 21-year equivalents, respectively, in our examples.

Acknowledgement

Supported by grant Nr. 32-33867.92 from the Swiss National Science Foundation and grants from Merck Sharp & Dohme-Chibret AG, Glattbrugg, Switzerland.

References

1. Goldstein JL, Kita T, Brown MS. Defective lipoprotein receptors and atherosclerosis: Lessons from an animal counterpart of familial hypercholesterolemia. N Engl J Med 1983;309:288-96.
2. Miller GJ, Miller NE. Plasma high-density lipoprotein concentration and development of ischemic heart disease. Lancet 1975;i:16-19.
3. Gordon DJ, Rifkind BM. High density lipoprotein - the clinical implication of recent studies. N Engl J Med 1989;321:1311-16.
4. Austin MA. Plasma triglyceride and coronary artery disease. Arterioscler Thromb 1991;11:2-13.
5. Fuster V, Badimon L, Badimon JJ, Chesebro JH. The pathogenesis of coronary artery disease and the acute coronary syndromes. N Engl J Med 1992;326:242-50.
6. Fuster V, Badimon L, Badimon JJ, Chesebro JH. The pathogenesis of coronary artery disease and the acute coronary syndromes. N Engl J Med 1992;326:310-18.
7. Drexel H, Amann FW, Rentsch K, et al. Relation of the level of high-density lipoprotein subfractions to the presence and extent of coronary artery disease. Am J Cardiol 1992;70:436-40.
8. Gotto AM, Gorry GA, Thompson JR, et al. Relationship between plasma lipid concentrations and coronary artery disease in 496 patients. Circulation 1977;56:875-83.
9. Warnick GR, Benderson J, Albers JJ. Quantitation of high-density-lipoprotein subclasses after separation by dextran sulfate and Mg2+ precipitation. (Abstract) Clin Chem 1982;28:74.
10. Friedewald WT, Levy RI, Fredrickson DS. Estimation of the concentration of low-density lipoprotein cholesterol in plasma without use of the preparative ultracentrifuge. Clin Chem 1972;18:499-502.
11. Drexel H, Amann FW, Beran J, et al. Plasma triglycerides and three lipoprotein cholesterol fractions are independent predictors of the extent of coronary atherosclerosis. Circulation, 1994;90:2230-35.
12. Hosmer DW, Lemeshow S. Applied logistic regression. New York: John Wiley & Sons, 1989:216-38.
13. Klag MJ, Ford DE, Mean LA, et al. Serum cholesterol in young men and subsequent cardiovascular disease. N Engl J Med 1993;328:313-18.
14. Phillips NR, Waters D, Havel RJ. Plasma lipoproteins and progression of coronary artery disease evaluated by angiography and clinical events. Circulation 1993; 88:2762-70.
15. Quinn MT, Parthasarathy S, Fong LG, Steinberg D. Oxidatively modified low density lipoproteins: A potential role in recruitment and retention of monocyte/ macrophages during atherogenesis. Proc Natl Acad Sci USA 1987;84:2995-98.
16. Hambly RI, Sherman L, Mehta J, Aintablian A. Reappraisal of the role of the diabetic state in coronary artery disease. Chest 1976;70:251-57.
17. Kukita H, Imamura Y, Hamada M, Joh T, Kokubu T. Plasma lipids and lipoproteins in Japanese male patients with coronary artery disease and in their relatives. Atherosclerosis 1982;42:21-29.

18. Barbir M, Wile D, Trayner I, Aber VR, Thompson GR. High prevalence of hypertriglyceridemia and apolipoprotein abnormalities in coronary artery disease. Br Heart J 1988;60:397-03.
19. Freedman DS, Gruchow HW, Anderson AJ, Rimm AA, Barboriak JJ. Relation of triglyceride levels to coronary artery disease: The Milwaukee Cardiovascular Data Registry. Am J Epidemiol 1988;127:1118-30.
20. Tall AR. Plasma lipid transfer proteins. J Lipid Res 1986;27:361-67.
21. Austin MA, King M-C, Vranizan KM, Krauss RM. Atherogenic lipoprotein phenotype: A proposed genetic marker for coronary heart disease risk. Circulation 1990;82:495-06.
22. Austin MA, Breslow JL, Hennekens CH, Buring JE, Willett WC, Krauss RM. Low density lipoprotein subclass patterns and risk of myocardial infarction. JAMA 1988;260:1917-21.
23. Assmann G, Schulte H. Role of triglycerides in coronary artery disease: Lessons from the Prospective Cardiovascular Münster Study. Am J Cardiol 1992;70:10H-13H.
24. Jacobs DR Jr, Mebane IL, Bangdiwala SI, Criqui MH, Tyroler HA. High density lipoprotein cholesterol as a predictor of cardiovascular disease mortality in men and women: The follow-up study of the Lipid Research Clinics Prevalence Study. Am J Epidemiol 1990;131:32-47.

TRIGLYCERIDES AS A RISK FACTOR FOR CORONARY HEART DISEASE: EPIDEMIOLOGIC STUDIES AND CLINICAL TRIALS

Michael H. Criqui
University of California, San Diego, School of Medicine, Departments of Family and Preventive Medicine and Medicine, 9500 Gilman Drive, La Jolla, California 92093-0607, USA

Epidemiologic Studies

Despite extensive analysis in numerous studies, controversy persists as to whether triglycerides are an independent risk factor for coronary heart disease (CHD). A new meta-analysis by Hokanson and Austin summarizes the information on triglycerides as a risk factor for cardiovascular disease (CVD) in population-based prospective studies [1]. The authors reviewed 16 studies in men: six from the USA, six from Scandinavia, and four from elsewhere in Europe. The univariate relative risk (RR) per mmol/liter of triglycerides in men was 1.32, with a 95% confidence interval (CI) of 1.26-1.39. Only six of these studies adjusted for the key covariate of high density lipoprotein (HDL) cholesterol. In these six studies the multivariate RR for triglycerides was attenuated to 1.14, but this result was still statistically significant, with a 95% CI of 1.05-1.28. Five studies in women (three from the USA and two from Scandinavia) gave a univariate RR per mmol/liter of triglycerides of 1.76, 95% CI 1.50-2.07, a stronger result than for men. Only two studies included HDL cholesterol in multivariate adjustment of the risk of triglycerides in women. Similar to men, the summary multivariate RR estimate for these two studies showed attenuation, but the RR of 1.37 remained significant, 95% CI 1.13-1.66.

One of the studies included in this meta-analysis, the Lipid Research Clinics (LRC) Follow-up Study, looked at the RR of triglycerides in subgroups of the study population [2]. The results indicated that triglycerides were a stronger risk factor in subjects less than 70 years of age, in subjects with a lower low density lipoprotein (LDL) cholesterol (< 160 mg/dl), and in subjects with a lower HDL cholesterol (< 35 mg/dl in men and < 45 mg/dl in women). A prospective study in Finland in 313 patients with noninsulin dependent diabetes mellitus (NIDDM) has reported similar stratified analyses for CHD events over a seven-year follow-up [3]. The lipoprotein strata cutpoints were quite similar to the LRC, 166 mg/dl for LDL cholesterol and 43 mg/dl for HDL cholesterol. Similar to the LRC Follow-up Study, they found very low density lipoprotein (VLDL) triglycerides to be a significant risk factor in the lower LDL cholesterol stratum and in the lower HDL

A. M. Gotto, Jr. et al. (eds.), Drugs Affecting Lipid Metabolism, 203–209.

cholesterol stratum, but not in either of the higher strata. In both the LRC and Finnish NIDDM studies, triglycerides were a much stronger risk indicator than HDL cholesterol at lower levels of LDL cholesterol and at lower levels of HDL cholesterol. A recent prospective study in an elderly population, age 65-94 years with a mean of 75 years, followed up an average of five years, showed triglycerides to similarly be more predictive of CHD death in elderly men and women in the lower LDL stratum (< 160 mg/dl), although risk of the triglycerides did not differ significantly by HDL strata [4].

Thus, although the study of an increased risk of triglycerides at lower levels of LDL cholesterol was seen in all three studies, the findings for HDL strata were somewhat less consistent. Two recent studies are relevant to this question. An analysis of the placebo group in the Helsinki Heart Study showed that the five-year risk of cardiac endpoints was elevated only in the subgroup with high triglycerides (≥ 204 mg/dl) and low HDL cholesterol (≤ 41.8 mg/dl) [5]. In this subgroup, adjusted for age and smoking, the RR was 2.7, 95% CI 1.6-4.6 compared to the normal HDL cholesterol-normal triglyceride reference group. In contrast, neither the normal-triglyceride, low-HDL cholesterol group (RR = 1.3, 95% CI 0.7-2.4) nor the high-triglyceride, normal-HDL cholesterol group (RR = 1.4, 95% CI 0.6-2.9) showed a significantly increased risk. In a study of 340 patients with nonfatal myocardial infarction and 340 matched controls, the strongest lipid/lipoprotein ratio predictor was the triglycerides to HDL cholesterol. After multivariate adjustment, the top quartile of this ratio compared to the lowest quartile gave a striking RR of 16.6, 95% CI 8.0-34.3 [6].

Although neither of the above studies specifically evaluated the risk of triglycerides within HDL (or LDL) cholesterol strata, both gave results quite consistent with the finding in the LRC [2] and Finnish NIDDM [3] studies that, in the setting of low-HDL cholesterol, triglycerides are a strong risk factor for CHD.

Another consideration in evaluating triglycerides as a risk factor in epidemiologic studies is that, unlike HDL and LDL cholesterol, there may be a threshold level at which risk no longer increases and may even decrease. Data on this question are sparse, but there is a clinical consensus that Type 1 hyperlipidemic patients, who are deficient in lipoprotein lipase or apoprotein C-II and often have triglycerides over 1000 mg/dl, do not have an increased risk of CHD. Some authors believe there is a linear increase up to about 400 mg/dl, some increased CHD risk in at least some persons with triglycerides in the 400 mg/dl to 1000 mg/dl range, and little if any increase in CHD risk above 1000 mg/dl, although at this high level there is an increased risk of certain other conditions such as pancreatitis [7].

Clinical Trials

Of particular relevance to this meeting focusing on drugs affecting lipid metabolism is the evidence on the efficacy of lowering triglycerides in clinical trials. Trials intervening on lipids to prevent CVD events have typically focused on changes in total or LDL cholesterol, particularly when the dietary or pharmacologic therapy employed had little effect on triglycerides or HDL cholesterol levels, or when the study population was restricted to subjects with "normal" triglycerides. Nonetheless, at least five trials have reported the correlation between lowering of triglycerides compared to cholesterol, or other lipid or lipoprotein fractions, and reduction in the risk of CHD events or progression.

The Coronary Drug Project began in 1966. A 1986 paper reported 15-year follow-up results and showed a significant 11% reduction in total mortality in the niacin group, who had been on active treatment for the first six years of the follow-up period [8]. There were 1,119 men in the niacin group and 2,789 men in the placebo group. Total cholesterol decreased 10.1% from baseline to year 1 in the niacin group. The authors state that "within the niacin group, patients with the largest decrease in serum cholesterol at 1 year experienced a lower subsequent mortality than did those with an increase in serum cholesterol. There was no significant correlation between change in serum triglyceride and mortality in the niacin group." However, the authors did not show any data, and no comment was made about the change in cholesterol and triglycerides at any other time point. In addition, no comment was made about cause-specific mortality.

The Stockholm Ischaemic Heart Disease Prevention Study began in 1972. A 1988 paper reported results in the treatment group stratified by the degree of lipid lowering [9]. The treatment group received both clofibrate and niacin. The trial was not blinded. Table 1 shows the results for the percentage of patients dying of CHD over five years by strata of changes in triglycerides and total cholesterol. There was a significant association between the degree of triglyceride lowering and the reduction in the CHD deaths, but there was no such association for cholesterol lowering.

Table 1. CHD death over 5 years by strata of triglycerides and cholesterol reduction, Stockholm Ischaemic Heart Disease Secondary Prevention Study.

N	TG ↓, %	CHD Deaths %	N	Chol ↓, %	CHD Deaths %
49	<0	24.5	61	<0	13.1
109	0-29	21.1	123	0-14	20.3
121	≥ 30	9.9	95	≥ 15	14.7
Total 279			Total 279		

(adapted from [9])

The Helsinki Heart Study began in 1980. The treatment group received gemfibrozil. A paper in 1988 reported the multivariate Cox proportional hazards coefficients for changes in various lipids and lipoproteins and CHD risk over five years [10]. The lipid and lipoprotein predictors were two-year average changes adjusted for baseline values and other CVD risk factors. The results are shown in Table 2. In the gemfibrozil group, changes in HDL and LDL cholesterol were both individually significant, while changes in triglycerides were not. However, the coefficient for triglycerides was in the expected direction, and interestingly, while no lipid or lipoprotein change in the placebo group was significantly associated with CHD incidence, the strongest association was for triglycerides. It is likely the greater variability in triglycerides makes it more difficult to demonstrate an association between changes in triglycerides and outcome than for changes in the other lipids and lipoproteins. A paper in 1989 from this same study evaluated reduction with gemfibrozil by lipid phenotype [11]. Interestingly, the reduction in risk was highly significant in Type IIb patients (with triglycerides ≥ 177 mg/dl), a 43% risk reduction, $p = .02$, but not in Type IIa patients (with triglycerides < 177 mg/dl), a 24% risk reduction, p = NS.

Table 2. Changes in lipids and lipoprotein and 5-year risk of CHD by treatment group, Helsinki Heart Study.

	Gemfibrozil N = 2046		Placebo N = 2035	
Lipid/Lipoprotein	coeff	p value	coeff	p value
Total Cholesterol	.025	.12	.012	.45
HDL Cholesterol	-.032	< .01	-.004	.72
Non-HDL Cholesterol	.025	< .05	.016	.23
LDL Cholesterol	.023	< .04	.010	.37
Triglycerides	.005	.28	.006	.12
HDL/Total Cholesterol	-.019	< .01	-.006	.47

(adapted from [10])

The Cholesterol Lowering Atherosclerosis Study (CLAS) was begun in 1980. An abstract published in 1993 stratified the treatment versus placebo results by baseline level of triglycerides and looked at angiographic benefit by change in lipids and lipoproteins [12]. The treatment regimen in CLAS was colestipol plus niacin, and global angiographic change score was evaluated at two years of follow-up. Table 3 shows the results. In the lower triglycerides stratum, treatment sharply decreased LDL cholesterol and increased HDL cholesterol, but there was only a small decrease in triglycerides, -14 mg/dl. Global angiographic change scores in the treatment group were not significantly different from placebo. In the high-triglycerides stratum, changes in the treatment group for LDL and HDL cholesterol were similar to the low-triglycerides stratum, but the decrease in triglycerides was much greater, -65 mg/dl. In contrast to the low-triglycerides stratum, there was a marked benefit in global angiographic score in the treatment group compared to the placebo group. Thus, despite employing a combination drug regimen with marked beneficial effects on both LDL and HDL cholesterol, benefit was limited to patients who had both higher triglycerides at baseline and a sharp decline in triglycerides with therapy.

Table 3. CHD progression by angiographic global change scores in treatment versus placebo group stratified by baseline triglycerides, CLAS.

		Lower Triglycerides Stratum (median = 98, range 49-128)		Higher Triglycerides Stratum (median = 187, range 129-517)	
		Rx	Placebo	Rx	Placebo
Angio	Yes(N)	17	22	14	28
Progression	No(N)	21	21	27	12
p value		0.56		0.001	
Δ Trig		-14	-1	-65	-27
Δ LDL		-82	-12	-67	-6
Δ HDL		+18	0	+15	+1

(adapted from [12])

The Monitored Atherosclerosis Regression Study (MARS) was begun in 1985. A paper in 1993 reported that diet plus a large dose of lovastatin, 80 mg/day, had a beneficial effect on coronary stenoses ≥ 50%, but not on < 50% stenoses [13]. The average LDL cholesterol in the treatment group decreased from 151 mg/dl to 93 mg/dl. A 1994 paper evaluated changes in lipid and lipoproteins as predictors of progression in both the placebo and in the lovastatin groups comparing the highest and lowest quartiles of lipids and lipoproteins [14]. The results from the multivariate analysis, stratified by the degree of coronary artery stenosis, are shown in Table 4. In the placebo group, where LDL levels remained high, the change in total cholesterol to HDL cholesterol ratio was the only predictor of lesion progression in both smaller and larger stenoses. In the lovastatin group with sharply lowered LDL, the LDL cholesterol to HDL cholesterol ratio was the only significant predictor for larger stenosis progression. However, for the smaller stenoses, which may be more unstable and more likely to precipitate CHD events [15], the only significant predictor of progression was apo-CIII heparin precipitate, a marker for triglyceride-rich lipoproteins. This latter result is consistent with the finding in epidemiologic studies that a significant risk for triglycerides is limited to persons with lower levels of LDL cholesterol

Conclusions

The best evidence now available suggests triglycerides are an independent risk factor for CHD, independent of confounding variables including HDL cholesterol. Although the overall association is modest, in subgroups of persons with lower levels of LDL cholesterol

Table 4. Significant relative risks and 95% confidence intervals for coronary artery stenosis progression in highest versus lowest quartile, multivariate analysis, MARS.

	Lovastatin				Placebo			
	Degree of Stenosis				Degree of Stenosis			
	< 50%		≥ 50%		< 50%		≥ 50%	
	RR	95% CI	RR	95% CI	RR	95% CI	RR	95% CI
Δ Chol /HDL	-	-	-	-	3.6	(1.0-12.7)	8.7	(2.0-38.3)
LDL/HDL	-	-	6.4	(1.5-27.9)	-	-	-	-
ApoCIII - HP*	5.0	(1.4-17.1)	-	-	-	-	-	-

*heparin precipitate.
(adapted from [14])

and lower levels of HDL cholesterol, the association is considerably stronger, and in these subgroups triglycerides usually are a better predictor than HDL cholesterol. There is some evidence that triglycerides may be a stronger risk factor in women than in men and also a stronger risk factor in noninsulin dependent diabetics than in nondiabetics.

The limited data available from clinical trials support the concept that reduction of triglycerides may provide benefit both for atherosclerotic progression and for clinical events. Similar to the epidemiologic data, such benefit may be greater in persons with higher levels of triglycerides, lower levels of HDL cholesterol, and lower levels of LDL cholesterol. The mechanism by which lowering of triglycerides results in angiographic and clinical benefit is uncertain and remains an important area for investigation.

References

1. Hokanson JE, Austin MA. Plasma triglyceride is a risk factor for cardiovascular disease independent of high-density lipoprotein cholesterol: A meta-analysis of population-based prospective studies. J Cardiovascular Risk 1996; in press.
2. Criqui MH, Heiss G, Cohn R, et al. Plasma triglyceride level and mortality from coronary heart disease. New Engl J Med 1993;328:1220-25.
3. Laakso M, Lehto S, Penttilä I, Pyörälä K. Lipids and lipoproteins predicting coronary heart disease mortality and morbidity in patients with non-insulin-dependent diabetes. Circulation 1993;88:1421-30.
4. Criqui MH, Langer RD, Denenberg JO, Scheidt-Nave C, Barrett-Connor E, Klauber MR. Triglycerides and coronary heart disease death in the elderly. Circulation 1995;91:923 (abstract).
5. Tenkanen L, Pietila K, Manninen V, Manttari M. The triglyceride issue revisited. Findings from the Helsinki Heart Study. Archives Intern Med 1994;154:2714-20.
6. Gaziano JM, Buring JE, Breslow J, Hennekens CH. Fasting triglycerides (TG), high density

lipoprotein cholesterol (HDL), and risk of myocardial infarction (MI). Circulation 1994;90: I-510 (abstract).

7. Handbook on the management of lipid disorders. McKenney JM, Hawkins DW, editors. National Pharmacy Cholesterol Council 1995.

8. Canner PL, Berge KG, Wenger NK, et al. for the Coronary Drug Project Research Group. Fifteen year mortality in Coronary Drug Project patients: Long-term benefit with niacin. J Am Coll Cardiol 1986;8:1245-55.

9. Carlson LA, Rosenhamer G. Reduction of mortality in the Stockholm Ischaemic Heart Disease Secondary Prevention Study by combined treatment with clofibrate and nicotinic acid. Acta Med Scand 1988;223:405-18.

10. Manninen V, Elo MO, Frick MH, et al. Lipid alterations and decline in the incidence of coronary heart disease in the Helsinki Heart Study. JAMA 1988;260:641-51.

11. Manninen V, Huttunen JK, Heinonen OP, Tenkanen L, Frick MH. Relation between baseline lipid and lipoprotein values and the incidence of coronary heart disease in the Helsinki Heart Study. Am J Cardiol 1989;63:42H-47H.

12. Miller BD, Krauss RM, Cashin-Hemphill L, Blankenhorn DH. Baseline triglyceride levels predict angiographic benefit of colestipol plus niacin therapy in the Cholesterol-Lowering Atherosclerosis Study (CLAS). Circulation 1993;88(I), I-363 (abstract).

13. Blankenhorn DH, Azen SP, Kramsch DM, et al. and the MARS Research Group. Coronary angiographic changes with lovastatin therapy: the Monitored Atherosclerosis Regression Study (MARS). Ann Intern Med 1993;119:969-76.

14. Hodis HN, Mack WJ, Azen SP, et al. Triglyceride- and cholesterol-rich lipoproteins have a differential effect on mild/moderate and severe lesion progression as assessed by quantitative coronary angiography in a controlled trial of lovastatin. Circulation 1994;90:42-9.

15. Brown BG, Zhao XQ, Sacco DE, Albers JJ. Lipid lowering and plaque regression: New insights into prevention of plaque disruption and clinical events in coronary disease. Circulation 1993;87:1781-91.

TRIGLYCERIDES AS A SIGNAL OF INCREASED CORONARY HEART DISEASE RISK DUE TO ADVERSE LIFESTYLE

Leena Tenkanen[1], Matti Mänttäri[2], Kati Pietilä[3], and Vesa Manninen[4]
Helsinki Heart Study[1], Divisions of Cardiology[4] and Emergency Medicine[2], University of Helsinki, and Tampere School of Public Health[3], University of Tampere, Finland

Introduction

Today every patient knows that smoking, a sedentary lifestyle, and obesity increase the risk of coronary heart disease (CHD) and thus should be avoided. Nevertheless more than every second patient has one or more of these adverse lifestyle indicators; therefore all means for better evaluating the CHD risk associated with them are useful.

Several studies have shown that obesity and a sedentary lifestyle enhance the development of insulin resistance [1,2], which precipitates the development of a series of CHD risk factors, such as high level of serum triglycerides (TG), low level of high density lipoprotein cholesterol (HDL-C), and hypertension [3]. In a previous study [4], the central mediating role of TG among the factors included in the insulin resistance syndrome emerged clearly. With elevated levels of TG, there was a significantly greater probability of having simultaneously low levels of HDL-C and hypertension, with an accompanying high CHD risk. This is consistent with findings in clinical praxis: TG is considered a signal of CHD risk [5].

The aim of the present study was to evaluate this signal value of high TG in the context of adverse lifestyle indicators, such as obesity, sedentary lifestyle, and smoking. As our previous studies indicated that subjects with several simultaneous risk factors contributing to the insulin resistance syndrome benefit from treatment with gemfibrozil [6], we also evaluated the extent to which subjects with these adverse lifestyle factors benefit from this treatment.

Subjects and Methods

The Helsinki Heart Study was a 5-year, placebo-controlled, double-blind clinical trial designed to test the hypothesis that lowering serum LDL cholesterol and triglyceride levels and elevating serum HDL-C level with gemfibrozil, reduces the incidence of CHD in middle-aged dyslipidemic men. The design and conduct of the trial have been described in

A. M. Gotto, Jr. et al. (eds.), Drugs Affecting Lipid Metabolism, 211–217.

detail elsewhere [7,8]. Briefly, the participants for the study were selected from 23,531 men, aged 40 to 55 years, who were registered as employed by two state agencies and five industrial companies in Finland. Volunteers were eligible for the trial if their serum non-HDL-C (i.e. LDL cholesterol plus VLDL cholesterol) was ≥ 5.2 mmol/l at two successive measurements and if they had no evidence of CHD or other major diseases. The trial participants were randomly allocated either to gemfibrozil (n=2,046) or placebo (n=2,035).

The follow-up examinations, performed at three-month intervals, included laboratory measurements and an interview on possible adverse effects, hospitalizations, major illnesses, and any symptoms suggesting myocardial infarction. Routine electrocardiograms were taken annually and whenever the participants reported symptoms suggesting myocardial infarction. Definite fatal and nonfatal myocardial infarctions and cardiac death were the trial end-points. End-point assessments were made without knowledge of the treatment.

MEASUREMENT OF LIPID, LIPOPROTEIN, AND GLUCOSE LEVELS

Serum samples were collected and mailed daily to the central laboratory at the National Public Health Institute in Helsinki. The HDL-C concentration was measured after precipitation of VLDL and LDL with dextran sulphate/magnesium chloride by an enzymatic method (Boehringer Mannheim, kit No 236691).

Fasting serum samples were collected at the second screening visit and the concentration of triglycerides was measured as glycerol after enzymatic hydrolysis with lipase/esterase (Boehringer Mannheim, kit No 124966). For most of the analyses we used a dichotomized variable for TG with 2.3 mmol/l as the cut-off point according to European recommendations for treatment practice [5]. Blood glucose concentrations were also determined from fasting samples at the second screening visit.

MEASUREMENT AND CATEGORIZATION OF THE LIFESTYLE INDICATORS

Data on the lifestyle indicators were recorded at the first screening visit. Smoking habits were classified using the reported number of cigarettes smoked per day, but for the analyses in the present paper the subjects were classified as nonsmokers or smokers. All ex-smokers who had stopped more than 3 months before the beginning of the study were categorized as nonsmokers. Spare time physical activity was recorded with the Gothenburg scale [9] into four categories, but for the analyses we used a dichotomized scale: sedentary (categories I and II) and active (categories III and IV).

STATISTICAL METHODS

To explore the associations of the lifestyle factors with some factors related to the insulin resistance syndrome, we calculated mean levels of the latter by categories of the lifestyle factors and we tested the significance of the differences using ANOVA. To compare the relative risks of CHD at different levels of the lifestyle factors and triglycerides, we used

Cox's proportional hazards models, with appropriate covariates, mostly age and smoking.

Results

INTERDEPENDENCIES AMONG THE LIFESTYLE INDICATORS AND ASSOCIATIONS WITH FACTORS RELATED TO THE INSULIN RESISTANCE SYNDROME

Spare time physical activity was highly significantly ($p < 0.001$) associated with body mass index (BMI); among sedentary subjects 59% had BMI > 26 kg/m^2, while among active subjects the figure was 44% (Table 1). Smokers tended to be slightly leaner than nonsmokers.

All these lifestyle indicators, especially obesity, were closely associated with components of the insulin resistance syndrome (Table 2). Triglycerides and HDL-C were associated distinctively and significantly with all the indicators considered, while systolic blood pressure (SBP) and glucose were significantly associated only with BMI. When the groups formed on the basis of categories of the lifestyle indicators were further split by TG level (Table 3), SBP and glucose also showed significantly different mean levels by category of TG.

TG AS A SIGNAL OF INCREASED CHD RISK

With both obesity and sedentary lifestyle, elevated TG levels indicated those at increased risk of CHD (Figure 1 A and B). In both cases the risk was reduced by treatment with gemfibrozil to the level of a lean/active placebo subject with low TG. With smoking (Figure 1 C) the risk pattern was different. Even though high TG delineated a high risk group among smokers (RR=5.2 $p < 0.001$) compared to nonsmokers with normal TG, there remained some excess risk due to smoking which was not completely removed by treatment with gemfibrozil.

Discussion

The main finding of this study was the central mediating role of triglycerides in the context of adverse lifestyle indicators and factors related to the insulin resistance syndrome, as well as in the CHD risk due to adverse lifestyle. Firstly, high levels of TG indicated that low levels of HDL-C and hypertension tended to be present. Secondly, obese and sedentary subjects had a substantially increased CHD risk only if they also had high levels of TG, while smoking entailed some excess risk even when TG level was normal. All excess risk associated with obesity or sedentary lifestyle was eliminated by treatment with gemfibrozil, but some excess risk associated with smoking remained.

It is tempting to speculate that most of the effect of obesity and sedentary lifestyle on CHD risk may be mediated through an accumulation of risk factors belonging to the insulin resistance syndrome. High level of TG and low level of HDL-C, dyslipidemia characteristics of insulin resistance syndrome, respond well to treatment with gemfibrozil

Table 1. Percentage (%) distribution of categories of BMI, spare time physical activity, and smoking. The distributions were calculated from the placebo group baseline measurements.

Level of Other Indicator	N	BMI kg/m² < 26 (%)	26-30 (%)	> 30 (%)	Total %
Spare Time Physical Activity					
Active	748	56	37	7	100
Sedentary	1273	41	44	15	100
Smoking					
Non/Past	1305	45	43	12	100
Current	730	51	38	11	100

Table 2. Mean (SD) baseline levels in the placebo group of some CHD risk factors by categories of lifestyle indicators.

Lifestyle Indicator		Mean TG mmmol/l	HDL-C mmol/l	Systolic BP mmHg	Glucose mmol/l
BMI kg/m²					
	≤ 26	1.8 (1.1)	1.28 (0.3)	135 (16)	4.3 (0.7)
	26 - 30	2.1 (1.4)	1.20 (0.3)	137 (16)	4.5 (0.8)
	> 30	2.7 (2.0)	1.14 (0.3)	141 (16)	4.8 (1.2)
Spare Time Physical Activity					
	Active	1.9 (1.2)	1.28 (0.3)	136 (16)	4.4 (0.7)
	Sedentary	2.1 (1.5)	1.20 (0.3)	137 (16)	4.5 (0.8)
Smoking					
	Non/Past	1.9 (1.3)	1.25 (0.3)	137 (16)	4.5 (0.9)
	Current	2.2 (1.6)	1.19 (0.3)	137 (16)	4.4 (0.7)

Table 3. Mean (SD) baseline levels in the placebo group, of some CHD risk factors by combined levels of triglycerides (TG) and lifestyle indicators.

		Mean		
Level of TG mmol/l	Level of the Other Indicator	HDL-C mmol/l	Systolic BP mmHg	Glucose mmol/l
	BMI kg/m^2			
< 2.3	≤ 26	1.30 (0.28)	134 (16)	4.3 (0.6)
	26 - 30	1.25 (0.27)	136 (15)	4.4 (0.6)
	> 30	1.22 (0.26)	141 (16)	4.5 (0.7)
≥ 2.3	≤ 26	1.12 (0.29)	136 (17)	4.5 (0.8)
	26 - 30	1.07 (0.23)	138 (16)	4.6 (1.1)
	> 30	1.02 (0.23)	143 (16)	4.9 (1.4)
	Spare Time Physical Activity			
< 2.3	Active	1.32 (0.27)	135 (15)	4.3 (0.6)
	Sedentary	1.26 (0.28)	136 (16)	4.4 (0.6)
≥ 2.3	Active	1.12 (0.25)	140 (16)	4.6 (1.2)
	Sedentary	1.04 (0.23)	139 (16)	4.7 (1.1)
	Smoking			
< 2.3	Non/Past	1.31 (0.28)	136 (16)	4.4 (0.6)
	Current	1.25 (0.28)	136 (16)	4.4 (0.6)
≥ 2.3	Non/Past	1.07 (0.24)	140 (16)	4.7 (1.3)
	Current	1.05 (0.24)	139 (16)	4.6 (0.9)

[6]. In addition, several studies have shown that the components of this syndrome exert an unfavorable effect on the fibrinolytic system predisposing to thrombosis and increased CHD risk [10-12], while Fujii and Sobel [13] have shown that gemfibrozil potentiates fibrinolysis, thereby protecting from thrombosis.

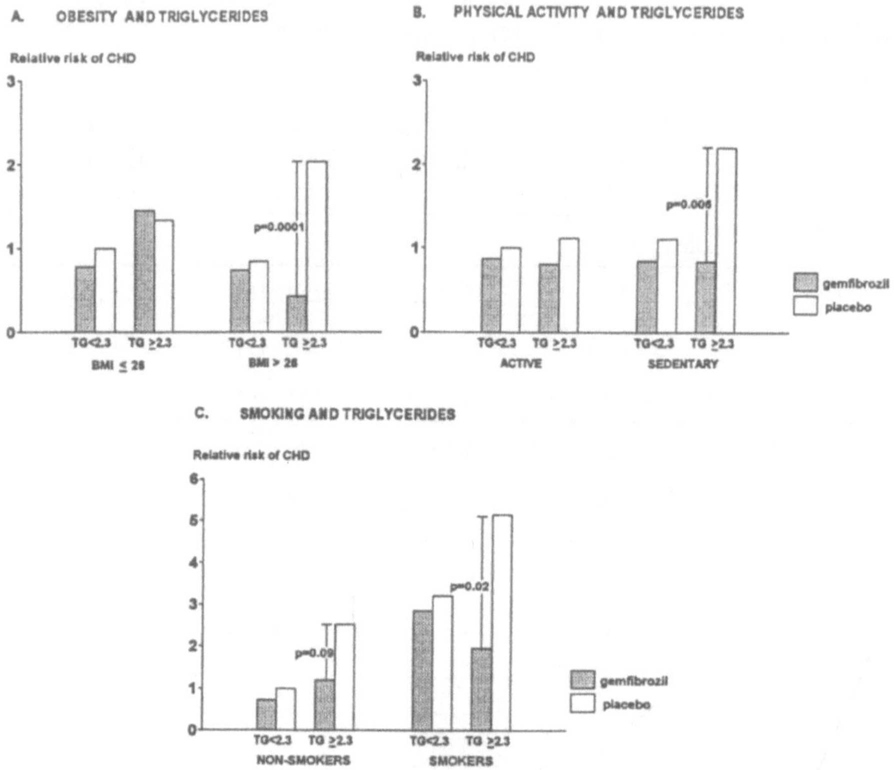

Figure 1. Relative risk of cardiac end-point by level of TG and category of lifestyle indicator. The relative risks were derived using Cox's proportional hazards models with age and smoking (Figures 1 A and B) and age (Figure 1 C) as covariates.

However, there are two caveats which emerge from the design of the study. Firstly, all the study participants were dyslipidemic at baseline, with high low density lipoprotein cholesterol (LDL-C) levels; less than 20% of the subjects had LDL-C < 4 mmol/l. Whether or not our results can be generalized to a normolipidemic population is far from clear. Secondly, the trial lasted only 5 years and the participants were selected to have no signs or symptoms of actual CHD. It is thus possible that the fibrinolytic component in the development of infarction was somewhat overrepresented at the beginning of the study and that the role of high LDL-C emerged only later, perhaps after the 5-year trial. These considerations suggest that in a normolipidemic population and with a longer follow-up time the results might be less dramatic. Nevertheless, high level of TG is a good signal of increased short term CHD risk among obese, sedentary, or smoking patients.

References

1. Pouliot M-C, Després J-P, Nadeau A, et al. Visceral obesity in men: Associations with glucose, plasma insulin, and lipoprotein levels. Diabetes 1992;41:826-34.
2. Barnard RJ, Ugianskis EJ, Martin DA, Inkeles SB. Role of diet and exercise in the management of hyperinsulinemia and associated atherosclerotic risk factors. Am J Cardiol 1992;69:440-44.
3. Reaven GM. Role of insulin resistance in human disease. Diabetes 1988;37:1595-1607.
4. Tenkanen L, Pietilä K, Manninen V, Mänttäri M. The triglyceride issue revisited. Findings from the Helsinki Heart Study. Arch Intern Med 1994;154:2714-20.
5. Study Group, European Atherosclerosis Society. The recognition and management of hyperlipidaemia in adults: A policy statement of European Atherosclerosis Society. Eur Heart J 1988;9:571-600.
6. Tenkanen L, Mänttäri M, Manninen V. Some coronary risk factors related to the insulin resistance syndrome and treatment with gemfibrozil: Experience from the Helsinki Heart Study. Circulation 1995;92:1779-85.
7. Frick MH, Elo O, Haapa K, et al. The Helsinki Heart Study: Primary prevention trial with gemfibrozil middle-aged men with dyslipidemia: Safety of treatment, changes in risk factors, and incidence of coronary heart disease. N Engl J Med 1987;317:1237-45.
8. Manninen V, Elo O, Frick H, et al. Lipid alterations and decline in the incidence of coronary heart disease in the Helsinki Heart Study. JAMA 1988;260:641-51.
9. Wilhelmsen L, Tibblin G, Fodor J, Werkö L. A multifactorial primary preventive trial in Gothenburg, Sweden. In: Larson OA, Malmborg RO, editors. Coronary heart disease and physical fitness. Copenhagen, Munksgaard, 1971:266-70.
10. Juhan-Vague I, Vague P, Alessi MC, Badier C, Valadier Aillaud MF, Atlan C. Relationships between plasma insulin, triglyceride, body mass index, and plasminogen activator inhibitor 1. Diabetes Metab 1987;13:331-36.
11. Juhan-Vague I, Thompson SG, Jespersen J. on behalf of the ECAT Angina Pectoris Study Group. Involvement of the hemostatic systems in the insulin resistance syndrome. A study of 1500 patients with angina pectoris. Arterioscler Thromb 1993;13:1865-73.
12. Mussoni L, Mannucci L, Sirtori M, et al. Hypertriglyceridemia and regulation of fibrinolytic activity. Arterioscler Thromb 1992;12:19-29.
13. Fujii S, Sobel BE. Direct effects of gemfibrozil on the fibrinolytic system: diminution of synthesis of plasminogen activator inhibitor type 1. Circulation 1992;85:1888-93.

HYPERCOAGULABILITY AND HYPOFIBRINOLYSIS IN SUBJECTS WITH HYPERLIPOPROTEINEMIA

Tamotsu Matsuda, Eriko Morishita*, Masahide Yamazaki, Hiroshi Jokaji, Hidesaku Asakura, and Masanori Saito
*Kanazawa University School of Medicine, Department of Internal Medicine (III), *Department of Laboratory Medicine, Takaramachi 13-1, Kanazawa, Japan 920*

Introduction

In atherosclerosis, it has been postulated that hypercoagulability, in a broad since, exists and play some role on the development of thrombosis and/or the progress of atherosclerosis. We studied disorders of coagulation and fibrinolysis in 76 hyperlipidemic subjects and compared to those in 39 control subjects.

Methods

Levels of tissue factor antigen, tissue factor pathway inhibitor (TFPI), prothrombin fragment (F1+2), and tissue-type plasminogen activator (t-PA) antigen, which mainly reflects the complex of t-PA and its inhibitor, plasminogen activator inhibitor-1, in plasma were determined using enzyme immunoassay (ELISA).

Factor VII activity, which reflects active factor VII as well as inactivated factor VII was determined using one stage method.

Determination of the level of active plasminogen activator inhibitor-1 (PAI-1), which does not form complex with t-PA, is fundamentally determined using ELISA. First, the level of t-PA-PAI complex, which does not reflect active PAI-1, was determined. Next, an excess amount of t-PA was added to the plasma to convert all active PAI-1 in the plasma into t-PA-PAI complex. Then, the level of t-PA-PAI complex in the plasma was determined. The difference between the former and the latter denotes the level of active PAI-1. Active PAI-1 was determined at 10 a.m. taking into consideration daytime fluctuations of this fibrinolytic inhibitor.

Subjects

Table 1 indicates mean values and standard deviations of age, body mass index, total cholesterol, triglyceride, and HDL-cholesterol levels, in the control and hyperlipidemic

A. M. Gotto, Jr. et al. (eds.), Drugs Affecting Lipid Metabolism, 219–225.

subjects. The body mass index was significantly higher in the type IV subjects. Levels of total cholesterol in serum were significantly higher in the type IIa and type IIb subjects. The level of HDL-cholesterol was significantly lower in the type IV subjects. Subjects with history of myocardial infarction, stroke, or diabetes mellitus, were excluded.

Table 1. Age, sex, body mass index, and levels of serum lipid in normal control and hyperlipidemic subjects.

	Control (n = 39)	IIa (n = 31)	IIb (n = 14)	IV (n = 31)
Age (years)	50 ± 11	52 ± 12	50 ± 12	49 ± 7
Sex (M/F)	30/9	14/17	10/4	30/1
BMI (Kg/m^2)	22.7 ± 2.2	22.7 ± 2.6	24.0 ± 2.1	25.6 ± 3.4**
TC(mg/dl)	180 ± 22	253 ± 26**	265 ± 36**	188 ± 27
TG(mg/dl)	94 ± 30	102 ± 25	283 ± 90**	247 ± 91**
HDL-C(mg/dl)	53 ± 11	56 ± 19	47 ± 9	401 ± 3*

Values are means ± SD. *$p < 0.0005$; **$p < 0.0001$. BMI, body mass index; TC, total cholesterol; TG, triglyceride; HDL-C, HDL-cholesterol.

Results

Mean values and standard deviations of tissue factor antigen, factor VII activity, factor VII antigen, F1+2, t-PA antigen, and active PAI-1 in plasma in the control subjects and the subjects with hyperlipoproteinemia are shown in Table 2.

In type IIa and IIb subjects, the levels of tissue factor were higher than those of the control subjects. Levels of TFPI were significantly higher in the type IIa and IIb subjects than in the control subjects. There was a statistically significant positive correlation between TFPI and cholesterol level ($n = 76$, $r = 0.50$, $p < 0.0001$). In the subjects with hyperlipoproteinemia, factor VII activity was significantly higher than that of the control subjects. There was a statistically significant positive correlation between factor VII activity and cholesterol level (Figure 1). The correlation coefficient between factor VII and total cholesterol level was 0.46 and between factor VII and triglyceride level, 0.32. Levels of F1+2 in plasma were significantly higher in the type IIa and IIb subjects than those of the control subjects. The levels of t-PA antigen were higher in the type IIb subjects. The levels of PAI-1 were significantly elevated in the type IIb and the type IV subjects. There was a positive correlation between level of triglyceride and of active PAI-1 (Figure 2).

Table 2. Coagulability of blood and fibrinolysis in normal control and hyperlipidemic subjects.

	Control (n = 39)	IIa (n = 31)	IIb (n = 14)	IV (n = 3)
TF(pg/ml)	72 ± 55	97 ± 55	98 ± 57	64 ± 68
TFPI(ng/ml)	120 ± 27	173 ± 53**	176 ± 50*	130 ± 36
F VII activity (%)	100 ± 21	107 ± 22†	128 ± 31**	106 ± 19†
F1+2(nmol/l)	0.7 ± 0.4	1.0 ± 0.3††	1.0 ± 0.5	0.9 ± 0.3
t-PA(ng/ml)	9.9 ± 4.6	9.7 ± 3.0	14.7 ± 3.5#	14.6 ± 3.4**
active PAI-1(ng/ml)	11.7 ± 9.5	14.4 ± 11.0	34.2 ± 23.1*	31.5 ± 21.0**

Values are means ± SD. †$p < 0.05$; ††$p < 0.01$; #$p < 0.001$; *$p < 0.0005$; **$p < 0.0001$. TF, tissue factor antigen; TFPI, tissue factor pathway inhibitor; F VII, factor VII; F1+2, prothrombin fragment; t-PA, tissue type plasminogen activator antigen; PAI-1, plasminogen activator inhibitor-1.

Recently, lipid-lowering effect of HMG-CoA reductase inhibitor has called attention. We determined factor VII activity six months after the administration of HMG-CoA reductase inhibitor. Factor VII activity and levels of F1+2 decreased significantly was observed following administration of HMG-CoA reductase inhibitor (Table 3).

Discussion

In the hyperlipidemic subjects without history of myocardial infarction, stroke, or diabetes mellitus, levels of tissue factor in plasma were increased. Although the mechanism of releasing tissue factor into blood is not known, elevation of tissue factor concentration in plasma enhances thrombotic tendency in these subjects because the complex formation of

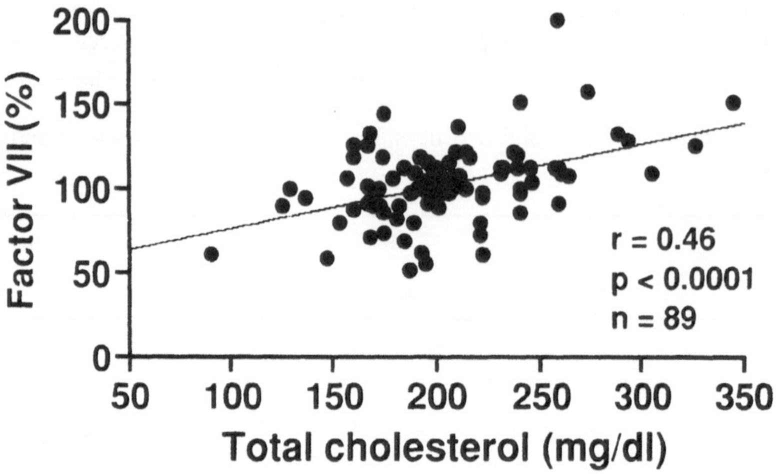

Figure 1. Relationship between serum cholesterol and factor VII activity.

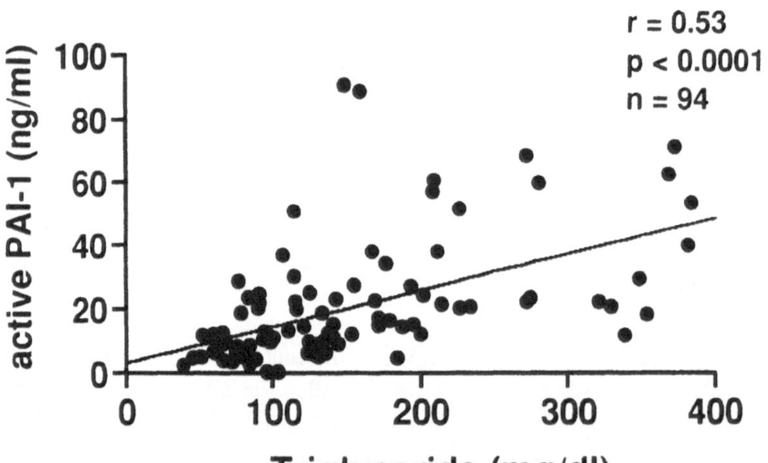

Figure 2. Relationship between serum triglyceride and active PAI-1.

activated factor VII and tissue factor triggers the coagulation cascade.

Table 3. Changes in factor VII activity and F1+2 levels six months after the administration of HMG-CoA reductase inhibitor.

	Before	After the administration of HMG-CoA reductase inhibitor
F VII activity (%)	111 ± 32	101 ± 23†
F1+2 (nmol/l)	1.3 ± 0.5	1.0 ± 0.5†

Values are means ± SD. $^{\dagger}p < 0.05$

A positive correlation between factor VII activity and total cholesterol levels also enhances thrombotic tendency in the hyperlipidemic subjects. The mechanism of the correlation has not been elucidated; however, it is possible that factor VII is activated in the hyperlipidemic subjects, because factor VII antigen is not so remarkably elevated in these subjects (data not shown). A statistically significant correlation between factor VII activity or antigen and serum lipid was observed in this study, and the similar results have already been reported [1-5].

However, TFPI levels also correlated with cholesterol levels. TFPI combines with activated factor X (Xa), and neutralizes it. Then, this complex combines the VIIa-tissue factor complex and neutralizes the procoagulant activity of VIIa-tissue factor complex, which activates factors IX and X. In other words, TFPI inhibits coagulation cascade by neutralizing Xa, and in the case in which a large amount of Xa is formed, TFPI also neutralizes VIIa-tissue factor complex. Because the close relationship between TFPI and lipoprotein [6] has been known since the discovery of this Kunitz-type inhibitor of blood coagulation, TFPI was once called as lipoprotein associated coagulation inhibitor (LACI). Our investigation also confirmed the correlation of plasma TFPI with total cholesterol.

Therefore, we cannot simply conclude that hypercoagulability or hypocoagulability is present in the subjects with hyperlipoproteinemia, but there is an unstable condition of coagulability in these subjects and the tendency to cause thrombosis is easily caused by various stimuli, for example, vascular damage by atherosclerosis. Moreover, it is possible that an increase in TFPI level in plasma may result from the release of TFPI from endothelial cells which causes impairment of the endothelial cell protecting mechanism against thrombosis.

If, activation of the coagulation cascade occurs, various inhibiting systems of blood coagulation other than TFPI, namely the antithrombin-heparinoid system, the protein C-thrombomodulin system, and the heparin cofactor II-dermatan system also block the progression of the coagulation cascade. But, if large amounts of some activated blood clotting factor are formed, thrombosis may occasionally occur. When the prothrombin molecule is activated by Xa and thrombin is formed, an activation peptide called prothrombin fragment (F1+2) is released from prothrombin molecule. Therefore, the presence of an increased amount of F1+2 in plasma indicates *in vivo* production of thrombin, which does not always reflect the presence of hypercoagulability in a narrow sense, but rather indicates the impairment of blood vessels which activates the blood clotting system, and suggests the presence of thrombotic tendency.

An increase in levels of F1+2 in the type IIa and IIb subjects is regarded as important evidence of thrombotic tendency. Almost all of the clot formed on the blood vessel wall disappears before occlusing blood vessels by activation of fibrinolytic system. Following the production of thrombin, t-PA is formed and released from the endothelial cells of blood vessels, and triggers activation of the fibrinolytic system. The fibrinolytic system is simpler than the coagulation system. Plasmin formed by t-PA from plasminogen absorbed onto fibrin digested fibrin. Active PAI-1, which is regarded as a most important inhibitor of fibrinolytic system, increased with an elevation of triglycerides. There have been reports that active PAI-1 or total PAI-1, reflecting both active PAI-1 and t-PA-PAI complex, correlates with triglyceride [7,8], similar to our results. Therefore, it would be reasonable to conclude that an increase in triglyceride levels impairs fibrinolysis and causes thrombotic tendency.

It seems that an increase in cholesterol is important in causing hypercoagulability, while an elevation of triglyceride level causes hypofibrinolysis. Factor VII activity and levels of F1+2 in plasma decreased following the administration of an HMG-CoA reductase inhibitor. From these results, it is concluded that the HMG-CoA reductase inhibitor does not only decrease liquid levels but also protects against the thrombotic tendency seen in subjects with hyperlipoproteinemia, although the mechanism and clinical effects of improvement of thrombotic tendency in these subjects remains to be elucidated.

Conclusion

In the subjects with hyperlipoproteinemia, an elevation in the levels of tissue factor, tissue factor pathway inhibitor (TFPI), factor VII activity, prothrombin fragment (F1+2), t-PA, and active plasminogen activator-1 were observed. Both factor VII activity and TFPI levels significantly correlated with total cholesterol levels. There were also positive correlations between active PAI-1 levels and triglyceride levels. Administration of an HMG-CoA reductase inhibitor improved hypercoagulability in the hyperlipidemic subjects. From these results, it is suggested that hyperlipoproteinemia causes hypercoagulability and hypofibrinolysis, although further study on its mechanism and clinical implication is needed.

References

1. Negri M, Argliano PL, Talamini G, Carlini S, Manzato F, Bonadonna G. Levels of plasma factor VII activated forms as a function of plasma triglyceride levels. Atherosclerosis 1993;99:55-61.

2. Hoffman C, Miller RH, Hultin MB. Correlation of factor VII activity and antigen with cholesterol and triglycerides in healthy young adults. Arterioscler Thromb 1992;12:262-70.
3. Humphries SE, Lane A, Green FR, Cooper J, Millers GJ. Factor VII coagulant activity and antigen levels in healthy men are determined by interaction between factor VII genotype and plasma triglyceride concentration. Arterioscler Thromb 1994;14:193-98.
4. Hoffman CJ, Lawson WE, Miller RH, Hultin MB. Correlation of vitamin K-dependent clotting factors with cholesterol and triglycerides in healthy young adults. Arterioscler Thromb 1994;14:1737-40.
5. Väisänen S, Rankinen T, Penttilä I, Rauramaa R. Factor VII coagulant activity in relation to serum lipoproteins and dietary fat in middle aged men. Thromb Haemostas 1995;73:435-38.
6. Hansen JB, Huseby NE, Sandset PM, Svensson B, Lyngmo V, Nordøy A. Tissue-factor pathway inhibitor and lipoproteins: Evidence for association with and regulation by LDL in human plasma. Arterioscler Thromb 1994;14:223-29.
7. Moussoni L, Mannucci L, Sirtori M, et al. Hypertriglyceridemia and regulation of fibrinolytic activity. Arterioscler Thromb 1992;12:19-27.
8. Cigolini M, Targher G, Seidell JC, et al. Relationships of plasminogen activator inhibitor-1 to anthropometry, serum insulin, triglycerides and adipose tissue fatty acids in healthy men. Atherosclerosis 1994;106:139-47.

POSTPRANDIAL LIPOPROTEINS AND THEIR RELATIONSHIP TO ATHEROSCLEROSIS AND THROMBOSIS

Jeffrey S. Cohn and Jean Davignon
Hyperlipidemia and Atherosclerosis Research Group, Clinical Research Institute of Montreal, 110 Pine Avenue West, Montreal, Quebec, Canada H2W 1R7

Introduction

By eating plentiful meals at regular intervals, people in affluent societies are in a metabolically postprandial or "fed" state throughout most of the day. The ingestion of 20 to 70 grams of fat with each meal results in a six-to-eight hour increase in plasma triglyceride concentration. Plasma lipoproteins are thus directly under the influence of the previous meal for the majority of the day, and only in the early hours of the morning are individuals in a truly "fasted state." Diagnosis of hyperlipidemia and subsequent assessment of coronary artery disease are however dependent upon a blood sample taken after a 12-hour overnight fast [1]. The use of a fasting blood sample is justified for three reasons: 1) day-to-day variability in plasma lipids due to the size and composition of the previous meal is reduced; 2) comparisons can be made with population "norms" established in fasting individuals; and 3) a relatively accurate estimation of LDL cholesterol can be made with a formula which depends on a fasting triglyceride concentration [2,3]. Despite the existence of a strong correlation between plasma lipid levels in the fed and fasting state, it has often been suggested that this approach may overlook an independent effect of postprandial lipoproteins on atherosclerosis and thrombosis.

Evidence for an Independent Role of Postprandial Lipoproteins in the Development of Coronary and Carotid Artery Disease

A number of studies have shown that patients with coronary artery disease (CAD) tend to have increased postprandial triglyceridemia [4,5]. Only recently however has evidence been presented showing that postprandial plasma triglyceride concentration is independently associated with CAD. Patsch et al. [6] investigated 101 angiographically characterized male patients, 61 who were classified as having severe CAD and 40 who were classified as control subjects without CAD. The patients with CAD had a greater and more prolonged increase in postprandial triglyceride concentration, which was most evident by the statistically significant elevation in plasma triglyceride concentration 6 and 8 hours after the

A. M. Gotto, Jr. et al. (eds.), Drugs Affecting Lipid Metabolism, 227–235.

test meal. Postprandial triglyceride levels had an accuracy of 68% in predicting the presence or absence of CAD. By multivariate logistic-regression analysis, postprandial but not fasting triglyceride levels were independently associated with disease. Postprandial triglyceride, fasting HDL_2-cholesterol, fasting apoB levels, and age were all identified as independent risk factors and together they predicted the presence or absence of CAD with an accuracy of 82%.

A similar case-control study has recently been conducted by Ginsberg et al. [7]. Plasma lipids were measured in 92 men and 113 women (evaluated for CAD by exercise-testing) in the fasted state and also for 8 hours following the ingestion of a liquid-formula fat load (53 gm/m^2 fat). Postprandial triglyceridemia was significantly greater in male cases than in controls, after statistical adjustment for age, race, and smoking status. A similar association was not evident for the women.

Postprandial triglyceridemia has also been independently associated with the presence of carotid atherosclerosis. Ryu et al. [8] studied 47 moderately hyper-cholesterolemic subjects (including 23 women) and correlated extent of alimentary lipemia with carotid artery wall thickness as measured by B-mode ultrasound. Peak postprandial triglyceride response was significantly correlated with B-mode score in multivariate analysis, and was able to account for 28% of the total variation in mean maximum intima-media wall thickness, in addition to the 10% of variation accounted for by such variables as total and HDL cholesterol, fasting triglyceride concentration, age, body mass index, and plasma insulin.

Postprandial Lipoproteins and Their Relationship to Atherosclerosis

The aforementioned evidence suggests that postprandial triglyceride-rich lipoproteins (TRL) can directly or indirectly affect the development of atherosclerosis. Although there are a large number of complex lipoprotein interactions and alterations in the postprandial state, it is possible to identify five of these as having particular atherogenic potential.

Increase in the Plasma Concentration of ApoB-48-Containing Chylomicrons and Their Remnants

It was originally proposed by Zilversmit [9], that atherosclerosis could be viewed as a process involving the binding of chylomicrons to the arterial surface, the hydrolysis of triglyceride by arterial lipoprotein lipase and the subsequent internalization of cholesterol-enriched chylomicron remnants by cells of the artery wall. This concept has been supported by case-control studies demonstrating that postprandial plasma levels of retinyl palmitate are significantly higher in CAD patients compared to healthy controls [10,11]. In the early stages of postprandial triglyceridemia, the majority of plasma retinyl esters (derived from vitamin A in the test meal) are found in chylomicrons of intestinal origin and their presence in plasma has been used as a measure of plasma chylomicrons and their remnants. It is important to realize however that newly synthesized chylomicrons are not themselves atherogenic, as reflected by the lack of premature atherosclerosis in patients with familial chylomicronemia [12]. These patients have greatly increased plasma levels of chylomicrons in the fasting state due to a genetic deficiency of lipoprotein lipase. Large triglyceride-rich chylomicrons are probably too large to enter the artery wall and it is only when their size is decreased by the hydrolytic action of lipoprotein lipase that they become atherogenic. This is best exemplified by the premature CAD observed in patients with type III dyslipidemia, who have normal lipoprotein lipase activity but have a plasma accumulation of remnant lipoproteins due to defective remnant lipoprotein clearance [13]. Recent methods to quantitate plasma apoB-48 [14], the principle structural protein of chylomicrons, has greatly facilitated our ability to assess the role of intestinally-derived TRL in atherosclerosis. Using one such technique, Karpe et al. have measured the postprandial increase in plasma apoB-48 concentration in large and small TRL in normolipidemic subjects with and without CAD, and in hypertriglyceridemic patients with CAD[15]. Rate of progression of coronary lesions, determined by two coronary angiographies at an interval of about five years, was significantly related to the plasma concentration of apoB-48 in small TRL [16], providing support for the concept that apoB-48-containing chylomicron remnants are potentially atherogenic.

INCREASE IN THE PLASMA CONCENTRATION OF APOB-100-CONTAINING TRL OF HEPATIC ORIGIN

Postprandial increase in the concentration of plasma triglyceride is predominantly due to an increase in the plasma concentration of apoB-48-containing TRL from the intestine [17]. However, hepatic TRL containing apoB-100 also make a significant contribution to postprandial triglyceridemia [18]. In normolipidemic individuals, TRL apoB-100 increase 50% after ingestion of a fatty meal, in association with a six- to eight-fold increase in TRL apoB-48 concentration [18]. A similar increase is observed in TRL apoB-100 in hypertriglyceridemic individuals [15]. Postprandial increase in TRL apoB-100 concentration is believed to be due to reduced clearance of VLDL caused by the postprandial presence in plasma of chylomicrons, which compete with VLDL for lipoprotein lipase and associated apolipoproteins required for TRL catabolism and clearance [15]. However, increased postprandial secretion of TRL apoB-100 by the liver may also make an important contribution [19]. It remains to be determined to what extent these postprandial increases in apoB-100 TRL contribute to atherogenesis. *In vitro* tissue culture experiments have clearly shown that triglyceride-rich VLDL and their remnants are potentially atherogenic as demonstrated by their ability to cause lipid accumulation in cultured macrophages [20]. Accumulating evidence from coronary angiographic studies also suggest that apoB-100 TRL play a role in the progression of coronary artery atherosclerosis [21].

INCREASE IN THE TRANSFER OF CHOLESTERYL ESTERS FROM HDL TO POSTPRANDIAL TRL

Irrespective of the intestinal or hepatic origin of postprandial TRL, the potential atherogenicity of these lipoproteins can be viewed in terms of their ability to affect the plasma metabolism of free and esterified cholesterol. As reviewed by Miesenböck and

Patsch [22], an individual's triglyceride metabolic capacity is a strong determinant of his or her HDL cholesterol concentration, particularly HDL_2. Efficiency of plasma TRL catabolism also determines the extent of TRL cholesteryl ester enrichment and the size of circulating LDL and HDL. The critical element responsible for these effects is the plasma cholesteryl ester transfer protein (CETP), which transfers triglycerides from TRL to LDL and HDL, and transfers cholesteryl esters from LDL and HDL to TRL [23]. Cholesterol esterification activity [24] and cholesteryl ester transfer activity [24,25] are both increased in the fed compared to the fasted state, and patients with fasting chylomicronemia have a marked elevation in plasma CETP concentration [26]. For relatively normal plasma triglyceride concentrations (up to approximately 270 mg/100ml), the activity of CETP is dependent on the concentration of CE-acceptor particles (TRL) rather than the concentration of CE-donor particles or the mass of CETP [27]. This suggests that under normal physiological circumstances, the transfer of plasma cholesteryl esters out of LDL and HDL into TRL is determined by circulating amounts of TRL. In individuals with poor capacity to clear postprandial TRL, CETP will promote the enrichment of TRL with cholesteryl esters and will enrich LDL and HDL with triglycerides, leading to the formation of small LDL and HDL. These features are characteristic of the atherogenic lipoprotein profile of patients with insulin resistance and premature coronary disease [28], and this mechanism therefore provides a possible explanation for the link between defective postprandial TRL metabolism and potentially atherogenic alterations in cholesterol metabolism.

INCREASE IN THE SUSCEPTIBILITY OF POSTPRANDIAL LDL TO OXIDATION

Leichleitner et al. [29] have recently suggested an additional mechanism to explain the increased atherogenicity of the postprandial state. Using the murine macrophage cell line P388, cellular cholesterol accumulation and esterification were measured in cells incubated with LDL isolated from plasma obtained in the fed and fasted state from healthy normolipidemic individuals. Cellular cholesterol accumulation and esterification were significantly greater in the presence of postprandial compared to postabsorptive (fasting) LDL. In addition, the lipid peroxide content of LDL (as determined by measuring the thiobarbituric acid-reacting substances) was found to be significantly higher in postprandial compared to postabsorptive LDL, after incubation of lipoprotein preparations with copper sulphate or cultured macrophages. Although additional studies are required to substantiate these findings, they suggest that postprandial LDL have increased atherogenicity due to their greater susceptibility to oxidative modification.

INCREASE IN THE ASSOCIATION OF PLASMA APO(A) WITH POSTPRANDIAL TRL

Apo(a) is a large highly glycosylated hydrophilic protein which has been implicated in the pathogenesis of both atherosclerosis and thrombosis, due to its covalent association with cholesterol-rich Lp(a) and its sequence homology with plasminogen [30,31]. The majority of apo(a) in plasma is characteristically associated with Lp(a) having a buoyant density of 1.05-1.08 g/ml (intermediate between LDL and HDL). However, in the fed state a proportion of plasma apo(a) is associated with larger and less dense triglyceride-rich lipoproteins [32]. In a group of normo- and hyperlipidemic male subjects, 16.0 $\pm$ 4.6% of total plasma apo(a) was found associated with postprandial TRL [33]. It has been proposed that the association of apo(a) with TRL increases the atherothrombogenicity of these lipoproteins, however, the complete pathophysiological relevance of TRL apo(a) remains to be elucidated.

Postprandial Lipoproteins and Their Relationship to Thrombosis

The significance of thrombosis in the pathogenesis of unstable angina pectoris, myocardial infarction and sudden death has been clearly documented [34]. Normal blood hemostasis is maintained by complex coagulation and fibrinolytic systems, and increasing evidence suggests that these systems can be affected by the composition and concentration of circulating plasma lipoproteins (see excellent reviews by Hamsten [35] and Mitropoulos [36]). Only recently has research focused on postprandial lipoproteins, and both direct and indirect evidence suggests that these lipoproteins can affect the coagulation and fibrinolytic systems, platelet aggregability and blood viscosity.

POSTPRANDIAL TRL AND COAGULATION

Hypertriglyceridemia has been described as a procoagulent state because elevated levels of plasma triglyceride are associated with increased levels of fibrinogen and factor VII coagulant activity (VIIc) [35,36]. Chylomicron and VLDL cholesterol concentrations and VLDL triglyceride concentration have been directly correlated with VIIc [37], and diurnal changes in plasma triglyceride concentration have been found to be positively related to changes in VIIc with a delay of about 160 mins [38]. Plasma VIIc is also increased after the ingestion of a fat-rich meal, due to an increase in circulating activated factor VII but no increase in factor VII protein [39]. *In vivo* activation of factor VII is apparently dependent on triglyceride-rich lipoprotein lipolysis, since patients with lipoprotein lipase deficiency (with pronounced hypertriglyceridemia and chylomicronemia) do not have elevated levels of VIIc or VII protein [40]. It has thus been proposed that during lipolysis, a negatively charged environment is created by fatty acids accumulating on the surface of triglyceride-rich lipoproteins, which activates the intrinsic coagulation pathway, which in turn activates factor VII [36]. It is therefore TRL lipolysis resulting in the formation of TRL remnants, rather than newly secreted TRL themselves, which has the ability to influence blood coagulability.

POSTPRANDIAL TRL AND FIBRINOLYSIS

Although few studies have specifically focused on the effect of postprandial TRL on fibrinolysis, a number of studies have shown that hypertriglyceridemia is associated with elevated levels of plasminogen activator inhibitor-1 (PAI-1) and impaired fibrinolysis in individuals with CAD [41,42]. Diet or drug therapy designed to lower plasma triglyceride concentration in turn improves or even normalizes PAI-1 levels and fibrinolytic capacity [43]. PAI-1 is a serine protease which is able to inactivate plasminogen activators. These activators in turn control the conversion of plasminogen to plasmin, a key enzyme in the dissolution of fibrin clots and in the maintenance of the antithrombotic properties of the endothelium. Increased PAI-1 secretion by endothelial cells may be of critical importance in controlling the development of atheroma, as suggested by studies with human autopsy material, showing that PAI-1 levels are elevated in atherosclerotic lesions relative to healthy endothelium [44]. Stiko-Rahm et al. have shown that VLDL stimulates PAI-1 secretion from endothelial cells and that hypertriglyceridemic VLDL is a more potent stimulus than normotriglyceridemic VLDL [45]. This effect is apparently mediated through binding of VLDL to the LDL receptor. VLDL-mediated secretion of PAI-1 from HepG2 cells (an hepatic cell line) has also been demonstrated [46]. Since hypertriglyceridemic VLDL is enriched with apoE, and since apoE has a higher affinity for the LDL receptor than apoB, it is likely that hypertriglyceridemic VLDL (and postprandial TRL) can more effectively bind to endothelial cells and can induce a greater increase in PAI-1 secretion.

Platelet Aggregability and Hemorheology

Platelet aggregability and reactivity can affect atherothrombosis and is influenced by circulating lipoproteins [47]. Chylomicrons isolated in the fasted [48] and fed state [49] have been shown to affect platelet function, but the relevance of these observations to the *in vivo* pathophysiology of CAD needs to be further defined.

Impaired blood flow due to increased plasma viscosity promotes hypercoagulability and has been suggested to play a role in atherothrombogenesis [50]. In a recent study, Schütz et al. [51] have demonstrated that plasma viscosity and erythrocyte aggregation is significantly increased in plasma isolated from healthy normolipidemic subjects in the fed state. This effect was not apparent in plasma or serum when TRL were removed, and was not dependent on the presence of fibrinogen, suggesting that postprandial TRL can have a direct effect on hemorheological parameters. In extreme cases (severe familial hyperchylomicronemia), chylomicron accumulation is associated with impaired plasma viscosity and microcirculatory disturbances [52].

Therapeutic Implications

Clearly, considerable research is still required to identify which factor or factors are primarily responsible for the increased atherogenicity and thrombogenicity of the postprandial state. New and more sophisticated assay techniques are required to quantitate the plasma concentration of remnant lipoproteins and additional clinical studies are required to establish the prognostic value of measuring plasma lipids and lipoproteins in the fed state. In the meantime, it is reassuring to know that therapeutic manipulations which reduce the fasting triglyceride concentration, also have a beneficial effect on postprandial lipoprotein metabolism. Aerobic exercise, weight reduction, and triglyceride-lowering drugs [53,54] have all been shown to reduce postprandial triglyceridemia, and they potentially reduce the associated risk of atherosclerosis and thrombosis.

References

1. Expert Panel on Detection, Evaluation, and Treatment of High Blood Cholesterol in Adults. Summary of the Second Report of the National Cholesterol Education Proram (NCEP) Expert Panel on Detection, Evaluation, and Treatment of High Blood Cholesterol in Adults (Adult Treatment Panel II). JAMA 1993;269:3015-23.
2. Friedewald WT, Levy RI, Fredrickson DS. Estimation of the concentration of low-density lipoprotein cholesterol in plasma without use of the preparative ultracentrifuge. Clin Chem 1972;18:499-502.
3. Cohn JS, McNamara JR, Schaefer EJ. Lipoprotein cholesterol concentrations in the plasma of human subjects as measured in the fed and fasted states. Clin Chem 1988; 34:2456-59.
4. Cohn JS. Postprandial lipid metabolism. Curr Opin Lipidol 1994;5:185-90.
5. Karpe F, Hamsten A. Postprandial lipoprotein metabolism and atherosclerosis. Curr Opin Lipidol 1995;6:123-29.
6. Patsch JR, Miesenböck G, Hopferwieser T, et al. Relation of triglyceride metabolism and coronary artery disease. Studies in the postprandial state. Arterioscler Thromb 1992;12:1336-45.
7. Ginsberg HN, Jones J, Blaner WS, et al. Association of postprandial triglyceride and retinyl palmitate responses with newly diagnosed exercise-induced myocardial ischemia in middle-aged men and women. Arterioscler Thromb 1995;15:1829-38.
8. Ryu JE, Howard G, Craven TE, Bond MG, Hagaman AP, Crouse J III. Postprandial triglyceridemia and carotid atherosclerosis in middle-aged subjects. Stroke 1992;23: 823-28.
9. Zilversmit DB. Atherogenesis: A postprandial phenomenon. Circulation 1979;60: 473-85.
10. Simpson HS, Williamson CM, Olivecrona T, et al. Postprandial lipemia, fenofibrate and coronary artery disease. Atherosclerosis 1990;85:193-202.
11. Groot PHE, Van Stiphout WAHJ, Krauss XH, et al. Postprandial lipoprotein metabolism in normolipidemic men with and without coronary artery disease. Arterioscler Thromb 1991;11:653-62.
12. Brunzell JD, Schroll HG, Motulsky AG, Bierman EL. Myocardial infarction in the familial forms of hypertriglyceridemia. Metabolism 1976;25:313-20.
13. Mahley RW, Rall SC Jr. Type III hyperlipoproteinemia (dysbetalipoproteinemia): the role of apolipoprotein E in normal and abnormal lipoprotein metabolism. In: Scriver CR, Beaudet AL, Sly WS, Valle D, editors.The metabolic basis of inherited disease. New York: McGraw-Hill Publishing Co, 1989:1195-1213.
14. Havel RJ. Postprandial hyperlipidemia and remnant lipoproteins. Curr Opin Lipidol 1994;5:102-109.
15. Karpe F, Steiner G, Olivecrona T, Carlson LA, Hamsten A. Metabolism of triglyceride-rich lipoproteins during alimentary lipemia. J Clin Invest 1993;91:748-58.
16. Karpe F, Steiner G, Uffelman K, Olivecrona T, Hamsten A. Postprandial lipoproteins and progression of coronary atherosclerosis. Atherosclerosis 1994;106:83-97.
17. Cohn JS, Johnson EJ, Millar JS, et al. Contribution of apoB48 and apoB100 triglyceride-rich lipoproteins (TRL) to postprandial increases in the plasma concentration of TRL triglycerides and retinyl esters. J Lipid Res 1993;34: 2033-40.

18. Cohn JS, McNamara JR, Cohn SD, Ordovas JM, Schaefer EJ. Plasma apolipoprotein changes in the triglyceride-rich lipoprotein fraction of human subjects fed a fat-rich meal. J Lipid Res 1988;29:925-36.
19. Cohn JS, Wagner DA, Cohn SD, Millar JS, Schaefer EJ. Measurement of very low density and low density lipoprotein apolipoprotein (apo) B100 and high density lipoprotein apoA-I production in human subjects using deuterated leucine. J Clin Invest 1990;85:804-811.
20. Gianturco SH, Bradley WA. Triglyceride-rich lipoproteins and their role in atherogenesis. Curr Opin Lipidol 1991;2:324-28.
21. Hodis HN, Mack WJ. Triglyceride-rich lipoproteins and the progression of coronary artery disease. Curr Opin Lipidol 1995;6:209-14.
22. Miesenböck G, Patsch JR. Postprandial hyperlipidemia: the search for the atherogenic lipoprotein. Curr Opin Lipidol 1992;3:196-201.
23. Tall AR. Plasma cholesteryl ester transfer protein. J Lipid Res 1993;34:1255-74.
24. Castro GR, Fielding CJ. Effects of postprandial lipemia on plasma cholesterol metabolism. J Clin Invest 1985;75:874-82.
25. Tall A, Sammett D, Granot E. Mechanisms of enhanced cholesteryl ester transfer from high density lipoproteins to apolipoproteinB-containing lipoproteins during alimentary lipemia. J Clin Invest 1986;77:1163-72.
26. McPherson R, Mann CJ, Tall AR, et al. Plasma concentrations of cholesteryl ester transfer protein in hyperlipoproteinemia. Relation to cholesteryl ester transfer protein activity and other lipoprotein variables. Arterioscler Thromb 1991;11:797-804.
27. Mann CJ, Yen FT, Grant AM, Bihain BE. Mechanism of plasma cholesterol ester transfer in hypertriglyceridemia. J Clin Invest 1991;88:2059-66.
28. Després J-P, Marette A. Relation of components of insulin resistance syndrome to coronary disease risk. Curr Opin Lipidol 1994;5:274-89.
29. Lechleitner M, Hoppichler F, Föger B, Patsch JR. Low-density lipoproteins of the postprandial state induce cellular cholesteryl ester accumulation in macrophages. Arterioscler Thromb 1994;14:1799-1807.
30. Utermann G. The mysteries of lipoprotein(a). Science 1989;246:904-10.
31. Scanu AM, Fless GM. Lipoprotein(a): Heterogeneity and biological relevance. J Clin Invest 1990;85:1709-15.
32. Bersot TP, Innerarity TL, Pitas RE, Rall SC Jr, Weisgraber HH, Mahley RW. Fat feeding in humans induces lipoproteins of density less than 1.006 that are enriched in apoprotein (a) and that cause lipid accumulation in macrophages. J Clin Invest 1986; 77:622-30.
33. Cohn JS, Lam CWK, Sullivan DR, Hensley WJ. Plasma lipoprotein distribution of apolipoprotein(a) in the fed and fasted states. Atherosclerosis 1991;90:59-66.
34. Fuster V, Badimon L, Badimon JJ, Chesebro JH. The pathogenesis of coronary artery disease and the acute coronary syndromes. New Eng J Med 1992;326:242-250,310-318.
35. Hamsten A. The hemostatic system and coronary heart disease. Thromb Res 1993; 70:1-38.
36. Mitropoulos KA. Lipid-thrombosis interface. Brit Med Bull 1994; 50:813-32.
37. Mitropoulos KA, Miller GJ, Reeves BEA, Wilkes HC, Cruickshank JK. Factor VII coagulent activity is strongly associated with the plasma concentration of large lipoprotein particles in middle-aged men. Atherosclerosis 1989;76:203-208.
38. Miller GJ, Martin JC, Mitropoulos KA, et al. Plasma factor VII is activated by postprandial triglyceridaemia, irrespective of dietary fat composition. Atherosclerosis 1991;86:163-71.
39. Silveira A, Karpe F, Blombäck M, Steiner G, Walldius G, Hamsten A. Activation of coagulation factor VII during alimentary lipemia. Arterioscler Thromb 1994;14:60-69.

40. Mitropoulos KA, Miller GJ, Watts GF, Durrington PN. Lipolysis of triglyceride-rich lipoproteins activates coagulant factor XII: A study in familial lipoprotein-lipase deficiency. Atherosclerosis 1992;94:119-25.
41. Hamsten A, DeFaire U, Walldius G. Plasminogen activator inhibitor in plasma: risk factor for recurrent myocardial infarction. Lancet 1986; ii:533-37.
42. Resch KL, Ernst E, Matrai A, Buhl M, Schlosser P, Paulsen HF. Can rheologic variables be of prognostic relevance in atherosclerotic disease? Angiology 1991;42: 963-70.
43. Andersen P, Smith P, Seljeflot I, Brataker S, Arnesen H. Effects of gemfibrozil on lipids and haemostasis after myocardial infarction. Thromb Haemostas 1990;63: 174-77.
44. Lupu F, Bergonzelli GE, Heim DA, et al. Localization and production of plasminogen activator inhibitor-1 in healthy and atherosclerotic arteries. Arterioscler Thromb 1993;13:1090-1100.
45. Stiko-Rahm A, Wiman B, Hamsten A, Nilsson J. Secretion of plasminogen activator inhibitor-1 from cultured human umbilical vein endothelial cells is induced by very low density lipoprotein. Arteriosclerosis 1990;10:1067-73.
46. Mussoni L, Mannucci L, Sirtori M, et al. Hypertriglyceridemia and regulation of fibrinolytic activity. Arterioscler Thromb 1992;12:19-27.
47. Brook JG, Aviram M. Platelet lipoprotein interaction. Semin Thromb Hemost 1988; 14:258-65.
48. Aviram M, Furman B, Brook JG. Chylomicrons from patients with type V hyperlipoproteinemia inhibit platelet function. Atherosclerosis 1985;56:157-67.
49. Nordoy A, Lagarde M, Renaud S. Platelets during alimentary hyperlipaemia induced by cream and cod liver oil. Eur J Clin Invest 1984;14:339-45.
50. Koenig W, Ernst E. The possible role of hemorheology in atherothrombogenesis. Atherosclerosis 1992;94:93-107.
51. Schütz E, Schuff-Werner P, Güttner Y, Schulz S, Armstrong VW. Investigations into the haemorheological significance of postprandial and fasting hypertriglyceridemia. Eur J Clin Invest 1993;23:270-76.
52. Chazan BI, Ferguson BD, Castelli WP, Tonborg JNF, Balodimos MC, Rutstein DD. Lipemic retinalis: Microcirculatory changes and lipid studies in a family. Metabolism 1969;18:978-85.
53. Weintraub MS, Rosen Y, Otto R,Eisenberg S, Breslow JL. Physical exercise conditioning in the absence of weight loss reduces fasting and postprandial triglyceride-rich lipoprotein levels. Circulation 1989;79:1007-14.
54. Weintraub MS, Eisenberg S, Breslow JL. Different patterns of postprandial metabolism in normals, and type IIa, type III and type IV hyperlipoproteinemics: Effects of treatment with cholestyramine and gemfibrozil. J Clin Invest 1987;79: 1110-19.

ATHEROGENIC DYSLIPIDEMIA AND THE METABOLIC SYNDROME: PATHOGENESIS AND CHALLENGE OF THERAPY

Scott M. Grundy
Departments of Clinical Nutrition, Internal Medicine, and Biochemistry and the Center for Human Nutrition, University of Texas Southwestern Medical Center at Dallas, 5323 Harry Hines Boulevard, Dallas, Texas 75235-9052, USA

Introduction

There is growing evidence that atherosclerosis develops because of injury to the arterial wall. Several injurious agents have been discovered. These are called risk factors. The major risk factors for atherosclerotic coronary heart disease (CHD) are cigarette smoking, hypertension, high serum cholesterol, and diabetes mellitus. All of these risk factors presumably inflict some form of injury upon the arterial wall that in turn promotes development of atherosclerosis. Epidemiological data indicate that most excess deaths from CHD can be attributed to the known risk factors [1]. Undoubtedly, other injurious factors contribute to atherogenesis; but it is unlikely that these will diminish the importance of the major risk factors.

Role of Risk Factors in Development of Atherosclerosis

The mechanisms whereby risk factors promote atherogenesis are not fully understood. Their role nonetheless is currently a topic of intense investigation. This research has been stimulated by advances in the study of vascular biology. Application of vascular biology research to the atherosclerosis field is largely a study of how the known risk factors influence atherogenesis. Investigation focuses on the arterial-wall response to the various injuries induced by risk factors. An important concept behind this research is that it may be possible to modify the response to injury and thereby retard development of atherosclerosis and its complications. However, enthusiasm for study of the vascular wall responses to risk factors should not divert attention away from the risk factors themselves. These are the true causes of atherosclerosis and CHD. In the absence of injurious risk factors, atherosclerosis will not develop. At least equal investment in effort and resources therefore should still be given to learning the origins of the CHD risk factors and how to modify them.

A few comments about what is known about the nature of the arterial injury produced by the risk factors nonetheless is warranted. Of particular importance is the

A. M. Gotto, Jr. et al. (eds.), Drugs Affecting Lipid Metabolism, 237–247.

temporal nature of the risk factors, i.e., in what sequence they act to promote atherogenesis. The initial injury appears to be the penetration of low density lipoproteins (LDL) and other apolipoprotein B (apo B)-containing lipoproteins into the arterial intima. These lipoproteins pass between endothelial cells into the intima of the artery. Although many of these lipoproteins seemingly pass out of the intima and return to the blood stream, a small amount is retained within the intima. Here they become entrapped by binding to the extracellular matrix of the intima [2]. Entrapped lipoproteins can undergo various modifications that can initiate cellular responses. One apparent modification is oxidation [3]; oxidized LDL produces a series of cellular responses of a type that are typically seen within atherosclerotic lesions [4]. Other active LDL modifications also may occur. Some modified LDL is incorporated into macrophages producing foam cells. Accumulation of cholesterol-filled foam cells gives rise to the fatty streak, the first stage of atherosclerosis. The injurious action of LDL appears to be mitigated by high density lipoproteins (HDL). Among several protective actions, HDL may prevent interaction of LDL with the extracellular matrix thereby reducing entrapment of LDL.

The second stage of atherogenesis is the fibrous plaque; in this stage, a fibrous cap forms over the fatty streak [5]. Lesion progression results from proliferation of smooth muscle cells and their extrusion of fibrous connective tissue. The rate of conversion of the fatty streak into fibrous plaque appears to affected by other risk factors, particularly hypertension and diabetes mellitus [6]. Smoking may play a role at this stage as well [6]. Thus the nonlipid risk factors seemingly promote lesion growth by accelerating formation of the fibrous cap.

It was once thought that LDL and other apo B-containing lipoproteins exert their influence only at the stage of the fatty streak; thereafter other risk factors determine the course of development of plaques. Recent evidence however suggests that lipoproteins effect injury throughout atherogenesis. Lipoprotein injury apparently continues at the edge of lesions and promotes their extension and progression. This is suggested by the finding of zones of cholesterol-filled macrophages at the margins of plaques [7]. These zones probably represent sites of active lesion extension.

"Active" areas of plaques are significant for another reason as well. They represent sites of lesion instability. Recent data suggest that lipid-filled regions of plaques are those most prone to plaque rupture and thrombosis. Of note, most acute coronary events (myocardial infarction and unstable angina) result from an occluding thrombosis developing from plaque rupture at sites of plaque instability [7]. This finding is of immense significance because it raises the possibility that acute coronary events might be prevented by modifying areas of plaque instability. The recent findings of risk reduction in cholesterol-lowering clinical trials in high-risk patients supports the hypothesis that plaque stability can be restored [8-10].

Cigarette smoking likewise appears to predispose to plaque rupture. Unstable regions of plaques probably have an "inflammatory" component characterized by increased macrophage activity. Oxidized LDL may induce increased macrophage activity leading to plaque instability; cigarette smoking may do the same. Thus both high LDL levels and cigarette smoking appear to predispose to acute coronary syndromes by creating plaque instability.

Although instability of lesions may reside mainly in lipid-enriched zones, these zones typically are present in advanced plaques. Acute coronary syndromes rarely result from rupture of fatty streaks. Thus lesion progression seemingly creates the substrate upon which zones of plaque instability develops. Consequently all of the risk factors, regardless of how they affect the process of atherosclerosis, ultimately raise the risk for CHD.

Multiple Risk Factors and the Metabolic Syndrome

Epidemiological studies show that several risk factors tend to cluster in single individuals [11]. Two to four risk factors often occur together. This clustering is commonly referred to as "multiple risk factors." Moreover, the majority of risk factors derive from metabolic abnormalities. When multiple "metabolic" risk factors occur together, the condition can be called the "metabolic syndrome." Four categories of risk factors typically comprise the metabolic syndrome. These are (a) insulin resistance and/or noninsulin dependent diabetes mellitus (NIDDM), (b) elevated blood pressure, (c) various and often multiple lipoprotein abnormalities, and (d) a tendency towards thrombosis (procoagulant state). In many patients, these four categories of risk factors occur together and thereby predispose to premature CHD.

The causes of the metabolic syndrome are a subject of intense interest. One hypothesis holds that "insulin resistance" underlies multiple risk factors [12]. This hypothesis derives from the observation that patients having multiple risk factors frequently have high plasma insulin levels, an indicator of insulin resistance. High insulin levels seemingly are the result of decreased utilization of glucose in peripheral tissues, especially skeletal muscle. Insulin resistance is known to predispose to NIDDM [12]. Investigators further speculate that insulin resistance raises blood pressure and can induce various lipoprotein abnormalities. Moreover, high insulin levels may influence the arterial wall response to injurious risk factors in a way to accelerate atherogenesis.

Whether insulin resistance and high insulin levels constitute a final common pathway for initiation of the metabolic syndrome is uncertain; however, the various components of this syndrome are subject to several types of influences. At least five different factors are known to modify the expression of risk-factors. These are (a) diet composition, (b) obesity, (c) lack of physical activity, (d) aging, and (e) genetics. Some of these factors could act by inducing insulin resistance. Others probably act through other pathways. Thus the etiology of each of the risk factors may have a complex basis. The concept of multiple risk factors arising out of a single metabolic aberration nonetheless is intriguing and worthy of further investigation. This is a particularly important hypothesis because if true a more direct therapeutic approach to controlling multiple risk factors by single agents might be possible.

In this paper, major attention will be given to the lipoprotein component of the metabolic syndrome. Multiple lipoprotein abnormalities often occur in single individuals having the metabolic syndrome. Again the possibility that several lipoprotein abnormalities can result from one metabolic abnormality must be considered. Since an abnormal lipoprotein pattern can occur in the absence of definite hyperlipidemia (i.e., raised serum cholesterol and triglycerides), the term "dyslipidemia" may be more appropriate. Further, since the dyslipidemia associated with the metabolic syndrome often is present in patients with premature CHD, the term "atherogenic dyslipidemia" seems justified. Other investigators [13] have employed the term "atherogenic lipoprotein phenotype" to denote this lipoprotein pattern. In this paper, the term "atherogenic dyslipidemia" will be applied to the form of dyslipidemia observed in patients with the metabolic syndrome.

The Metabolic Syndrome and Atherogenic Dyslipidemia

Four lipoprotein abnormalities are commonly recognized in atherogenic dyslipidemia. They consist of (a) borderline-high levels of serum cholesterol (mild hypercholesterolemia), (b) mildly elevated triglycerides, (c) high levels of small, dense LDL particles, and (d) low levels of HDL cholesterol. Each of these lipoprotein abnormalities may contribute independently to the development of atherosclerosis. Borderline-high cholesterol levels (total cholesterol 200 to 239 mg/dl) typically reflect increased LDL cholesterol [14]. Mechanisms whereby raised LDL cholesterol promote atherogenesis were considered earlier. Mildly elevated triglycerides usually denote increases in different atherogenic, apo B-containing lipoproteins, namely, intermediate density lipoproteins (IDL) and remnants of very low density lipoproteins (VLDL). Small LDL particles, which are characteristic of this form of dyslipidemia [13], probably filter more readily into the arterial intima, resulting in more entrapment of LDL. And a low serum HDL cholesterol signifies a deficiency of HDL to protect against the injurious effects of atherogenic lipoproteins. Consequently, each of the components of atherogenic dyslipidemia likely acts independently but in concert to accelerate atherosclerosis.

FACTORS UNDERLYING ATHEROGENIC DYSLIPIDEMIA

Lipoprotein risk factors are multifactorial in origin. Lipoprotein metabolism is complex and subject to many influences. The question to be addressed here is whether there are certain metabolic changes that will elicit the atherogenic lipoprotein phenotype and simultaneously induce the other abnormalities of the metabolic syndrome. At present there are two candidates for underlying metabolic abnormalities. One of these is insulin resistance; the other is a high level of free fatty acids (FFA). Both of these abnormalities will be considered later, along with other possibilities. But it will be necessary to discuss as well as the basic aberrations that ultimately underlie the metabolic syndrome, namely, the composition of the diet, obesity, lack of physical activity, aging, and genetics. Each can be briefly reviewed.

DIET COMPOSITION

Saturated fatty acids and cholesterol. These two dietary factors act jointly to raise the LDL-cholesterol level. Both apparently suppress LDL-receptor activity [15]. Dietary cholesterol suppresses LDL receptor synthesis; this action is accentuated by saturated fatty acids [15]. Thus, diets high in meat fats, dairy fat, and eggs, which are the major sources of saturated fatty acids and cholesterol in the diet, contribute importantly to mild-to-moderate elevations of LDL cholesterol. Recently another category of fatty acid, trans monounsaturated fatty acids, has been observed to raise LDL cholesterol levels [16]. Although intakes of trans fatty acids are typically considerably less than those of saturated fatty acids, the former must be considered as another form of cholesterol-raising fatty acid. These two types of fatty acids must be distinguished from those that do not raise LDL cholesterol, namely, the polyunsaturated acid, linoleic acid, and the monounsaturated acid, oleic acid [17]. Unsaturated fatty acids are an important source of dietary fatty acids and are potential replacements for cholesterol-raising fatty acids. Of interest, one saturated fatty acid, stearic acid, does not raise LDL levels; apparently stearic acid is rapidly converted into oleic acid in the body and therefore has the action of oleic acid on LDL levels.

Dietary carbohydrate. Whereas dietary fat has its major effects on LDL metabolism, dietary carbohydrate influences lipoprotein metabolism in other ways. These effects are seen at high-carbohydrate intakes, i.e., with low-fat diets [17]. High-carbohydrate intakes lead to mild hypertriglyceridemia, low HDL-cholesterol levels, and small, dense LDL particles. These changes represent the other components of the atherogenic lipoprotein phenotype. There is considerable dispute whether the lipoprotein changes induced by carbohydrate are atherogenic. Populations that typically consume low-fat, high-carbohydrate diets usually have relatively low rates of CHD; however, whether the effects of high-carbohydrate diets in the presence of other risk factors are harmless is uncertain.

The mechanisms whereby high-carbohydrate diets induce the atherogenic lipoprotein phenotype are not fully understood. It is possible that certain causes of this phenotype are less atherogenic than others. The elevated triglycerides accompanying high-carbohydrate intakes may be due both to overproduction of triglyceride-rich lipoproteins by the liver and by sluggish lipolysis of triglyceride-rich lipoproteins. These changes in triglyceride metabolism may be partially responsible for the presence of small, dense LDL particles and for low HDL-cholesterol levels. On the other hand, a low HDL level may be due in part to a decreased secretion of apolipoprotein AI (apo AI) [18].

OBESITY

Obesity has two influences on lipoprotein metabolism that may accentuate atherogenic dyslipidemia. These are high levels of FFA and insulin resistance. Adipose tissue stores excess triglycerides and constantly releases FFA into the circulation. In the presence of obesity, the release of FFA is increased; consequently obese patients have high FFA levels [19]. High FFA levels have a direct action on hepatic lipid metabolism. They enhance synthesis of triglycerides that provide more triglyceride for incorporation into VLDL particles [20]. In addition, obesity apparently increases the number of apo B-containing lipoproteins secreted into the circulation [21,22]. This may be the result of overproduction of both triglyceride and cholesterol by the liver. For reasons not understood, obesity further reduces HDL-cholesterol levels [21]. This response may be due in part to changes in triglyceride metabolism, but other, undefined actions on HDL metabolism may be at work as well.

A second effect of obesity is insulin resistance [22]. In fact, the effect also is due in large part to high FFA levels. Excess circulating FFA convert skeletal-muscle metabolism into predominant fat utilization. This occurs at the expense of glucose oxidation (the Randle effect) [23]. The result is peripheral insulin resistance, and secondarily, high insulin levels. Seemingly resistance to insulin-mediated uptake of glucose by muscle raises the plasma glucose level; this in turn stimulates the secretion of insulin by beta-cells of pancreatic islets and restores normoglycemia. This stimulation of insulin secretion may be further enhanced by high FFA levels [24].

High plasma levels of FFA not only induce insulin resistance in skeletal muscle but also in liver. Similar mechanisms lead to decreased glucose oxidation and hepatic insulin resistance [25]. Insulin seemingly suppresses the formation of lipoproteins by the liver [26]. Failure of this usual action in the insulin-resistant liver allows for enhanced formation of apo B-containing lipoproteins, and hence to atherogenic dyslipidemia.

An unresolved question is whether high insulin levels per se have untoward metabolic effects. Some investigators have speculated that high insulin levels cause an overproduction of lipoproteins leading to atherogenic dyslipidemia. More likely, hepatic insulin resistance, and not hyperinsulinemia, is primarily responsible for this phenomenon. On the other hand, high insulin levels directly contribute to the development of hypertension, although the mechanisms are uncertain.

Even though obese individuals typically have high FFA levels and high insulin levels, there is considerable variability in absolute levels. This variability goes beyond variations in total body fat content. One factor that influences FFA concentrations and degree of insulin resistance is the distribution of body fat. When the distribution favors a truncal location, the metabolic complications are worse [22,27-29]. Apparently truncal adipose tissue more readily releases FFA than does adipose tissue in peripheral locations. This form of adipose tissue appears to be more "active" in its release of FFA; it contrasts to the more "inactive" form of adipose tissue found in the lower body (gluteofemoral region). The precise location of fat in the truncal region that is more prone to release FFA is uncertain. Some investigators believe that intraperitoneal fat is the most active; recent studies from our laboratory however suggest that subcutaneous fat in the truncal region imparts the greatest adverse impact on metabolism [22]. This may be explained by the fact that subcutaneous truncal fat exceeds amounts of intraperitoneal fat by about four fold.

Physical Inactivity

A third "cause" of the metabolic syndrome and atherogenic dyslipidemia is physical inactivity. Lack of exercise accentuates the metabolic abnormalities brought about by obesity. The preferred type of physical activity, namely, "aerobic" or dynamic activity, enhances FFA utilization and lowers circulating FFA levels. In this case, increased FFA oxidation does not interfere with glucose metabolism. Seemingly exercise lowers FFA levels and reduces insulin resistance at the same time. The effect apparently is prolonged, going beyond the time of immediate exercise. This state might be called "metabolic fitness." In spite of these apparently favorable actions of exercise, more research is needed on the metabolic consequences of various types and amounts of exercise.

AGING

The prevalence of atherogenic dyslipidemia increases with aging [14]. A question of considerable interest is whether the onset of dyslipidemia is a result of the aging process *per se*, or is indirectly the result of changes in body weight and body composition with aging. The possibility exists that intracellular metabolic changes do occur with aging. These could alter lipoprotein metabolism leading to dyslipidemia. For example, it has been claimed that LDL-receptor activity decreases with age [30-32]. If so, this decrease could partially explain a rise of LDL-cholesterol levels with aging.

A second cause of atherogenic dyslipidemia with aging is weight gain. For example, average American adult gains approximately 20 pounds from age 20 to age 50 [33]. Much of this excess weight accumulates in the trunk where adipose tissue is more active in releasing FFA. This weight gain corresponds and correlates with increasing cholesterol and triglyceride levels [33]. It is widely believed that some weight gain with aging is "normal" and without adverse consequences; in many people however it probably is sufficient to elicit the atherogenic lipoprotein phenotype [33].

Finally, even in the absence of weight gain there is a change in body composition with aging. Typically fat stores increase and skeletal muscle decline. This change represents an unfavorable change in the adipose tissue-skeletal muscle axis. It could contribute significantly to the increase in insulin resistance and the increased prevalence of atherogenic dyslipidemia with aging.

GENETICS

A final factor contributing to atherogenic dyslipidemia is genetics. Most genetic investigations [34-36], such as those in twins, indicate that about 50% of the variability in a given lipoprotein trait (e.g. LDL cholesterol, HDL cholesterol, or triglycerides) is determined by heredity. The remainder is acquired. Thus within populations, only people who are genetically susceptible will develop atherogenic dyslipidemia in the presence of aggravating acquired factors. Moreover, most lipoprotein abnormalities occurring in the atherogenic lipoprotein phenotype are polygenic in origin. Multiple genes are known to affect concentrations of all the different lipoprotein species; their interplay most likely is responsible for atherogenic dyslipidemia.

Numerous monogenic defects have been identified that cause various forms of hyperlipidemia or dyslipidemia. In the population as a whole, however, monogenic forms of dyslipidemia are relatively rare. Most of the lipoprotein abnormalities typically observed in atherogenic dyslipidemia are polygenic in origin. This accounts for the failure of previous attempts to define a common monogenic causes of the atherogenic lipoprotein phenotype. Most previous genetic studies [37-39] have examined the statistical associations between DNA sequence polymorphisms in candidate genes and plasma concentrations of lipoproteins or apolipoproteins in populations of unrelated individuals. Polymorphisms in gene alleles have been used to group individuals according to the occurrence of a particular DNA sequence. By comparing plasma levels of the trait between the groups, the influence of a polymorphic sequence on the concentration of the trait can be assessed. However, on the basis of the data obtained to date in these association studies, the proportion of the variation in levels of various lipoproteins has been small. A major reason for this likely is that the power of association studies in unrelated individuals is limited because DNA polymorphisms do not unambiguously distinguish alleles. Alleles considered to be "identical-by-state" according to the presence or absence of a restriction site may be highly heterogeneous. Expansion of this approach to the defining of haplotypes by using several different polymorphisms appear to add little additional power. The limitations of this approach are well illustrated by a recent report in which various DNA polymorphisms were determined in a large number of patients with and without CHD [40]; in this study, no consistent allelic associations were noted between those with and without the disease.

Recently however a new conceptual approach has been employed to resolve this problem [41-43]. This is the use of sibling-pair analysis. This analysis typically makes use of genetic testing in a large number of families in which several family members are present. By linking the inheritance of specific candidate genes with variation of a given trait in the siblings of a large number of families, it is possible to determine whether particular genes affect the expression of a trait; in addition, an estimate can be made of how much they contribute to variation in gene expression. This approach has been made possible by the identification of many polymorphic DNA markers through the Human Genome Project and by the development of technology to analyze large number of DNA samples. Although sibling-pair analysis was early limited by availability of informative DNA sequence polymorphisms, data from the Human Genome Project now provides highly informative microsatellite polymorphisms that allow for unambiguous identification of parental alleles for any candidate locus in almost all nuclear families. Recently innovations [42-43] in statistical analysis have increased the power of this approach.

Recently, Cohen et al. [44] evaluated candidate genes affecting one component of atherogenic dyslipidemia, namely, low HDL-cholesterol levels, using the sibling-pair approach. These studies revealed that two gene loci, hepatic lipase and the AI/CIII/AIV gene complex, account for about 50% of the genetic contribution to variation in HDL-cholesterol levels in the general Caucasian population. In the future it will be possible to apply this method to the study of other candidate genes affecting other components of the atherogenic lipoprotein phenotype.

THERAPEUTIC IMPLICATIONS

Since both genetic and acquired factors contribute to the development of atherogenic dyslipidemia, the therapeutic approach must attack both categories of causes. For treatment of acquired causes, attention should be given mainly to modification of life habits. For the most part, this will include reducing intakes of cholesterol and saturated fatty acids, weight control, and regular exercise. Moreover, education directed towards life-habit modification should be directly predominantly to the general public. This requires the public health approach to risk reduction. In contrast, treatment of the genetic component of atherogenic dyslipidemia may need drug treatment. Since elevated LDL-cholesterol lies at the heart of this lipoprotein phenotype, statin drugs will be necessary for many patients [45], particularly those at high risk or having established CHD [9,10]. Patients who have low HDL-cholesterol levels with or without hypertriglyceridemia will respond well to nicotinic acid therapy [46]. This drug can be given either with or without concomitant statin therapy. Unfortunately, many patients are not able to tolerate nicotinic acid; moreover, there are no good alternatives to this agent. Fibric acids are effective triglyceride-lowering drugs; but they have little influence on HDL-cholesterol levels [47]. The future thus presents a challenge for the development of new pharmaceutical approaches to the management of atherogenic dyslipidemia.

References

1. Stamler J, Wentworth D, Neaton JD for the MRFIT Research Group. Is relationship between serum cholesterol and risk of premature death from coronary heart disease continuous or graded? JAMA 1986;256:2823-28.
2. Wight TN. The vascular extracellular for matrix. In: Fuster V, Ross R, Topol EJ, editors. Atherosclerosis and coronary artery disease. Philadelphia: Lippincott-Fraven Pub, 1986:421-40.
3. Steinberg D, Witztum JL. Lipoproteins and atherogenesis: Current concepts. JAMA 1990; 264:3047-52.
4. Chisolm GM III and Penn MS. Oxidized lipoproteins and atherosclerosis. In: Fuster V, Ross R, Topol EJ, editors. Atherosclerosis and coronary heart disease. Philadelphia: Lippincott-Fraven Pub, 1996:129-49.
5. Stary HC. The histological classification of atherosclerotic lesions in human coronary arteries. In: Fuster V, Ross R, Topol EJ, editors. Atherosclerosis and coronary heart disease. Philadelphia: Lippincott-Fraven Pub, 1996:436-74.
6. Wissler RW, Hiltscher I, Oinuma T, PDAY Research Groups. In: Fuster V, Ross R, Topol EJ, editors. Atherosclerosis and coronary heart disease. Philadelphia: Lippincott-Fraven Pub, 1996:475-879.
7. Davies MJ, Richardson PD, Woolf N, Katz DR, Mann J. Risk of thrombosis in human atherosclerotic plaques: Role of extracellular lipid, macrophage, and smooth muscle cell content. Br Heart J 1992;69:377-81.
8. Brown BG, Zhao X-Q, Sacco DE, Albers JJ. Lipid lowering and plaque regression: New insights into prevention of plaque disruption and clinical events in coronary disease. Circulation 1993;87:1781-91.
9. Scandinavian Simvastatin Survival Study Group. Randomized trial of cholesterol lowering in 4444 patients with coronary heart disease; the Scandinavian Simvastatin Survival Study (4S). Lancet 1994;344:1383.
10. Shepherd J, Cobbe SM, Ford I, et al. for the West of Scotland Coronary Prevention Study Group. Prevention of coronary heart diseases with pravastatin in men with hypercholesterolemia. N Engl J Med 1995;333:1301-7.
11. Stokes J III, Kannel WB, Wolf PA, Cupples LA, D'agostino RB. The relative importance of

selected risk factors for various manifestations of cardiovascular disease among men and women from 35 to 64 years old: 30 years of follow-up in the Framingham Study. Circulation 1987;75:V-65-V-73.
12. Reaven GM. Insulin resistance and compensatory hyperinsulinemia: Role in hypertension, dyslipidemia, and coronary heart disease. Am Heart J 1991;121:1283-88.
13. Austin MA, King M-C, Vranizan KM, Krauss RM. Atherogenic lipoprotein phenotype. A proposed genetic marker for coronary heart disease risk. Circulation 1990;82:495-506.
14. Expert Panel on Detection, Evaluation, and Treatment of High Blood Cholesterol in Adults: National Cholesterol Education Program. Second report of the expert panel on detection, evaluation, and treatment of high blood cholesterol (Adult Treatment Panel II) Circulation 1994;89:1329-445.
15. Daumeri CM, Woolett LA, Dietschy JM. Fatty acids regulate hepatic low density lipoprotein receptor activity through redistribution of intracellular cholesterol pools. Proc Natl Acad Sci USA 1992;89:10797-801.
16. Mensink RP and Katan MB. Effect of dietary trans fatty acids on high density and low density lipoprotein cholesterol levels in healthy subjects. N Engl J Med 1990;323:439-45.
17. Grundy SM and Denke MA. Dietary influence on serum lipids and lipoproteins. J Lipid Res 1990;31:1149-92.
18. Brinton EA, Eisenberg S, Breslow JL. A low-fat diet decreases high density lipoprotein (HDL) cholesterol levels by decreasing HDL apolipoprotein transport rates. J Clin Invest 1990;85: 144-51.
19. Bjorntorp P, Bergman H, Varnauskas E, Lindholm B. Lipid mobilization in relation to body composition in man. Metabolism 1969;18:841-51.
20. Grundy SM. Metabolism of very low density lipoprotein-triglycerides in man. In: Gotto AM Smith LC, Allen B, editors. Atherosclerosis V. New York: Springer-Verlag, 1980:586-90.
21. Denke MA, Sempos CT, Grundy SM. Excess body weight: An underrecognized contributor to high blood cholesterol levels in white American men. Arch Intern Med 1993;153:1093-103.
22. Abate N, Garg A, Peshock RM, Stray-Gundersen J, Grundy SM. Relationship of generalized and regional adiposity to insulin sensitivity in men. J Clin Invest 1995;96:88-98.
23. Randle PJ, Garland PB, Hales CN, Newsholme EA. The glucose fatty acid cycle. Its role in insulin sensitivity and metabolic disturbances of diabetes mellitus. Lancet 1963;I:785-89.
24. Crespin SR, Greenbough III WB, Steinberg D. Stimulation of insulin secretion by infusion of free fatty acids. J Clin Invest 1969;48:1934-37.
25. Randle PJ, Priestman DA, Mistry S, Halsall A. Mechanisms modifying glucose oxidation in diabetes mellitus. Diabetologia 1994;37:2155-61.
26. Pullinger CR, North JD, Teng B-B, Rifici VA, Ronhild de Brito AE, Scott J. The apolipoprotein B gene is constitutively expressed in HepG2 cells: Regulation of secretion by oleic acid, albumin, and insulin, and measurement of the mRNA half-life. J Lipid Res 1989; 30:1065-77.
27. Despres J-P, Marette A. Relation of components of insulin resistance syndrome to coronary disease risk. Current Opinion in Lipidology 1994;5:274-89.
28. Evans DJ, Murray R, Kissebah AH. Relationship between skeletal muscle insulin resistance, insulin-mediated glucose disposal, and insulin binding. Effects of obesity and body fat topography. J Clin Invest 1984;74:1515-25.
29. Landin K, Lonnroth P, Krotkiewski M, Holm G, Smith U. Increased insulin resistance and fat cell lipolysis in obese but not lean women with a high waist/hip ratio. Eur J Clin Invest 1990; 20:530-35.

30. Miller NE. Why does plasma low density lipoprotein concentration in adults increase with age? Lancet 1984;1:263-66.
31. Grundy SM, Vega GL, Bilheimer DW. Kinetic mechanisms determining variability in low density lipoprotein levels and their rise with age. Arteriosclerosis 1985; 5:623-30.
32. Ericsson S, Eriksson M, Vitrols S, Einarsson E, Berglund L, Angelin B. Influence of age on the metabolism of plasma low density lipoproteins in healthy males. J Clin Invest 1991;87: 591-96.
33. The Lipid Research Clinics Population Studies Data Book. The Prevalence Study. Bethesda, Maryland, NIH Publication No. 79-1527, 1979.
34. Bucher KD, Friedlander Y, Kaplan EB, et al. Biological and cultural sources of familial resemblance in plasma lipids: A comparison between North America and Israel--the Lipid Research Clinics Program. Genetic Epidemiol 1988;5:17-33.
35. Austin MA, King MC, Bawol RD, Huley SB, Friedman GD. Risk factors for coronary heart disease in adult female twins. Genetic heritability and shared environmental influences. Am J Epidemiol 1987;125:308-18.
36. Heller DA, De Faire D, Pedersen NL, Dahlen G, McClearn GE. Genetic and environmental influences on serum lipid levels in twins. N Engl J Med 1993;328:1150-56.
37. Humphries SE. DNA polymorphisms of the apolipoprotein genes--their use in the investigation of the genetic component of hyperlipidaemia and atherosclerosis. Atherosclerosis 1988;72:89-108.
38. Lussi AJ. Genetic factors affecting blood lipoproteins: The candidate gene approach. J Lipid Res 1988;29:397-429.
39. Kessling A, Ouellette S. Bouffard O, et al. Patterns of association between genetic variability in apolipoprotein (apo) B, apo AI-CIII-AIV, and cholesterol ester transfer protein gene regions and quantitative variation in lipid and lipoprotein traits: Influence of gender and exogenous hormones. Am J Human Gen 1992;50:92-106.
40. Marshall HW, Morrison LC, Wu LL, et al. Apolipoprotein polymorphisms fail to define risk of coronary artery disease. Results of a prospective, angiographically controlled study. Circulation 1994;89:567-77.
41. Haseman JK, Elston RC. The investigation of linkage between a quantitative trait and a marker locus. Behavior Genetics 1972;2:3-19.
42. Kruglyak L, Lander ES. A nonparametric approach for mapping quantitative trait loci. Genetics 1972;139:1421-28.
43. Amos CI. Robust variance-components approach for assessing genetic linkage in pedigrees. Am J Human Gen 1994;54:535-43.
44. Cohen JC, Wang Z, Grundy SM, Stoesz MR, Guerra R. Variation at the hepatic lipase and apolipoprotein AI/CIII/AIV loci is a major cause of genetically determined variation in plasma HDL cholesterol levels. J Clin Invest 1994; 94:2377-84.
45. Grundy SM. HMG-CoA reductase inhibitors for treatment of hypercholestesrolemia. N Engl J Med 1988;319:24-33.
46. Vega GL, Grundy SM. Lipoprotein responses to treatment with lovastatin, gemfibrozil, and nicotinic acid in normolipidemic patients with hypoalphalipoproteinemia. Arch Intern Med 1994;154:73-82.
47. Vega GL, Grundy SM. Comparison of lovastatin and gemfibrozil in normolipidemic patients with hypoalphalipoproteinemia. JAMA 1989;262:3148-53.

VERY LOW DENSITY LIPOPROTEIN RECEPTOR GENE THERAPY IN A MOUSE MODEL OF FAMILIAL HYPERCHOLESTEROLEMIA

Lawrence Chan and Kunihisa Kobayashi
Departments of Cell Biology and Medicine, Baylor College of Medicine, One Baylor Plaza, Houston, Texas 77030-3498, USA

Somatic gene therapy is an experimental form of treatment that was initially developed for the management of monogenic diseases. It was rapidly expanded and used for the treatment of cancer and infectious diseases as well as polygenic disorders. Familial hypercholesterolemia (FH) is the prototype monogenic disorder affecting lipoprotein metabolism that has been used as a model system for somatic gene therapy.

Familial hypercholesterolemia is an autosomal dominant disorder characterized by elevated plasma cholesterol and premature coronary artery disease [1]. Heterozygotes occur in the general population with a frequency of about 1 in 500 and homozygotes, with a frequency of about 1 in a million. Heterozygotes develop moderate hypercholesterolemia resulting in myocardial ischemia usually in early middle age. Homozygous patients present with angina pectoris, myocardial infarction, or sudden death between the ages of 5 and 30. FH is caused by defects in the low density lipoprotein receptor (LDLR). Conventional forms of treatment include exercise, diet therapy, and lipid-lowering drugs. Alternative modes of therapy that have been used for resistant cases include ileal bypass, protacaval shunt, and liver transplantation. The drastic nature of these last modes of therapy justifies the exploration of somatic gene therapy as an alternative form of treatment for this monogenic disease.

The standard approach to monogenic disorders is the replacement of the defective gene by somatic gene transfer. Therefore, the LDLR was used as a therapeutic gene in the initial trials of somatic gene therapy for FH. Chowdhury et al. transduced hepatocytes isolated from watanabe heritable hyperlipidemic (WHHL) rabbits (an FH animal model) with a retroviral vector containing the LDLR gene [2]. Transplantation of these genetically modified hepatocytes into the liver of WHHL rabbits resulted in a 30-50% decrease in total serum cholesterol that persisted for the duration of the experiment (4 months). Recently, Grossman et al. used the same *ex vivo* approach to treat five homozygous FH patients using retrovirus-mediated LDLR gene transfer [3]. They found that the patients showed a widely variable response with unequivocal improvement in only one of them. They concluded that substantial modification must be made on the *ex vivo* gene transfer protocol before such an approach should be applied as a therapeutic measure for FH patients.

A. M. Gotto, Jr. et al. (eds.), Drugs Affecting Lipid Metabolism, 249–253.

In contrast to *ex vivo* gene therapy which requires the transduction of target cells surgically removed from the patient, *in vivo* gene therapy involves the direct administration of the therapeutic gene to a patient. The *in vivo* route is the much preferred approach if gene therapy is to be applied routinely to large numbers of patients. As a gene transfer vehicle, adenoviral vectors efficiently deliver therapeutic genes to the liver of experimental animals *in vivo*. They have been found to be highly efficient in reversing the hypercholesterolemia in LDLR-deficient rabbits (WHHL rabbits) [4,5] and mice (LDLR knockout mice) [6].

In addition to the LDLR, a number of other genes have been tested for the treatment of hypercholesterolemia in experimental animals (reviewed in [7] and in [8]). Our laboratory has examined two genes, those for apobec-1 and the very low density lipoprotein receptor (VLDLR), as potential therapeutic genes in the treatment of hypercholesterolemia in LDLR knockout mice.

Apobec-1 is the catalytic subunit of an editosome complex that catalyzes the conversion of apoB-100 mRNA to apoB-48 mRNA (reviewed in [9]). Overexpression of apobec-1 mRNA in the liver of the mouse has been shown to markedly lower plasma apoB-100 and drastically reduce plasma low density lipoprotein (LDL) production [10]. Similar experiments in LDLR knockout mice indicate that apobec-1 can be used as a potential therapeutic gene in this FH animal model.

The VLDLR is a newly described receptor that belongs to the LDLR gene family. It is normally expressed at moderately high levels in heart, muscle, adipose tissue as well as other tissues. Its expression is extremely low in the liver. Its normal role in lipoprotein metabolism is unknown. However, cells transfected with the LDLR have been shown to recognize apoE-containing lipoproteins [11,12]. We have made use of this information and examined the use of the VLDLR as a therapeutic gene in the treatment of LDLR knockout mice [13].

We generated a replication-defective adenovirus (AdmVLDLR) containing mouse VLDLR cDNA driven by a cytomegalovirus promoter. Transduction of cultured Hepa (mouse hepatoma) cells and LDLR-deficient CHO-ldlA7 cells *in vitro* by the virus led to high-level expression of immunoreactive VLDLR proteins with M_r of 143 kDa and 161 kDa. Digestion of the cell extract with the enzymes neuraminidase, N-glycanase, and O-glycanase resulted in the stepwise lowering of the apparent size of the 161 kDa species toward the 143 kDa species. LDLR(-/-) mice fed a 0.2% cholesterol diet were treated with a single intravenous injection of 3×10^9 pfu AdmVLDLR. Control LDLR(-/-) mice received either phosphate-buffered saline or AdLacZ, a similar adenovirus containing the LacZ cDNA instead of mVLDLR cDNA. Comparison of the plasma lipids in the 3 groups of mice indicates that in the AdmVLDL animals, total cholesterol is reduced by ~50% at days 4 and 9 and returned toward control values on day 21 (Figure 1). In these animals there was also a ~30% reduction in plasma apoE accompanied by a 90% fall in apoB-100 on day 4 of treatment. By FPLC analysis, the major reduction in plasma cholesterol in the AdmVLDLR animals was accounted for by a marked reduction in the intermediate density lipoprotein (IDL)/LDL fraction. Plasma VLDL, IDL/LDL and high density lipoprotein (HDL) were isolated from the three groups of animals by ultracentrifugal flotation. In the AdmVLDLR animals there was substantial loss (~65%) of protein and cholesterol mainly in the IDL/LDL fraction on days 4 and 9. Nondenaturing gradient gel electrophoresis indicates a preferential loss of the IDL peak although the LDL peak was also reduced. When ^{125}I-IDL was administered intravenously into animals on day 4, the AdmVLDLR animals cleared the ^{125}I-IDL at a rate 5-10 times higher than the AdLacZ animals.

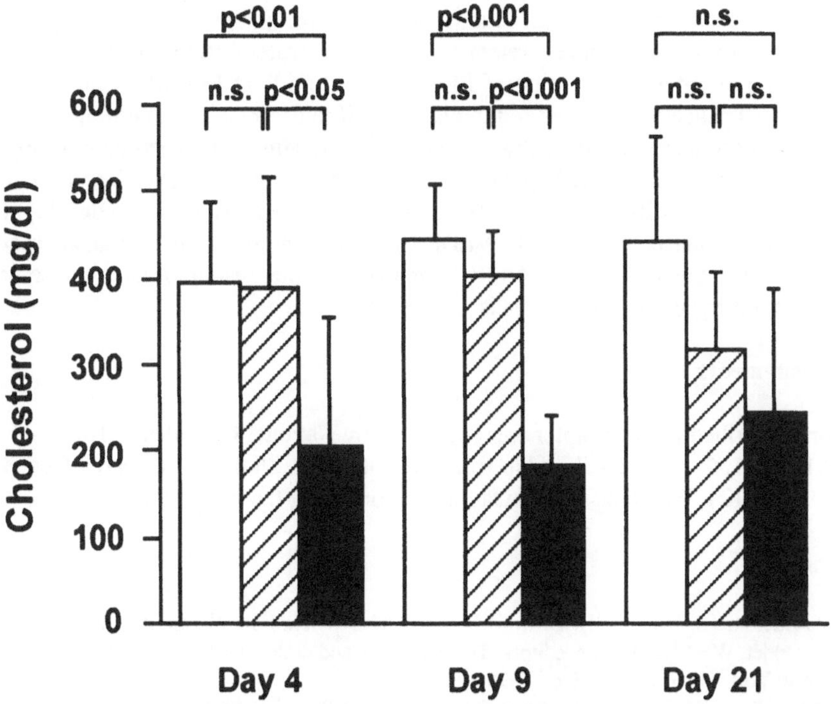

Figure 1. Plasma cholesterol in LDLR knockout mice on day 4, 9, and 21 following a single intravenous injection of phosphate-buffered saline (open bars), 3 x 10^9 pfu AdLacZ (hatched bars), or 3 x 10^9 pfu AdmLDLR (solid bars). Values represent mean ± standard deviation.

We conclude that adenovirus-mediated transfer of the VLDLR gene induces high-level hepatic expression of the VLDLR and results in a reversal of the hypercholesterolemia in 0.2% cholesterol diet-fed LDLR(-/-) mice. The VLDLR overexpression appears to greatly enhance the ability of these animals to clear IDL, resulting in a marked lowering of the plasma IDL/LDL.

Our observations raise the possibility that the VLDLR may be an effective therapeutic gene for the treatment of hypercholesterolemia. Use of this gene is especially attractive for the treatment of FH patients who have total absence of the LDLR or who have major abnormality in their LDLR. These patients are likely to be resistant to the usual hypolipidemic agents. Replacement of the normal LDLR gene in these patients may appear to be a rational approach and has been found to be efficacious in experimental animals in the short term. However, there are theoretical drawbacks to LDLR gene transfer that may be circumvented by the use of the VLDLR gene instead. The normal LDLR might be recognized as a foreign protein in LDLR-deficient patients and its expression on the liver cell surface could evoke an immunological response which may eventually cause the inactivation of the LDLR protein. The VLDLR, in contrast, is nonimmunogenic, because VLDLR is normally expressed in various tissues of the patient with FH and is not recognized by the host immune system as a foreign protein. Additional experiments comparing the long-term expression of LDLR and VLDLR in LDLR(-/-) animals, and eventually in FH patients, will be needed to determine if this is a valid concern. In any case, VLDLR appears to be a good alternative to LDLR in the treatment of hypercholesterolemia.

In conclusion, the LDLR gene appears to be effective in reversing the hypercholesterolemia in LDLR(-/-) animals. Its use in FH patients must await the development of improved gene transfer methods. The VLDLR gene has shown promise as an alternative therapeutic gene in the treatment of LDLR(-/-) animals. Further testing of its use in somatic gene therapy for hypercholesterolemia is warranted.

Acknowledgments

The work described in this chapter was supported by National Institutes of Health Grant HL-16512 (to L.C.) and a fellowship from the Children's Nutrition Research Center in Houston (to K.K.). We thank Ms. Linda Phillips for typing the manuscript.

References

1. Goldstein JL, Hobbs HH, Brown MS. Familial hypercholesterolemia In: CR Scriver, AL Beaudet, WS Sly, D Valle, editors. The metabolic and molecular bases of inherited disease. New York:McGraw-Hill, Inc., 1995:1981-2030.
2. Chowdhury JR, Grossman M, Gupta S, Chowdhury NR, Baker JR Jr, Wilson JM. Long-term improvement of hypercholesterolemia after *ex vivo* gene transfer in LDLR-deficient rabbits. Science 1991;254:1802-1805.
3. Grossman M, Rader DJ, Muller DWM, et al. A pilot study of ex vivo gene therapy for homozygous familial hypercholesterolaemia. Nature Medicine 1995;1:1148-54.
4. Kozarsky KF, McKinley DR, Austin LL, Raper SE, Stratford-Perricaudet LD, Wilson JM. *In vivo* correction of low density lipoprotein receptor deficiency in the watanabe heritable hyperlipidemic rabbit with recombinant adenoviruses. J Biol Chem 1994;289:13695-702.
5. Li J, Fang B, Eisensmith RC, Li XHC, et al. *In vivo* gene therapy for hyperlipidemia: Phenotypic correction in watanabe rabbits by hepatic delivery of the rabbit LDL receptor gene. J Clin Invest 1995;95:768-73.
6. Ishibashi S, Brown MS, Goldstein JL, Gerard RD, Hammer RE, Herz J. Hypercholesterolemia in LDL receptor knockout mice and its reversal by adenovirus-mediated gene delivery. J Clin Invest 1993;92:883-93.
7. Chan L. Use of somatic gene transfer to study lipoprotein metabolism in experimental animals *in vivo*. Curr Opin Lipidol 1995;6:335-40.

8. Gerard RD, Chan L. Adenovirus-mediated gene transfer: Strategies and applications in lipoprotein research. Curr Opin Lipidol 1996; in press.
9. Chan L, Seeburg PH. RNA editing. Scientific American, Science and Medicine 1995;2:68-77.
10. Teng B, Blumenthal S, Forte T, et al. Adenovirus-mediated gene transfer of rat apolipoprotein B mRNA editing protein in mice virtually eliminates apolipoprotein B-100 and normal low density lipoprotein production. J Biol Chem 1994;269:29395-404.
11. Takahashi S, Kawarabayasi Y, Nakai T, Sakai J, Yamamoto T. Rabbit very low density lipoprotein receptor: A low density lipoprotein receptor-like protein with distinct ligand specificity. Proc Natl Acad Sci 1992;89:9252-56.
12. Takahashi S, Suzuki J, Kohno M, et al. Enhancement of the binding of triglyceride-rich lipoproteins to the very low density lipoprotein receptor by apolipoprotein E and lipoprotein lipase. J Biol Chem 1995;270:15747-54.
13. Kobayashi K, Oka K, Forte T, et al. Reversal of hypercholesterolemia in low density lipoprotein receptor knockout mice by adenovirus-mediated gene transfer of the very low density lipoprotein receptor. J Biol Chem 1996;271:6852-60.

STUDIES ON THE PATHOGENESIS OF ATHEROSCLEROSIS USING APOLIPOPROTEIN E-DEFICIENT MICE

Sunny H. Zhang, Robert L. Reddick, and Nobuyo Maeda
Department of Pathology, The University of North Caroline at Chapel Hill, NC 27599-7525, USA

Introduction

Atherosclerosis is a complex disease resulting from the interaction of diverse genetic and environmental factors. In order to study the contribution of each etiological factor to the development of atherosclerosis, suitable animal models are needed. With the progress in mouse genetics and the development of gene targeting techniques, recently it has become in vogue to use genetically engineered mouse models to study atherogenesis. The apolipoprotein E-deficient mouse model is one of such examples.

Development of Atherosclerosis in Apo E-Deficient Mice

The apolipoprotein (apo) E-deficient mice were generated by gene targeting in the embryonic stem cells [1]. The gene coding for apo E protein, an essential protein for lipoprotein clearance in mice, was inactivated in these mice. Mice homozygous for the genetic modification do not express apo E (apo E deficient). Apo E-deficient mice have spontaneously elevated plasma cholesterol levels, five times normal, even when fed a regular low fat diet [2,3]. The hypercholesterolemia in these mice is due to marked accumulation of cholesterol-rich remnant particles of very low density lipoprotein (VLDL) and chylomicrons. Apo B48 levels are elevated. Although high density lipoprotein (HDL) levels are reduced, plasma apo AI levels are not changed, and a significant amount of apo AI is found in the remnant lipoproteins in the apo E-deficient mice [2].

Atherosclerotic lesions develop in the aorta of the apo E-deficient mice without any addition of high fat/cholesterol to their diet. The lesions developed in these mice occur in a consistent and time-dependent manner [4]. The time course of lesion appearance in the aortic tree of apo E-deficient mice with C57BL/6 (B6) and 129 mixed genetic background is shown in Figure 1. In a 2-month-old animal, the lesions are initially seen in the proximal aorta close to the aortic sinus and around the valve attachment site [4]. At around 4-6 months of age, lesions can also be found in the aortic arch and the branch points of the common carotids and subclavian arteries. At 8 months old, plaques can be found mainly at

A. M. Gotto, Jr. et al. (eds.), Drugs Affecting Lipid Metabolism, 255–261.

the branch points of the vertebral arteries, renal and gonadal arteries. At 10-12 months of age, isolated plaques in the descending aorta and at the iliac bifurcation are present.

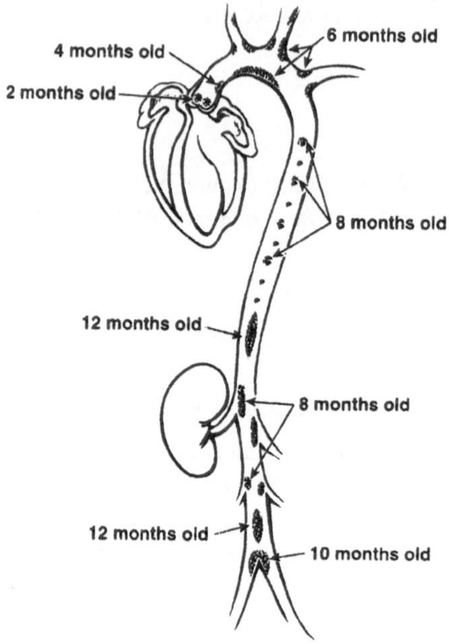

Figure 1. Illustration of the time-dependent and sequential appearance of atherosclerotic plaques in the aortic wall of the apo E deficient mice. This is the summary of 5-10 apo E-deficient mice at various ages with B6/129 mixed genetic background.

The composition of the lesions also change with time [4]. Early lesions are mainly composed of foam cells, similar to the fatty streaks found in humans. With time, smooth muscle cells in the tunica media proliferate and migrate to the intima to form a fibrous cap, which covers a necrotic lipid core and foam cell debris. Lipid infiltration into intimal smooth muscle cells and cholesterol crystal depositions in the acellular lipid core are commonly seen. At later stages, calcifications form in the necrotic centers of the lesions. All of these are typical characteristics seen in matured atherosclerotic lesions in humans [5]. Virtually complete occlusion of small coronary artery branches were seen in some old animals (> 8 months of age); however, no signs of cardiac muscle infarctions were found at the sites. Vascular thrombosis and embolism caused by plaques have not been observed in these mice. The close similarity of the atherosclerotic lesions in apo E-deficient mice to those of humans at all development stages, and produced without the necessity of feeding a high fat diet, make these mice an excellent and unique animal model to study the pathogenesis of atherosclerosis, especially in the areas of dietary and therapeutic manipulations.

Genetic Background and Gender Affect the Size of Atherosclerotic Lesions in the Apo E-Deficient Mice

The genetic background of the apo E-deficient mice contributes significantly to the size of their atherosclerotic lesions. For example, 5-6-month-old female mice that are backcrossed to B6 for six generations have larger lesions in the proximal aorta than the age-matched female mice having mixed B6/129 genetic background (Figure 2).

Significant differences in atherosclerotic lesion size between male and female mice were found in the apo E-deficient mice with B6 genetic background (Figure 3). Female mice have larger lesions than male mice. Similarly, Paigen et al. have previously noted that C57BL/6 strain of mice developed larger lesions that the 129 strain of mice in response to an atherogenic diet [6]. They also observed that female C57BL/6 mice are more susceptible to atherosclerosis than the males [7]. Therefore, the diet-induced atherosclerotic model is in agreement with the genetically generated apo E-deficient mouse model in these respects. It would be of interest to study why female mice tend to develop more severe atherosclerosis in contrast to the relatively lower risk of coronary heart disease in premenopausal human females.

Thrombogenic Potential of Atherosclerotic Plaques in Apo E-Deficient Mice

Thrombosis induced by the disruption or fracturing of atherosclerotic plaques is associated with the development of either mural or partial occlusive thrombi in the area of plaque injury, a main cause of cardiac infarction in humans. However, in the apo E-deficient mice, we have not been able to document thrombus formation in intact plaques. In order to investigate whether simple endothelial denudation and injury to atherosclerotic plaques promote thrombus formation, we applied injury to the aorta and aortic plaques of these mice by squeezing the abdominal portion of the aorta between forceps from outside the aorta. Animals were sacrificed 15-30 minutes after the injury. Two types of vascular damages may be produced by this type of injury. One is the denudation of endothelial cells without the disruption of the elastic lamina. We define this type of injury as simple injury. The second type of injury was the rupture of the plaques, resulting in the exposure of foam cell necrotic cores. We describe this type of injury as plaque injury.

We found that in the aorta of normal mouse and in the plaque-free segments of the aorta in the apo E-deficient mouse, at the point of simple injury, a monolayer of platelets attached to the subendothelium. This finding is similar to the normal response to endothelial cell damage in swine model [8]. However, in the apo E-deficient mice, large platelet fibrin aggregates were found in the simple-injured segments distal to injured plaques. These thrombi were not associated with injury to the media and most likely represent a heightened thrombogenicity associated with plaque disruption. At the site of the plaque injury, we observed thrombus formation containing degranulating platelets mixed with fibrin. By transmission electron microscopy, the thrombi were found to be attached to plaque matrix and foam cell debris.

From these studies, we provide direct evidence that the contents of atherosclerotic

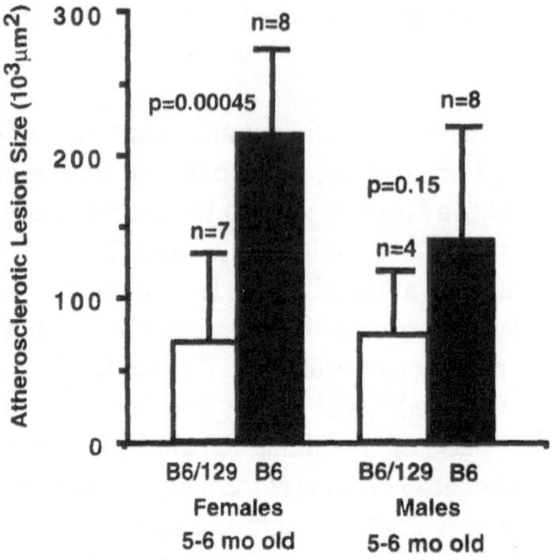

Figure 2. Genetic background affects atherosclerotic lesion size in the apo E-deficient mice. Mice with B6 backcrossed genetic background had been backcrossed 6 generations to B6. The ages of the mice at the time of being sacrificed are indicated. Lesion sizes were obtained by measuring the cross-sectional area of four different areas in the aortic sinus and proximal aorta as previously described [13]. Error bars stand for SD. P values were derived from Student t test of two sample means assuming equal variance.

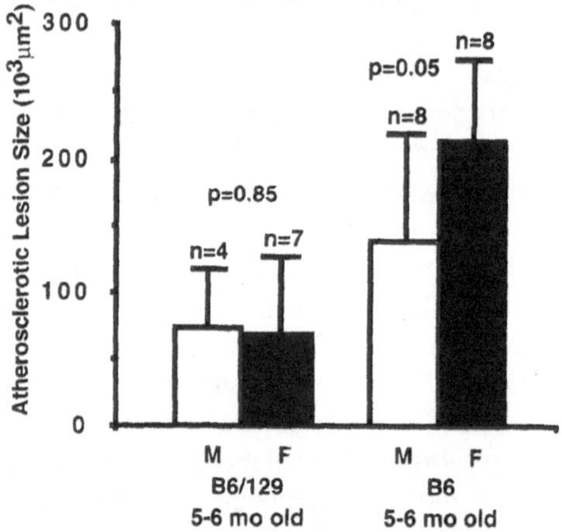

Figure 3. Gender affects atherosclerotic lesion size in apo E deficient mice. F, females; M, males. Lesion size were measured as described in Figure 2. The ages of the mice at the time of being sacrificed are indicated. Error bars stand for SD. P values were derived from Student t test of two sample means assuming equal variance.

plaques are thrombogenic, and provide attachment sites for developing thrombi. The ruptured plaque may also release thrombogenic substance (factors) which cause the platelet to aggregate distal to the disrupted plaques. Since the operation is fairly easy and the direct visualization of the plaque is possible, this injury model provides a simple procedure in which direct plaque injury is allowed to interact with blood flow and cellular components to investigate the atherothrombosis after injury (R.L. Reddick et al., submitted).

Effect of Probucol on Atherogenesis

Probucol is a drug with both cholesterol-reducing and antioxidant effects. Studies have indicated that probucol reduces LDL levels by enhancing LDL removal via an LDL receptor-independent pathway [9], since the drug can effectively reduce cholesterol levels in homozygous LDL receptor-deficient patients. Probucol reduces HDL levels to an even greater degree, which makes its use somewhat controversial. In experimental animal models, probucol effectively reduces lesion development when administered to Watanabe heritable hyperlipidemic (WHHL) rabbits in some but not all experiment [10,11,12].

In order to study the effect of probucol on cholesterol levels and the development of atherosclerosis in the apo E-deficient mice, probucol was administered to 2-3-month-old apo E-deficient mice in their food (0.5% w/w). Total plasma cholesterol levels were significantly reduced by 21-44% in the probucol treated apo E-deficient mice. Although this reduction was mainly in non-HDL cholesterol levels, HDL cholesterol was also reduced significantly (50% reduction), accompanied by a reduction of plasma apo AI levels (52% reduction compared to untreated animals).

However, despite the marked reduction of total cholesterol levels, we found that the aortic lesions in the apo E-deficient mice developed at a more accelerated rate after probucol treatment than in the untreated apo E-deficient mice. We have conducted three independent experiments, a total of 37 animals including both male and female mice with either C57BL/6 and 129 mixed genetic background or C57BL/6 backcrossed (6 generations) genetic background. When data were analyzed in 5 sets of age, sex, and genetic background-matched groups, we found that the lesion size were 2-4 times larger in the probucol-treated apo E-deficient mice in all groups. The combined P value of five sets of independent observations by Fisher's method was less than 0.0002. These results suggest that the proposed antiatherogenic effect of probucol may depend on an apo E-mediated mechanism, and that a reduction in plasma cholesterol is not by itself a good clinical indicator for the antiatherogenic effect of probucol (S.H. Zhang et al., submitted).

Final Remarks

The apo E-deficient mouse is undoubtably an excellent mouse model for studying the pathogenesis of atherosclerosis and therapeutic intervention. The uniqueness of this model is that

1) lesions develop early and rapidly and without the need for dietary induction, in contrast to most mouse models;

2) lesion composition has all the main characteristics seen in human lesions at all phases;

3) the homozygous mice reproduce actively and easily to be maintained; and

4) four to five times elevated cholesterol levels in these mice offer an unmistakable marker which allows these animals to be easily identified.

These latter two characteristics allow efficient breeding to apo E-deficient mice with other genetically modified mouse models, thus offering ample research opportunities to study the contribution of each defined genetic factor to atherogenesis.

While some results may only apply to mice and may be irrelevant to human diseases, it is important to keep our minds open to the unexpected results generated from studying this and other genetically manipulated mouse models, since a journey leading to the unravelling of the true pathogenesis of atherosclerosis may well start from here.

Acknowledgments

Authors thank Robert Jones, Lara K. Surles, and Jay Reynolds for their excellent technical help, to Merrell-Dow Pharmaceuticals and Chugai Pharmaceuticals Co. Japan for providing us with probucol, and to Dr. O. Smithies for continuous encouragement and help. This work was supported by NIH research grant HL-42630 to NM.

References

1. Piedrahita, JA, Zhang SH, Hagman JR, Oliver PM, Maeda N. Generation of mice carrying a mutant apolipoprotein E gene inactivated by gene targeting in embryonic stem cells. Proc Natl Acad Sci 1992;89:4471-75.
2. Zhang SH, Reddick RL, Piedrahita JA, Maeda N. Spontaneous hypercholesterolemia an arterial lesions in mice lacking apolipoprotein E. Science 1992;258:468-71.
3. Plump AS, Smith JD, Hayek K, et al. Severe hypercholesterolemia and atherosclerosis in apolipoprotein E-deficient mice created by homologous recombination in ES cells. Cell 1992; 71:343-53.
4. Reddick RL, Zhang SH, Maeda N. Atherosclerosis in mice lacking apolipoprotein E: Evaluation of lesion development and progression. Arterioscler Thromb 1994;14:141-47.
5. Strong JP. Atherosclerotic lesions: Natural history, risk factors and topography. Arch Pathol Lab Med 1992;116:1268-75.
6. Paigen B, Ishida BY, Verstuyft J, Winters RB, Albee D. Atherosclerosis susceptibility differences among progenitors of recombinant inbred strains of mice. Arteriosclerosis 1990; 10:316-23.
7. Paigen B, Holmes P, Mitchell D, Albee D. Comparison of atherosclerotic lesions and HDL-lipid levels in male, female, and testosterone-treated female mice from strains C57BL/6, BALB/c, and C3H. Atherosclerosis 1987;64:215-21.
8. Reddick RL, Grigg TG, Lamb MA, Brinkhous KM. Platelet adhesion to damaged coronary arteries: Comparison in normal and von Willbrand disease swine. Proc Natl Acad Sci USA 1982;79:5076-79.
9. Naruszewicz M, Carew TE, Pittman RC, Witztum JL, Steinberg D. A novel mechanism by which probocul lowers low density lipoprotein levels demonstrated in the LDL receptor-

deficient rabbit. J Lipid Res 1984;25:1206-13.
10. Kita T, Nagano Y, Yokode M, et al. Probucol prevents the progression of atherosclerosis in Watanabe heritable hyperlipidemic rabbit, an animal model for familial hypercholesterolemia. Proc Natl Acad Sci USA 1987;84:5928-31.
11. Nagano Y, Nakamura T, Matsuzawa Y, Cho M, Ueda Y, Kita T. Probucol and atherosclerosis in Watanabe heritable hyperlipidemic rabbit - long term antiatherogenic effect and effects on established plaques. Atherosclerosis 1992;92:131-40.
12. Daugherty A, Zweifel BS, Shonfeld G. The effects of probucol on the progression of atherosclerosis in mature Watanabe heritable hyperlipidemic rabbits. Br J Pharmacol 1991; 103:1013-18.
13. Zhang SH, Reddick RL, Burkey B, Maeda N. Diet-induced atherosclerosis in mice heterozygous and homozygous for apolipoprotein E gene disruption. J Clin Invest 1994;94: 937-45.

THE METABOLISM OF VLDL REMNANTS IN APOE*3-LEIDEN TRANSGENIC MICE

Louis M. Havekes, Bart J.M. van Vlijmen, Miek C. Jong, Pieter H.E. Groot, Rune R. Frants, and Marten H. Hofker
TNO-PG, Gaubius Laboratory and MGC-Dept. of Human Genetics, P.O. Box 2215, 2301 CE Leiden, The Netherlands

Introduction

Patients with familial dysbetalipoproteinemia (FD) are characterized by elevated plasma levels of VLDL- and chylomicron-remnant lipoproteins concomitant with a strongly increased risk for atherosclerosis. Even in healthy people of industrialized societies the plasma levels of remnant lipoproteins is rather high, since people live under nonfasting conditions during most of their lives. It is commonly assumed therefore that in Western societies increased levels of remnant lipoproteins is a main contributor to the high risk of atherosclerosis in these societies.

The aim of our study is to investigate the environmental and genetic factors that influence the remnant lipoprotein metabolism. A better insight in the mechanism of remnant lipoprotein metabolism will eventually lead to new strategies in lowering the prevalence of heart and vessel diseases, the main cause of death in Western societies.

Results

Plasma Lipid Levels in ApoE*3-Leiden Transgenic Mice

Since humans are heterogenous in both genetic and environmental background (nutrition), we decided to perform our studies with the use of transgenic mice. However, since mice display very low plasma lipid levels and the metabolism of remnant lipoproteins is very rapid, we decided first to generate transgenic mice carrying the gene for human apoE*3-Leiden [1]. ApoE*3-Leiden is known to inhibit remnant clearance, which is a prerequisite for studying remnant metabolism in mice. Three different apoE*3-Leiden transgenic lines were generated with different levels of expression of the transgene. The high expressing line (#2) shows hyperlipidemia, whereas a low expressor (#195) did not show a clear phenotype (Table 1). After feeding high cholesterol- and fat-containing diets the high expressor line #2 displayed a severe hypercholesterolemia (confined to the VLDL/LDL-sized fraction),

A. M. Gotto, Jr. et al. (eds.), Drugs Affecting Lipid Metabolism, 263–270.

Table 1. Serum lipid levels before and after dietary treatment.

Mouse Line	SRM-A		HFC Diet	
	Cholesterol	Triglycerides	Cholesterol	Triglycerides
	mmol/l		*mmol/l*	
Control	1.8 ± 0.2	0.4 ± 0.1	2.8 ± 0.2	0.1 ± 0.1
#195	2.3 ± 0.2[a]	0.7 ± 0.2[a]	3.9 ± 0.2[a]	0.2 ± 0.1[a]
#2	2.7 ± 0.5[a]	1.7 ± 0.5[a]	9.9 ± 1.4[a]	2.7 ± 0.6[a]
Control, apoE(+/-)	1.8 ± 0.2	0.2 ± 0.1[a]	3.0 ± 0.6	0.1 ± 0.1
#195, apoE(+/-)	2.4 ± 0.3[a]	0.7 ± 0.2[a]	4.9 ± 0.6[ab]	0.4 ± 0.2[ab]
#2, apoE(+/-)	2.6 ± 0.5[a]	1.5 ± 0.6[a]	15.8 ± 4.8[ab]	5.7 ± 2.5[ab]

SRM-A, standard rat/mouse A diet; HFC, mild high fat/cholesterol, containing 15 % cocoa butter and 0.25% cholesterol. Values are the mean serum levels ± SD of at least 12 mice. Mice were fed the HFC diet for 8 weeks. [a]Significant difference ($P < 0.05$) as compared with control mice on the same diet, using nonparametric Mann-Witney test. [b]Significant difference ($P < 0.05$) as compared with same transgenic line with two *apoE* genes on the same diet, using nonparametric Mann-Witney test

Table 2. Serum lipid levels before and after dietary treatment.

Mouse	Age (days)	SRM-A Cholesterol	SRM-A Triglycerides	HFC Diet Cholesterol	HFC Diet Triglycerides
		mmol/l		*mmol/l*	
Control ♂	45	2.5 ± 0.5	1.5 ± 1.0	3.8 ± 0.4	0.9 ± 0.2
Control ♀	45	1.8 ± 0.2^{a}	0.8 ± 0.2^{a}	3.2 ± 0.1	0.7 ± 0.1
#2 ♂	45	4.5 ± 1.3^{b}	4.0 ± 1.0^{b}	10.8 ± 2.6^{b}	4.9 ± 1.5^{b}
#2 ♀	45	2.8 ± 0.3^{ab}	2.8 ± 0.6^{ab}	9.1 ± 1.7^{ab}	4.5 ± 1.0^{b}
Control ♂	> 100	1.9 ± 0.2	0.4 ± 0.1	3.2 ± 0.7	0.6 ± 0.2
Control ♀	> 100	1.8 ± 0.2	0.5 ± 0.2	2.5 ± 0.2^{a}	0.3 ± 0.1^{a}
#2 ♂	> 100	2.1 ± 0.3^{b}	1.4 ± 0.2^{b}	7.3 ± 0.8^{b}	1.3 ± 0.1^{b}
#2 ♀	> 100	2.5 ± 0.5^{b}	2.0 ± 0.4^{ab}	10.0 ± 1.5^{ab}	1.6 ± 0.3^{a}_{b}

SRM-A, standard rat/mouse A diet; HFC, mild high fat/cholesterol, containing 15% cocoa butter and 0.25% cholesterol. Values are the mean serum levels ± SD of at least 12 mice. Mice were fed the HFC diet for 8 weeks. [a]P < 0.05. Indicating significant difference between male and female mice of the same genetic background on the same diet, using non-parametric Mann-Witney test. [b]P < 0.05. Indicating significant difference between apoE*3-Leiden and control mice of the same sex and on the same diet, using nonparametric Mann-Witney test whereas the low expressor #195 only showed a very weak hypercholesterolemia, indicating that the response to dietary treatment is related to the level of transgene expression.

By crossbreeding these apoE3-Leiden transgenic mice (#2, #195 and control) with homozygous apoE-deficient mice, we obtained apoE*3-Leiden transgenic mice with a reduced level of endogenous apoE. It appeared that a reduction of endogenous (wild type) apoE in apoE*3-Leiden transgenic mice leads to a more severe phenotype on chow diet and a more responsiveness to cholesterol feeding (Table 1). Analyses of the lipoprotein profiles of these mice showed that the increased plasma cholesterol levels is confined to the VLDL/LDL-sized lipoprotein fraction.

ATHEROSCLEROSIS IN APOE*3-LEIDEN TRANSGENIC MICE

Upon feeding cholesterol-containing diets the VLDL lipoprotein fraction accumulating in the plasma was highly enriched in cholesterol as compared to VLDL from chow-fed animals. Increased cholesterol-to-triglyceride ratios in the VLDL fraction is commonly assumed to be atherogenic and also occur in patients with familial dysbetalipoproteinemia. We wondered therefore whether cholesterol feeding leads to atherosclerosis in the mice of line #2. Feeding cholesterol to line #2 indeed resulted in the development of atherosclerotic lesions near the aortic arch [2]. Quantification of the atherosclerotic lesion areas in cross sections of the aortic sinus showed that in the apoE*3-Leiden mice the lesion area is 5-to-10 times greater than in control mice and increasing with duration of the diet administration and with the amount of cholesterol in the diet. We calculated a strong correlationship between plasma cholesterol exposure and lesion size ($r = 0.85$) [3].

EFFECT OF AGE AND GENDER ON PLASMA LIPID LEVELS IN APOE*3-LEIDEN TRANSGENIC MICE

As presented in Table 2, at young age transgenic mice showed higher plasma cholesterol and triglyceride levels (with an optimum at 45 days of age) than at older age (> 100 days). This phenomenon occurred more pronounced in males than in females [4]. We hypothesized that the transient hyperlipidemia in young animals is due to a relatively greater flux of nutrients which is needed during rapid growth. Since these transgenic mice have a reduced rate of clearance of remnant lipoproteins (due to the introduction of the binding defective apoE*3-Leiden protein), an increased production of either hepatic VLDL or intestinal chylomicrons will lead to an extra response in plasma lipid levels.

This hypothesis is sustained by VLDL turnover experiments. In young transgenic mice the fractional catabolic rate was reduced as compared to nontransgenic young mice (1.45 ± 0.34 versus 3.94 ± 1.22 pools/hour), whereas the VLDL synthetic rate was similar for both animals. This implies that the apoE*3-Leiden transgene indeed inhibits the clearance of VLDL remnant lipoproteins, as expected. We also found that young transgenic mice indeed have a significantly higher VLDL production rate than older mice (4.24 ± 0.95 versus 2.45 ± 1.05 μg apoB/hour/gr body weight), as measured by VLDL-apoB turnover experiments. Similar results were found following rise in plasma triglyceride levels after injection with Triton WR1339.

Female apoE*3-Leiden mice display significantly higher plasma cholesterol and triglyceride levels than males, when fed hyperlipidemic diets (Table 3). In line with this, injection of both male and female transgenic mice with estrogen leads to an enhanced plasma lipid level, whereas injection with apoE*3-Leiden mice with testosterone showed the opposite (Table 3). Lipoprotein profile analyses showed that this effect of sex steroid hormone on plasma lipid levels is confined to the VLDL/LDL-sized lipoprotein fraction. By Triton WR 1339 injection experiments we were able to show that estrogens increase the hepatic production of VLDL, whereas testosterone administration had no effect on VLDL production. We also found by VLDL-apoB turnover studies that in female mice the VLDL synthetic rate is increased as compared to male mice (2.13 ± 0.79 versus 1.65 ± 0.34 μg apoB/hour/gr body weight), and that administration of estrogen to male mice also leads to an increased VLDL synthesis.

Table 3. Serum lipid concentrations after 4 weeks of hormone treatment of apoE*3-Leiden transgenic mice.

Sex	Treatment	TC	TG
		mmol/liter	
Males	Placebo	6.2 ± 1.2	2.3 ± 0.3
	Estradiol decanoate (100 μg/mouse)	6.7 ± .03	4.5 ± 0.6[a]
	Testosterone decanoate (1250 μg/mouse)	5.1 ± .07	2.6 ± 0.4
Females	Placebo	9.4 ± 1.5	3.3 ± 0.7
	Estradiol decanoate (100 μg/mouse)	10.6 ± 1.5	5.1 ± 0.7[a]
	Testosteron decanoate (1250 μg/mouse)	6.6 ± 1.1[a]	2.3 ± 0.3[a]

TC, total cholesterol; TG, triglyceride. Total cholesterol and triglyceride values are the mean serum levels ± SD of five apoE*3-Leiden transgenic mice per group. [a]$P < 0.05$, indicating the difference between hormone and placebo treated groups of mice of the same sex, using nonparametric Mann-Witney tests.

In male mice without hormone treatment the fractional catabolic rate is equal to that in female mice without treatment. After injection male mice with testosterone, however, the fractional catabolic rate increased. We have experimental evidence that an increased VLDL clearance in male apoE*3-Leiden mice is the result of an inhibited expression of the apoE*3-Leiden transgene in these mice. Thus, the increase in plasma lipid levels by estrogen is due to an increase in hepatic VLDL production followed by a lower fractional catabolic rate of VLDL, whereas the hypolipidemic effect of testosterone can be explained by an increased fractional catabolic rate.

ROLE OF APOC1 IN REMNANT METABOLISM IN APOE*3-LEIDEN TRANSGENIC MICE

To investigate the role of apoC1 in remnant metabolism we first generated mice in which the apoC1 gene has been knocked out [5]. These mice display only a mild phenotype upon cholesterol feeding when compared with control mice. On cholesterol-containing diet the homozygous apoC1-deficient mice have elevated cholesterol levels as compared to control mice (10.6 versus 5.1 mmol/l). The fact that on normal standard diets these mice have no phenotype suggests that apoC1 is not playing a very crucial role in lipoprotein metabolism under normal dietary conditions. Only if the system of lipoprotein metabolism is severely stressed by high-fat high-cholesterol feeding, a defect by the absence of apoC1 becomes evident.

Table 4. Plasma lipid leves in apoE*3-Leiden, apoE*3-Leiden-apoC1 and apoC1 transgenic mice and control mice.

	Diet			
Mouse Strain	Chow		LFC	
	TC	TG	TC	TG
	mmol/l		mmol/l	
ApoE*3L-C1	2.97 ± 0.6*	1.88 ± 0.6**	4.33 ± 0.9*	4.38 ± 1.1**
ApoE*L	2.76 ± 0.6*	0.81± 0.3*	4.30 ± 0.6*	0.64 ± 0.2*
ApoC1	2.05 ± 0.4	0.49 ± 0.1	2.98 ± 0.1*	0.71 ± 0.1*
Control	1.78± 0.1	0.38 ± 0.1	2.13 ± 0.4	0.19 ± 0.2

Mice were either fed standard rat mouse diet (chow) or a low fat/cholesterol diet (LFC; containing 50.5% sucrose). Values are the mean serum levels ± SD of 8 mice per group. *P < 0.05, indicating the difference between control and transgenic mice on the same diet. **P < 0.05, indicating the difference between apoE*3L-C1 and apoE*3L mice on the same diet, using nonparametric Mann-Witney tests. TC, total cholesterol; TG, triglyceride.

In receptor binding competition experiments we have found that less apoC1 on VLDL particles is accompanied by a less efficient competition of these particles with LDL for binding to the LDL receptor. This is not expected from the results reported in the literature, claiming that excess of apoC1 inhibits apoE as ligand for binding to the LDL receptor and to LRP. It is observed that, similar to apoE-deficient VLDL, apoC1-deficient VLDL contains considerable amounts of apoA1 and apoA4. We hypothesize therefore that the presence on the apoC1-deficient VLDL particles of both apoA1 and apoA4 influences the conformation of apoE, thereby affecting the binding affinity of apoE to the receptor.

In another attempt to investigate the role of apoC1 in lipoprotein metabolism, we studied the effect of overexpression of the apoC1 gene. As presented in Table 4, transgenic mice that overexpress the apoE*3-Leiden gene exhibit elevated cholesterol levels, whereas simultaneous overexpression of the human apoC1 gene showed an elevated plasma triglyceride in addition to it. Transgenic mice overexpressing only the apoC1 gene also showed increased plasma triglyceride levels, in particular upon feeding the sucrose-containing LFC diet.

In order to explain this hypertriglyceridemia in apoC1 overexpressing mice, we performed turnover studies using VLDL endogenously labeled with ^{3}H-TG. We calculated that in the apoE*3-Leiden animals the VLDL-TG fractional catabolic rate is decreased when apoC1 gene is also overexpressed (11.0 versus 3.5 pools/hour), whereas the synthetic rate of VLDL was not affected by the expression of the apoC1 gene. If similar turnover experiments were performed in hepatectomized mice, we found that the lipolysis of ^{3}H-TG-labeled VLDL was not influenced by apoC1 overexpression. However, in both apoE*3-Leiden transgenic lines as compared to nontransgenic mice the lipolysis rate was severely defective (1.6 versus 6.3 pools/hour). Consequently, excess of apoC1 leads to a defect in hepatic clearance of VLDL, whereas overexpression of apoE*3-Leiden inhibited the extra-hepatic lipolysis of VLDL triglyceride. Further experimental evidence for this observation was obtained from studies with mice that overexpress only apoC1, thus without co-expression of the apoE*3-Leiden gene. In these mice also the fractional catabolic rate of VLDL was hampered (9.1 versus 13.9 pools/hour), whereas an effect on the extra-hepatic lipolysis was not observed.

Conclusion

In apoE*3-Leiden transgenic mice the atherosclerotic lesion size is correlated with plasma cholesterol. In these mice the plasma lipid levels are positively correlated with the relative amount of apoE3-Leiden protein on the VLDL particle. The plasma cholesterol levels are influenced by diet, age, and gender, mainly due to an effect of these factors on VLDL production rate. Excess of apoC1 protein does inhibit the hepatic clearance of VLDL remnant particles, whereas excess of apoE leads to a hampered extra-hepatic lipolysis of VLDL triglyceride.

Reference

1. van den Maagdenberg AM, Hofker MH, Krimpenfort PJ, et al. Transgenic mice carrying the apolipoprotein E3-Leiden gene exhibit hyperlipoproteinemia. J Bio

Chem 1993;268 (14):10540-45.

2. van Vlijmen B, van der Maagdenberg AMJM, Gijbels MJJ, et al. Diet-induced hyperlipoproteinemia and atherosclerosis in apolipoprotein E3-Leiden transgenic mice. J. Clin Invest 1994;93:1403-10.
3. Groot PHE, van Vljimen BJM, Benson GM, et al. Quantitative assessment of aortic atherosclerosis in apoE3Leiden transgenic mice and its relationship to serum cholesterol exposure. Art Thromb Vasc Biol 1996; in print.
4. van Vlijmen BJM, van't Hof HB, Mol MJTM, et al. Modulation of very low density lipoprotein production and clearance contributes to age and gender dependent hyperlipoproteinemia in apolipoprotein E3-Leiden transgenic mice. J Clin Invest 1996; in print.
5. Van Ree JH, Hofker MH, van den Broek WJAA, et al. Increased response to cholesterol feeding in apolipoprotein C1-deficiient mice. Biochem J 1995;305:905-11.

ROLES OF APOLIPOPROTEIN E IN LIPOPROTEIN METABOLISM AND ATHEROSCLEROSIS: INSIGHTS FROM TRANSGENIC MICE

Hitoshi Shimano, Junichi Ohsuga, Yoshio Yazaki, and Nobuhiro Yamada
The Third Department of Internal Medicine, University of Tokyo, 7-3-1 Hongo, Bunkyo-ku, Tokyo, Japan 113

Introduction

Apo E is a major component of mammalian lipoproteins and a ligand for low density lipoprotein (LDL) receptors, as well as apoB100, in catabolism of plasma lipoproteins through receptor-mediated endocytosis mainly in the liver. It is thought to be a specific ligand for the putative hepatic chylomicron remnant receptor (apoE receptor) that is probably the LDL receptor-related protein (LRP). ApoE is expressed in many tissues and plays a crucial role in cholesterol transport and redistribution in peripheral tissues [1]. Lipoproteins with several molecules of apoE have a higher affinity for LDL receptors than those without apoE [1,2]. We and another group have recently reported that intravenous administration of apoE causes the incorporation of exogenous apoE onto plasma lipoproteins, and enhances clearance of lipoproteins containing apoB100, resulting in a lowered plasma cholesterol level in hypercholesterolemic rabbits [3,4]. Exogenous addition of apoE *in vitro* increases uptake of lipoproteins by cultured cells [5,6]. These findings suggest that apoE acts as a regulator of the metabolism of lipoproteins containing apoB100.

The effect of apoE on atherosclerosis is an issue in a controversial debate. Lack of apoE causes severe hyperlipidemia and atherosclerosis in human and mice [7,8]. We have reported that chronic intravenous injection of purified apoE into Watanabe heritable hyperlipidemic (WHHL) rabbits inhibited progression of atheroma, although they did not show significant decrease in plasma cholesterol levels [9]. This suggests that apoE modulates the process of atherosclerosis through a mechanism other than plasma cholesterol-lowering effect.

To assess the multiple roles of apoE in lipoprotein metabolism and atheroma formation *in vivo*, we established different lines of apoE transgenic mice, and observed changes by overexpression of apoE. First, we intended to overproduce apoE in the liver under control metallothionein promoter and obtain a high level of apoE in the plasma to see the changes in plasma lipoprotein metabolism. Second, another line with the same transgene expressed apoE in the intestine and was used to investigate the effect on chylomicron metabolism. Last, we obtained another line under control of Ld promoter which is

A. M. Gotto, Jr. et al. (eds.), Drugs Affecting Lipid Metabolism, 271–279.

characterized by a high expression of apoE in the arterial wall to estimate a local effect of apoE on atherogenesis.

Transgenic Mice Overexpressing in the Liver

The construct of DNA for microinjection is shown in Figure 1. The highest liver-expressing

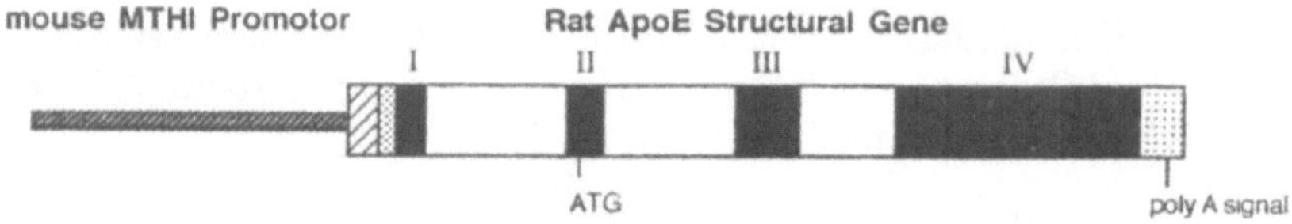

Figure 1. DNA construct for apoE transgenic mice overexpressing in the liver or intestine (modified from [10,11]). Mouse metallothionein I (MTHI) promoter containing heavy metal ion responsive element was fused to rat apoE structural gene containing four exons, and microinjected into nuclei of BDF1 fertilized eggs to generate transgenic mice.

line on Northern blot analysis was designated MAE4-20. To get higher expressors, homozygotes for the transgene were obtained by mating. The plasma level of rat apoE in these homozygotes was increased up to 17.4 mg/dl after induction by administration with zinc ion, which was five-fold higher than mouse endogenous apoE. Immunoblot analysis of the high performance liquid chromatography (HPLC) fraction of plasma from the MAE line demonstrated that apoE molecules from transgene were mainly associated with lipoproteins and distributed among all lipoprotein fractions. Changes in plasma cholesterol and triglycerides on normal and high-cholesterol diets were shown in Table 1. On normal diet, plasma levels of cholesterol, triglycerides, and apoB were decreased in transgenic homozygotes by 60%, 68%, and 79% as compared to controls, respectively. More strikingly, transgenic mice showed resistance against diet-induced hypercholesterolemia which was observed in control mice. As shown in Figure 2, HPLC analysis indicated that decreases in plasma lipids in transgenic mice were due to dramatic reduction in very low density lipoprotein (VLDL) and LDL on both diets. Heterozygotes showed intermediate levels in every parameter, suggesting dose-dependent effects of apoE. Turnover studies using iodinated VLDL and LDL showed that plasma disappearances of VLDL and LDL were 3-fold and 2.4-fold faster in transgenic mice than in controls, respectively. There were no differences in the levels of hepatic LDL receptor proteins and LRP message between transgenic and control animals on both diets (data not shown). These data suggest that apoE enhanced plasma clearance of lipoproteins containing apoB through hepatic lipoprotein receptors, and that this effect overcame accumulation of these lipoproteins which was induced by dietary cholesterol loading.

We also estimated the effect of hepatic overproduction of apoE on plasma clearance of chylomicron and its remnants. As shown in Figure 3, oral retinyl-palmitate challenge test

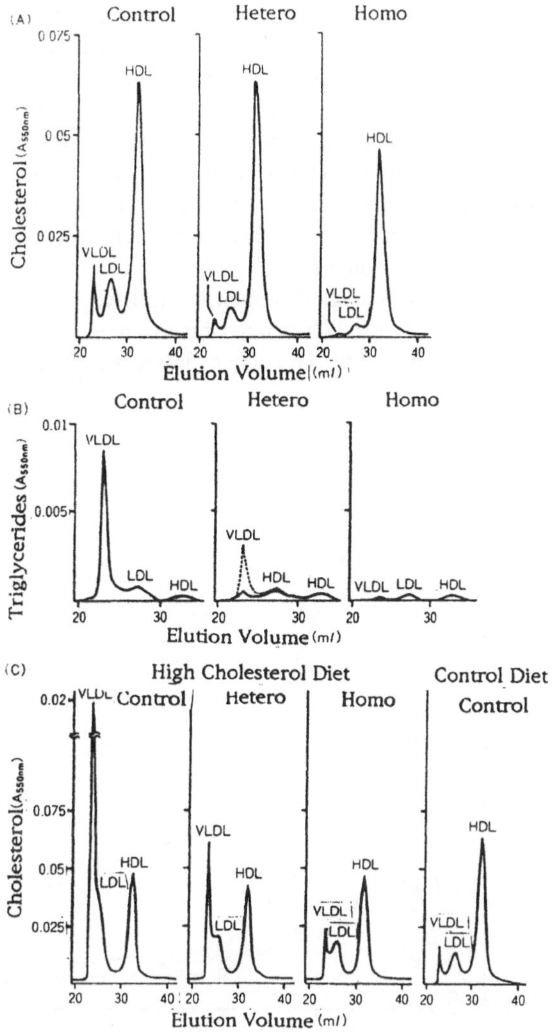

Figure 2. HPLC profile of plasma cholesterol (A, C) and triglycerides (B) (modified from [11,12]). Plasma samples from each group in Table 1 was pooled and subjected to gel filtration chromatography.

showed that the peak and the curve under the area in the time-coursed plasma levels of retinyl-palmitate of transgenic mice were 5-fold decreased as compared to controls, which was consistent with the turnover studies using iodinated chylomicrons. Presumably, hepatic uptake of chylomicron remnants was enhanced by excess of apoE in the liver or in the plasma. To see its mechanism, we performed immunohistochemistry of the liver for apoE in these animals. ApoE was specifically localized at the basolateral surface of hepatocytes of transgenic mice. After intravenous injection of a large amount of chylomicrons, the density of the cell-surface apoE was markedly reduced and vesicular staining appeared in the cytoplasm, suggesting that the cell-surface apoE was used for hepatic endocytosis of chylomicrons and remnants (Figure 4). This phenomenon was specific to chylomicrons and not observed after injection of VLDL or LDL. These results provide strong evidence for the secretion-recapture process of apoE whereby chylomicron remnants flow into the sinusoidal space, acquire apoE molecules on the surface of hepatocytes, and subsequently are endocytosed probably through both LDL receptor and LRP (Figure 5). Several lines of evidence suggest that capture of chylomicron remnants in sinusoidal space may be mediated by proteoglycans like heparan sulfate. The way of interaction between these cell surface molecules and apoE is not known.

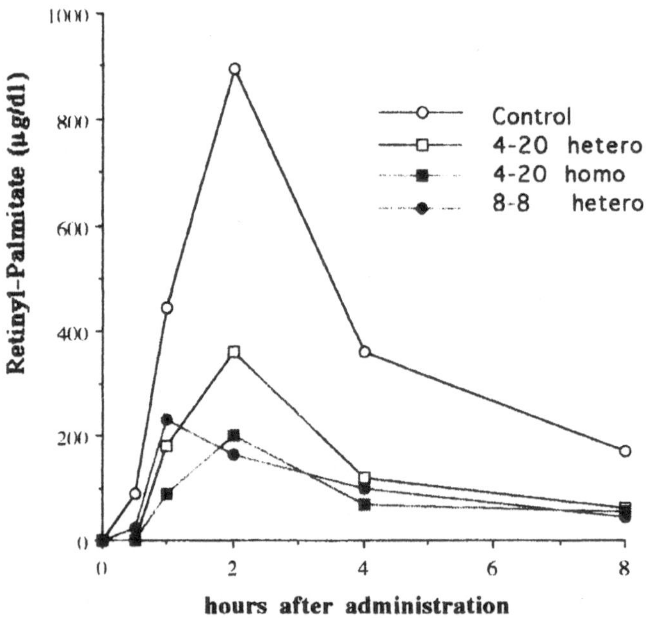

Figure 3. Oral retinyl-palmitate loading test on the liver-(MAE4-20) and intestine(MAE8-8)-producing types of apoE transgenic mice (modified from [13]). Retinyl-palmitate (4 mg) was orally administered to five animals from each group. At the specified times, blood samples were drawn. Plasma levels of retinyl-palmitate were determined.

Transgenic Mice Overexpressing ApoE in the Vascular Wall

Even after prolonged atherogenic diet, the liver-producing line of apoE transgenic mice

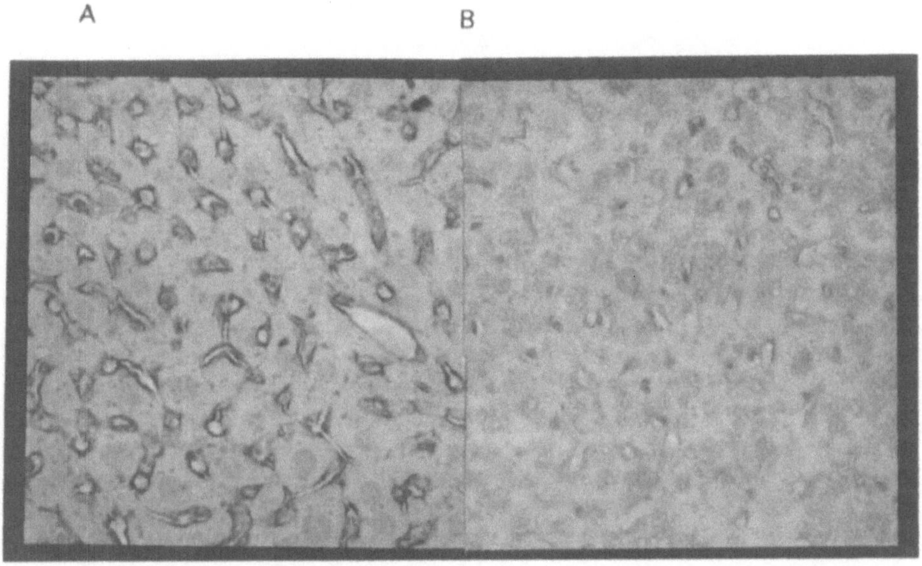

Figure 4 A. Hepatic localization of apoE in transgenic mice and B. changes after injection of chylomicrons on immunohistochemistry. (modified from [14]) A. Liver samples from transgenic (homozygous MAE 4-20) were processed for immunostaining with polyclonal anti-rat apoE antibodies. Human chylomicrons (0.3 mg protein / 100 μl PBS) were injected into transgenic mice (homozygous MAE 4-20) through the tail vein. Seven minutes later, the liver was perfused with ice-cold saline and dissected for immunohistochemistry . Magnification x 100.

showed no atheroma formation, while some considerable fatty streak lesion was observed in the aortic sinus in control mice on the same genetic background (unpublished data). This difference was likely to be due to the antihyperlipidemic effect of apoE since transgenic mice on the atherogenic diet had a plasma cholesterol level as low as that of the control mice on a normal diet. To test whether apoE in the vascular wall has a direct and local effect on the formation of atherosclerosis, we established transgenic mice expressing human apoE in the vascular wall under control of H2 Ld promoter. Studies on mRNA levels demonstrated that this line was characterized by high expression of human apoE in the arterial wall, while its expression was relatively low in other tissues as compared to the respective endogenous expression of mouse apoE [15]. Immunohistochemistry showed that both endothelial cells and medial smooth muscle cells produced apoE from the transgene[15]. They showed no difference in plasma cholesterol levels and lipoprotein profile from controls when fed both normal and atherogenic diets. However, after 24 weeks of an atherogenic diet, the formation of fatty streak lesions in the proximal aorta was markedly inhibited in transgenic mice as compared to those found in controls (Figure 7). Both the lesion area and the esterified

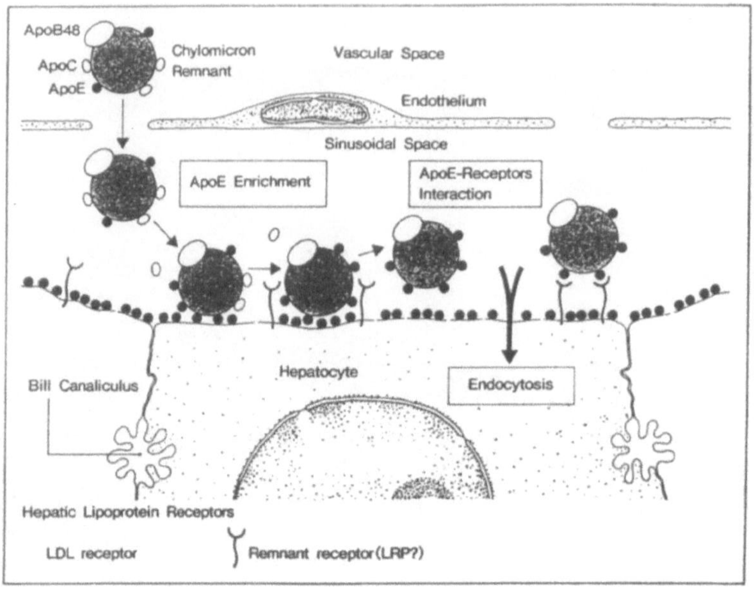

Figure 5. Secretion-recapture process of apoE in hepatic uptake of chylomicron remnants (modified from [13]). Proteoglycans like heparan sulfates may be involved in this process, although not shown.

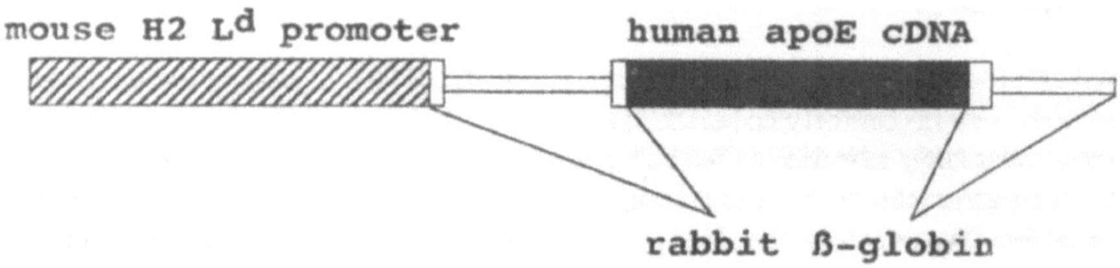

Figure 6. DNA construct for microinjection for ApoE transgenic mice overexpressing in the vascular wall (modified from [15]). The promoter of MHC class1 antigen Ld gene was fused to human apoE DNA with β-globin gene intron. The DNA was injected into nuclei of eggs from C57 Black6.

cholesterol content in the aorta were estimated to be less than 30% of those in controls. In a tissue cholesterol-labeling study with ^{3}H-cholesterol, the specific activity of aorta cholesterol was lower in transgenic mice, suggesting that apoE enhances cholesterol efflux from the aortic wall into plasma (Figure 8). These data indicate apoE has antiatherogenic action which is at least partially mediated via enhancing reverse cholesterol transport from

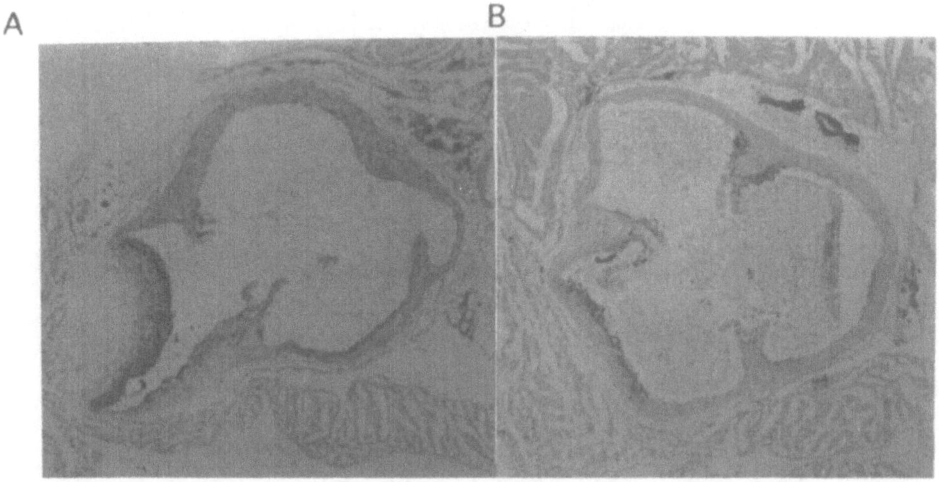

Figure 7. Fatty streak lesions in proximal aorta and aortic sinus after atherogenic diet (modified from [15]). After 24 weeks of atherogenic diet containing 1.25% cholesterol, 15% coconut butter, and 0.5% cholic acid, the hearts and aortae of transgenic mice (A) and non-transgenic littermates (B) were resected for evaluation of fatty streak lesions. Cross section of aortic sinus after Oil Red O and hematoxylin staining was shown. Magnification: x140.

arterial wall. Different kinds of cytokines are suggested to be involved in the early process of diet-induced atherogenesis. They could have enhanced apoE expression in the vascular cells including macrophages by the MHC class1 promoter.

Conclusion

The current studies on different lines of apoE transgenic mice demonstrated the multiple roles of apoE:

1. Plasma cholesterol lowering effect through enhanced plasma clearance of apoB-containing lipoproteins;
2. Secretion recapture process in hepatic uptake of chylomicron remnants; and
3. Antiatherogenic action via enhanced cholesterol efflux.

These data implicate potential possibilities of apoE as a therapeutic agent against hyperlipidemia and atherosclerosis.

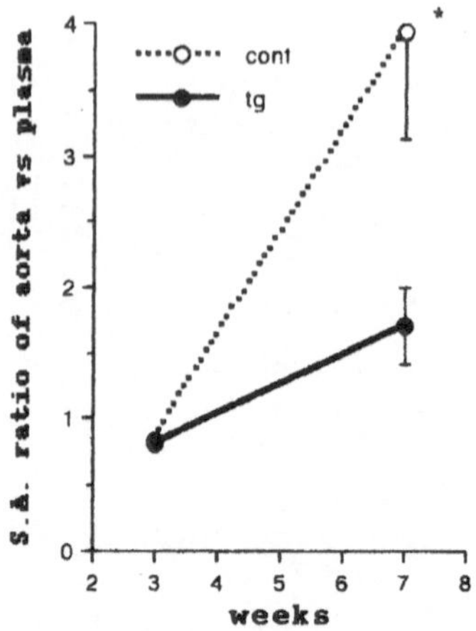

Figure 8. Cholesterol efflux from the aorta. Transgenic and control mice at 12 weeks of age were given atherogenic diet containing ^{3}H-cholesterol (1 mCi/1 g cholesterol, approximately 30 μCi/mouse) for two days. Then, the diet was switched to the atherogenic diet without radioisotopes. After 3 and 7 weeks of the atherogenic diet, the animals were sacrificed. Blood was drawn and the aorta was resected. Cholesterol was extracted from plasma and aortae. The cholesterol content and radioactivity of each sample were measured. The ratio of specific activity (dpm/mg cholesterol) in aorta to that in plasma was calculated. The mean value of each group at 3 and 7 weeks is shown ($n = 4$; bars, SD). The difference at 7 weeks between the two groups was significant at $p < 0.05$.

Acknowledgments

We are grateful to Dr. M. Katsuki for his great help in the generation of transgenic mice.

References

1. Mahley RW. Apolipoprotein E: Cholesterol transport protein with expanding role in cell biology. Science 1988;240:622-30.
2. Yamada N, Shames DM, Stoudmire JB, Havel RJ. Metabolism of lipoproteins containing apolipoprotein B-100 in blood plasma of rabbits: Heterogeneity related to the presence of apolipoprotein E. Proc Natl Acad Sci USA 1986;83:3479-83.
3. Yamada N, Shimano H, Mokuno H, et al. Increased clearance of plasma cholesterol after injection of apolipoprotein E into Watanabe heritable hyperlipidemic rabbits. Proc Natl Acad Sci USA 1989;86:665-69.
4. Mahley RW, Weisgraber KH, Hussain MM, et al. Intravenous infusion of apolipoprotein E accelerates clearance of plasma lipoproteins in rabbits. J Clin Invest 1989;83:2125-30.
5. Mokuno H, Yamada N, Shimano H, et al. The enhanced cellular uptake of very-low-density lipoprotein enriched in apolipoprotein E. Biochim Biophys Acta 1991;1082: 63-70.

6. Shimano H, Fukazawa C, Shibasaki Y, et al. The effect of apo E secretion on lipoprotein uptake in transfected cells. Biochim Biophys Acta 1991;1086:245-54.
7. Zhang SH, Reddick RL, Pierdrahita JA, Maeda N. Spontaneous hypercholesterolemia and arterial lesions in mice lacking apolipoprotein E. Science 1992;258:468-71.
8. Plump AS, Smith JD, Hayek H, et al. Severe hypercholesterolemia and atherosclerosis in apolipoprotein E-deficient mice created by homologous recombination in ES cells. Cell 1992;71:343-53.
9. Yamada N, Inoue I, Kawamura M, et al. Apolipoprotein E prevents the progression of atherosclerosis in WHHL rabbits. J Clin Invest 1992;89:706-11.
10. Shimano H, Yamada N, Shimada M, et al. Hepatic and renal expression of rat apolipoprotein E under control of the metallothionein promotor in transgenic mice. Biochim Biophys Acta 1991;1090:91-94.
11. Shimano H, Yamada N, Katsuki M, et al. Overexpression of apolipoprotein E in transgenic mice: A marked reduction in plasma lipoproteins except high density lipoprotein, and resistance against diet-induced hypercholesterolemia. Proc Natl Acad Sci 1992;89:1750-54.
12. Shimano H, Yamada N, Katsuki M, et al. Plasma lipoprotein metabolism in transgenic mice overexpressing apolipoprotein E: Accelerated clearance of lipoproteins containing apolipoprotein B J Clin Invest 1992;90:2084-91.
13. Shimano H, Namba Y, Ohsuga J, et al. Metabolism of chylomicron remnants in transgenic mice expressing apolipoprotein E in the intestine. Biochem Biophys Res Commun 1994;200:716-21.
14. Shimano H, Yamada N, Ohsuga J, et al. Secretion-recapture process of apolipoprotein E in hepatic uptake of chylomicron remnants in transgenic mice. J Clin Invest 1994;93:2215-23.
15. Shimano H, Ohsuga J, Shimada M, et al. Inhibition of diet-induced atheroma formation in transgenic mice expressing apolipoprotein E in the arterial wall. J Clin Invest 1995;95:469-76.

RECEPTORS FOR APOE-CONTAINING LIPOPROTEINS

Tokuo Yamamoto
Tohoku University Gene Research Center, 1-1 Tsutsumidori-Amamiya, Aoba, Sendai 981, Japan

Introduction

The receptor-mediated endocytosis of plasma lipoproteins is a massive transport system in higher animals. The best-characterized low density lipoprotein (LDL) receptor plays a key role in the uptake of LDL into cells thereby mediating the homeostasis of cholesterol metabolism [1]. The second lipoprotein receptor termed very low density lipoprotein (VLDL) receptor was identified by cDNA cloning [2,3]. The VLDL receptor consists of five functional domains that resemble the LDL receptor and binds only apoE-containing lipoproteins; the LDL receptor binds both apoB-containing LDL and apoE-containing lipoproteins. However, their expressions and roles in the lipoprotein metabolism are different. In this paper, I describe the structure, expression, and function of the VLDL receptor, and discuss its biological role in the metabolism of apoE-containing lipoproteins.

Structure of the VLDL Receptor

The VLDL receptor is a member of the LDL receptor family that includes the LDL receptor related protein (LRP), a giant kidney glycoprotein termed gp330/megalin, a LRP-like molecule in *C. elegans*, and a recently identified *Drosophila* vitellogenin receptor [4]. Among them, the VLDL receptor is most closely related to that of the LDL receptor [5]. The two receptors consist of five functional domains: an N-terminal ligand binding domain, an EGF precursor homology domain, an O-linked sugar domain, a transmembrane domain, and a cytoplasmic domain. Between the two receptors, the amino acids in the functionally important three domains (the ligand binding, epidermal growth factor [EGF] precursor, and cytoplasmic domains) are highly conserved. The key structural difference between the two receptors is the number of the cysteine-rich repeats in their ligand binding domains: the ligand binding domain of the VLDL receptor consists of 8-fold repeats, whereas that of the LDL receptor contains 7 repeats [2,3].

A striking feature of the VLDL receptor is its extremely high degree of amino acid conservation during evolution. Approximately 95% of the amino acids in human, rabbit, rat, and mouse VLDL receptors are identical and more than 80% of the amino acids in the

A. M. Gotto, Jr. et al. (eds.), Drugs Affecting Lipid Metabolism, 281–283.

mammalian receptors are conserved in the chicken receptor [6]. This suggests that the VLDL receptor is an essential protein in mammalian and avian species.

VLDL Receptor Gene

The human VLDL receptor gene is located on chromosome 9 and its gene organization is almost the same as that of the LDL receptor gene present on chromosome 19 [3]. The 5'-untranslated region of the VLDL receptor gene contains a unique polymorphic triplet (CGG) repeat sequence that is also found in the human fragile X syndrome gene. The polymorphism of the CGG repeat in the VLDL receptor gene displays at least 6 discrete alleles ranging from 4 to 10 repeat units in the normal Japanese population [3,7]. Since this triplet repeat sequence is considered to be highly unstable, we analyzed the VLDL receptor genes and the triplet repeat in patients with familial hyperlipidemia; however, we haven't found any abnormality. Recently, Okuizumi et al. have shown that the frequency of the 5-repeat allele was significantly higher in patients with Alzheimer's disease, suggesting that the VLDL receptor gene is a susceptibility gene for this disease [7].

Tissue Expression and Regulation of the VLDL Receptor

The VLDL receptor mRNA is most abundant in heart, skeletal muscle, and adipose tissue in mammals whereas the chicken receptor is expressed almost exclusively in oocytes. The tissue expression of the mRNA in mammals suggests that the basic function of the receptor in mammals is most likely to provide muscle and fat cells with fatty acids.

The promoter region of the VLDL receptor gene contains two copies of imperfect sterol regulatory element-1 (SRE-1) [3]. SRE-1 is present in the promoter regions of LDL receptor and HMG-CoA synthase genes and mediates the downregulation of these important genes for cholesterol metabolism [8]. Despite the presence of SRE-1 like sequences, the levels of the VLDL receptor mRNA in THP-1 cells are unaffected by excess LDL or β-VLDL [3]. The SRE-1 of the LDL receptor gene consists of a direct repeat that is believed to be the target of the SRE-binding protein 1 that controls the transcription of the LDL receptor gene. Since single nucleotide substitutions disrupt the function of the SRE-1, the SRE-1-like sequences that contain imperfect repeats in the VLDL receptor appear to be inactivated.

Biological Role of the VLDL Receptor

The biological role of the VLDL receptor in chicken has been revealed by the characterization of the mutant "restricted ovulator" (R/O) hen, which has a defect in the oocyte growth and exhibits severe hyperlipidemia and sterility [9]. Localized in coated pits, the VLDL receptor mediates the uptake of yolk precursors, VLDL, and vitellogenin into growing oocytes, thereby playing a pivotal role in the reproduction of avian species.

To elucidate the biological role of the mammalian VLDL receptor, Frykman et al. have produced homozygous mice lacking the VLDL receptor [10]. Despite the high degree of amino acid conservation of the VLDL receptor during evolution, the knockout mice in both sexes are viable and normally fertile. The plasma levels of cholesterol, triglyceride, and lipoprotein profiles were normal when they were fed normal, high-carbohydrate, and high-fat diets. The only abnormality was a modest decrease in the body weight due to the decreased triglyceride content in adipose tissue. These results suggest the presence of a backup mechanism in mammals.

Other Receptors for ApoE-Containing Lipoproteins

To demonstrate the presence of multiple apoE receptors, we have been working on the isolation of cDNAs-encoding receptors for apoE-containing lipoproteins. Recently, we have cloned an apoE-containing lipoprotein receptor that is expressed predominantly in the brain. Although the newly identified receptor is not found in the liver, heart, muscle, and fat cells, the isolation of the receptor suggests the presence of other unidentified apoE receptors that backup the VLDL receptor.

References

1. Brown MS, Goldstein JL. A receptor-mediated pathway for cholesterol homeostasis. Science 1986;232:34-47.
2. Takahashi S, Kawarabayasi Y, Nakai T, Sakai J, Yamamoto T. Rabbit very low density lipoprotein receptor: A low density lipoprotein receptor-like protein with distinct ligand specificity. Proc Natl Acad Sci USA 1992;89:9252-56.
3. Sakai J, Hoshino A, Takahashi S, Miura Y, Ishii H, Suzuki H, et al. Structure, chromosome location, and expression of the human very low density lipoprotein receptor gene. J Biol Chem 1994;269:2173-82.
4. Yamamoto T, Davis CG, Brown MS, Schneider WJ, Casey ML, Goldstein JL, et al. The human LDL receptor: A cysteine-rich protein with multiple Alu sequences in its mRNA. Cell 1984;39:27-38.
5. Jingami H, Yamamoto T. The VLDL receptor: Wayward brother of the LDL receptor. Cur Opin Lipidol 1995;6:104-108.
6. Bujo H, Hermann M, Kaderli MO, et al. Chicken oocyte growth is mediated by an eight ligand binding repeat member of the LDL receptor family. EMBO J 1994;13:5165-75.
7. Okuizumi K, Onodera O, Mamba Y, et al. Genetic association of the very low density lipoprotein (VLDL) receptor gene locus with sporadic Alzheimer's disease. Nature Genetics 1995;11:207-209.
8. Goldstein JL, Brown M S. Regulation of the mevalonate pathway. Nature 1990;343:425-30.
9. Bujo H, Yamamoto T, Hayashi K, Hermann M, Nimpf J, Schneider WJ. Mutant oocytic LDL receptor gene family member causes atherosclerosis and female sterility. Proc Natl Acad Sci USA 1995;92:9905-9909.
10. Frykman PL, Brown MS, Yamamoto T, Goldstein JL, Herz J. Normal plasma lipoproteins and fertility in gene-targeted mice homozygous for a disruption in the gene encoding very low density lipoprotein receptor. Proc Natl Acad Sci USA 1995;92:8453-57.

MODULATION OF *IN VIVO* FIBRINOLYSIS BY APOLIPOPROTEIN(A) EXPRESSION IN TRANSGENIC MICE

Theresa M. Palabrica[1], Alexander C. Liu[2], Mark Aronovitz[1], Bruce Furie[3], Richard M. Lawn[2], and Barbara C. Furie[3]
[1]*Division of Cardiology, New England Medical Center, 750 Washington Street, NEMC Box #70, Boston, Massachusetts 02111, USA, and the Department of Medicine, Tufts University School of Medicine, Boston, Massachusetts 02111, USA,* [2]*Falk Cardiovascular Research Center, Division of Cardiovascular Medicine, Stanford University School of Medicine, 300 Pasteur Drive, Stanford, California 94305, USA, and* [3]*Center for Hemostasis and Thrombosis Research, Division of Hematology-Oncology, New England Medical Center, 750 Washington Street, NEMC Box #832, Boston, Massachusetts 02111, USA, and the Departments of Medicine and Biochemistry, Tufts University School of Medicine, Boston, Massachusetts 02111, USA*

Introduction

Elevated plasma concentrations of Lp(a) correlate with an increased risk of developing atherosclerosis and coronary artery disease [1-3]. Lp(a) resembles low density lipoprotein, containing apolipoprotein B-100, cholesterol, and similar phospholipids. This similarity to low density lipoprotein may confer atherogenic properties to Lp(a). However, Lp(a) also contains the glycoprotein apo(a) which is linked to apolipoprotein B-100 and is a unique feature [3]. The apo(a) component of Lp(a) exhibits extensive structural homology to plasminogen, containing an identical secretion signal peptide and multiple copies of the fourth kringle domain [4]. However, apo(a) appears to lack an active protease domain thereby preventing fibrinolytic activity [4]. It has been postulated that this structural similarity to plasminogen may allow apo(a) to competitively inhibit fibrinolysis at sites of vascular injury and serve as a link between thrombosis and atherosclerosis. Previous *in vitro* studies and plasma lysis assays have shown that Lp(a) can inhibit plasminogen activation and this inhibition is more effective on cell surfaces [5]. However, *in vivo* studies testing this hypothesis have produced equivocal results [6].

An animal model is necessary to define the mechanisms by which Lp(a) contributes to the pathology of atherogenesis since in addition to subintimal lipid deposition, formation of focal thrombi at sites of shear induced vascular injury may also potentiate atherogenesis. Animal models to study these effects are limited since the apo(a) gene is absent from rodents

A. M. Gotto, Jr. et al. (eds.), Drugs Affecting Lipid Metabolism, 285–295.

and most subprimate species with the exception of the hedgehog and guinea pig [7,8]. Fortunately, a strain of transgenic mice that express an isoform of the human apo(a) gene containing 17 copies of a kringle domain homologous to the fourth kringle domain of plasminogen followed by a kringle 5 domain and an inactive protease-like domain has been established [9]. These transgenic mice were created in a hybrid mouse strain produced by crossing strains SJL and C57Bl/6. The transgenic mice express apo(a) in all tissues including liver, complexed with lipoproteins. Vascular fatty streaks, histologically similar to early human atherosclerotic lesions develop in these mice to a much greater extent than their control, nontransgenic litter mates and apo(a) has been found in lipid deposits within the arterial wall [9,10]. These mice provide an attractive model to study the mechanisms by which apolipoprotein(a) influences atherogenesis because the effects of a single gene product upon the complex pathophysiological processes that underlie thrombosis and atherosclerosis can be studied in a paired fashion with nontransgenic litter mate controls.

In this study, we adapted an experimental pulmonary thrombolysis model described by Collen and co-workers [11,12] to determine whether the expression of apo(a) in transgenic mice interferes with fibrinolysis mediated by tPA. We recently reported that the expression of apo(a) in male mice renders these animals refractory to fibrinolysis mediated by tPA in a dose-dependent manner [13]. We now demonstrate that this inhibition of fibrinolysis by apo(a) is attenuated in female mice expressing the transgene.

Methods

Preparation of Human Plasma Clots

Platelet-rich plasma clots containing a radiotracer were prepared by incorporating ^{99m}Tc-labeled F(ab')$_2$ fragments of T2G1s antifibrin antibodies (Centocor) into the clot. The T2G1s monoclonal antifibrin antibody, which does not bind to human fibrinogen or murine fibrin [14], was labeled with ^{99m}Tc as previously described [15]. The ^{99m}Tc-labeled F(ab')$_2$ fragment of T2G1s (500 μCi) was added to 0.5 ml of human platelet-rich plasma followed by addition of bovine thrombin (100 μl, 3 NIH units/ml, 0.5 M CaCl2, 0.9% NaCl; Sigma). This plasma mixture was immediately aspirated into two 10 cm lengths of silastic tubing (0.024/0.012",OD/ID) and allowed to clot for 10 minutes at 37° C. The radioactivity within each silastic catheter was measured and the tubing was cut so that each catheter contained approximately 8,000 c.p.m. of ^{99m}Tc.

Murine Pulmonary Embolus Model

Paired experiments were performed in apo(a) transgenic mice and their normal litter mates. Pulmonary emboli were generated in 17 male pairs [13] and 14 female pairs by injection of clotted human platelet-rich plasma as previously described [13]. Anesthesia was induced with an intraperitoneal injection of Nembutal (60 mg/kg) and Ketamine (10 mg/kg). A longitudinal incision was then made over the right jugular vein. The right jugular vein was cannulated with the silastic catheter containing the ^{99m}Tc-labeled plasma clot using x 8 loop magnification. The catheter was advanced 1 to 2 cm into the right atrium of the heart and secured with nylon ligatures. The clot was injected into the lung with 0.2 ml of 0.9% NaCl. Each animal received a bolus of heparin (1,000 IU/kg) through the right jugular vein catheter following clot embolization. Recombinant tPA was diluted to a total volume of 90 µl in 0.15 M NaCl, 0.01% Tween 80, 0.2 M arginine. The dose as indicated (0.13 mg/kg, 0.25 mg/kg, 0.50 mg/kg, 0.75 mg/kg or 1.0 mg/kg) was infused over 60 minutes via the right jugular vein catheter using a Harvard constant-rate infusion pump. Images of the embolized ^{99m}Tc-labeled plasma clots were obtained with an Ohio Nuclear series 100 gamma camera equipped with a medium-energy, high-resolution, parallel-hole collimator with a 20% window and were interfaced with a Macintosh computer equipped with Gamma 11 software (Strichman Medical) employing a 124 x 124 matrix mode. Four 5 minute baseline scans were obtained before the heparin injection and tPA infusion. Twelve serial 5 minute images were obtained during the course of tPA infusion. Upon completion of the experiment, infusion of ^{99m}Tc-labeled erythrocytes (1.0 mCi) allowed imaging of the blood pool to visualize anatomical landmarks and document the orientation of the animals in a single 5 minute static frame. Both animals were then euthanized by an intravenous overdose of Nembutal.

ANALYSIS OF FIBRINOLYSIS KINETICS

The kinetics of clot fibrinolysis were evaluated from the 5 minute dynamic images obtained over the course of each experiment as previously described [13]. The radioactivity, expressed as counts per 5 minute frame, was determined in 60 pixel regions overlying the embolus and adjacent lung tissue. The extent of fibrinolysis was calculated by comparing the activity at a given time point with the radioactivity present in the same region during the baseline frames and was expressed as percent thrombolysis. The data were processed using a moving average algorithm and three point intervals (Excel, version 4.0).

Results

In this murine model, human platelet-rich plasma clots containing radiolabeled antifibrin antibodies were injected into the right atrium of each animal's heart. Subsequent pulmonary embolization was achieved in 95% of the animals. Collen's original model detected the loss of ^{125}I-labeled fibrin from clots with an external gamma-ray counting crystal to quantitate thrombolysis. We utilized a gamma camera to visualize the clots and evaluate thrombolysis by measuring the loss of ^{99m}Tc-labeled T2G1s antibody from the site. In this model, the dose response, magnitude, and time course of thrombolysis produced by tPA in normal male and female mice were similar to data previously reported by other investigators in hamsters [11] and mice [12].

GAMMA SCINTIGRAPHY OF THROMBOLYSIS

Representative images obtained by gamma scintigraphy of a pair of male mice [13] have been reproduced in Figure 1. Radioactive thromboemboli were successfully deployed in the

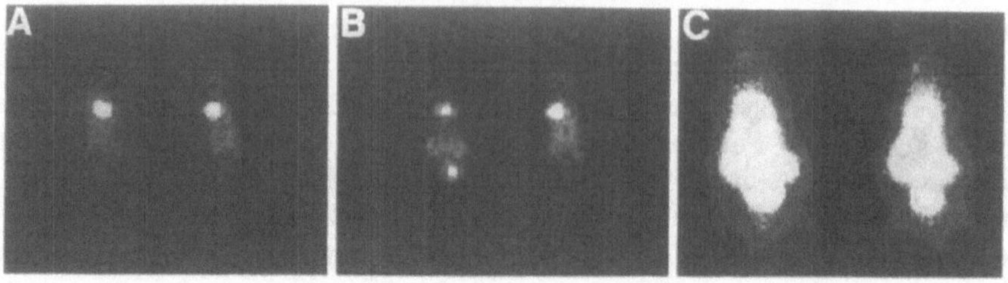

Figure 1. Gamma Scintigrams. A, Initial image at time zero of male mice with pulmonary emboli; normal mouse, left; transgenic mouse, right. B, Image of the same two animals 60 minutes after initiation of tPA infusion at a dose of 0.5 mg/kg. C, Image of the same two animals after injection of ^{99m}Tc-labeled erythrocytes to allow visualization of anatomical landmarks. (From Palabrica et al. [Ref. 13]; reproduced with permission)

lungs of both animals. Panel A shows the initial image obtained immediately following embolization of the radiolabeled clots and before tPA infusion. Panel B reveals the final image of the same two animals obtained 60 minutes after initiation of the tPA infusion. The image of the transgenic male on the right exhibits little change in the amount of radioactivity lodged within the thromboembolus. However, the image of the normal control animal on the left reveals diminished radioactivity within the pulmonary thromboembolus and a concurrent increase of radioactivity in the bladder and kidneys consistent with fibrinolysis. In Panel C, ^{99m}Tc-labeled erythrocytes were used to visualize the blood pool and identify murine orientation and anatomy. The heart, lungs, kidneys, and bladder exhibited the greatest radioactivity. Quantitative data from these images were used to compare the dose response for tPA mediated thrombolysis between normal and transgenic mice expressing human apo(a).

THROMBOLYTIC DOSE-RESPONSE TO TPA

^{99m}Tc-labeled pulmonary emboli were deployed in pairs of mice. Each pair consisted of a transgenic and a normal litter mate of the same gender. Upon successful collection of four baseline images, an infusion of the stated dose of tPA was started. We recently reported that the extent of thrombolysis was decreased in male mice carrying the apo(a) transgene relative to their sex matched normal litter mates at tPA doses of 0.13 mg/kg, 0.25 mg/kg and 0.75 mg/kg. However, at a dose of 1.0 mg/kg, thrombolysis was similar in both mice [13]. Data from several of these experiments in male mice have been reproduced in Figure 2. These experiments were repeated in pairs of female mice at each tPA dose originally used in the male experiments. Specifically, 0.13 mg/kg (n = 5), 0.25 mg/kg (n = 4), 0.50 mg/kg

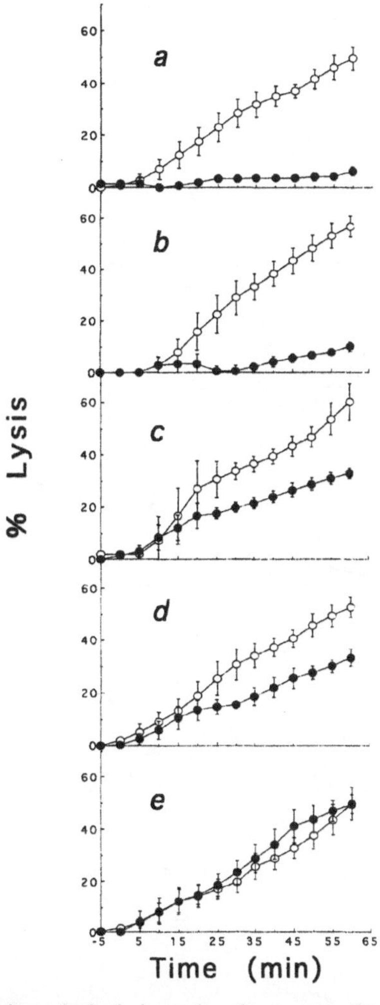

Figure 2. Time course of thrombolysis in male mice. *a - e*, Representative experiments at each of the tPA doses employed. *a*, 0.13 mg/kg; *b*, 0.25 mg/kg; *c*, 0.5 mg/kg; *d*, 0.75 mg/kg; *e*, 1.0 mg/kg. Normal mouse (○); transgenic mouse (●). Percent lysis values are derived from a moving average analysis; data indicate means ± SEM values. (From Palabrica et al. [Ref. 13]; reproduced with permission)

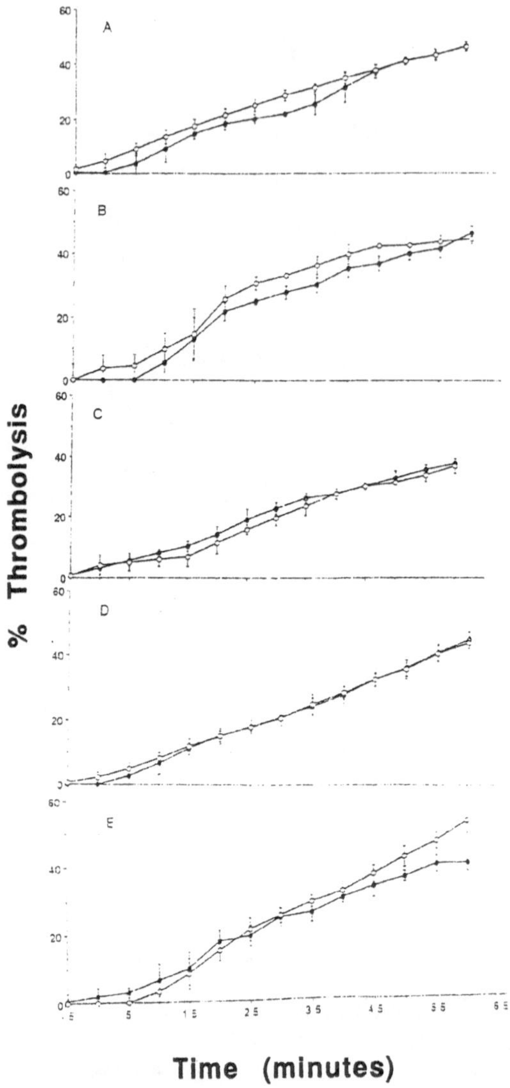

Figure 3. Time course of thrombolysis in female mice. A - E, Representative experiments at each of the tPA doses employed. A, 0.13 mg/kg; B, 0.25 mg/kg; C, 0.5 mg/kg; D, 0.75 mg/kg; E, 1.0 mg/kg. Normal mouse (○); transgenic mouse (●). Percent thrombolysis values are derived from a moving average analysis; data indicate mean ± SEM values. thrombolysis were exhibited by the transgenic female mice compared to their normal litter mates at any of the tPA doses.

(n = 2), 0.75 mg/kg (n = 2), and 1.0 mg/kg (n = 1) of tPA were infused in a total of 14 experiments. Figure 3 shows the data from a representative experiment at each tPA dose. In contrast to the male mice expressing the apo(a) transgene, no significant differences in thrombolysis were exhibited by the transgenic female mice compared to their normal litter mates at any of the tPA doses.

The average difference in thrombolysis, 60 minutes after initiation of the tPA infusion was ascertained in multiple pairs of animals at each tPA dose and are shown in Figure 4. The difference in the extent of thrombolysis between transgenic and normal male mice was 24% and 28% at tPA doses of 0.13 mg/kg and 0.25 mg/kg, respectively. This difference was reduced to 2.0% at a tPA dose of 1.0 mg/kg. In contrast, the mean differences observed in the female mice were 5%, 7%, 0.9%, and 6% at tPA doses of, 0.13 mg/kg, 0.25 mg/kg, 0.5 mg/kg, and 0.75 mg/kg, respectively. A single experiment was performed at a dose of 1.0 mg/kg tPA. These results were similar to previous results from control experiments performed in pairs of normal mice which revealed an average difference of 6.0 $\pm$ 5.1% between animals at 60 minutes [13]. We therefore conclude that the expression of apo(a) in transgenic male mice decreases fibrinolysis mediated by tPA at doses up to 0.75 mg/kg. In addition, a dose of 1.0 mg/kg is sufficient to overcome this effect. However, this inhibition of fibrinolysis by apo(a) expression is significantly attenuated in female mice carrying the transgene.

Discussion

Lipoprotein(a) is a homologue of plasminogen and as such, has been postulated to inhibit plasminogen activation and substrate binding [6]. This may impair fibrinolysis of arterial thrombi and result in abnormal inflammatory and proliferative responses at sites of arterial injury thereby promoting the development of atherosclerotic plaques in the presence of high concentrations of Lp(a). This hypothesis has been supported by several compelling *in vitro* studies which have demonstrated that Lp(a) and apo(a) can compete with plasminogen binding to substrates, i.e. fibrin and endothelial cell surfaces, and inhibit plasmin activation [5,16-18]. There is also evidence that Lp(a) may exert a prothrombotic influence by increasing levels and activity of plasminogen activator inhibitor [19].

However, *in vitro* studies have yielded inconsistent evidence that Lp(a) plasma concentration is inversely related to thrombolysis of clots formed from withdrawn blood samples as measured by several different assays [20-26]. These findings may be due to the difficulty inherent in controlling for all possible variables in human population studies, or variations in the assay systems utilized. Or, perhaps, the inhibitory effects of Lp(a) upon fibrinolysis may be limited to localized areas such as atherosclerotic plaques where Lp(a) and apo(a) are concentrated [9,27-31] since plasminogen in blood is usually present in molar excess. Finally, the myriad of interactions between vessel wall constituents and Lp(a) may be difficult to duplicate using *in vitro* assays of withdrawn blood samples.

In human plasma, the majority of apo(a) is complexed with apo B-100 in Lp(a). However, the inability of low density lipoprotein to bind fibrinogen [32] as well as the recent finding that a mutant apo(a) with a single point mutation in kringle 4-37 is not capable of

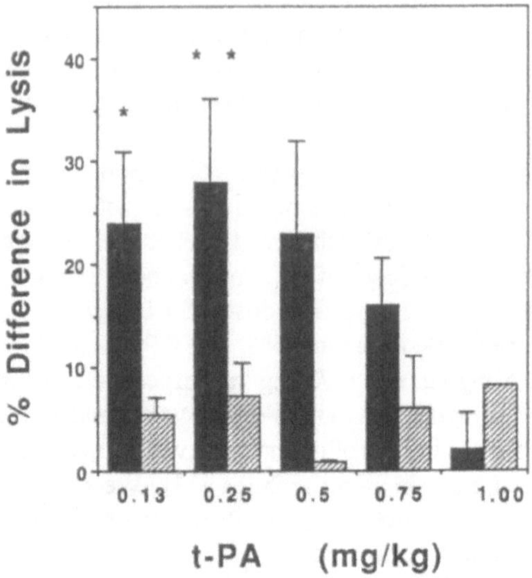

Figure 4. Differences in percent thrombolysis between normal and transgenic mice. The average differences in thrombolysis at 60 minutes after initiation of tPA infusion between normal and transgenic mice are shown for each tPA dose used. Male mice (solid bars); 0.13 mg/kg (n = 5), 0.25 mg/kg (n = 6), 0.50 mg/kg (n = 2), 0.75 mg/kg (n = 2), 1.0 mg/kg (n = 2). Female mice (striped bars); 0.13 mg/kg (n = 5), 0.25 mg/kg (n = 4), 0.50 mg/kg (n = 2), 0.75 mg/kg (n = 2), 1.0 mg/kg (n = 1). Data indicate mean ± SEM values. * p = 0.026 in a paired two-tail test, ** p = 0.035 in a paired two-tail test.

binding to lysine residues of fibrinogen and fibrin [33] suggest that it is the apo(a) component of this molecule that is the critical determinant of Lp(a) interactions in the fibrinolytic pathway. Our paired transgenic model allowed us to visualize and evaluate thrombolysis of a single clot, and attribute observed differences in thrombolysis to the expression of apo(a). Our results demonstrated that this protein exerts antifibrinolytic activity in male mice expressing this transgene.

Our observation that apo(a) inhibition of thrombolysis in male transgenic mice was most prominent at low doses of tPA is consistent with the findings of two recent human studies. Moliterno et al. found mean Lp(a) levels of 49 mg/dl in patients surviving myocardial infarction who did not spontaneously recannalize the infarct related artery. The mean Lp(a) levels were lower (18 mg/dl) in the infarction survivors who exhibited spontaneous thrombolysis. None of the patients in this study received thrombolytic therapy [34]. Von Hodenberg et al. failed to demonstrate that Lp(a) levels were inversely related to the success rates of thrombolytic therapy in myocardial infarction patients treated with urokinase and 60 mg of tPA [35]. The results of these two studies and our data suggest that the antifibrinolytic effects of apo(a) may be overwhelmed by supraphysiologic doses of plasminogen activator and could play an important pathophysiologic role at sites of intravascular injury.

The presence of elevated Lp(a) levels in women has proven to be a strong independent predictor of atherosclerotic cardiovascular disease [36]. Therefore, the finding that the inhibition of fibrinolysis observed in the transgenic male mice was attenuated in female mice carrying the transgene was surprising. This gender difference could not be attributed to variable apo(a) expression since plasma concentrations of apo(a) were similar in both sexes. We suspect hormonal influences may play an important role in modulating apo(a) effects upon fibrinolysis in females and additional experiments are planned to explore this further. We conclude that apo(a) inhibits *in vivo* fibrinolysis in males and believe that this murine model provides a valuable tool to study the mechanisms by which apolipoprotein(a) contributes to the progression of atherosclerosis.

References

1. Untermann G. The mysteries of lipoprotein(a). Science 1989;246:904-10.
2. Scanu AM, Fless GM. Lipoprotein(a): Heterogeneity and biological significance. J Clin Invest 1990;85:1709-15.
3. Scanu AM, Lawn RM, Berg K. Lipoprotein(a) and atherosclerosis: Davis Conference. Ann Intern Med 1991;115:209-18.
4. McLean JW, et al. Human apolipoprotein(a): cDNA sequence of apolipoprotein(a) is homologous to plasminogen. Nature 1987;300:132-39.
5. Hajjar KA, Gavish D, Breslow JL, Nachman RL. Lipoprotein(a) modulation of endothelial cell surface fibrinolysis and its potential role in atherosclerosis. Nature 1989;339:303-305.
6. Zysow BR, Lawn RM. The relationship of lipoprotein(a) to hemostasis. Curr Opin Lipidology 1993;4:484-89.
7. Laplaud PM, Beaubatie L, Rall SJ, Luc G, Saboureau M. Lipoprotein(a) is the major apo B-containing lipoprotein in the plasma of a hibernator, the hedgehog. J Lipid Res 1988;29:1157-70.
8. Rath M, Pauling L. Immunological evidence for the accumulation of lipoprotein(a) in the atherosclerotic lesion of the hypoascorbemic guinea pig. Proc Natl Acad Sci USA 1990;87:9388-90.
9. Lawn RM, et al. Atherogenesis in transgenic mice expressing human apolipoprotein(a). Nature 1992;360:670-72.
10. Chiesa G, et al. Reconstitutio of lipoprotein(a) by infusion of human LDL into transgenic mice expressing human apolipoprotein(a). J Biol Chem 1992;267:24369-74.
11. Stassen J, Lignin HR, Kiekens L, Collen D. Small animal thrombosis models for the evaluation of thrombolytic agents. Circulation 1991;83(IV):65-72.
12. Carmelliet P, et al. Plasminogen activator inhibitor-1 gene deficient mice. Effects on hemostasis, thrombosis and thrombolysis. J Clin Invest 1993;92:2756-60.
13. Palabrica TM, Liu AC, Aronovitz MJ, Furie B, Lawn RM, Furie BC. Antifibrinolytic activity of apolipoprotein(a) in vivo: Human apolipoprotein(a) transgenic mice are resistant to tissue plasminogen activator-mediated thrombolysis. Nature Medicine 1995;1(3):256-59.
14. Kudryk B, Rohoza A, Ahadi M, Nechtin J, Wiebe ME. The specificity of a monoclonal

antibody for the NH_2-terminal region of fibrin. Molec Immun 1984;21: 89-94.
15. Rosenbrough SF, et al. Thrombus imaging with indium-111 and iodine-131-labeled fibrin-specific monoclonal antibody and its $F(ab)'_2$ and Fab fragments. J Nucl Med 1988;29:1212-22.
16. Miles LA, Fless GM, Levin EG, Scanu AM, Plow EF. A potential basis for the thrombotic risks associated with lipoprotein(a). Nature 1989;339:301-303.
17. Edelberg J, Gonzales-Gronow M, Pizzo SV. Lipoprotein(a) inhibition of plasminogen activation by tissue-type plasminogen activator. Thromb Res 1990;57: 155-62.
18. Loscalzo J, Weinfeld M, Fless GM, Scanu AM. Lipoprotein(a), fibrin binding, and plasminogen activation. Arteriosclerosis 1990;10:240-45.
19. Ettingin OR, Hajjar DP, Hajjar KA, Harpel PC, Nachman RL. Lipoprotein(a) regulates plasminogen activator inhibitor-1 expression in endothelial cells. J Biol Chem 1991;266:2459-65.
20. Terres W, Krewitt M, Hamm CW. Effects of lipoprotein(a) on *in vitro* lysis of whole blood thrombi from healthy volunteers. Thromb Res 1993;69:479-87.
21. Anzar J, Estelles A, Breto M, Espana F, Alos T. Euglobulin clot lysis induced by tissue-type plasminogen activator is reduced in subjects with increased levels of lipoprotein(a). Thromb Res 1992;66:569-82.
22. Halvorsen S, Skjonsberg OH, Berg K, Ruyter R, Godal HC. Does Lp(a) lipoprotein inhibit the fibrinolytic system? Thromb Res 1992;68:223-32.
23. Garcia-Frade LJ, et al. Fibrinolytic parameters and lipoprotein(a) levels in plasma of patients with coronary artery disease. Thromb Res 1991;63:407-18.
24. Heinrich H, Sandkamp M, Kokott R, Schulte H, Assmann G. Relationship of lipoprotein(a) to variables of coagulation and fibrinolysis in a healthy population. Clin Chem 1991;37:19500-54.
25. Oshima S, et al. Transient increase of plasma lipoprotein(a) in patients with unstable angina pectoris. Does lipoprotein(a) alter fibrinolysis. Arterioscler Thromb 1991;11: 1772-77.
26. Glueck CJ, et al. Relationship between lipoprotein(a), lipids, apolipoproteins, basal and stimulated fibrinolytic regulators, and D-dimer. Metabolism 1993;42:236-46.
27. Rath M, Niendorf A, Reblin T, Dietel M, Krebber HJ, Beisiegel U. Detection and quantification of lipoprotein(a) in the arterial wall of 107 coronary bypass patients. Arteriosclerosis 1989;9:579-92.
28. Cushing GL, et al. Quantitation and localization of apolipoprotein(a) and B in coronary artery bypass vein grafts resected at re-operation. Arteriosclerosis 1989; 9:593-603.
29. Smith EB, Cochran S. Factors influencing the accumulation in fibrous plaques of lipid derived from low density lipoprotein. II Preferential immobilization of lipoprotein(a) Lp(a). Atherosclerosis 1990;84:173-81.
30. Pepin J, O'Neil JA, Hoff HF. Quantitation of apo(a) and apoB in human atherosclerotic lesions. J Lipid Res 1991;32:317-27.
31. Smith EB, Crosbie L. Does lipoprotein(a) Lp(a) compete with plasminogen in human atherosclerotic lesions and thrombi? Atherosclerosis 1991;89:127-36.
32. Harpel PC, Gordon BR, Parker TS. Plasmin catalyzes binding of lipoprotein(a) to immobilized fibrinogen and fibrin. Proc Natl Acad Sci USA 1989;86:3847-51.
33. Scanu AM, Praffinger D, Lee JC, Hinman J. A single point mutation (Trp72 → Arg) in human apo(a) kringle 4-37 associated with a lysine binding defect in Lp(a). Biochim Biophys Acta 1994;1227:41-45.
34. Moliterno JD, et al. Relation of plasma lipoprotein(a) to infarct artery patency in survivors of

myocardial infarction. Circulation 1993;88:935-40.
35. Von Hodenberg E, et al. Effects of lipoprotein(a) on success rate of thrombolytic therapy in acute myocardial infarction. Am J Cardiol 1991;67:1349-53.
36. Bostom AG, et al. A prospective investigation of elevated lipoprotein(a) detected by electrophoresis and cardiovascular disease in women. Circulation 1994;90:1688-95.

ROLE OF GENE THERAPY IN THE TREATMENT OF THE GENETIC DYSLIPOPROTEINEMIAS

H. Bryan Brewer, Jr., Silvia Santamarina-Fojo, and Jeffrey M. Hoeg
The Molecular Disease Branch, National Heart, Lung and Blood Institute, National Institutes of Health, Bethesda, Maryland 20892, USA

Introduction

Over the last several years the precise molecular basis of the gene defects in the genetic dyslipoproteinemias have been elucidated. The major molecular defects which result in the human genetic dyslipoproteinemias may be classified into gene mutations either in apolipoproteins, enzymes, or lipoprotein receptors. The identification of the specific genes responsible for the genetic dyslipoproteinemias provides the opportunity for the ultimate definitive correction of these genetic defects by somatic gene therapy. There are two conceptual approaches to the application of gene therapy for the treatment of patients with the genetic dyslipoproteinemias particularly in those patients with premature cardiovascular disease. The first approach involves gene replacement to correct the known molecular defect in a specific gene which leads to a dyslipoproteinemic lipoprotein profile and premature atherosclerosis. The second approach is to use gene therapy to overexpress a gene which will reduce the atherosclerosis process regardless of the underlying genetic defect which is responsible for initiating the accelerated atherosclerosis. The latter approach requires the search for candidate genes which are effective in decreasing the progression and inducing regression of atherosclerosis. The development of dyslipoproteinemic animal models resulting from gene knockouts developed by homologous recombination and the current availability of transgenic mice and rabbits which develop spontaneous or diet-induced atherosclerosis permits the testing of selected candidate genes to prevent atherosclerosis.

The present report will summarize the available information on the initial gene therapy studies on correction of the molecular defects in genetic dyslipoproteinemias in man and the results in two animal models we have chosen to evaluate the feasibility of gene replacement for genetic defects in an apolipoprotein and lipolytic enzyme. In addition, data will be presented on the quest for a candidate gene for reducing atherosclerosis which may ultimately have a potential therapeutic benefit for the treatment of cardiovascular disease in man.

A. M. Gotto, Jr. et al. (eds.), Drugs Affecting Lipid Metabolism, 297–309.

Gene Therapy for the Correction of the Molecular Defects Resulting in the Genetic Dyslipoproteinemias

GENE THERAPY FOR GENETIC DEFECTS IN LIPOPROTEIN RECEPTORS

LDL Receptor. The initial pilot study on the correction of the LDL receptor defect in patients [1] with familial hypercholesterolemia (FH) has recently been reported [2,3]. The protocol developed by Wilson and colleagues for gene therapy of FH utilizes an *ex vivo* approach with autologous hepatocytes. In this protocol the left lateral segment of the liver is removed, perfused with collagenase to release the hepatocytes, and the hepatocytes are cultured *in vitro*. The LDL receptor defect in the cultured hepatocytes was corrected using a recombinant retrovirus expressing the LDL receptor. The genetically corrected transduced hepatocytes were harvested and infused back into the patient via a catheter in the inferior mesenteric vein. Five patients with FH have participated in this protocol. LDL kinetic studies have been performed on four of the patients before and following LDL receptor gene therapy. One of the four FH patients studied had a significant increase in LDL fractional catabolic rate from 0.182 day^{-1} to.0280 day^{-1} and the LDL cholesterol levels decreased from 737 mg/dl to 595 mg/dl after LDL receptor gene therapy [3].

The combined results from this initial gene therapy trial established that primary hepatocytes obtained from partial hepatectomy from FH patients could be corrected *in vitro*. The genetically corrected hepatocytes could be effectively infused back into the patients for seeding of the transduced cells in the liver. The major limitation of this *ex vivo* gene therapy approach is the small number of cells that can be safely and effectively delivered back to the patient. Using the current *ex vivo* approach there is not sufficient delivery of transduced cells to the liver in the FH patient to totally correct the plasma lipoprotein profile. Thus, the *ex vivo* approach has significant limitations for gene therapy of FH patients since only partial correction of the severe hypercholesterolemia can be achieved using this methodology.

GENE THERAPY FOR GENETIC DEFECTS IN PLASMA APOLIPOPROTEINS

Apolipoprotein E. In our studies we selected apoE gene replacement in the apoE knockout mouse to test the feasibility of replacing a deficient plasma apolipoprotein present in the plasma at a concentration in the mg/dl range. ApoE plays a key role in lipoprotein metabolism by facilitating the cellular uptake of remnants of triglyceride rich chylomicrons and VLDL [4,5] by serving as a ligand on lipoprotein particles for the LDL receptor and LRP, the putative remnant receptor [6-11]. The important role that apoE plays in lipoprotein transport has been established both by the identification of patients with apoE deficiency [12-16] and by patients with a structural defect in apoE which results in decreased affinity of plasma lipoproteins for lipoprotein receptors [17-20]. A defect in the function of apoE leads to delayed plasma clearance of remnants of triglyceride rich lipoproteins and the development of dysbetalipoproteinemia or type III hyperlipoproteinemia. Kindreds with apoE deficiency and type III hyperlipoproteinemia have been extensively studied and are characterized by elevated plasma levels of cholesterol, triglycerides, cholesterol rich remnants of chylomicrons and VLDL as well as by xanthomas and premature cardiovascular disease [12-16].

A mouse model for apoE deficiency has been developed using homologous recombination with apoE targeted gene disruption in embryonic stem cells. The apoE knockout mice develop marked hypercholesterolemia with total cholesterol levels five to six fold greater than control mice [21,22]. These apoE-deficient mice have a dramatic shift in plasma lipoproteins from HDL, the major lipoprotein in control mice, to cholesterol-enriched remnants of chylomicrons and VLDL. Of particular interest in the apoE-deficient mice is the development of spontaneous atherosclerosis on a normal chow diet [22,23].

The apoE-deficient mouse represents a unique model to study gene replacement of a plasma apolipoprotein for correction of a genetic dyslipoproteinemia with marked atherosclerosis. The correction of the apoE deficiency in the apoE-deficient mouse model presented several interesting challenges [24]. For apoE to function in facilitating the clearance of lipoprotein remnants, gene replacement must be followed by synthesis and secretion of the apolipoprotein in a pathway which will permit it to become associated with both hepatic endothelial cell proteoglycans as well as plasma lipoproteins. In addition, to achieve physiological replacement of apoE, the transgene must be expressed in the mg/dl level in plasma which has not been readily achieved in previous gene replacement studies.

When compared to control C57 black mice, the apoE-deficient mice were markedly hyperlipidemic with plasma total cholesterol, cholesteryl esters, and free cholesterol levels approximately six fold greater than control mice, and plasma triglycerides two fold greater. Furthermore, HDL is reduced to one third of the plasma levels present in control mice. We have successfully corrected the apoE deficiency in the apoE-knockout mice utilizing an adenovirus vector containing the human apoE cDNA [24]. The apoE cDNA was subcloned into a shuttle vector (pAd12 apoE) containing a CMV enhancer and promoter elements, a SV40 polyadenylation signal, and the E1 region of the human adenovirus (Ad5). The recombinant virus was propagated in 293 cells and purified by cesium chloride density ultracentrifugation.

Following apoE-adenovirus infusion the hypercholesterolemia in the apoE-deficient mice decreased at day 4 from 739 ± 165 mg/dl in animals infused with luciferase as control to 103 ± 18 mg/dl similar to control mice of 103 ± 13 mg/dl (Table 1). The lipoprotein profile was normalized for a period of up to three weeks with plasma apoE levels ranging from a physiological level of 3-4 mg/dl to 650 mg/dl. After apoE-adenovirus gene therapy the lipoprotein profile analyzed by FPLC of the apoE-deficient mice normalized and demonstrated a striking shift from the profile of increased VLDL-IDL-LDL to a normal pattern of predominately HDL. Quantitation of aortic atherosclerosis 4 weeks after adenoviral infusion demonstrated a marked reduction in the mean lesion area of mice infused with rAdv.apoE ($58 \pm 8 \times 10^3$ μm^2) when compared to control mice infused with rAdv.luc ($161 \pm 19 \times 10^3$ μm^2, $p < 0.0001$) (Figure 1). Thus, apoE expression for 1 month was sufficient to markedly reduce the atherosclerosis demonstrating the feasibility of gene therapy for correction of genetic hyperlipidemias resulting in atherosclerosis. Successful replacement of apoE in apoE-deficient mice also demonstrates the feasibility of replacing an apolipoprotein at physiological plasma levels which may ultimately be applicable for gene therapy in patients with genetic dyslipoproteinemias due to apolipoprotein deficiencies and atherosclerosis.

Other laboratories have also now reported on additional studies on the successful correction of the apoE deficiency in apoE knockout mice using bone marrow transplant [25,26], and adenovirus vectors [27].

Table 1. Plasma lipoprotein profiles in control and apoE-deficient mice following the infusion of adenovirus containing apoE.

	TC mg/dl	TG mg/dl	HDL-C mg/dl
ApoE Def. (n = 8)	739 ± 165	130 ± 44	21 ± 6
rAdv.apoE (n = 7)	103 ± 18*	97 ± 32	85 ± 44*
Controls (n = 15)	103 ± 13	76 ± 17	69 ± 3

*$p < 0.002$
Plasma samples were obtained four days after infusion of control apoE deficient mice with rAdv.luc or rAdv.apoE in apoE deficient mice.

GENE THERAPY FOR GENETIC DEFECTS IN ENZYMES

Hepatic Lipase. Hepatic lipase plays a key role in lipoprotein metabolism in the conversion of IDL to LDL and HDL_2 to HDL_3. Patients with a deficiency of hepatic lipase have a type III like lipoprotein phenotype with increased plasma levels of cholesterol, triglycerides, IDL, and HDL_2 [28-33]. Clinically these patients may have palmar and tuberous xanthomas, as well as an increased risk of premature cardiovascular disease. A hepatic lipase-deficient mouse model has been developed by gene disruption using homologous recombination [34]. When compared to control mice, hepatic lipase-deficient animals have approximately two fold increased plasma levels of total cholesterol, phospholipids, cholesteryl esters, and HDL cholesterol.

The successful replacement of the hepatic lipase gene in the hepatic lipase-deficient mice using the adenovirus vector system has several requirements. The human hepatic lipase gene must be delivered to the liver, hepatic lipase must be synthesized as well as undergo post-translational processing and secretion from the cell. Following secretion the active HL enzyme must be transported and then bound to the endothelial glycosaminoglycans where it is effective in hydrolyzing plasma lipoprotein triglycerides and phospholipids.

The complete correction of the lipoprotein profile in the hepatic lipase-deficient mouse has been achieved using the human cDNA HL recombinant adenovirus under the control of the CMV promoter and enhancer, an SV40 spice donor and acceptor, and an SV40 polyadenylation signal sequence [35]. Plasma hepatic lipase mass by immunoblot

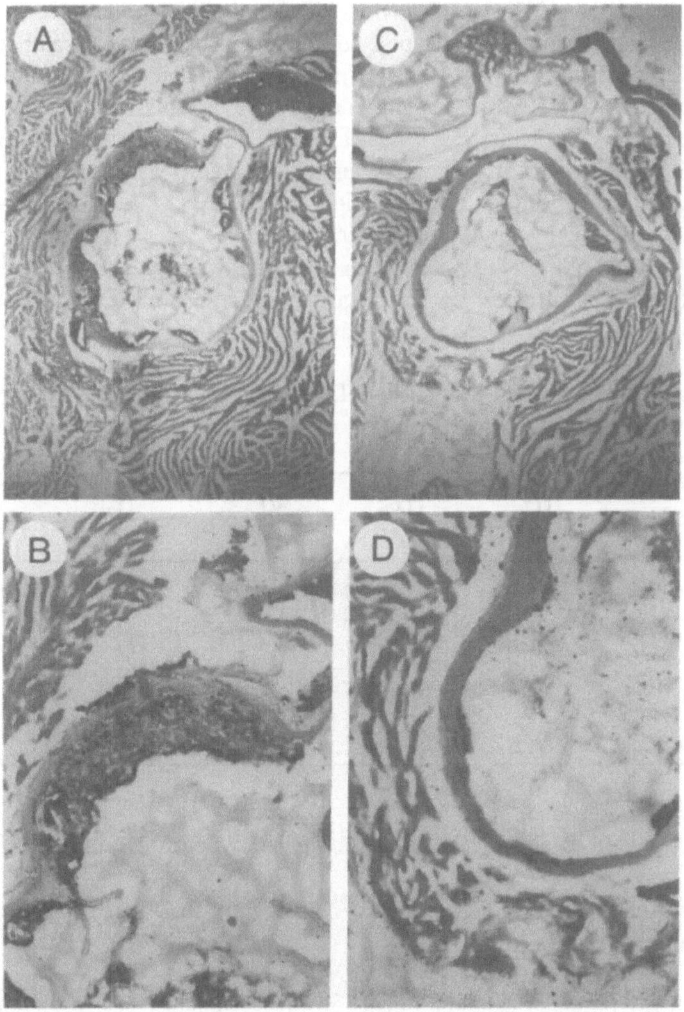

Figure 1. Proximal aortic sections from control apoE-deficient mice (left) and apoE-deficient mice after receiving rAdv.apoE for one month (right). All sections were stained with oil-red-O and hematoxylin and then counter stained with light green. ApoE-deficient mice have significant atherosclerotic changes with marked lipid accumulation and fibrosis (A, B). ApoE-deficient mice after rAdv.apoE treatment had a marked reduction in atherosclerosis with an absence of complex lesions and minimal lipid staining of the intima. (A, C X30; B, D X75)

analysis and enzymic activity were used to quantitate gene replacement in the hepatic lipase-deficient mouse after hepatic lipase adenovirus infusion. Following intravenous injection of the hepatic lipase-adenovirus vector the post-heparin plasma hepatic lipase activity increased 100 times over pretreatment values. Hepatic lipase activity reached a maximum at days 4-6 and could be detected in 50% of the animals at 30 days. The plasma lipoprotein profile in hepatic lipase-deficient mice following hepatic lipase adenovirus infusion returned to normal on days 4-6 and was similar to control mice. The post-treatment FPLC profile was normalized with total cholesterol, phospholipids, and cholesteryl esters decreased by 80%, and triglycerides reduced by approximately 50% (Table 2). Post-heparin injection revealed that greater than 90% of the human hepatic lipase enzyme was heparin-releasable indicating that the enzyme was attached to the capillary endothelium where it bound to the glycosaminoglycans and was enzymically active.

Table 2. Plasma lipids and lipoproteins in HL-deficient mice before and after infusion of HlrAdV.

	TC mg/dl	TG mg/dl	PL mg/dl	CE mg/dl	HDL-C mg/dl
HL Def (n = 7)	176 ± 9*	58 ± 4	314 ± 12*	122 ± 8*	129 ± 9*
rAdv.HL (n = 5)	94 ± 10	51 ± 5	207 ± 16	35 ± 12	62 ± 8
Controls (n = 13)	101 ± 2	63 ± 2	211 ± 4	66 ± 2	78 ± 3‡

*$p < 0.001$ versus control; ‡n = 10
Plasma samples were obtained eight days after infusion of rAdv.HL in HL deficient mice.

Identification of Candidate Genes for Gene Therapy for Patients with Premature Cardiovascular Disease

In the search for potential candidate genes to protect against atherosclerosis we have focused our attention on genes which regulated plasma HDL levels. HDL have been the focus of great interest during the last two decades since elevated and reduced plasma HDL levels are associated with decreased and increased risk of premature cardiovascular disease, respectively [36-38]. Several lines of evidence now indicate that HDL are heterogeneous and contain several separate lipoprotein particles which may have different functions in lipoprotein metabolism and reverse cholesterol transport [39-42]. The major lipoprotein particles within HDL classified by apolipoprotein composition include LpA-I, LpA-I:A-II and nascent lipoproteins containing LpA-I. The E, C, and A-IV apolipoproteins and other minor apolipoproteins are also present on the major lipoproteins particles within HDL. The clinical importance of separating HDL into its major component lipoprotein particles, LpA-I and LpA-I:A-II, is based on the increasing body of data which suggests that LpA-I and LpA-I:A-II may have separate metabolic functions and different potentials to efflux cellular cholesterol as well as protection against the development of premature cardiovascular disease. Based on clinical, metabolic, as well as cell culture studies *in vitro*, LpA-I has been proposed to be metabolic distinct and a more effective antiatherogenic lipoprotein particle in HDL than LpA-I:A-II (for review see [39,43]).

We have performed a series of kinetics studies of the LpA-I and LpA-I:A-II lipoprotein particles present in HDL in normal controls [43]. A detailed characterization of the lipid and protein composition of LpA-I in normolipidemic men and women has recently been reported [44,45]. Based on these studies we have developed a schematic working model of HDL metabolism and reverse cholesterol transport including LpA-I and LpA-I:A-II and the interrelationship of the lipolytic enzymes, receptors and CETP (Figure 2). HDL has been proposed to modulate the risk of premature cardiovascular disease by facilitating the removal of excess cholesterol from peripheral tissues and transporting the cholesterol back to the liver. This hypothetical process of HDL-mediated transport of cholesterol from peripheral tissues back to the liver has been termed reverse cholesterol transport [46,47]. The cholesterol esters present in HDL may be transported to the liver by two pathways. HDL cholesteryl esters may be carried directly to the liver or the cholesteryl esters may be exchanged for triglycerides by CETP and returned to the liver via the apoB-containing lipoproteins, IDL and LDL. Increasing plasma HDL has been proposed to reduce the risk of atherosclerosis. Infusion of HDL resulted in decreased atherosclerosis in cholesterol-fed rabbits [48], and transgenic mice overexpressing apoA-I have increased plasma HDL levels and are protected against diet-induced atherosclerosis [49], as well as the atherosclerosis in the apoE-deficient mouse model [50] as outlined above. These and other results have led to the concept that raising HDL and more specifically LpA-I will be an effective way to reduce atherosclerosis and thus may be an effective strategy for the treatment of atherosclerosis in man regardless of the genetic defect leading to the atherosclerosis.

LCAT plays a key role in the transport of cholesterol by the HDL pathway. LCAT catalyzes the esterification of lipoprotein free cholesterol to cholesteryl esters which can be carried in the core of the lipoprotein particle converting nascent disc-shaped particles into mature, spherical HDL [51,52]. Thus, LCAT in conjunction with CETP, hepatic lipase, and apoA-I are required for efficient reverse cholesterol transport [53-56] (Figure 2).

In order to gain insight into the potential pivotal role that LCAT may play in modulating plasma HDL levels, we have developed transgenic mice [57] and rabbits [58] overexpressing human LCAT. The construct used to develop the transgenic animals was a 6.2 kb DNA fragment consisting of 0.851 and 1.134 kb of the 5' and 3' flanking regions as well as the entire human LCAT gene. Transgenic mice overexpressing human LCAT had increased plasma total cholesterol and HDL-cholesterol levels of 124-218% and 123-194%, respectively, when compared to control mice. Plasma apoA-I (63 ± 14 mg/dl), apoA-II (54 ± 11 mg/dl), and apoE (16 ± 2 mg/dl) were increased in LCAT transgenic mice when compared to control mice apoA-I (47 ± 15mg/dl), apoA-II (40 ± 12 mg/dl), and apoE (7 ± 2 mg/dl). FPLC analysis of plasma lipoproteins of high expresser LCAT transgenic mice revealed increased levels of HDL which were larger, cholesteryl ester and phospholipid enriched with two distinct subclasses of HDL lipoprotein particles, an apoE-rich HDL_1, and an apoA-I:apoA-II containing HDL. The results obtained with LCAT transgenic mice established that LCAT increases plasma HDL levels, a hyperalphalipoproteinemia profile that would be anticipated to be associated with a reduced risk of atherosclerosis.

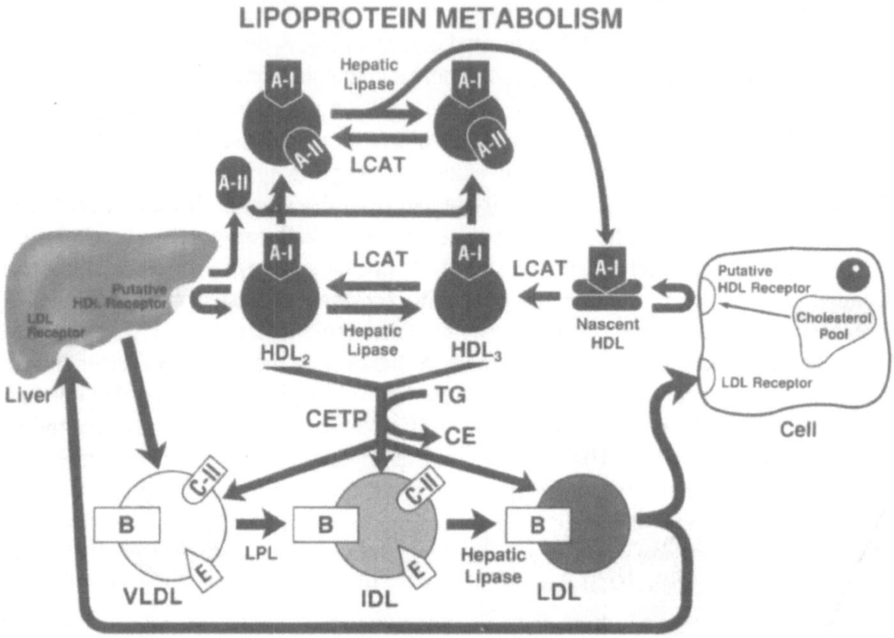

Figure 2. Schematic model of human plasma lipoprotein metabolism (see text for details).

The effects of overexpression of LCAT on HDL metabolism has also been investigated in transgenic rabbits. Lipoprotein metabolism in rabbits differs from mice in the presence of CETP, the absence of apoA-II, and lack of apoB editing in the liver. LCAT transgenic rabbits had an increased plasma total cholesterol and HDL cholesterol levels when compared to control rabbits (Table 3). FPLC analysis of LCAT transgenic rabbit plasma revealed a marked increase in apoA-I:apoE-enriched HDL and decreased apoB-containing lipoproteins. Thus both the LCAT transgenic rabbit and the LCAT transgenic mouse develop hyperalphalipoproteinemia and a lipoprotein profile which is associated with protection against the development of atherosclerosis.

In order to test the protective effect of LCAT on diet-induced atherosclerosis, rabbits were placed on a high cholesterol diet (0.3% cholesterol) for 16 weeks after which the animals were sacrificed and the extent of atherosclerosis quantitated in control and LCAT transgenic rabbits. The atherosclerosis by quantitative planimetry was reduced in the LCAT rabbit by 86% ($p < .003$). The marked reduction in the atherosclerosis in the LCAT transgenic rabbit when compared to control rabbits is illustrated in Figure 3.

Table 3. Plasma lipoprotein profile and LCAT activities in control and LCAT transgenic rabbits.

	LCAT Activity nmol/ml/h	Total Cholesterol	Triglycerides	HDL Cholesterol
Control (n = 10)	101 ± 11	29 ± 3	39 ± 4	24 ± 1
LCAT TG (n = 9)	1593 ± 101*	179 ± 7*	43 ± 4	161 ± 5*

*$p < 0.05$

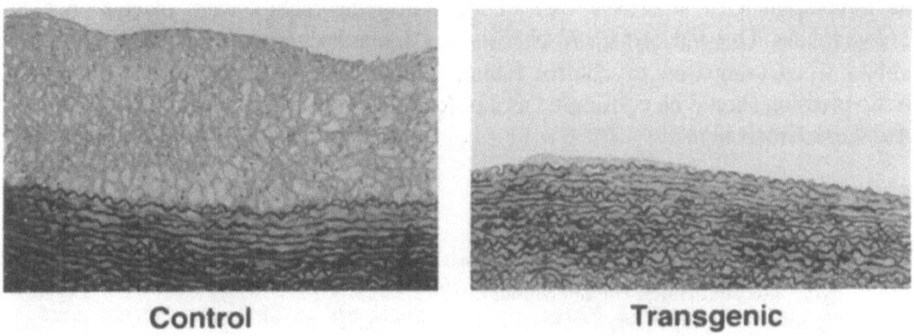

Figure 3. 1 mm sections of the descending thoracic aorta of cholesterol-fed control rabbits (left) and LCAT transgenic rabbits (right) stained with PAS. The increased intimal thickness with extensive foam cell accumulation in the controls (left) was markedly decreased in the LCAT transgenic rabbits (right).

Summary

The studies reviewed in this report summarize the initial approaches that have been used for gene therapy for familial hypercholesterolemia in man and animal models for the genetic dyslipoproteinemias. Limited success has been achieved using the *ex vivo* hepatic retroviral mediated approach to the correction of the genetic defect in patients with FH and indicate that other *in vivo* vector delivery systems may be required to totally correct the genetic defect in FH.

Current results indicate that the molecular defects in the genetic dyslipoproteinemias can be effectively corrected using adenovirus vectors. The complete correction of the apoE- and hepatic lipase-deficiencies in the knockout mice models established that it will be possible in the future to correct gene defects in both apolipoproteins and lipolytic enzymes. The major limitation of the currently employed first generation adenovirus vectors is the limited time of expression of the transgene. Future studies on the feasibility of adenovirus gene therapy for the genetic dyslipoproteinemias will continue using second and third generation adenovirus vectors in which the E2 and E4 regions have been deleted as well as attempts to modulate the immune system. Other new vectors as well as nonviral vectors are currently being developed and tested by several pharmaceutical companies and laboratories. The continued development of improved vectors and basic research in the biology of gene transfer will ultimately provide the information and technology for gene therapy of the genetic dyslipoproteinemias in man in the future.

Our search to identify a candidate gene that would be useful to reduce atherosclerosis has focused on genes involved in HDL metabolism. Of particular interest have been the results obtained with transgenic mice and rabbits overexpressing LCAT. LCAT overexpression in mice and rabbits leads to increased HDL levels and a hyperalphalipoproteinemia profile. To test the protective effect of LCAT overexpression on the development of atherosclerosis LCAT transgenic rabbits were placed on a high cholesterol diet. Diet-induced atherosclerosis was dramatically reduced in LCAT transgenic rabbits when compared to control rabbits. These initial results indicate that LCAT overexpression should be considered as a potential therapeutic approach for gene therapy of atherosclerosis in man.

References

1. Hobbs HH, Brown MS, Goldstein JL. Molecular genetics of the LDL receptor gene in familial hypercholesterolemia. Human Mutation 1992;1:445-46.
2. Grossman M, Raper SE, Kozarsky K, et al. Successful ex vivo gene therapy directed to liver in a patient with familial hypercholesterolaemia. Nature Genetics 1994;6:335-41.
3. Grossman M, Rader DJ, Muller DWM, et al. A pilot study of ex vivo gene therapy for homozygous familial hypercholesterolaemia. Nature Medicine 1995;1:1148-54.
4. Brewer HB, Jr, Gregg RE, Hoeg JM. Apolipoproteins, lipoproteins, and atherosclerosis. In: Braunwald E, editor. Heart disease: A textbook of cardiovascular medicine. 3rd ed. New York: WB Saunders, Co., 1989:121-44.
5. Mahley RW. Apolipoprotein E: Cholesterol transport protein with expanding role in cell biology. Science 1988;240:622-30.
6. Mahley RW, Innerarity TL, Weisgraber KH, et al. Cellular and molecular biology of lipoprotein metabolism: Characterization of lipoprotein receptor-ligand interactions. Cold Spring Harb Symp Quant Biol 1986;51:821-28.
7. Nykjaer A, Bengtsson-Olivecrona G, Lookene A, et al. The α_2-macroglobulin receptor/low density lipoprotein receptor-released protein binds lipoprotein lipase and β-migrating very low density lipoprotein associated with the lipase. J Biol Chem 1993;268:15048-55.
8. Mulder M, Lombardi P, Jansen H, Van Berkel TJC, Frants RR, Havekes LM. Low density lipoprotein receptor internalizes low density and very low density lipoproteins that are bound to heparin sulfate proteoglycans via lipoprotein lipase. J Biol Chem 1993;268:9369-75.
9. Mahley RW, Ji ZS, Brecht WJ, Miranda RD, He D. Role of heparan sulfate proteoglycans and the LDL receptor-related protein in remnant lipoprotein metabolism. Ann NY Acad Sci 1994;

737:39-52.

10. Santamarina-Fojo S, Dugi K. Structure, function and role of lipoprotein lipase in lipoprotein metabolism. Curr Opin Lipidol 1994;5:117-25.
11. Takahashi S, Kawarabayasi Y, Nakai T, Sakai J, Yamamoto T. Rabbit very low density lipoprotein receptor: A low density lipoprotein receptor-like protein with distinct ligand specificity. Proc Natl Acad Sci USA 1992;89:9252-56.
12. Ghiselli G, Schaefer EJ, Gascon P, Brewer HB, Jr. Type III hyperlipoproteinemia associated with apolipoprotein E deficiency. Science 1981;214:1239-41.
13. Schaefer EJ, Gregg RE, Ghiselli G, et al. Familial apolipoprotein E deficiency. J Clin Invest 1986;78:1206-19.
14. Mabuchi H, Itoh H, Takeda M, et al. A young type III hyperlipoproteinemic patient associated with apolipoprotein E deficiency. Metabolism 1989;38:115-19.
15. Kurosaka D, Teramoto T, Matsushima T, et al. Apolipoprotein E deficiency with a depressed mRNA of normal size. Atherosclerosis 1991;88:15-20.
16. Lohse P, Brewer HB, III, Meng MS, Skarlatos SI, LaRosa JC, Brewer HB, Jr. Familial apolipoprotein E deficiency and type III hyperlipoproteinemia due to a premature stop codon in the apolipoprotein E gene. J Lipid Res 1992;33:1583-90.
17. Zannis VI, Breslow JL. Characterization of a unique human apolipoprotein E variant associated with type III hyperlipoproteinemia. J Biol Chem 1980;255:1759-62.
18. Brewer HB, Jr, Zech LA, Gregg RE, Schwartz D, Schaefer EJ. Type III hyperlipoproteinemia: Diagnosis, molecular defects, pathology, and treatment. Ann Intern Med 1983;98:623-40.
19. Brewer HB, Jr, Santamarina-Fojo S, Hoeg JM. Disorders of lipoprotein metabolism. In: DeGroot LJ, Besser M, Jameson JL, et al., editors. Endocrinology. 3rd ed. Philadelphia: WB Saunders Company, 1995:2731-53.
20. Mahley RW, Rall SC, Jr. Type III hyperlipoproteinemia (dysbetalipoproteinemia): The role of apolipoprotein E in normal and abnormal lipoprotein metabolism. In: Scriver CR, Beaudet AL, Sly WS, et al., editors. The metabolic and molecular bases of inherited disease. 7th ed. New York: McGraw-Hill, Inc., 1995:1953-80.
21. Piedrahita JA, Zhang SH, Hagaman JR, Oliver PM, Maeda N. Generation of mice carrying a mutant apolipoprotein E gene inactivated by gene targeting in embryonic stem cells. Proc Natl Acad Sci USA 1992;89:4471-75.
22. Plump AS, Smith JD, Hayek T, et al. Severe hypercholesterolemia and atherosclerosis in apolipoprotein E-deficient mice created by homologous recombination in ES cells. Cell 1992; 71:343-53.
23. Zhang SH, Reddick RL, Piedrahita JA, Maeda N. Spontaneous hypercholesterolemia and arterial lesions in mice lacking apolipoprotein E. Science 1992;258:468-71.
24. Kashyap VS, Santamarina-Fojo S, Brown DR, et al. Apolipoprotein E deficiency in mice: Gene replacement and prevention of atherosclerosis using adenovirus vectors. J Clin Invest 1995;69:1612-20.
25. Linton MF, Atkinson JB, Fazio S. Prevention of atherosclerosis in apolipoprotein E deficient mice by bone marrow transplantation. Science 1995;267:1034-37.
26. Boisvert WA, Spangenberg J, Curtiss LK. Treatment of severe hypercholesterolemia in apolipoprotein E-deficient mice by bone marrow transplantation. J Clin Invest 1995;96: 1118-24.
27. Stevenson SC, Marshall-Neff J, Teng B, Lee CB, Roy S, McClelland A. Phenotypic correction of hypercholesterolemia in apoE-deficient mice by adenovirus mediated in vivo gene transfer. Arterioscler Thromb Vasc Biol 1995;15:479-84.

28. Breckenridge WC, Little JA, Alaupovic P, et al. Lipoprotein abnormalities associated with a familial deficiency of hepatic lipase. Atherosclerosis 1982;45:161-79.
29. Carlson LA, Holmquist L, Nilsson-Ehle P. Deficiency of hepatic lipase activity in post-heparin plasma in familial hyper-α-triglyceridemia. Acta Med Scand 1986;219:435-47.
30. Auwerx JH, Marzetta CA, Hokanson JE, Brunzell JD. Large buoyant LDL-like particles in hepatic lipase deficiency. Arteriosclerosis 1989;9:319-25.
31. Auwerx JH, Babirak SP, Hokanson JE, et al. Coexistence of abnormalities of hepatic lipase and lipoprotein lipase in a large family. Am J Hum Genet 1990;46:470-77.
32. Ikeda Y, Takagi A. Hypertriglyceridemia in a deficiency of lipoprotein lipase and hepatic lipase. Tanpakushitsu Kakusan Koso 1988;33:783-90.
33. Connelly PW, Maguire GF, Lee M, Little JA. Plasma lipoproteins in familial hepatic lipase deficiency. Arteriosclerosis 1990;10:40-48.
34. Homanics GE, De Silva HV, Osada J, et al. Mild dyslipidemia in mice following targeted inactivation of the hepatic lipase gene. J Biol Chem 1995;270:2974-80.
35. Applebaum-Bowden D, Kobayashi J, Kashyap VS, et al. Hepatic lipase gene therapy in hepatic lipase-deficient mice: Adenovirus-mediated replacement of a lipolytic enzyme to the vascular endothelium. J Clin Invest 1996;97:799-805.
36. Miller NE, Miller GJ. Clinical and metabolic aspects of high density lipoproteins. New York: Elsevier, 1984:1-459.
37. Gordon DJ, Probstfield JL, Garrison RJ, et al. High-density lipoprotein cholesterol and cardiovascular disease: Four prospective American studies. Circulation 1989;79:8-15.
38. Gordon DJ, Rifkind BM. High-density lipoprotein--the clinical implications of recent studies. N Engl J Med 1989;321:1311-16.
39. Fruchart JC, Ailhaud G. Apolipoprotein A-containing lipoprotein particles: Physiological role, quantification, and clinical significance. Clin Chem 1992;38:793-97.
40. Schultz JR, Verstuyft JG, Gong EL, Nichols AV, Rubin EM. Protein composition determines the anti-atherogenic properties of HDL in transgenic mice. Nature 1993;365:762-24.
41. Tall AR. Plasma cholesteryl ester transfer protein. J Lipid Res 1993;34:1255-74.
42. Cheung MC, Albers JJ. Characterization of lipoprotein particles isolated by immunoaffinity chromatography. Particles containing A-I and A-II and particles containing A-I but no A-II. J Biol Chem 1984;259:12201-209.
43. Rader DJ, Castro G, Zech LA, Fruchart JC, Brewer HB, Jr. In vivo metabolism of apolipoprotein A-I on high density lipoprotein particles LpA-I and LpA-I, A-II. J Lipid Res 1991;32:1849-59.
44. Duverger N, Rader DJ, Duchateau P, Fruchart JC, Castro G, Brewer HB, Jr. Biochemical characterization of the three major subclasses of lipoprotein A-I (LpA-I) preparatively isolated from human plasma. Biochem 1993;32:12373-79.
45. Duverger N, Rader D, Brewer HB, Jr. Distribution of subclasses of HDL containing ApoA-I without ApoA-II (LpA-I) in normolipidemic men and women. Arterioscler Thromb 1994;14: 1594-99.
46. Glomset JA, Janssen ET, Kennedy R, Dobbins J. Role of plasma lecithin:cholesterol acyltransferase in the metabolism of high density lipoproteins. J Lipid Res 1966;7:638-48.
47. Glomset JA, Assmann G, Gjone E, Norum KR. Lecithin:cholesterol acyltransferase deficiency and fish eye disease. In: Scriver CR, Beaudet AL, Sly WS, et al., editors. The metabolic and molecular bases of inherited disease. 7th ed. New York: McGraw-Hill, Inc., 1995:1933-51.
48. Badimon JJ, Badimon L, Fuster V. Regression of atherosclerotic lesions by high density lipoprotein plasma fraction in the cholesterol-fed rabbit. J Clin Invest 1990;85:1234-41.

49. Rubin EM, Krauss RM, Spangler EA, Verstuyft JG, Clift SM. Inhibition of early atherogenesis in transgenic mice by human apolipoprotein AI. Nature 1991;353:265-67.
50. Plump AS, Scott CJ, Breslow JL. Human apolipoprotein A-I gene expression increases high density lipoprotein and suppresses atherosclerosis in the apolipoprotein E-deficient mouse. Proc Natl Acad Sci USA 1994;91:9607-11.
51. Francone OL, Gurakar A, Fielding C. Distribution and functions of lecithin: cholesterol acyltransferase and cholesteryl ester transfer protein in plasma lipoproteins. Evidence for a functional unit containing these activities together with apolipoproteins A-I and D that catalyzes the esterification and transfer of cell-derived cholesterol. J Biol Chem 1989; 264:7066-72.
52. Castro GR, Fielding CJ. Early incorporation of cell-derived cholesterol into pre-beta-migrating high-density lipoprotein. Biochem 1988;27:25-29.
53. Glomset JA. The plasma lecithins:cholesterol acyltransferase reaction. J Lipid Res 1968;9: 155-67.
54. Miller NE, La Ville A, Crook D. Direct evidence that reverse cholesterol transport is mediated by high-density lipoprotein in rabbit. Nature 1985;314:109-11.
55. Marzetta CA, Meyers TJ, Albers JJ. Lipid transfer protein-mediated distribution of HDL-derived cholesteryl esters among plasma apo B-containing lipoprotein subpopulations. Arteriosclerosis and Thrombosis 1993;13:834-41.
56. Huang Y, von Eckardstein A, Wu S, Assmann G. Cholesterol efflux, cholesterol esterification, and cholesteryl ester transfer by LpA-I and LpA-I/A-II in native plasma. Arterioscler Thromb Vasc Biol 1995;15:1412-18.
57. Vaisman BL, Klein H-G, Rouis M, et al. Overexpression of human lecithin cholesterol acyltransferase leads to hyperalphalipoproteinemia in transgenic mice. J Biol Chem 1995; 270:12269-75.
58. Hoeg JM, Vaisman BL, Demosky SJ, Jr., et al. Lecithin-cholesterol acyltransferase overexpression generates hyperalphalipoproteinemia and a nonatherogenic lipoprotein pattern in transgenic rabbits. J Biol Chem 1996;271:4396-402.

THE GENETICS OF LIPOPROTEIN DISORDERS

Jean Davignon, Jeffrey S. Cohn, Madeleine Roy, and Anne Minnich
Clinical Research Institute of Montreal, 110 Pine Avenue, West, Montreal, QC, Canada H2W 1R7

Introduction

This selective review will focus on atherogenic forms of primary dyslipoproteinemias. We will consider in turn familial hypercholesterolemia (FH), familial ligand-defective apo B-100 and phytosterolemia (two conditions which may be manifested by the FH clinical phenotype), familial combined hyperlipidemia, familial dysbetalipoproteinemia (type III), familial endogenous hypertriglyceridemia (type IV), and hypoalphalipoproteinemia. Most of these conditions are heterogeneous. The genetic etiology is not established for all, but even the known genetic defects represent only a fraction of the genetic variations responsible for atherogenic dyslipoproteinemias. There are many susceptibility/variability genes [1] that not only can confer a predisposition to the development of dyslipoproteinemia and atherosclerosis, but that can also modulate the onset, severity, and progression of these inherited conditions. We will emphasize the context dependency of primary dyslipoproteinemias (i.e. effect of gender, age, environment, and other genes), consider new developments, and give attention to potential candidate genes when the etiology of the disorder is unknown. We will also give examples of gene-gene and gene-environment interactions modulating the lipoprotein phenotypes of these primary disorders. Familial hypercholesterolemia will be discussed in more detail as it is a focus of our research group and stands out among the atherogenic dyslipoproteinemias because of its severity and pathophysiological consequences.

Familial Hypercholesterolemia

Heterozygous FH is often associated in adults with the presence of tendon xanthomas (extensor tendons of the fingers, Achilles' tendons), premature atherosclerosis, and a family history of coronary artery disease (CAD). Other skin and ocular manifestations (which are florid and present at birth in the homozygote) may include tuberous xanthomas, prepatellar, tricipital or plantar xanthomas, xanthelasmas, and arcus corneae. Association of these diagnostic clues with high plasma levels of LDL-cholesterol (LDL-C) transmitted with an autosomal codominant pattern usually confirms the diagnosis. This monogenic disorder is

A. M. Gotto, Jr. et al. (eds.), Drugs Affecting Lipid Metabolism, 311–327.

due to an LDL-receptor defect resulting in delayed clearance of plasma LDL and intermediate density lipoproteins (IDL) and an increased conversion of IDL into LDL. Typically plasma cholesterol concentration is greater than 350 mg/dL (9 mmol/L), and LDL-C is greater than 250 mg/dL (6.4 mmol/L) in the heterozygote (see [2,3] for review). Triglyceride concentration is normal unless a second genetic defect (or predisposition) adds hypertriglyceridemia to the biochemical phenotype [4]. A "type IIb" lipoprotein pattern may thus be present in patients with FH. Hence, type IIa hyperlipoproteinemia is not a synonym for FH, particularly since this phenotype is also found in patients with familial combined hyperlipidemia (FCH).

Table 1. French-Canadian LDL-receptor mutations.

Mutation*	Site	Defect	Frequencies (number of subjects)			
			130[a]	376[b]	343[c]	88[d]
FC-1. 10 kb deletion	Promoter Exon 1	No expression	59%	60%	56%	57%
FC-2. Cys_{646} → Tyr	Exon 14	Transport	5%	6%	6%	9%
FC-3. Glu_{207} → Lys	Exon 4	Transport	2%	3%	<1%	1%
FC-4. Trp_{66} → Gly	Exon 3	Binding	7%	12%	18%	3%
FC-5. 5 kb deletion	Exons 2 & 3	Binding	3%	2%	0%	1%
FC-6. Tyr_{468} → Stop	Exon 10	Truncation		<1%	4%	
			76%	84%	85%	71%

* The nomenclature for mutations among French Canadians (FC) 1-5 corresponds to that of Hobbs et al. [5] except for FH-6 [6]

a. Original cohort of FH subjects from the Montreal area unrelated to the second degree [7]
b. FH cohort with strict exclusion criteria from the Montreal area [8]. The exon 10 mutation was determined *a posteriori* on the 63 subjects without the first 5 mutations, revealing 2 cases with Tyr_{468} - Stop.
c. Children from the Quebec City area [6]. The exon 10 mutation was probably overestimated as the 14 subjects with this mutation originated from two kindreds and were related.
d. FH children in the Montreal area [9]

The frequency of FH is about 1:500 and over 200 mutations of the LDL-R gene have been reported [3,5,10]. In areas where a founder effect is present such as Finland, South Africa, Norway, Israel, Lebanon and Canada, the frequency can be as high as 1:80. In Quebec, Canada, 6 mutations have been reported (Table 1) which account for 70 to 85% of FH cases [6,8,9,11]. One of these, a > 10 kb deletion (Δ > 10 kb) of the promoter and exon 1 of the LDL-receptor gene (resulting in a null allele), is found in as many as 60% of cases [12] due to a founder effect [13]. There are important regional differences in the frequency distribution of these mutations; for instance, in adults as well as in children, the prevalence of LDL-R exon 3 Trp_{66}→Gly is greater in Quebec City than in Montreal, whereas the Δ5 kb observed in Montreal is absent from the Quebec City area (Table 1). There are also wide phenotypic variations among patients sharing the same LDL-receptor mutation

[14] and preliminary results from our laboratory indicate that approximately 6% of total variability (or 12% of the genetic variability) in LDL-cholesterol is accounted for by variations in the normal LDL-R allele in FH heterozygotes with the $\Delta > 10$ kb [15,16]. Some of these mutations, such as the $\Delta > 10$ kb, and the exon 14 $Cys_{646} \rightarrow Tyr$, result in a more severe LDL-R defect *in vitro* than for example the exon 3 $Trp_{66} \rightarrow Gly$. In homozygotes, the $\Delta > 10$ kb is associated with higher plasma LDL-C levels (26.7 mmol/L versus 16.1 mmol/L) and a more severe phenotype in terms of onset of CAD and CAD mortality than the exon 3 mutation [17]. In contrast, LDL-C levels in heterozygotes do not differ greatly (7.25 ± 1.47 mmol/L, n = 80, versus 6.94 ± 1.69 mmol/L, n = 55, N.S., Figure 1), indicating compensatory mechanisms in the presence of one normal LDL-R allele. Studies of FH patients with the same receptor defect have shown that the LDL-receptor gene has a sex-specific pleiotropic effect (i.e. one gene producing multiple effects) on plasma lipid and lipoprotein traits [14].

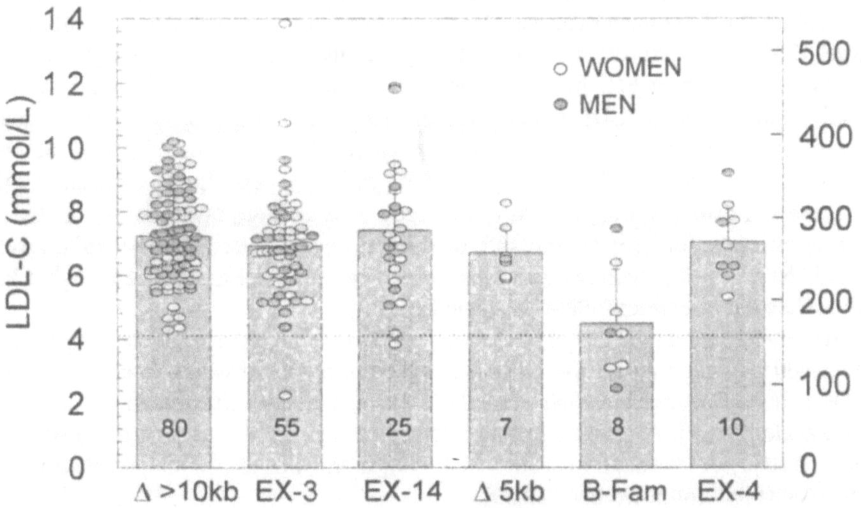

Figure 1. Age-adjusted plasma LDL-C concentrations in probands with familial hypercholesterolemia due to 5 different LDL-receptor mutations and in the B-kindred (B-FAM) where the 5 kb deletion (Δ5 kb) segregates. The sample size was limited to 40 men and 40 women for the 10 kb deletion ($\Delta > 10$kb) randomly selected from our lipid clinic database in Montreal. The means and standard deviations were 7.25 ± 1.47 mmol/L for the $\Delta > 10$kb, 6.94 ± 1.69 mmol/L for the exon 3 mutation (Ex-3), 7.42 ± 2.03 mmol/L for the exon 14 mutation (Ex-14), 6.73 ± 0.85 for the Δ5 kb versus 4.47 ± 1.71 mmol/L in the B-kindred where the presence of the apo E $\epsilon 2$ allele lowered LDL-C in the Δ5 kb subjects, and 7.59 ± 2.03 mmol/L for the exon 4 (Ex-4) mutation. The dotted line represents the upper limit of normal for LDL-cholesterol (4.14 mmol/L).

Gene-gene and gene-environment interactions contribute to the wide phenotypic variability between FH heterozygotes sharing the same LDL-R defect. Some mutations are particularly vulnerable to such interactions. In one family, the B-kindred (Figure 1), some carriers of the LDL-R Δ5 kb had normal LDL-C levels [18,19]. This occurred despite the severity of the Δ5 kb as demonstrated *in vitro* [20]. A similar situation was reported with another mutation in a Puerto Rican family [21]. Within the B-kindred, the normal cholesterol levels in carriers of the Δ5 kb were associated with the ϵ2 allele of the apolipoprotein E (apo E) gene which seemed to be the major contributor to this LDL-lowering effect [19].

Apo E polymorphism appears, indeed, to be a major modulator of the phenotypic expression of FH. In patients with the more severe Δ > 10 kb of the LDL-R gene, in contrast to what is observed in carriers of the Δ5 kb in the B-kindred, the cholesterol-lowering effect of the ϵ2 allele is evident but does not normalize plasma lipoprotein levels [22]. The effect is stronger in women than in men [23]. Furthermore, in women, the E3/2 phenotype is associated with a large effect on the concatenated multivariate measures of mean levels of adjusted lipid and lipoprotein traits with little influence on total variance. In men, in contrast, the E3/2 phenotype has a large effect on total variance with little influence on levels [23]. The lipoprotein lipase (LPL) gene may also impact strongly on the phenotypic expression of FH. In one member of a family where both the mild exon 3 Trp_{66}→Gly mutation of the LDL-R gene and the Pro_{207}→Leu mutation of the LPL gene segregated, the homozygous LPL defect prevented the LDL-raising effect of the heterozygous LDL-receptor defect [24]. The LPL deficiency also lowered plasma HDL levels in the FH heterozygote. Recently, the study of four large kindreds that included double heterozygotes for both FH and LPL deficiency, demonstrated that low HDL levels in FH could be ascribed to heterozygosity for an LPL gene mutation, but that a single LPL defective allele did not affect LDL-C levels in FH [25].

It is interesting to note that in FH, even the response to cholesterol-lowering agents may be genetically determined; this has been shown for probucol which is more effective [26,27] and HMG-CoA reductase inhibitors (HCRI) which are less effective in the presence of the ϵ4 allele [28,29]. A gene by gender interaction was noted in two of these studies, such that the ability of lovastatin to reduce LDL-cholesterol was less in the presence of the ϵ4 allele in men but not in women [28,30].

Familial Ligand-Defective Apo B

In this condition, a mutation in the apo B gene is responsible for impaired ligand-receptor interaction (20-30% of normal binding to fibroblast LDL-receptors *in vitro*) and delayed clearance of defective LDL particles. Familial ligand-defective apo B (FLDB) was proposed as a preferred term to designate this disease [31], formerly called familial defective apo B-100 [32]. It is inherited as an autosomal dominant trait (i.e. the phenotype is not more severe in the homozygote [33,34]). At least three apo B mutations are associated with FLDB: Arg_{3500}→Gln [32]; Arg_{3500}→Trp [35]; and Arg_{3531}→Cys [36]. Recent methodological developments facilitate screening for these mutations [37,38]. The most predominant mutation, apo B Arg_{3500}→Gln, occurs on the same haplotype in several populations. The clinical manifestations of FLDB range from no evidence of disease, to the full features of heterozygous FH. The disorder is associated with normocholesterolemia, or with moderate to severe hypercholesterolemia. Typically, plasma LDL-C concentrations range from 100 to 400 mg/dL (2.7-10.3 mmol/L) in FLDB heterozygotes; homozygosity for FLDB is not as severe as homozygosity for FH phenotype caused by an LDL-receptor defect [33,34]. Plasma triglyceride and HDL-C concentrations tend to be higher and lower, respectively, than levels observed in unaffected first degree relatives [39]. The prevalence of FLDB was approximately 1:500 in a United States population sample [32], 2% to 5% in patients with the FH phenotype [40] and as high as 8% in hypercholesterolemic patients [41], but this depends of country of origin. The phenotypic expression is variable and context-dependent which may be related to genetic variation at the apo E and the LDL-receptor loci [42]. In one kindred, including 5 FLDB affected relatives, the E3/2 phenotype was associated with normocholesterolemia, the E3/3 phenotype with moderate hypercholesterolemia and the E4/2 and E4/4 phenotypes with severe hypercholesterolemia and tendon xantomatosis typical of FH. The severity of the phenotype was further associated with a particular haplotype of the LDL-receptor gene [42]. In this family, care was taken to exclude the concomitant presence of an LDL-receptor defect. Recently, the extent of phenotypic variability in FLDB was systematically studied and compared to that observed in FH [43]. Although FH and FLDB affected subjects may share the same clinical and biochemical phenotype, in most instances, FLDB is associated with a less severe phenotype than FH. LDL isolated from FLDB patients have an increased susceptibility to oxidation *in vitro* [44], another factor which may modulate the atherogenic potential of this condition.

Familial Phytosterolemia

Familial phytosterolemia (familial sitosterolemia) is a rare condition presenting clinically with an FH phenotype [45]. Xanthomatosis, developing in childhood, may be severe and indistinguishable from that of homozygous FH. This may be accompanied by arthralgia and arthritis (knees and ankle joints), hypersplenism, and hemolysis. Premature atherosclerosis and coronary artery disease are typical (CAD death at age 13 has been reported). Familial phytosterolemia (FP) is characterized primarily by an increased intestinal absorption and a reduced biliary secretion of plant sterols, resulting in plasma levels of sitosterol and campesterol that are about 50-fold higher than normal (0.3-1.0 mg/dL versus 14-65 mg/dL for β-sitosterol). Plasma cholestanol, sitostanol, and campestanol are also elevated. This disease is also characterized by abnormally high neutral sterol absorption, reduced biliary cholesterol excretion and decreased synthesis of cholesterol. Plasma cholesterol concentrations may be normal to moderately elevated; plasma triglycerides are normal. Plasma apo B concentrations have been reported to be inherited as an autosomal codominant trait in this disease with very high levels in homozygotes and intermediates levels in heterozygotes [46]; however, using phytosterolemia as the marker phenotype, its inheritance appears to be controlled by a rare autosomal recessive gene [45]. In heterozygotes, increased sitosterol absorption is offset by a rapid elimination of plant sterols

[47]. Seventy-five to 85% of plasma phytosterols and stanols are transported by LDL, the remainder by HDL.

The genetic defect underlying FP is not known and is probably heterogeneous. The absorption defect has been reported occasionally in association with cerebrotendinous xanthomatosis and with pseudohomozygous FH [48]. The latter is a rare condition of unknown etiology which may mimic homozygous FH, but in which the parents are normolipidemic. In a recent study of the pathophysiology of FP, overproduction of LDL in the absence of a functional LDL-receptor abnormality was described [49]. Following the discovery that shellfish sterols were overabsorbed and poorly concentrated in the bile, it has been proposed that phytosterolemia results from a general loss of discrimination between various sterols for esterification [50], such that increased esterification by acyl-CoA:cholesterol acyltransferase (ACAT) causes enhanced absorption in the intestinal mucosa and reduced sterol secretion by the liver into the bile. However, this hypothesis has not been substantiated by evidence of alteration of ACAT activity in phytosterolemia. Alternatively, it has been suggested that the primary defect could be inadequate cholesterol synthesis due to reduced production of HMG-CoA reductase (HCR), resulting in a compensatory enhancement of sterol absorption and retention [51]. Demonstration that HCR activity is reduced in mononuclear leucocytes, liver and ileal mucosa supports this hypothesis, but it has not been established whether this is a primary or secondary phenomenon [45,52]. Results of a recent sterol balance study with stable isotopes have confirmed reduced cholesterol synthesis in phytosterolemia but failed to find a difference in absolute absorption rate of different sterols between affected and controls [53]. This study also demonstrated that ingestion of sitostanol (an unabsorbable sterol, 0.5 g t.i.d.) resulted in reduced cholesterol absorption, increased fecal output of cholesterol and plant sterols, and a marked reduction in serum sterols, providing a new approach to treatment of this disease. A low plant sterol diet and administration of cholestyramine is the current treatment of choice. Unexpectedly, the sitostanol effect was not accompanied by an increase in endogenous sterol synthesis in the two patients where this was tested. Among candidate genes for FP are the following: ACAT, sterol carrier proteins, and HCR.

Familial Combined Hyperlipidemia

The clinical manifestations of familial combined hyperlipidemia (FCH, multiple phenotype disease, hyperapobetalipoproteinemia), if any, are usually mild. The presence of xanthelasmas, arcus corneae, or manifestations of atherosclerotic vascular disease (singly or in combination) are often the only diagnostic clues. A mild-to-moderate elevation of plasma cholesterol (or LDL-C), triglycerides, or both and low HDL-C with an increased plasma LDL-apo B determine the variety of lipoprotein phenotypes characterizing FCH [31]. Typically, the lipoprotein phenotype (IIa, IIb, IVB, NB, rarely V) differs among family members and may vary with time in the same subject ("B" denotes a relative increase in LDL-apo B and "N" denotes normolipidemia: a nomenclature which we have adopted in our lipid clinic). Presence of small dense LDL, which are prone to oxidation *in vitro* [54,55], are part of the biochemical phenotype. FCH is inherited as an autosomal dominant trait, and although it is reported in childhood, delayed expression in adulthood and/or incomplete penetrance is more common. The prevalence of FCH is estimated to range between 1:50 to 1:30. The atherogenic pattern B phenotype [55], also with dominant inheritance, bears resemblance to, but is distinct from FCH; FCH individuals expressing pattern B tend to have plasma triglyceride and apo B concentrations which are higher than those with pattern B alone, whereas those expressing phenotype pattern A have elevated levels of apo B but normal triglycerides [31,56]. A gene-gene interaction could thus be responsible for the phenotypic heterogeneity of FCH. Furthermore, FCH is often associated with hypertension, insulin resistance, hyperinsulinemia, and abdominal obesity which could also modulate its phenotypic expression. So far, attempts to link FCH to the apo B, LDL-receptor, apo AI-CIII-AIV, or LPL genes have been either negative or not reproducible.

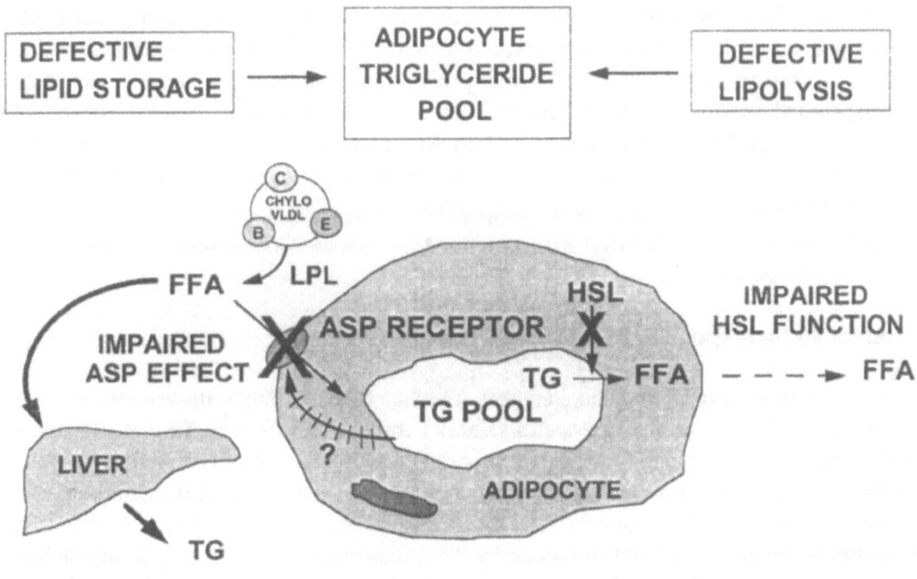

Figure 2. Adipose tissue metabolism in familial combined hyperlipidemia: a combined defect in lipid storage and lipolysis. Diagram of a hypothesis raised from the results of work carried out by Teng et al. [57], Cianflone et al. [58], and Reynisdottir et al. [59] (see text). CHYLO-VLDL represent remnants of chylomicrons and very low density lipoproteins. ASP: acylation stimulating protein; FFA: free fatty acids; HSL: hormone sensitive lipase; LPL: lipoprotein lipase; TG: triglycerides.

FCH is characterized by hepatic overproduction of apo B, delayed chylomicron remnant clearance, and prolonged postprandial elevation of plasma free fatty acids. The recent discovery of two new metabolic abnormalities may constitute a breakthrough in the understanding of the pathophysiology of FCH. One is the demonstration of impaired acylation stimulating protein (ASP)-mediated cellular triglyceride synthesis in cells obtained from FCH patients [58] and the other is impaired activation of adipose tissue lipolysis [59]. Subcutaneous adipocytes from patients with FCH are less responsive to stimulation of lipolysis by noradrenaline and isoprenaline (β-adrenoceptor agonists), forskolin (an adenylyl cyclase activator) and dibutyryl-cyclic AMP (a direct activator of the protein-kinase-hormone sensitive lipase [HSL] complex) [59]. Furthermore, the maximum HSL activity of subcutaneous adipocytes *in vitro* was significantly lower in FCH than in controls [59]. When impaired ASP receptor and HSL activities are linked together as in Figure 2, a general scheme can be developed to account for the hypertriglyceridemia and apo B overproduction in FCH. A defective HSL would prevent lipolysis and FFA release by adipocytes, leading to increased intracellular TG. Expansion of the intracellular TG pool could in turn downregulate the ASP receptor which would reduce FFA entry for further TG synthesis by the cell and increase plasma FFA and ASP levels. Alternatively, a primary defect in ASP action could be responsible. In either situation, FFA flux into the liver and direct hepatic uptake of small chylomicron remnants would increase substrate for enhanced TG synthesis and VLDL formation, resulting in a secondary overproduction of apo B. The primary defect underlying FCH remains to be determined. Among potential candidate genes are the ASP receptor gene and the genes coding for the HSL complex. It is likely that a contribution from variability at the LPL gene locus or at a locus responsible for susceptibility to the phenotype pattern B could account for some of the heterogeneity in phenotypic expression. A gene coding for a factor regulating apo B gene expression could also contribute to this complex phenotype.

Familial Dysbetalipoproteinemia

Familial dysbetalipoproteinemia (remnant disease, type III hyperlipoproteinemia) is a relatively rare condition (frequency from about 1 to 5 per 5000) [60]. Skin manifestations are typical and xanthoma striata palmaris, orange pigmentation of the palmar or plantar creases, and orange yellow tubero-eruptive xanthomas are virtually pathognomonic of the disease, but arcus corneae, xanthelasmas, tuberous xanthomas, and even tendon xanthomas may also be present. Peripheral and coronary atherosclerosis usually develop in middle-aged patients but occasionally occur prematurely. Apo E2 has 1% of the affinity of apo E3 or apo E4 for the LDL-receptor. The apo E2/2 phenotype in type III, in the presence of a second factor interfering with triglyceride-rich lipoprotein (TRL) metabolism (a "second hit"), results in delayed chylomicron remnant and VLDL-remnant (IDL) removal by the liver, impaired conversion of IDL into LDL, and an overproduction of VLDL. The resulting remnant accumulation in plasma is associated with high levels of cholesterol, triglyceride, and apo E, low LDL-C concentrations and normal or low HDL-C. Because remnants are enriched in cholesteryl esters, the VLDL-C/TG ratio is typically high (> 0.3, if mg/dL are used, or > 0.7, if mmol/L are used).

Type III has a recessive mode of inheritance because it segregates with the E2/2 phenotype (not with a single ε2 allele) and is expressed when a second factor intervenes to promote remnant accumulation [61]. Conditions that promote overproduction of triglycerides may be responsible. Familial hypertriglyceridemia, hypothyroidism, obesity, diabetes, and pregnancy (among others) may act as the second factor. Recently, heterozygosity for mutations in the LPL gene has been shown to contribute to increased plasma triglyceride levels in pregnant women with one ϵ2 allele [62], a phenomenon which has also been reported in one kindred with FCH, where an increase in β-VLDL in the presence of one ϵ2 allele was associated with accelerated atherosclerosis [63]. Type III is also manifested in apo E deficiency [64]. In one family this was found to be due to an acceptor splice site mutation in intron 3 [65], in another a point mutation ($Trp_{210} \rightarrow$ Stop) caused the truncated apo $E3_{WASHINGTON}$ [66]. Several mutations of apo E are associated with dominant transmission of type III (see [67] for review). Hepatic lipase (HL) deficiency also reproduces many of the biochemical characteristics of type III, since HL plays a role in the catabolism of IDL into LDL. One condition of as yet unknown etiology, pseudo type III, occurs in the absence of the E2/2 phenotype. It is characterized by hyperlipidemia with a high plasma VLDL-apo B and mimics many of the features of type III [68,69]. There is no evidence so far that this condition is due to an apo E receptor defect [70]. Fibrates are the drug of choice in the treatment of type III and striking regression of even the most severe xanthomas can be observed.

Familial Hypertriglyceridemia

Familial hypertriglyceridemia (FHT, carbohydrate-induced endogenous hypertriglyceridemia, type IV hyperlipoproteinemia) is also associated with few clinical signs, such as arcus corneae and xanthelasmas. Tuberous or eruptive xanthomas are rare and mostly seen in severe cases. Triglycerides and VLDL-C are moderately to markedly increased, LDL-C is normal or low, and HDL-C is usually decreased. Plasma cholesterol is normal or increased, depending on the VLDL-C elevation. The hyperlipidemia is markedly context-dependent (alcohol ingestion, dietary carbohydrates, caloric intake), resulting in large fluctuations in plasma TG. FHT is often associated with obesity, hyperuricemia, glucose intolerance, and insulin resistance. Its prevalence is estimated to be between 1:100 and 1:50. An increased risk for atherosclerosis may [71] or may not be present [72], reflecting the heterogeneity of the disease. The metabolic defect may be an overproduction and/or an impaired removal of VLDL, associated with impaired bile acid absorption. The hypertriglyceridemia is inherited as an autosomal dominant trait with delayed expression, and should be distinguished from that associated with FCH. An attempt to establish a linkage between FHT and the apo B, apo CIII or lipoprotein lipase genes has not been successful [73]. Fibrates are effective at lowering triglycerides in FHT. It has recently been demonstrated that fibrates inhibit transcription of apo CIII via the peroxisome proliferator activated receptor (PPAR) system [74], probably by suppression of HNF-4 [75], a hepatic nuclear factor needed for the interaction of the activated PPAR-retinoic acid receptor (RXR) complex with the peroxisome proliferator responsive element (PPRE). This constitutes a breakthrough in our understanding of the action of fibrates and emphasizes the importance of the role of apo CIII in hypertriglyceridemia.

An impaired bile acid absorption has been postulated to be the primary defect in some patients with primary hypertriglyceridemia [76]. A recent kinetic study in patients with FHT demonstrated a two-fold increase in fractional turnover rate of cholic and chenodeoxycholic acid in comparison to normolipidemic controls matched for age and gender [77]. This was associated with increased bile acid synthesis and no change or a small decrease in bile acid pools. Bile acid absorption was significantly lower in hypertriglyceridemic subjects than in controls, but the rate of enterohepatic cycling was normal. An increased rate of cholesterol secretion into the bile resulted in a significant increase in the cholesterol saturation index of the bile. This work further supports a defect in bile acid absorption in FHT and suggests candidate genes for linkage studies in FHT. They include the ileal lipid binding protein gene (ILBP) on chromosome 5 (which encodes in humans a 128 amino acid protein), a member of the fatty acid binding protein family and a candidate for transcellular transport of bile acids from the apical to the basolateral membranes of the enterocyte [78]. The ileal sodium bile acid cotransporter gene (ISBT) is another candidate. It encodes a 348 amino acid glycoprotein which is a member of a new family of sodium/solute symporters, which binds bile acids at the brush border membrane and is involved in the enterohepatic recirculation of bile salts [79,80]. Finally, consideration should also be given to the multi-drug-resistance-2 (MDR2) gene which plays a role in phospholipid transport into bile, according to gene targeting studies in transgenic mice [81]. Some patients respond to cholestyramine with a marked rise in triglycerides, leading to contraindication of this drug in FHT. This effect has been attributed to an enhanced activity of phosphatidate phosphohydrolase [82], a key enzyme in TG synthesis, apparently sensitive to interruption of the enterohepatic circulation of bile salts. It would be interesting to determine if a gene defect could lead to overexpression of this enzyme.

Familial Hypoalphalipoproteinemia

Many syndromes associated with LDL-deficiency are grouped under familial hypoalphalipoproteinemia. They have been recently reviewed [83,84] and were discussed at this meeting by Prof. G. Assmann. The clinical phenotype varies with the underlying condition responsible for the low plasma HDL levels. Clinical manifestations may include planar xanthomas, arcus corneae or corneal clouding, renal insufficiency, orange tonsils, neuropathy, and hepatosplenomegaly. Severe premature atherosclerosis may be present in some forms whereas the absence of coronary artery disease and even longevity characterizes some of the others (apo AI_{MILANO}). Plasma concentrations of HDL-C and apo AI are below the 5th percentile or absent, and the levels of apo CIII, apo AIV, TG, and apo B are variably affected. Lipoprotein composition may also be altered as a consequence of the metabolic defect, including TG enrichment of HDL. Inherited hypoalphalipoproteinemia may be secondary to mutations in the apo AI-CIII-AIV gene cluster (deletions, inversions, missense and nonsense mutations), apo CII, LPL, and LCAT genes. The genetic defect may be unknown such as in Tangier disease where normal apo AI is produced but is rapidly cleared from plasma [85]. The mode of inheritance is usually codominant. The apparently atherogenic forms include AI-CIII deficiency [86], AI-CIII-AIV deficiency [87], and the apo AI $Gln_{84} \rightarrow Stop$ mutation [88]. The Δ Lys_{107} ($Lys_{107} \rightarrow 0$) mutation (apo $AI_{MARBURG}$ or apo

$AI_{MÜNSTER2}$) has been associated with premature CAD and low LpAI:AII in one Finnish kindred (apo $AI_{HELSINKI}$) [89]. CAD is rarely observed in fish eye disease and LCAT deficiency (consequence of renal failure with secondary hyperlipidemia and hypertension) [90] or Tangier disease [91]. CAD may aggregate in families in which hypoalpha-lipoproteinemia of unknown etiology segregates [84,92].

Genetic Predisposition to Atherogenic Lipoprotein Abnormalities

The inherited atherogenic lipoprotein disorders identified as "diseases" represent only a fraction of the genetic contribution to atherogenic lipoprotein abnormalities. Variation in a gene may confer susceptibility to disease due to environmental factors or by interaction with another gene (epistasis). Susceptibility genes may determine variations in the onset, severity, and progression of diseases due to a major gene defect and may account for the wide variation in its phenotypic expression. Their effects are often pleiotropic (affect more than one system) and are often gender-dependent. Virtually all genes involved in lipid and lipoprotein metabolism can act as susceptibility genes. Prime examples include: apo E, apo(a), LPL, apo AI, enzymes of oxidation, and the gene(s) for the pattern B atherogenic phenotype. These gene-gene interactions are numerous and only a few have been alluded to above. They should be given due consideration in practice as potential determinants of the mildness or severity of an atherogenic lipoprotein defect caused by a major gene. Importantly, they should be considered as part of complex multifactorial interactions which take place in the etiology of atherosclerosis which should encourage physicians to proceed with a global approach in the cardiovascular disease risk assessment of patients.

Conclusion

Genetic defects have been identified for approximately half of the known primary atherogenic lipoprotein disorders. Diagnosis is still primarily based on a clinical/biochemical phenotype which often represents a diversity of genetic defects. Phenotypic expression is context-dependent and modulated by gene-gene and gene-environment interactions which may vary throughout life. Many susceptibility genes are probably involved in determining the onset, severity, and progression of disease and their pleiotropic effects and context-dependency should be given consideration. It is important to remember that response to treatment is also genetically determined.

References

1. Berg K. Gene-environment interaction:Variability gene concept. In: Goldbourt U, de Faire U, Berg K, editors. Genetic factors in coronary heart disease. First ed. Dordrecht: Kluwer Academic Publishers, 1994:373-83.
2. Davignon J, Roy M, Dufour R, Roederer G. Familial hypercholesterolemia. In: Steiner G, Shafrir E, editors. Primary hyperlipoproteinemias. New York: McGraw-Hill Inc., 1991:201-34.

3. Goldstein JL, Hobbs HH, Brown MS. Familial hypercholesterolemia. In: Scriver CR, Beaudet AL, Sly WS, Valle D, editors. The metabolic and molecular bases of inherited disease. Seventh ed. New York: McGraw-Hill Inc., 1995:1981-2030.
4. Davignon J, Lussier-Cacan S, Gattereau A, Moll PP, Sing CF. Interaction of two lipid disorders in a large French-Canadian kindred. Arteriosclerosis 1983;3:13-22.
5. Hobbs HH, Russell DW, Brown MS, Goldstein JL. The LDL receptor locus in familial hypercholesterolemia: Mutational analysis of a membrane protein. Annu Rev Genet 1990;24:133-70.
6. Simard J, Moorjani S, Vohl M-C, et al. Detection of a novel mutation (stop 468) in exon 10 of the low-density lipoprotein receptor gene causing familial hypercholesterolemia among French Canadians. Hum Mol Genet 1994;3:1689-91.
7. Leitersdorf E, Tobin EJ, Davignon J, Hobbs HH. Common low-density lipoprotein receptor mutations in the French-Canadian population. J Clin Invest 1990;85:1014-23.
8. Minnich A, Roy M, Chamberland A, Lavigne J, Davignon J. New methods for rapid detection of low-density lipoprotein receptor and apolipoprotein B gene mutations causing familial hypercholesterolemia. Clin Biochem 1995;28:277-84.
9. Assouline L, Levy E, Feoli-Fonseca JC, Godbout C, Lambert M. Familial hypercholesterolemia: Molecular, biochemical, and clinical characterization of a French-Canadian pediatric population. Pediatrics 1995;96:239-46.
10. Shachter NS, Weinberger J. Mutations of the low-density-lipoprotein receptor gene and familial hypercholesterolemia. Trends Endocrinol Metab 1994;5:245-49.
11. Ma Y, Bétard C, Roy M, Davignon J, Kessling A. Identification of a second "French-Canadian" LDL receptor gene deletion and a rapid method to detect both deletions. Clin Genet 1989;36:219-28.
12. Hobbs HH, Brown MS, Russell DW, Davignon J, Goldstein JL. Deletion in the gene for the low-density lipoprotein receptor in a majority of French Canadians with familial hypercholesterolemia. N Engl J Med 1987;317:734-37.
13. Bétard C, Kessling AM, Roy M, Chamberland A, Lussier-Cacan S, Davignon J. Molecular genetic evidence for a founder effect in familial hypercholesterolemia among French Canadians. Hum Genet 1992;88:529-36.
14. Roy M, Sing CF, Bétard C, Davignon J. Impact of a common mutation of the LDL receptor gene, in French-Canadian patients with familial hypercholesterolemia, on means, variances and correlations among traits of lipid metabolism. Clin Genet 1995;45:59-67.
15. Minnich A, Lussier-Cacan S, Sass C, Roy M, Davignon J. Allele-specific expression of the low density lipoprotein receptor. Circulation 1995;92(I):494[Abstract]
16. Bétard C, Kessling AM, Roy M, Davignon J. Influence of genetic variability in the nondeletion LDL-receptor allele on phenotypic variation in French-Canadian familial hypercholesterolemia heterozygotes sharing a 'null' LDL-receptor gene defect. Atherosclerosis 1996;119:43-55.
17. Moorjani S, Roy M, Torres A, et al. Mutations of low-density-lipoprotein-receptor gene, variation in plasma cholesterol, and expression of coronary heart disease in homozygous familial hypercholesterolaemia. Lancet 1993;341:1303-06.
18. Davignon J, Roy M. Familial hypercholesterolemia in French-Canadians: Taking advantage of the presence of a "founder effect". Am J Cardiol 1993;72:6D-10D.
19. Sass C, Giroux L-M, Ma Y, et al. Evidence for a cholesterol-lowering gene in a French-Canadian kindred with familial hypercholesterolemia. Hum Genet 1995;96: 21-26.
20. Sass C, Giroux L-M, Lussier-Cacan S, Davignon J, Minnich A. Unexpected consequences of deletion of the first two repeats of the ligand-binding domain from the low density lipoprotein

receptor. Evidence from a human mutation. J Biol Chem 1995;270:25166-71.
21. Hobbs HH, Leitersdorf E, Leffert CC, Cryer DR, Brown MS, Goldstein JL. Evidence for a dominant gene that suppresses hypercholesterolemia in a family with defective low density lipoprotein receptors. J Clin Invest 1989;84:656-64.
22. Dallongeville J, Roy M, Leboeuf N, Xhignesse M, Davignon J, Lussier-Cacan S. Apolipoprotein E polymorphism association with lipoprotein profile in endogenous hypertriglyceridemia and familial hypercholesterolemia. Arteriosclerosis 1991;11: 272-78.
23. Ferrières J, Sing CF, Roy M, Davignon J, Lussier-Cacan S. Apolipoprotein E polymorphism and heterozygous familial hypercholesterolemia: Sex-specific effects. Arterioscler Thromb 1994;14:1553-60.
24. Zambon A, Torres A, Bijvoet S, et al. Prevention of raised low-density lipoprotein cholesterol in a patient with familial hypercholesterolaemia and lipoprotein lipase deficiency. Lancet 1993;341:1119-21.
25. Pimstone SN, Gagné SE, Gagné C, et al. Mutations in the gene for lipoprotein lipase - A cause for low HDL cholesterol levels in individuals heterozygous for familial hypercholesterolemia. Arterioscler Thromb Vasc Biol 1995;15:1704-12.
26. Nestruck AC, Bouthillier D, Sing CF, Davignon J. Apolipoprotein E polymorphism and plasma cholesterol response to probucol. Metabolism 1987;36:743-47.
27. Eto M, Sato T, Watanabe K, Iwashima Y, Makino I. Effects of probucol on plasma lipids and lipoproteins in familial hypercholesterolemic patients with and without apolipoprotein E4. Atherosclerosis 1990;84:49-53.
28. Carmena R, Roederer G, Mailloux H, Lussier-Cacan S, Davignon J. The response to lovastatin treatment in patients with heterozygous familial hypercholesterolemia is modulated by apolipoprotein E polymorphism. Metabolism 1993;42:895-901.
29. Ordovas JM, Lopez-Miranda J, Perez-Jimenez F, et al. Effect of apolipoprotein E and A-IV phenotypes on the low density lipoprotein response to HMG CoA reductase inhibitor therapy. Atherosclerosis 1995;113:157-66.
30. O'Malley JP, Illingworth DR. Apolipoprotein ϵ4 and coronary artery disease. Lancet 1992;340:1350
31. Kane JP, Havel RJ. Disorders of the biogenesis and secretion of lipoproteins containing the B apolipoproteins - Familial combined hyperlipidemia. In: Scriver CR, Beaudet AL, Sly WS, Valle D, editors. The metabolic and molecular bases of inherited disease. Seventh ed. New York: McGraw-Hill Inc., 1995:1872-74.
32. Innerarity TL, Mahley RW, Weisgraber KH, et al. Familial defective apolipoprotein B-100: A mutation of apolipoprotein B that causes hypercholesterolemia. J Lipid Res 1990;31:1337-49.
33. Funke H, Rust S, Seedorf U, et al. Homozygosity for familial defective apolipoprotein B-100 (FDB) is associated with lower plasma cholesterol concentrations than homozygosity for familial hypercholesterolemia (FH). Circulation 1992;86(I):I-691.
34. Gallagher JJ, Myant NB. The affinity of low-density lipoproteins and of very-low-density lipoprotein remnants for the low-density lipoprotein receptor in homozygous familial defective apolipoprotein B-100. Atherosclerosis 1995;115:263-72.
35. Gaffney D, Reid JM, Cameron IM, et al. Independent mutations at codon 3500 of the apolipoprotein B gene are associated with hyperlipidemia. Arterioscler Thromb Vasc Biol 1995;15:1025-29.
36. Pullinger CR, Hennessy LK, Chatterton JE, et al. Familial ligand-defective apolipoprotein B. Identification of a new mutation that decreases LDL receptor binding affinity. J Clin Invest

1995;95:1225-34.
37. Mamotte CDS, Van Bockxmeer FM. A robust strategy for screening and confirmation of familial defective apolipoprotein B-100. Clin Chem 1993;39:118-21.
38. Schewe CK, Schuster H, Hailer S, Wolfram G, Keller C, Zöllner N. Identification of defective binding of low density lipoprotein by the U937 proliferation assay in German patients with familial defective apolipoprotein B-100. Eur J Clin Invest 1994;24:36-41.
39. Hansen PS, Meinertz H, Jensen HK, et al. Characteristics of 46 heterozygous carriers and 57 unaffected relatives in five Danish families with familial defective apolipoprotein B-100. Arterioscler Thromb 1994;14:207-13.
40. Myant NB. Familial defective apolipoprotein B-100: A review, including some comparisons with familial hypercholesterolaemia. Atherosclerosis 1993;104:1-18.
41. Kotze MJ, Peeters AV, Langenhoven E, Wauters JG, Van Gaal LF. Phenotypic expression and frequency of familial defective apolipoprotein B-100 in Belgian hypercholesterolemics. Atherosclerosis 1994;111:217-25.
42. Davignon J, Dufour R, Roy M, et al. Phenotypic heterogeneity associated with defective apolipoprotein B-100 and occurrence of the familial hypercholesterolemia phenotype in the absence of an LDL-receptor defect within a Canadian kindred. Eur J Epidemiol 1992;8(1):10-17.
43. Miserez AR, Keller U. Differences in the phenotypic characteristics of subjects with famillial defective apo B-100 and familial hypercholesterolemia. Arterioscler Thromb Vasc Biol 1995;15:1719-29.
44. Stalenhoef AFH, Defesche JC, Kleinveld HA, Demacker PNM, Kastelein JJP. Decreased resistance against in vitro oxidation of LDL from patients with familial defective apolipoprotein B-100. Arterioscler Thromb 1994;14:489-93.
45. Björkhem I, Muri Boberg K. Inborn errors in bile acid biosynthesis and storage of sterols other than cholesterol -Phytosterolemia (sitosterolemia). In: Scriver CR, Beaudet AL, Sly WS, Valle D, editors.The metabolic and molecular bases of inherited disease. Seventh ed. New York: McGraw-Hill Inc., 1995:2088-93.
46. Kwiterovich PO, Jr., Bachorik PS, Smith HH, et al. Hyperapobetalipoproteinaemia in two families with xanthomas and phytosterolaemia. Lancet 1981;1:466-69.
47. Salen G, Tint GS, Shefer S, Shore V, Nguyen L. Increased sitosterol absorption is offset by rapid elimination to prevent accumulation in heterozygotes with sitosterolemia. Arterioscler Thromb 1992;12:563-68.
48. Low LCK, Lin HJ, Lau KS, Kung AWC, Yeung CY. Phytosterolemia and pseudohomozygous type II hypercholesterolemia in two Chinese patients. J Pediatr 1991;118:746-49.
49. Masana L, Joven J, Rubiés-Prat J, Lewis B. Low density lipoprotein metabolism and receptor studies in a patient with pseudohomozygous familial hypercholesterolaemia. Acta Paediatr Scand 1990;79:475-76.
50. Gregg RE, Connor WE, Lin DS, Brewer HB, Jr. Abnormal metabolism of shellfish sterols in a patient with sitosterolemia and xanthomatosis. J Clin Invest 1986; 77:1864-72.
51. Nguyen LB, Shefer S, Salen G, et al. A molecular defect in hepatic cholesterol biosynthesis in sitosterolemia with xanthomatosis. J Clin Invest 1990;86:923-31.
52. Nguyen LB, Salen G, Shefer S, Tint GS, Shore V, Ness GC. Decreased cholesterol biosynthesis in sitosterolemia with xanthomatosis: Diminished mononuclear leukocyte 3-hydroxy-3-methylglutaryl coenzyme A reductase activity and enzyme protein associated with increased low-density lipoprotein receptor function. Metabolism 1990;39:436-43.
53. Lütjohann D, Björkhem I, Beil UF, Von Bergmann K. Sterol absorption and sterol balance in

phytosterolemia evaluated by deuterium-labeled sterols: Effect of sitostanol treatment. J Lipid Res 1995;36:1763-73.
54. Dejager S, Bruckert E, Chapman MJ. Dense low density lipoprotein subspecies with diminished oxidative resistance predominate in combined hyperlipidemia. J Lipid Res 1993;34:295-308.
55. Krauss RM. Heterogeneity of plasma low-density lipoproteins and atherosclerosis risk. Curr Opin Lipidol 1994;5:339-49.
56. Austin MA, Brunzell JD, Fitch WL, Krauss RM. Inheritance of low density lipoprotein subclass patterns in familial combined hyperlipidemia. Arteriosclerosis 1990;10:520-30.
57. Teng B, Forse A, Rodriguez A, Sniderman A. Adipose tissue glyceride synthesis in patients with hyperapobetalipoproteinemia. Can J Physiol Pharmacol 1988;66:239-42.
58. Cianflone KM, Maslowska MH, Sniderman AD. Impaired response of fibroblasts from patients with hyperapobetalipoproteinemia to acylation-stimulating protein. J Clin Invest 1990;85:722-30.
59. Reynisdottir S, Eriksson M, Angelin B, Arner P. Impaired activation of adipocyte lipolysis in familial combined hyperlipidemia. J Clin Invest 1995;95:2161-69.
60. Mahley RW, Rall SC, Jr. Type III hyperlipoproteinemia (dysbetalipoproteinemia): The role of apolipoprotein E in normal and abnormal lipoprotein metabolism. In: Scriver CR, Beaudet AL, Sly WS, Valle D, editors. The metabolic and molecular bases of inherited disease. Seventh ed. New York: McGraw-Hill Inc., 1995:1953-80.
61. Brown BG, Maher VMG. Reversal of coronary heart disease by lipid-lowering therapy - Observations and pathological mechanisms. Circulation 1994;89:2928-33.
62. Ma Y, Ooi TC, Liu M-S, et al. High frequency of mutations in the human lipoprotein lipase gene in pregnancy-induced chylomicronemia: Possible association with apolipoprotein E2 isoform. J Lipid Res 1994;35:1066-75.
63. Haffner SM, Kushwaha RS, Hazzard WR. Metabolism of apolipoprotein B in members of a family with accelerated atherosclerosis: Influence of apolipoprotein E-3/E-2 pattern. Metabolism 1992;41:241-45.
64. Schaefer EJ, Gregg RE, Ghiselli G, et al. Familial apolipoprotein E deficiency. J Clin Invest 1986;78:1206-19.
65. Cladaras C, Hadzopoulou-Cladaras M, Felber BK, Pavlakis G, Zannis VI. The molecular basis of familial apo E deficiency: an acceptor splice site mutation in the third intron of the deficient apo E gene. J Biol Chem 1987;262:2310-15.
66. Lohse P, Brewer HB, III, Meng MS, Skarlatos SI, LaRosa JC, Brewer HB, Jr. Familial apolipoprotein E deficiency and type III hyperlipoproteinemia due to a premature stop codon in the apolipoprotein E gene. J Lipid Res 1992;33:1583-90.
67. Davignon J. Apolipoprotein E polymorphism and atherosclerosis. In: Schwartz CJ, Born GVR, editors. New horizons in coronary heart disease. London: Current Science 1993:5.1-5.21.
68. Davignon J, Dallongeville J, Roederer G, et al. A phenocopy of type III dysbetalipoproteinemia occurring in a candidate family for a putative Apo E receptor defect. Ann Med 1991;23:161-67.
69. Davignon J, Dallongeville J, Fortin LJ, et al. Apolipoprotein E and atherosclerosis: Quest for an Apo E receptor defect leads to the discovery of pseudo type III dyslipoproteinemia in a family. In: Stein O, Eisenberg S, Stein Y, editors. Atherosclerosis IX. Tel Aviv, Israel: R & L Creative Communications Ltd 1992:199-203.
70. Giroux L-M, LaMarre J, Cohn JS, Davignon J. Pseudo type III dyslipoproteinemia is not

associated with an identifiable lipoprotein receptor defect. Atherosclerosis 1994;109:133-34 [Abstract].

71. Goldstein JL, Schrott HG, Hazzard WR, et al. Hyperlipidemia in coronary heart disease. II. Genetic analysis of lipid levels in 176 families and delineation of a new inherited disorder, combined hyperlipidemia. J Clin Invest 1973;52:1544-68.
72. Austin MA. Plasma triglyceride and coronary heart disease. Arteriosclerosis 1991;11:2-14.
73. Heliö T, Palotie A, Sane T, Tikkanen MJ, Kontula K. No evidence for linkage between familial hypertriglyceridemia and apolipoprotein B, apolipoprotein C-III or lipoprotein lipase genes. Hum Genet 1994;94:271-78.
74. Staels B, Vu-Dac N, Kosykh VA, et al. Fibrates downregulate apolipoprotein C-III expression independent of induction of peroxisomal acyl coenzyme A oxidase. A potential mechanism for the hypolipidemic action of fibrates. J Clin Invest 1995; 95:705-12.
75. Hertz R, Bishara-Shieban J, Bar-Tana J. Mode of action of peroxisome proliferators as hypolipidemic drugs. Suppression of apolipoprotein C-III. J Biol Chem 1995; 270:13470-75.
76. Angelin B, Hershon KS, Brunzell JD. Bile acid metabolism in hereditary forms of hypertriglyceridemia: Evidence for an increased synthesis rate in monogenic familial hypertriglyceridemia. Proc Natl Acad Sci USA 1987;84:5434-38.
77. Duane WC. Abnormal bile acid absorption in familial hypertriglyceridemia. J Lipid Res 1995;36:96-107.
78. Oelkers P, Dawson PA. Cloning and chromosomal localization of the human ileal lipid-binding protein. Biochim Biophys Acta Lipids Lipid Metab 1995;1257:199-202.
79. Dawson PA, Oelkers P. Bile acid transporters. Curr Opin Lipidol 1995;6:109-14.
80. Shneider BL, Dawson PA, Christie D, Hardikar W, Wong MH, Suchy FJ. Cloning and molecular characterization of the ontogeny of a rat ilial sodium-dependent bile acid transporter. J Clin Invest 1995;95:745-54.
81. Smit JJM, Schinkel AH, Oude Elferink RPJ, et al. Homozygous disruption of the murine mdr2 p-glycoprotein gene leads to a complete absence of phospholipid from bile and to lliver disease. Cell 1993;75:451-62.
82. Angelin B, Björkhem I, Einarsson K. Influence of bile acids on the soluble phosphatidic acid phosphatase in rat liver. Biochem Biophys Res Commun 1981; 100:606-12.
83. Schonfeld G, Krul ES. Genetic defects in lipoprotein metabolism. In: Goldbourt U, de Faire U, Berg K, editors. Genetic factors in coronary heart disease. First ed. Dordrecht: Kluwer Academic Publishers, 1994:239-66.
84. Breslow JL. Familial disorders of high-density lipoprotein metabolism. In: Scriver CR, Beaudet AL, Sly WS, Valle D, editors. The metabolic and molecular bases of inherited disease. Seventh ed. New York: McGraw-Hill Inc., 1995:2031-52.
85. Assmann G, Von Eckardstein A, Brewer HB, Jr. Familial high density lipoprotein deficiency: Tangier Disease. In: Scriver CR, Beaudet AL, Sly WS, Valle D, editors. The metabolic and molecular bases of inherited disease. Seventh ed. New York: McGraw-Hill Inc., 1995:2053-72.
86. Norum RA, Lakier JB, Goldstein S, et al. Familial deficiency of apolipoproteins A-I and C-III and precocious coronary heart disease. N Engl J Med 1982;306:1513-19.
87. Ordovas JM, Cassidy DK, Civeira F, Bisgaier CL, Schaefer EJ. Familial apoplipoprotein A-I, C-III, and A-IV deficiency and premature atherosclerosis due to deletion of a gene complex on chromosome 11. J Biol Chem 1989;264:16339-42.
88. Matsunaga T, Hiasa Y, Yanagi H, et al. Apolipoprotein A-I deficiency due to a codon 84 nonsense mutation of the apolipoprotein A-I gene. Proc Natl Acad Sci USA 1991;88:2793-97.

89. Tilly-Kiesi M, Qiuping Z, Ehnholm S, et al. ApoA-$I_{Helsinki}$(Lys_{107}-->0) associated with reduced HDL cholesterol and LpA-I:A-II deficiency. Arterioscler Thromb Vasc Biol 1995;15:1294-306.
90. Glomset JA, Assmann G, Norum KR. Lecithin:cholesterol acyltransferase deficiency and fish eye disease. In: Scriver CR, Beaudet AL, Sly WS, Valle D, editors. The metabolic and molecular bases of inherited diseases. Seventh ed. New York: McGraw-Hill Inc., 1995:1933-51.
91. Mautner SL, Sanchez JA, Rader DJ, et al. The heart in Tangier disease: Severe coronary atherosclerosis with near absence of high-density lipoprotein cholesterol. Am J Clin Pathol 1992;98:191-98.
92. Marcil M, Boucher B, Krimbou L, et al. Severe familial HDL deficiency in French-Canadian kindreds: Clinical, biochemical, and molecular characterization. Arterioscler Thromb Vasc Biol 1995;15:1015-24.

REPLACEMENT OF ENDOTHELIAL-BOUND LIPOLYTIC ENZYMES IN LIPASE-DEFICIENT MICE USING RECOMBINANT ADENOVIRUS

Silvia Santamarina-Fojo, Deborah Applebaum-Bowden, Junji Kobayashi, Klaus A. Dugi, and Nobuyo Maeda*
*Molecular Disease Branch, National Heart, Lung and Blood Institute, National Institutes of Health, Bethesda, Maryland 20892 and *The University of North Carolina, School of Medicine, Chapel Hill, North Carolina 37599, USA*

Introduction

Hepatic lipase (HL) and lipoprotein lipase (LPL) are lipolytic enzymes which play a major role in lipoprotein metabolism by hydrolyzing triglycerides and phospholipids present in circulating plasma chylomicrons, very low density lipoproteins (VLDL), intermediate density lipoproteins (IDL), and high density lipoproteins (HDL) [1,2]. As members of the lipase family, both enzymes share a high degree of homology [3]. Thus, both LPL and HL are organized into an amino terminal domain, which confers the catalytic properties of the enzymes [4-6], and a carboxyl terminal domain that may mediate the initial interaction of the lipase with lipoprotein substrates [7-9]. In addition, both enzymes are anchored to the capillary endothelium via glycosaminoglycans and are released into the circulation by intravenous administration of heparin [1,2].

Despite their similarities, LPL and HL exhibit major differences in their structure and function. Thus, HL is synthesized in the liver while LPL is primarily made in adipocytes, smooth muscle cells, and macrophages [10]. Unlike HL, LPL is salt sensitive and requires the presence of apolipoprotein C-II as a cofactor for full activation [11,12]. The two enzymes also differ markedly in their substrate specificities. The preferred substrate for LPL are large triglyceride-rich chylomicrons and VLDL [1] whereas HL functions in the hydrolysis of smaller lipoproteins including IDL and HDL_2 [13-18]. In addition, relative to LPL, HL is the more active phospholipase, a function which may be essential for normal IDL metabolism [1,15,19-21].

Interestingly, there is very little homology between the amino acid sequences of the LPL and HL lids [3,22]. By analogy to pancreatic lipase, the LPL and HL lids appear to cover the catalytic site and may require repositioning to permit access of the lipid substrate to the site of hydrolysis [23,24]. Secondary structural analysis of the LPL and HL lids have identified the presence of two-helical structures which are highly amphipathic [22]. We have recently demonstrated that the lids of LPL and HL are essential for the hydrolysis of

A. M. Gotto, Jr. et al. (eds.), Drugs Affecting Lipid Metabolism, 329–335.

emulsified, long chain fatty acid triglyceride substrate [22]. Our present studies also demonstrate an important role of the lipase lid in mediating the different phospholipase activities of the two enzymes.

Results and Discussion

In order to investigate the role of the lipase lid in mediating the different phospholipase activities between HL and LPL, mutant lipases in which the HL and LPL lids had been exchanged were expressed *in vitro* in human embryonal kidney 293 cells. Figure 1 summarizes the effect of exchanging the HL and LPL lids on the ability of the mutant lipases to hydrolyze triolein, versus phospholipid substrates. Compared to wild-type LPL (Figure 1, construct 1), the mutant LPL lipase containing the HL lid (Figure 1, construct 2) showed a decreased ability to hydrolyze triolein but a marked increase in its phospholipid hydrolyzing properties. Conversely, compared to native HL (Figure 1, construct 3), the mutant enzyme which contained the HL backbone and the LPL lid (Figure 1, construct 4) demonstrated an enhanced ability to hydrolyze triolein but markedly reduced phospholipase activity. These studies demonstrate that exchange of the HL lid with the LPL lid modifies the ability of the lipase, *in vitro*, to hydrolyze phospholipids.

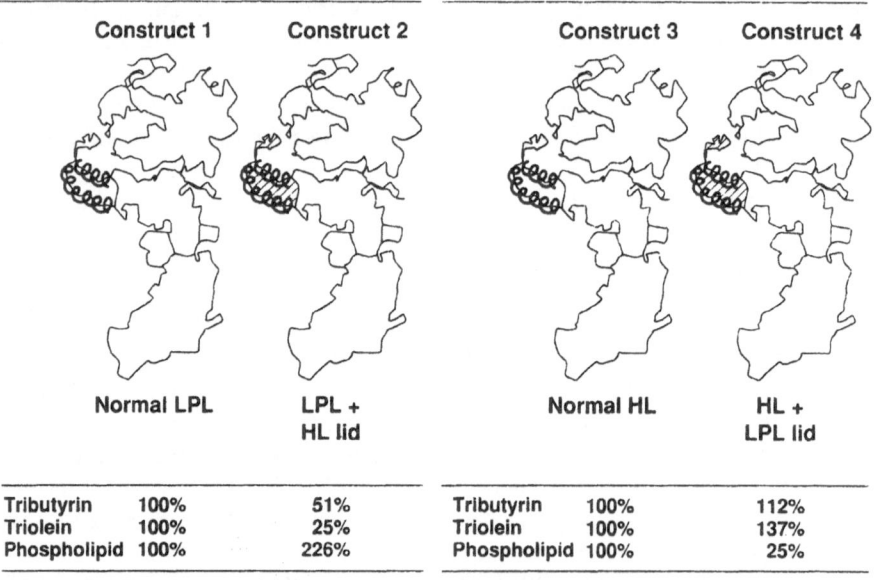

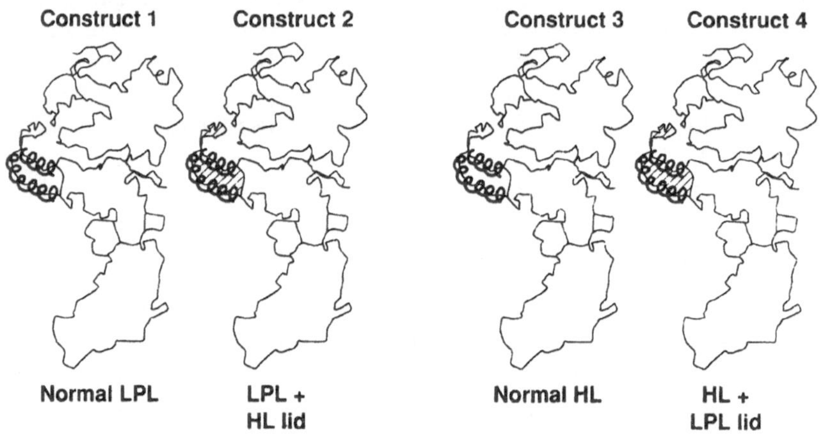

Tributyrin	100%	51%	Tributyrin	100%	112%
Triolein	100%	25%	Triolein	100%	137%
Phospholipid	100%	226%	Phospholipid	100%	25%

Figure 1. Schematic representation of the structure of normal LPL (construct 1) and mutant LPL in which the LPL lid has been replaced with the HL lid (construct 2), as well as native HL (construct 3) and mutant HL in which the HL lid has been replaced by the LPL lid (construct 4). The activity of the mutant lipases using tributyrin [25], triolein [26] and phospholipid [27] substrates is presented as a percent of the respective native lipase activity.

To extend these *in vitro* studies to an *in vivo* system we used recombinant adenovirus to replace normal human HL in HL-deficient mice [28], HL-deficient mice have a deficiency of HL as well as moderately increased plasma concentrations of total-cholesterol, HDL-cholesterol, and phospholipids. Infusion of 1-5 x 10^8 pfu of recombinant adenovirus per animal [29] resulted in significant HL expression (day 5) as assayed in mouse post-heparin plasma (Table 1). Unlike the mouse enzyme, most of the expressed human HL was heparin-releasable (Table 1) indicating successful delivery of the human enzyme to the vascular endothelium.

Table 1. HL activity in pre- and post-heparin plasma of HL-deficient mice after infusion of HlrAdV. Plasma HL activity was determined using triolein substrate [26] in the presence of high salt and absence of apoC-II. Post-heparin human HL activities prior to infusion with HL-rAdV (day 0) as well as pre- and post-heparin plasma HL activity 5 days after virus delivery are shown. For comparison, the pre- and post-heparin plasma HL activities of nonvirus treated control mice with normal mouse HL activity are included. Data is presented as mean ± SEM.

	Day 0	Day 5	
	Post-Heparin	Pre-Heparin	Post-Heparin
		nmoles/min/ml	
HL-rAdV (n = 7)	10 ± 2	918 ± 228	25,700 ± 4,810*
Controls (n = 4)	-	344 ± 36	649 ± 45

*p < 0.001

The results of adenoviral gene transfer of human HL on the plasma lipid profile of HL-deficient mice are summarized in Table 2. Relative to pretreatment values, animals injected with the recombinant adenovirus expressing normal HL had a significant reduction of plasma cholesterol and phospholipids which resulted in normalization of their plasma lipid profile demonstrating successful adenovirus-mediated HL gene replacement. The marked changes in phospholipid levels achieved as late as 15 days after replacement of the human HL gene using recombinant adenovirus confirms the important role of HL as a phospholipase.

Having demonstrated correction of the gene defect in HL-deficient mice [29], studies were initiated to perform *in vivo* analysis of lipase lid function. Thus, recombinant adenovirus vectors expressing the reporter gene luciferase (rLucif-AdV) [30], native human HL (rHL-AdV) [31,32] and LPL (rLPL-AdV) [33] as well as lipase mutants in which the lids of HL and LPL were exchanged as previously described [34], were generated. Systemic infusion of recombinant adenovirus via saphenous vein injection resulted in significant expression of both native and chimeric lipases by day 5 in HL-deficient mice (Table 3).

Table 2. Plasma lipid profile of hepatic lipase-deficient mice after infusion of HlrAdV. Total cholesterol (TC), triglycerides (TG), phospholipids (PL), and cholesteryl ester (CE) concentrations in the plasma of HL-deficient mice before and after HL-rAdV infusion are shown. For comparison, the plasma lipid values in control mice with normal HL activity are included. Data is presented as mean ± SEM.

	TC	TG	PL	CE
			mg/dl	
HL-Def pre-tx (n = 7)	176 ± 9	58 ± 4	314 ± 12	122 ± 8
HL-Def post-tx (n = 5)	94 ± 10*	51 ± 5	207 ± 16*	35 ± 12*
Controls (n = 13)	101 ± 2	63 ± 2	211 ± 4	66 ± 7

*p < 0.01

Table 3. Post-heparin Plasma lipase activity and phospholipid changes in hepatic lipase-deficient mice after infusion of recombinant adenovirus. HL and LPL activities presented as mean ± SEM were measured using triolein substrate [26].

Construct	Activity nmoles/min/ml		PL Reduction %
	Day 0	Day 5	
LPL			
rLPL-AdV (n = 4)	549 ± 209	4,495 ± 534**	32%
rLPL +HL lid AdV (n = 4)	575 ± 120	4,844 ± 1,336*	81%
rLucif-Adv (n = 3)	203 ± 41	217 ± 29	-
HL			
rHL-AdV (n=4)	4 ± 3	9,806 ± 915**	70%
rHL + LPL lid AdV (n=4)	13 ± 5	9,677 ± 2,033*	32%
rLucif-AdV (n=3)	9 ± 2	7 ± 2	-

*p < 0.05; **p < 0.01 paired t-analyses, (compared to day 0). PL = phospholipid.

Adenovirus-mediated expression of all four lipases led to decreases in plasma phospholipids concentrations on day 4 compared to baseline (day 0) values (paired t-test, p < 0.01). However, despite expression of similar post-heparin lipolytic activities on day 5 (9,806 ± 915 and 9,677 ± 2,033 nmoles/min/ml, respectively, Table 3), injection of the recombinant virus expressing native HL (rHL-AdV) resulted in a much more significant reduction in plasma phospholipid concentrations (70% decrease from baseline) than infusion of adenovirus expressing a mutant lipase containing the HL backbone and the LPL lid (rHL + LPL lid-AdV) which reduced baseline phospholipids by only 32% ($p < 0.01$). Similarly (Table 3), injection of adenovirus expressing either native LPL (rLPL-AdV) or a mutant lipase containing the LPL backbone and the HL lid (rLPL + HL lid-AdV) resulted in post-heparin lipolytic activities of 4,495 ± 534 and 4,844 ± 1336 nmoles/min/ml, respectively and phospholipid reduction of 32% versus 81%, respectively ($p < 0.01$). Thus, the simple exchange of the lids between LPL and HL, without other structural modifications, markedly altered the ability of the lipases to hydrolyze phospholipids *in vivo*. These combined studies demonstrate that the presence of the HL lid markedly enhances the ability of native or mutant lipases to hydrolyze phospholipid substrates *in vitro* as well as *in vivo*. Thus, the lipase lid may be a major structural motif which modulates the distinct *in vivo* physiological roles of these two highly homologous lipolytic enzymes in lipoprotein, and especially HDL, metabolism.

Our studies demonstrate, for the first time, successful gene replacement of an endothelial-based lipolytic enzyme using recombinant adenovirus vectors, and establishes the feasibility of performing gene therapy in human lipase deficiency syndromes as well as other genetics disorders of lipid metabolism. The use of recombinant adenovirus vectors to express mutant proteins in animal models for human genetic deficiencies provides a powerful new approach for performing protein structure-function analysis *in vivo*.

References

1. Jackson RL, Boyer PD, editors.The enzymes. Vol XVI. New York:Academic Press, 1983: 141-86.
2. Brunzell JD. Familial lipoprotein lipase deficiency and other causes of the chylomicronemia syndrome. In: Scriver CR, Beaudet AL, Sly WS, Valle D, editors.The metabolic and molecular bases of inherited disease. 7th ed. New York: McGraw-Hill, Inc., 1995:1913-32.
3. Hide WA, Chan L, Li WH. Structure and evolution of the lipase superfamily. J Lipid Res 1992;33:167-78.
4. Davis RC, Stahnke G, Wong H, et al. Hepatic lipase: Site-directed mutagenesis of a serine residue important for catalytic activity. J Biol Chem 1990;265:6291-95.
5. Faustinella F, Smith LC, Semenkovich CF, Chan L. Structural and functional roles of highly conserved serines in human lipoprotein lipase. J Biol Chem. 1991;266:9481-85.
6. Emmerich J, Beg OU, Peterson J, et al. Human lipoprotein lipase. Analysis of the catalytic triad by site-directed mutagenesis of Ser-132, Asp-156, and His-241. J Biol Chem 1992;267: 4161-65.
7. Davis RC, Wong H, Nikazy J, Wang K, Han Q, Schotz MC. Chimeras of hepatic lipase and lipoprotein lipase. Domain localization of enzyme-specific properties. J Biol Chem 1992;267: 21499-504.
8. Dichek HL, Parrott C, Ronan R, Brunzell JD, Brewer HB Jr, Santamarina-Fojo S. Functional characterization of a chimeric protein genetically engineered from human lipoprotein lipase and human hepatic lipase. J Lipid Res 1993;34:1393-401.
9. Wong H, Davis RC, Nikazy J, Seebart KE, Schotz MC. Domain exchange: Characterization of a chimeric lipase of hepatic lipase and lipoprotein lipase. Proc Natl Acad Sci USA 1991;88:

11290-94.
10. Semenkovich CF, Chen SH, Wims M, Luo CC, Li WH, Chan L. Lipoprotein lipase and hepatic lipase mRNA tissue specific expression, developmental regulation, and evolution. J Lipid Res 1989;30:423-31.
11. LaRosa JC, Levy RI, Herbert P, Lux SE, Fredrickson DS. A specific apoprotein activator for lipoprotein lipase. Biochem Biophys Res Commun 1970;41:57-62.
12. Havel RJ, Fielding CJ, Olivecrona T, Shore VG, Fielding PE, Egelrud T. Cofactor activity of protein components of human very low density lipoproteins in the hydrolysis of triglycerides by lipoproteins lipase from different sources. Biochem 1973;12:1828-33.
13. Kuusi T, Kinnunen PK, Nikkila EA. Hepatic endothelial lipase antiserum influences rat plasma low and high density lipoproteins in vivo. FEBS Lett 1979;104:384-88.
14. Jansen H, van Tol A, Hulsmann WC. On the metabolic function of heparin-releasable liver lipase. Biochem Biophys Res Commun 1980;92:53-59.
15. Shirai K, Barnhart RL, Jackson RL. Hydrolysis of human plasma high density lipoprotein 2-phospholipids and triglycerides by hepatic lipase. Biochem Biophys Res Commun 1981;100: 591-99.
16. Nozaki S, Kubo M, Sudo H, Matsuzawa Y, Tarui S. The role of hepatic triglyceride lipase in the metabolism of intermediate-density lipoprotein--postheparin lipolytic activities determined by a sensitive, nonradioisotopic method in hyperlipidemic patients and normals. Metabolism 1986;35:53-58.
17. Auwerx JH, Marzetta CA, Hokanson JE, Brunzell JD. Large buoyant LDL-like particles in hepatic lipase deficiency. Arteriosclerosis 1989;9:319-25.
18. Connelly PW, Maguire GF, Lee M, Little JA. Plasma lipoproteins in familial hepatic lipase deficiency. Arteriosclerosis 1990;10:40-48.
19. Ehnholm C, Shaw W, Greten H, Brown WV. Purification from human plasma of a heparin-released lipase with activity against triglyceride and phospholipids. J Biol Chem 1975;250:6756-61.
20. van Tol A, van Gent T, Jansen H. Degradation of high density lipoprotein by heparin-releasable liver lipase. Biochem Biophys Res Commun 1980;94:101-108.
21. Deckelbaum RJ, Ramakrishnan R, Eisenberg S, Olivecrona T, Bengtsson-Olivecrona G. Triacylglycerol and phospholipid hydrolysis of human plasma lipoproteins: Role of lipoprotein and hepatic lipase. Biochem 1992;31:8544-51.
22. Dugi KA, Dichek HL, Talley GD, Brewer HB, Jr, Santamarina-Fojo S. Human lipoprotein lipase: The loop covering the catalytic site is essential for interaction with lipid substrates. J Biol Chem 1992;267:25086-91.
23. Winkler FK, D'Arcy A, Hunziker W. Structure of human pancreatic lipase. Nature. 1990;343: 771-74.
24. Van Tilbeurgh H, Egloff MP, Martinez C, Rugani N, Verger R, Cambillau C. Interfacial activation of the lipase-procolipase complex by mixed micelles revealed by X-ray crystallography. Nature 1993;362:814-20.
25. Shirai K, Saito Y, Yoshida S. Post-heparin plasma hepatic triacylglycerol lipase-catalyzed tributyrin hydrolysis. Effect of trypsin treatment. Biochem Biophys Acta 1984;795:9-14.
26. Iverius P-H, Brunzell JD. Human adipose tissue lipoprotein lipase: Changes with feeding and relation to postheparin plasma enzyme. Am J Physiol 1985;249:E107-14.
27. Chen CH, Albers JJ. Characterization of proteoliposomes containing apoprotein A-I: A new substrate for the measurement of lecithin: cholesterol acyltransferase activity. J Lipid Res 1982;23:680-91.

28. Homanics GE, DeSilva HV, Osada J, et al. Mild dyslipidemia in mice following targeted inactivation of the hepatic lipase gene. J Biol Chem 1995;270:2974-80.
29. Applebaum-Bowden D, Kobayashi J, Kashyap VS, et al. Hepatic lipase gene therapy in hepatic lipase-deficient mice: Adenovirus-mediated replacement of a lipolytic enzyme to the vascular endothelium. J Clin Invest 1996;97:1-7.
30. de Wet JR, Wood KV, DeLuca M, Helinski DR, Subramani S. Firefly luciferase gene: structure and expression in mammalian cells. Mol Cell Biol 1987;7:725-37.
31. Datta S, Luo C-C, Li W-H, et al. Human hepatic lipase. Cloned cDNA sequence, restriction fragment length polymorphisms, chromosomal localization, and evolutionary relationships with lipoprotein lipase and pancreatic lipase. J Biol Chem 1988;263:1107-10.
32. Stahnke G, Sprengel R, Augustin J, Will H. Human hepatic triglyceride lipase: cDNA cloning, amino acid sequence and expression in a cultured cell line. Differentiation 1987;35:45-52.
33. Wion KL, Kirchgessner TG, Lusis AJ, Schotz MC, Lawn RM. Human lipoprotein lipase complementary DNA sequence. Science 1987;235:1638-41.
34. Dugi KA, Dichek HL, Santamarina-Fojo S. Human hepatic and lipoprotein lipase: The loop covering the catalytic site mediates lipase substrate specificity. J Biol Chem 1995;270:25396-401.

NONVIRAL GENE DELIVERY USING DNA: SYNTHETIC PEPTIDE COMPLEXES

Louis C. Smith[2], Stephen Gottschalk[1], Jochen Hauer[2], Savio L. C. Woo[1,3] and James T. Sparrow[2]
Departments of Cell Biology[1] and Medicine[2], Howard Hughes Medical Institute[3], Baylor College of Medicine, One Baylor Plaza, Houston, Texas 77030, USA

Introduction

Somatic gene therapy is recognized [1] as "a logical and natural progression in the application of fundamental biomedical science to medicin ...[with]...extraordinary potential, in the long-term, for the management and correction of human disease, including inherited and acquired disorders. Significant problems remain in all basic aspects of gene therapy, [including] shortcomings in all current gene transfer vectors and an inadequate understanding of the biological interaction of these vectors with the host." The panel recommends "greater focus on basic aspects of gene transfer and gene expression...[by]...improving vectors for gene delivery, enhancing and maintaining high level expression of genes transferred to somatic cells, achieving tissue-specific and regulated expression of transferred genes, and directing gene transfer to specific cell types."

The mechanisms by which DNA and RNA viruses deliver exogenous genes to cells *in vivo* are being elucidated, as are the biological mechanisms that limit effective gene expression using this route of delivery. The major challenge is to understand humoral and cell-mediated immune responses to viruses. Major efforts in other gene therapy laboratories are directed toward modifying viruses to avoid the host defenses against viruses without compromising the long-term well being of the patient. The complex and redundant antiviral defenses of mammalian systems have stimulated interest in alternative approaches with nonviral DNA delivery vehicles that are either non- or weakly immunogenic. Our long-term goal is to develop synthetic nonviral DNA complexes containing human therapeutic genes.

The effectiveness of a direct gene delivery system *in vivo* depends on (i) the route of administration, (ii) interaction with biofluids, (iii) uptake by a specific cell type, (iv) escape from lysosomal degradation, (v) vectorial transit through the cytoplasm, (vi) transport through the nuclear membrane, (vii) recognition and utilization by nuclear enzymes and transcription factors for expression, and, when desired, (viii) persistence in an episomal form or by integration into genomic DNA for long-term expression [2].

The ideal nonviral DNA delivery system should have the following properties:

A. M. Gotto, Jr. et al. (eds.), Drugs Affecting Lipid Metabolism, 337–345.

(i) The composition and structure is known;
(ii) The stability of the delivery system in biofluids is controlled by the composition of the complex;
(iii) Cellular uptake is controlled by cell specific plasma membrane receptors;
(iv) There is rapid, pH dependent release from the endosome;
(v) There is efficient uncoating and transport of the DNA through the cytoplasm;
(vi) There is efficient nuclear uptake of the DNA; and
(vii) Persistent expression can be achieved, if desired.

This sequence is illustrated in Figure 1.

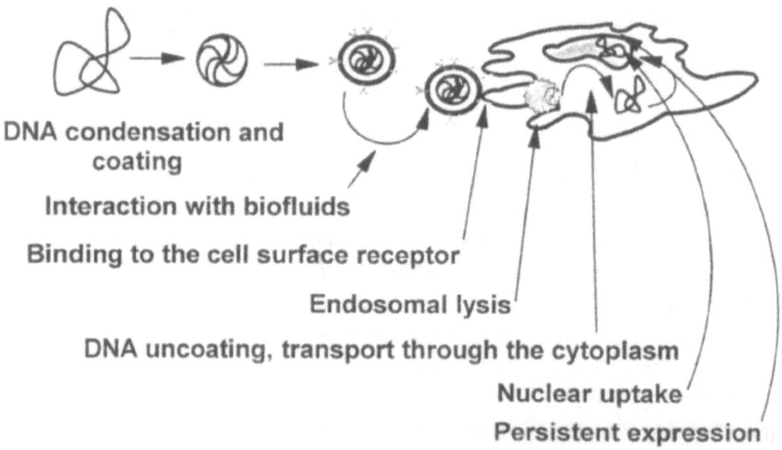

Figure 1. The sequence of processes required for gene expression using nonviral DNA delivery systems.

Cationic DNA delivery systems, naked DNA, and DNA: poly-L-lysine conjugated with asialoglycoprotein give detectable but extremely low expression *in vivo* [3-6]. Since the mechanisms and routes of nonviral DNA uptake and expression are poorly understood, either *in vitro* or *in vivo*, it is impossible to identify what leads to poor expression using these gene delivery systems since only the final step is measured.

Our rationale of the design of a nonviral DNA delivery system is based on the fact that active sites of enzymes, receptors, and antibodies involve about 5-20 amino acids. Thus, it should be possible to use small synthetic peptides to emulate the active site regions of viral proteins and construct synthetic DNA complexes that are as efficient as viruses, but without their limitations. These peptides should be either weakly or nonimmuogenic [2]. Our strategy for improving delivery systems has been to define the parameters for the individual processes with measurements appropriate for that process. When each step is understood mechanistically it can be optimized and thereby the overall process of gene delivery with nonviral DNA delivery system can be optimized systematically. With this information from biophysical and cell culture studies, it is more likely that experiments with rigorously defined DNA delivery systems in the unique *in vivo* environments can be interpreted.

Our objective is to create a biochemically homogeneous DNA delivery vehicle with reproducible stability, and then to define the mechanism of cellular compositional uptake and intracellular transport of the DNA to the nucleus *in vitro* and *in vivo*. Our model for the first generation peptide based DNA delivery system is shown in Figure 2. Our premise is that cell-specific, high level expression of exogenous genes *in vivo* can be achieved by receptor-mediated delivery of synthetic DNA complexes. We now have efficient gene delivery *in vitro* by both receptor and nonreceptor-mediated uptake.

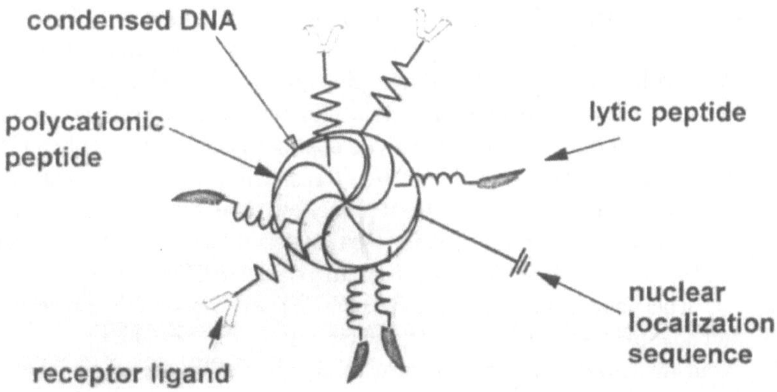

Figure 2. Schematic representation of a DNA delivery system based on synthetic peptides. The DNA is usually an expression vector between 6 to 30 kb. The peptides contain polycationic, lytic and nuclear localization sequences of 12 to 50 amino acids. The receptor ligand can be a peptide or a carbohydrate.

The principal limitation of existing approaches is the inability to prepare reproducible proteinaceous DNA complexes in a consistent manner for gene delivery [7,8]. The covalent coupling of polylysine or ligands with proteins is nonspecific and gives a random mixture of conjugates. The actual site of ligation is unknown. Commercially available poly-L-lysine used for direct DNA delivery is heterogeneous [9]. The poly-L-lysine sample, separated by capillary electrophoresis, contained more than 30 molecular species. Moreover, because the conformation of positively charged surfaces is formed by chance, binding of DNA to the charged template is also variable. High molecular weight and variable stoichiometry of the components in the complex has made it difficult to prepare the complexes either consistently well or in sufficient quantity for *in vivo* delivery [8]. The complexity of the mixtures precludes a molecular definition of the biologically active reagent and accounts for the meager *in vivo* results

To improve gene expression *in vitro*, a replication-defective adenovirus has been used [10-13]. One effect of adenovirus is to lyse the endosome before the contents can be either routed to the lysosomes or recycled to the cell surface. When present either as free virus or as a component of the DNA complex, the transfection rate *in vitro* was increased to 100%. The size of the clathrin-coated pit also constrains uptake of conjugates of adenovirus and a DNA complex, probably a limit of one virus in a DNA complex [13].

An alternative approach to achieve endosome rupture is to induce lysis by specific peptide sequences in viral coat proteins [14,15]. After binding to sialic acid-containing receptors on the plasma membrane, influenza virus is taken up into its host cell by receptor-mediated endocytosis [16]. The low pH of the endosomal compartment activates influenza virus hemagglutinin (HA), which produces fusion of viral and endosomal membranes and release of the viral nucleocapsid into the cytoplasm. The fusion activity of HA occurs only at pH 5-6. At 37° C, fusion half-times are generally < 30 seconds, and fusion is usually complete within 2 to 5 minutes. Short synthetic peptides from HA_2 subunit of influenza HA have been studied extensively with artificial lipid membranes [17]. Although the rates are slower, peptides with amino acid substitutions give both fusion and leakage of liposomal contents, similar to whole hemagglutinin molecules with the corresponding sequence changes. More than 100 different fusiogenic/lytic peptides have been described [18].

Complexes containing plasmid DNA, transferrin-polylysine conjugates, and polylysine-conjugated peptides derived from the N-terminal sequence of the influenza hemagglutinin subunit HA_2 have been used for the transfer of luciferase or β-galactosidase marker genes [14,15]. In HeLa cells, expression of β-galactosidase occurred in about 5-10% of all cells. This value is low compared to controls performed in the presence of free or DNA-bound adenoviruses, which give transfection frequencies > 90%.

To avoid these problems associated with complex mixtures of proteins, poly-L-lysine, and viruses, we have designed and synthesized [19] two peptides which emulate viral functions--a DNA condensing agent, $YKAK_8WK$, and an amphipathic, pH-dependent endosomal releasing agent, GLFEALLELLESLWELLLEA, JTS-1, shown in Figure 3. The hydrophobic face contains only strongly apolar amino acids, while the hydrophilic face is dominated by negatively charged glutamic acid residues at physiological pH values.

The active gene delivery complex was constructed stepwise through a spontaneous self assembly process involving oppositely charged, electrostatic interactions [20]. To assemble DNA/peptide complexes with different overall net charges, only the negative charges of DNA phosphate, the positive charges of the 10 ϵ-amino groups of $YKAK_8WK$ and the negative charges of the 5 γ-carboxyl groups of GLFEALLELLESLWELLLEA were considered. In the first step, negatively charged DNA was rapidly mixed with excess of $YKAK_8WK$ to form positively charged DNA/$YKAK_8WK$ complexes, which gave very little gene transfer. In the second step and to form the active complex, the cationic DNA complex was rapidly mixed with negatively charged GLFEALLELLESLWELLLEA which spontaneously incorporated through electrostatic interactions. JTS-1 enhances transduction with synthetic DNA complexes about 6300 fold in HepG2 cells. Transfection using these complexes of CMV-luciferase, $YKAK_8WK$, and GLFEALLELLESLWELLLEA gave high levels of gene expression in more than 20 cell lines.

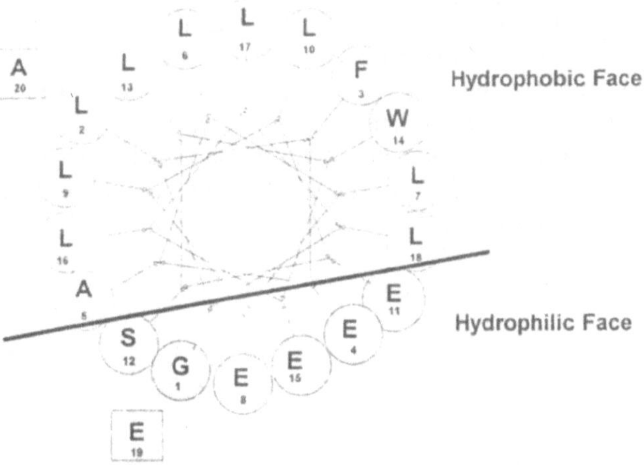

Figure 3. A synthetic lytic peptide, JTS-1, represented as a helical wheel. The hydrophilic amino acids are shaded circles, while the hydrophobic amino acids are open circles.

Ding et al. has described the use of the malaria circumsporozoite (CS) protein as a specific ligand for gene targeting to hepatocytes and other cell lines in culture [21]. The CS protein covers the entire surface of sporozoites of malaria parasites and *in vivo* binds specifically to the basolateral surface of hepatocytes within minutes. To provide proof of principle for the use of a bifunctional peptide, we chose to synthesize a 35 amino acid peptide from region II+, an evolutionarily conserved amino acid sequence conferring the binding of CS protein to its receptor, linked with a glycyl-seryl spacer as an amino terminal extension of $YKAK_8WK$ (Figure 4). Expression was quantified with a chemiluminescence assay of β-galactosidase activity. This composite peptide was about 8-fold more effective than K8 in transduction of Hep1a. The relative light units for DNA alone were 287, for DNA:K8:JTS-1 (1:3:2 charge ratio) 3,640,000, and for DNA: CS-35-K8:JTS-1 (1:3:2 charge ratio) 27,750,000.

Early studies found that random linear homopolymers of amino acids were rarely antigenic [22]. McDevitt and Benacerraf note that the antigenicity of these polypeptides has been evaluated in animals after repeated immunizations with complete Freund's adjuvant [23]. The immunogenicity of the polypeptides depends primarily upon the degree of their complexity. Nonantigenic homopolymers are excellent carriers for haptens, if the polypeptide is long enough. For example, studies of ε-N-DNP-poly-L-lysine in responder and nonresponder guinea pigs show that α-N-DNP-hexalysine and lower polymers are not immunogenic and are not able to elicit delayed hypersensitivity reactions in animals immunized with the higher polymers [24]. Except in guinea pig strains that possess the poly-L-lysine response gene [25,26] several groups have been unable to elicit antibody formation with either poly-L-lysine or poly-L-glutamic acid [27-30], although aggregates containing both poly-L-lysine and poly-L-glutamic acid are immunogenic in rabbits [31]. The ionic aggregates are about 10% as active as the linear polypeptide containing 60% glutamic acid and 40% lysine. The majority of the antibodies elicited by the aggregate are directed against poly-L-lysine. By contrast, the $glu_{60}lys_{40}$ copolymer does not give an immune response in humans [32] or in mice [33]. The existing literature suggests that the immune response to synthetic DNA delivery systems will be species specific and is likely to give a minimal, if any, response when the DNA-poly-L-lysine is injected intravenously or into the portal vein, particularly if the complex is formed with hexalysine derivatives.

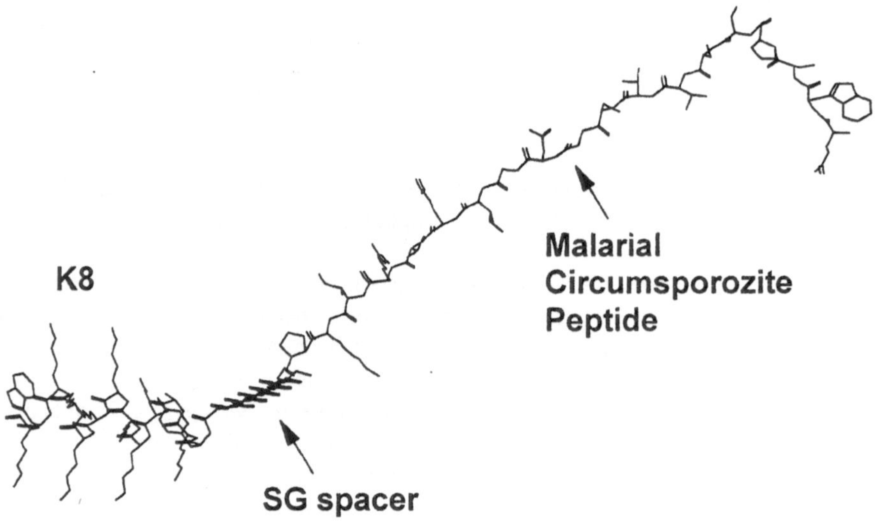

Figure 4. Molecular model of the hepatocyte ligand. The 35 amino acid Circumsporozite ligand domain is linked through a seryl-glycyl spacer to the DNA condensing peptide, K8.

We conducted a series of experiments to determine whether or not our peptid- based DNA complexes produce a significant immune response, i.e. one sufficiently strongly to preclude the repetitive use of the peptides for gene delivery. Two conditions were compared. The first protocol used Freund's adjuvant intraperitoneally, which usually gives a strong immune response. In the second protocol, the DNA: peptide complex was injected subcutaneously, similar to the procedure used for gene therapy. The reagents were JTS-1-GGGC-BSA conjugate, K8-GSGSGSGSGSC-BSA conjugate, DNA:K8:JTS-1 (1:4:1 charge ratio of phosphate, amino, and carboxyl groups), JTS-1-GGGC-SS-CGGG-JTS-1 aggregate and Freund's adjuvant for the standard immunization protocol. The reagents were K8, JTS-1, DNA, JTS-1-GGGC-BSA conjugate, K8-GSGSGSGSGSC-BSA conjugate, and DNA:K8:JTS-1 (1:4:1 charge ratio) in 250 mM sucrose for the gene therapy protocol. The ELISA reagents were JTS-1-GGGC-ovalbumin conjugate, K8-GSGSGSGSGSC-ovalbumin conjugate, DNA:K8:JTS-1 (1:4:1 charge ratio), K8, JTS-1 and DNA. The test animals for each antigen were 4 Balb/c female mice, 5-7 weeks old. After priming, samples were collected at 13, 28, 42, 56, and 90 days, with boosts at 21 and 50 days. $YKAK_8WK$, alone, in a complex, or conjugated, does not give a detectable antigenic response, with or without adjuvant. A weak response was seen for JTS-1, about a 1,000 times weaker than the titer (10^6) for bovine serum albumin to which it was conjugated, but only when coadministered with Freund's adjuvant. Consistent responses were seen with the JTS-1-GGGC-BSA conjugate and JTS-1-GGGC-SS-CGGG-JTS-1 aggregate. With DNA:K8:JTS-1 and only with Freund's adjuvant, just 2 of 4 animals gave a detectable immune response to JTS-1. Data are shown in Figure 5 for the highest responder. There were no observable effects, either acute or long term, on the health of the animals.

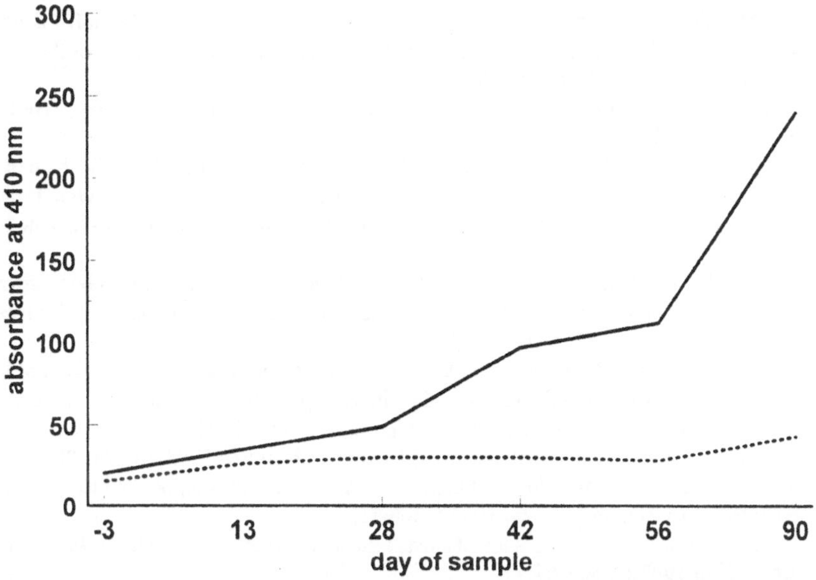

Figure 5. Weak immune response to DNA: peptide complex in mice. The dashed line is the immune response to JTS-1 in mice immunized with the DNA complexes without adjuvant; while the solid line is the immune response to JTS-1 in mice immunized with the DNA complexes and adjuvant.

In summary, these simple DNA complexes, which contain only 3 molecularly defined components, have general utility for gene delivery and can replace viral vectors and cationic lipids for some applications in gene therapy [19]. We conclude there is little immune response to these DNA formulations and that the observed response is not sufficient to preclude their repetitive use in gene delivery *in vivo*. Clearly, these DNA: peptide delivery systems are at an early stage of characterization. The conceptual approach has been validated, and only technical obstacles remain before the overall objective of nonviral peptide based DNA delivery systems can be achieved.

Acknowledgements

The work was supported in part by Cystic Fibrosis Foundation Z995, HL-50422, HL-51754 and contracts from GeneMedicine, Inc. (JTS, LCS). Stephen Gottschalk was a recipient of a Deutsche Forschungsgemeinschaft training fellowship. Savio L.C. Woo is an Investigator of the Howard Hughes Medical Institute.

References

1. Orkin SH, Motulsky AG. Report and recommendations of the panel to assess the NIH investment in research on gene therapy, December 7, 1995. http://www.nih.gov/news/panelrep.html.
2. Eck SL, Wilson JM. Gene-based therapy. In: Hardman JG, Limbird LE, Molinoff PB, Ruddon RW, Gilman AG, editors. Goodman & Gilman's the pharmacological basis of therapeutics. 9th edition. McGraw-Hill: New York, 1995:77-95.
3. Wu GY, Wu CH. Receptor-mediated gene delivery and expression *in vivo*. J Biol Chem 1988;263:14621-24.
4. Chowdhury NR, Wu CH, Wu GY, Yerneni PC, Bommineni VR, Chowdhury JR. Fate of DNA targeted to the liver by asialoglycoprotein receptor-mediated endocytosis in vivo. Prolonged persistence in cytoplasmic vesicles after partial hepatectomy. J Biol Chem 1993;268:11265-71.
5. Ferkol T, Lindberg GL, Chen J, et al. Regulation of the phosphoenolpyruvate carboxykinase/human factor IX gene introduced into the livers of adult rats by receptor-mediated gene transfer. FASEB J 1993;7:1081-91.
6. Stankovics J, Crane AM, Andrews E, Wu CH, Wu GY, Ledley FD. Overexpression of human methylmalonyl CoA mutase in mice after in vivo gene transfer with asialoglycoprotein/polylysine/DNA complexes. Human Gene Therapy 1994;5:1095-104.
7. Behr J-P. Synthetic gene transfer vectors. Accounts Chem Res 1993;26:274-78.
8. McKee TD, DeRome ME, Wu GY, Findeis MA. Preparation of asialoorosomucoid-polylysine conjugates. Bioconjugate Chem 1994;5:306-11.
9. Dolník V, Novotny MV. Separation of amino acid homopolymers by capillary electrophoresis. Anal Chem 1993;65:563-67.
10. Curiel DT, Agarwal S, Wagner E, Cotten M. Adenovirus enhancement of transferrin polylysine mediated gene delivery. Proc Natl Acad Sci USA 1991;88:8850-54.
11. Cotten M, Wagner E, Zatloukal K, Phillips S, Curiel DT, Birnsteil ML. High-efficiency receptor-mediated delivery of small and large (48 kilobase) gene constructs using the endosome-disruption activity of defective or chemically inactivated adenovirus particles. Proc Natl Acad Sci USA 1992;89:6094-98.
12. Cristiano R, Smith LC, Woo SLC. Hepatic Gene Therapy: Receptor-mediated gene delivery and elevated expression in primary hepatoctyes. Proc Natl Acad Sci USA 1993;90:2122-27.
13. Cristiano RJ, Smith LC, Kay MA, Brinkley B, Woo SLC. Hepatic gene therapy: Efficient gene delivery and expression in primary hepatocytes utilizing a conjugated adenovirus/DNA complex. Proc Natl Acad Sci USA 1993;90:11548-52.
14. Wagner E, Plank C, Zatloukal K, Cotten M, Birnstiel ML. Influenza virus hemagglutinin HA-2 N-terminal fusogenic peptides augment gene transfer by transferrin-polylysine-DNA complexes: Toward a synthetic virus-like gene-transfer vehicle. Proc Natl Acad Sci USA

1992;89:7934-38.
15. Plank C, Oberhauser B, Mechtler K, Koch C, Wagner E. The influence of endosome-disruptive peptides on gene transfer using synthetic virus-like gene transfer systems. J Biol Chem 1994;269:12918-24.
16. White JM. Membrane fusion. Science 1992;258:917-24.
17. Wharton SA, Martin SR, Ruigrok RWH, Skehel JJ, Wiley DC. Membrane fusion by peptide analogues of influenza virus haemagglutinin. J Gen Virol 1988;69:1847-57.
18. Ojcius DM, Young JDE. Cytolytic pore-forming proteins and peptides: A common structural motif? Trends in Biochem Sci 1991;16:225-29.
19. Gottschalk S, Sparrow JT, Hauer J, Leland FE, Mims MP, Woo SLC, Smith LC. A novel DNA/peptide complex for efficient gene transfer and expression in mammalian cells. Gene Therapy 1996; in press.
20. Kabanov AV, Kabanov VA. DNA complexes with polycations for the delivery of genetic material into cells. Bioconjugate Chem 1995;6:7-20.
21. Ding ZM, Cristiano RJ, Wroth JA, Tacks B, Kuo MT. Malarial circumsporozoite protein is a novel gene delivery vehicle to primary hepatocyte cultures and cultured cells. J Biol Chem 1995;270:3667-76.
22. Sela M. Immunological studies with synthetic polypeptides. Adv Immunol 1966;5: 29-129.
23. McDevitt HO, Benacerraf B. Genetic control of specific immune responses. Adv Immunol 1963;11:31-74.
24. Schlossman SF, Yaron A, Ben-Efraim S, Sober HA. Immunogenicity of a series of α,N-DNP-L-lysines. Biochemistry 1965;4:1638-45.
25. Kantor FS, Ojeda A, Benacerraf B. Studies on artificial antigens. I. Antigenicity of DNP-polylysine and DNP copolymer of lysine and glutamic acid in guinea pigs. J Exper Med 1963; 117:55.
26. Green I, Paul WE, Benacerraf B. The behavior of hapten-poly-L-lysine conjugates as complete antigens in genetic responder and as haptens in non-responder guinea pigs. J Exper Med 1966; 123:859-79.
27. Stahmann MA, Tsuyuki H, Weinke K, Lapresle C, Grabar P. L'antigénicitié des polypeptides synthéques. C R Soc Biol, Paris 1955;241:1928-29.
28. Maurer PH. Attempts to produce antibodies to a preparation of polyglutamic acid. Proc Soc Exptl Biol Med 1957;96:394.
29. Buchanan-Davidson DJ, Stahmann MA, Lapresle C, Grabar P. Immunochemistry of synthetic polypeptides and polypeptidyl proteins. III. Antigenicity of the synthetic polypeptides. J Immunol 1959;83:552.
30. Gill TJ III, Doty P. Studies on synthetic polypeptide antigens. II. The immunochemical properties of a group of linear synthetic polypeptides. J Biol Chem 1961;236:2677-83.
31. Gill TJ III, Doty P. Studies on synthetic polypeptide antigens. VII. The immunogenicity of an aggregate of poly-L-glutamic acid and poly-L-lysine. Biochem Biophys Acta 1962;60:450-51.
32. Mauer PH. Antigenicity of polypeptides (poly-α-amino acids). II. J Immunol 1962; 88:330-38.
33. Pinchuck P, Maurer PH. Antigenicity of polypeptides (poly-alpha-amino acids). XXVI. Studies of the ability of homo- and copolymers to act as hapten carriers in mice. J Immunol 1968;100:384-94.

RECOMBINANT APOLIPOPROTEIN A-I_{Milano} FOR THE TREATMENT OF VASCULAR DISEASE

Guido Franceschini, Laura Calabresi, Hans Ageland*, Franco Bernini, Maurizio Soma, and Cesare R. Sirtori
*Center E. Grossi Paoletti and Institute of Pharmacological Sciences, University of Milan, Milan, Italy, and *Pharmacia Therapeutics, Stockholm, Sweden*

Introduction

High density lipoproteins (HDL) play a major role in the so-called reverse cholesterol transport [1], the process by which excess cholesterol in peripheral tissues, including the arterial wall, is transported to the liver for elimination from the body. This major function of HDL is believed to explain the strong inverse correlation between plasma HDL levels and coronary heart disease found in many prospective and case-control studies [2]. Apolipoprotein A-I (apoA-I), the primary protein component of HDL, seems to be the major entity responsible for the antiatherogenic activity of HDL. Indeed, apoA-I participates in reverse cholesterol transport, being a cofactor in LCAT activation [3] and a ligand for the putative HDL receptor [4], and stimulating cholesterol efflux from lipid-loaded cells [5]. In addition, apoA-I displays peculiar properties not directly related to its major activities in lipoprotein metabolism but possibly involved in HDL protection against vascular disease, i.e. prostacyclin stabilization [6], activation of fibrinolysis [7], and modulation of complement function [8].

The growing number of contributions showing the dramatic effectiveness of infusions of HDL fractions or of extractive apoA-I on atheromatous lesions have certainly strengthened the working hypothesis that increasing HDL/apoA-I levels may provide a beneficial effect on atheroma formation and possibly induce a regression. Studies have ranged from repeated injections of homologous lipoproteins of d >1.125 g/ml (HDL-VHDL) in cholesterol-fed rabbits, to the infusion of isolated human apoA-I in these same animals. Infusions of homologous HDL-VHDL can both prevent atheroma formation and also induce regression of established lesions [9,10], with human apoA-I being as effective as rabbit HDL on plaque removal in cholesterol-fed rabbits [11]. These animal studies provide a very useful background to therapeutic approaches to atherosclerosis involving extractive or recombinant apoA-I. In a first clinical study, synthetic HDL containing recombinant proapoA-I has been injected into four patients with primary hypoalphalipoproteinemia [12]. HDL-cholesterol levels rapidly increased and stayed elevated for at least 3 days after injection. The shortcut

A. M. Gotto, Jr. et al. (eds.), Drugs Affecting Lipid Metabolism, 347–354.

to the development of a recombinant protein for therapeutic use, i.e. by reducing preclinical testing, might likely accelerate the development of other recombinant apolipoproteins, e.g. apoE [13] and the apoA-I_{Milano} mutant.

ApoA-I_{Milano}: Background

The apoA-I_{Milano} (A-I_M) is the first described mutant of human apolipoproteins [14]. The original clinical observation dates back 20 years, to the clinical evaluation of a 43-year-old man who presented with a severe hyperlipoproteinemia. Further analysis of his plasma lipid profile disclosed a remarkably low HDL-cholesterol level, ranging from 7 mg/dl to 12-13 mg/dl. Extensive investigations on the original carrier failed to detect any notable abnormalities in the vascular system. A considerable effort into the determination of the molecular defect led to the definition, in 1980, of a mayor change in the amino acid composition of apoA-I, i.e. the presence of a cysteine residue in the mutant apolipoprotein [14]. This leads to the formation of disulfide-linked dimers with itself or with apoA-II.

With definition of the molecular origin of the abnormality, interest rose to the mode of genetic transmission and the possible "beneficial" role of the mutation in maintaining normal cardiovascular health despite dramatic reduction of the putative protective lipoprotein fraction. The mode of genetic transmission of apo A-I_M was established by a population study in Limone sul Garda, a small community on Lake Garda in northern Italy, where the proband was born. A survey of the whole population (about 1,000 citizens), established the presence of 33 carriers (the number has increased to 38 in the past 12 years), all descending from a couple who lived in Limone in the second half of the eighteenth century [15]. Careful analysis of the genealogy tree failed to detect records of sudden deaths among the carriers (with the exception of a 54-years-old hypertensive, heavy smoker, who died around 1950). There was clear evidence, by examining the lifespan of the carriers in the past 2 centuries, of a tendency to relative longevity. Among the 38 apo A-I_M carriers, most are characterized by mild to severe hypertriglyceridemia, HDL-cholesterol levels in the range of 7-25 mg/dl, some with elevation of low density lipoprotein (LDL)-cholesterol. Although a systematic analysis of vascular conditions in these subjects has never been performed, occasional investigations by noninvasive methodologies revealed perfectly patent arteries, which are morphologically normal and free of arterial lipid deposition [15]. The mutation in apoA-I_M thus results in low HDL but no increased risk for cardiovascular disease. This suggests that the apoA-I_M mutant might possess unique structural and functional properties which confer to the carriers a high degree of protection against vascular disease.

The molecular error was recognized as a Cys for Arg substitution at position 173 [16], i.e. in one of the predicted amphipathic helical segments characterizing apoA-I and allowing its interaction with lipids [17]. A series of *in vitro* studies comparing apoA-I_M monomer with wild-type apoA-I indicated that the mutant protein is characterized by enhanced spatial flexibility in solution, resulting in an accelerated interaction with phospholipids and a more rapid release from lipid complexes [18]. This enhanced flexibility is probably consequent to structural alterations induced in apoA-I by the Arg → Cys mutation. When analyzed by circular dichroism, the apoA-I_M monomer displays a 10% less α-helical content, compared to normal apoA-I [18]. ApoA-I in solution is about 50% α-helical, which would accommodate approximately seven helical domains of 18 residues. Arg_{173} is exposed on the surface of the amphipathic helix comprising residues 167 to 184, and is able to form a salt bridge with an oppositely charged residue on an adjacent helix [19]. Based on the homology between apoA-I and apoE, which crystal structure has been recently described [20], we built a model for the spatial organization of lipid-free apoA-I in which the central portion of the molecule forms a four helices bundle, while the N-terminal and C-terminal portions are structured into independent, but interacting domains (Figure 1). We hypothesize that Arg_{173} is actively involved in the interaction between the central helical bundle and the C-terminal domain, and that its substitution with a cysteine in apoA-I_M results in the disruption of this interaction, with a net loss of α-helical structure in the C-terminal domain (Figure 1). Since the C-terminal domain of apoA-I has been recently involved in the initial binding of apoA-I to lipid structures [21] and in the modulation of apolipoprotein catabolism [22], the enhanced structural flexibility in apoA-I_M would explain both the increased affinity for lipids [18] and the accelerated *in vivo* catabolism of monomeric apoA-I_M versus wild-type apoA-I [23].

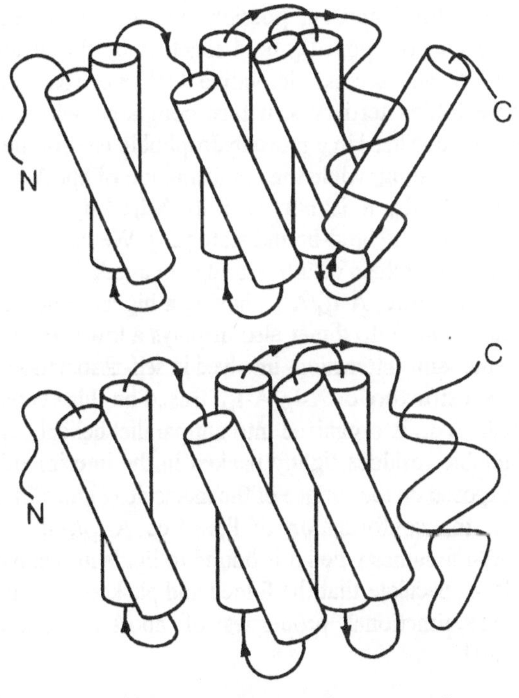

Figure 1. Proposed structure of apoA-I (top) and monomeric apoA-I_M (bottom). For simplicity the amphipathic helical segments are depicted here as straight cylinders.

In contrast, the A-I_M homodimer (A-I_M/A-I_M) is characterized by a tight binding to lipids and a slow turnover *in vivo* (half-life more than double that of apoA-I). These observations prompted the development of A-I_M/A-I_M as a therapeutic tool for the treatment of vascular disease, the apoA-I_M dimer seeming more promising than the monomer for clinical use, in view of the prolonged plasma half-life.

Expression and Characterization of Recombinant A-I_M/A-I_M

A-I_M/A-I_M was expressed in the *E. coli* K12 derivative strain BC 0050, by using an expression vector derived form pTrc99A [24]. The A-I_M cDNA was prepared by site-directed mutagenesis of apoA-I cDNA and placed immediately downstream of an *OmpA* signal sequence, where the second-to-last amino acid was changed from Gln to Asn. Two transcription terminators were placed downstream of the A-I_M gene and the ampicillin resistance marker of pTrc99A was replaced with kanamycin resistance marker. A-I_M/A-I_M is secreted to the growth medium at a concentration of 4-5 g/l. The recombinant product proved to be identical to the plasma-derived protein [24].

In the attempt to characterize the molecular architecture of A-I_M/A-I_M, its secondary and tertiary structures have been analyzed by a variety of spectroscopic techniques. Circular dichroism in the far-UV region revealed that A-I_M/A-I_M has a high content of α-helical structure compared to normal apoA-I, possibly because of protein-protein interaction between the two molecules of apoA-I_M, hold together by the disulfide bridge. Circular dichroism in the near-UV and second derivative UV spectroscopy demonstrated that A-I_M/A-I_M has a more folded tertiary structure compared with wild-type apoA-I, the aromatic residues being immobilized in a more hydrophobic environment in A-I_M/A-I_M than in apoA-I. Even more interesting, while the conformation of apoA-I is drastically affected by the interaction with lipids, it is not so with A-I_M/A-I_M which displays a similar conformation in the lipid-free and lipid-bound state [24]. We concluded from these studies that the introduction of an interchain disulfide bridge in apoA-I markedly alters the protein secondary and tertiary structure, A-I_M/A-I_M having a higher helical structure and a more folded tertiary structure. The A-I_M dimer also displays a lower tendency to self-associate [24], possibly because the same interactions involved in self-association are already effective in maintaining the folded structure of A-I_M/A-I_M. Based on this evidence we built a model in which lipid-free A-I_M/A-I_M is organized into antiparallel helical segments, with the side chains of the hydrophobic residues tightly packed in the interior of the molecule, while charged residues are exposed on the surface of the molecule (Figure 2). As suggested by the spectroscopic studies, the conformation of lipid-free A-I_M/A-I_M is very close to the conformation that apoA-I assumes when it is bound to lipids in reconstituted HDL (Figure 2). It seems reasonable to speculate that the folded and packed structure of A-I_M/A-I_M may significantly affect the functional properties of apoA-I, potentially increasing its antiatherogenic potential.

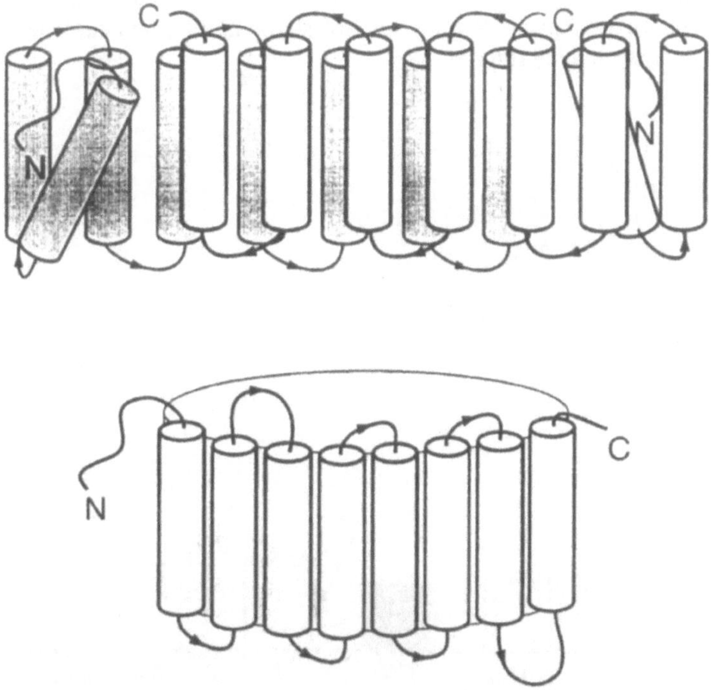

Figure 2. Proposed structure of lipid-free A-I_M/A-I_M (top) and lipid-bound apoA-I in reconstituted discoidal HDL (bottom). For simplicity the amphipathic helical segments are depicted here as straight cylinders.

The Antiatherogenic Properties of A-I_M/A-I_M

The limited availability up until now of a highly purified recombinant A-I_M/A-I_M has somewhat restricted the *in vivo* evaluation of its antiatherogenic properties. However, at least two studies should be mentioned. Treatment with A-I_M/A-I_M-containing synthetic HDL in cholesterol-fed rabbits inhibited by more than 50% neointimal hyperplasia caused by periarterial manipulation [25]. A-I_M/A-I_M was effective in preventing lesion initiation and progression only when treatment was started before lesion induction, and the effect was independent of an effect on plasma cholesterol levels. In a peripheral angioplasty model, treatment with the same synthetic HDL, given five times before and after the surgical procedure, resulted in < 40% stenosis of the operated arteries versus > 80% involvement in control animals [26].

The mechanism responsible for the inhibitory effect of A-I_M/A-I_M on development of intimal lesions remains to be clarified. Two major *in vitro* properties of the recombinant

A-I_M/A-I_M have become clearly apparent, which may contribute to the antiatherogenic effect: a) an enhanced capacity to promote cholesterol efflux from lipid-laden cells, and b) a direct fibrinolytic activity (Figure 3).

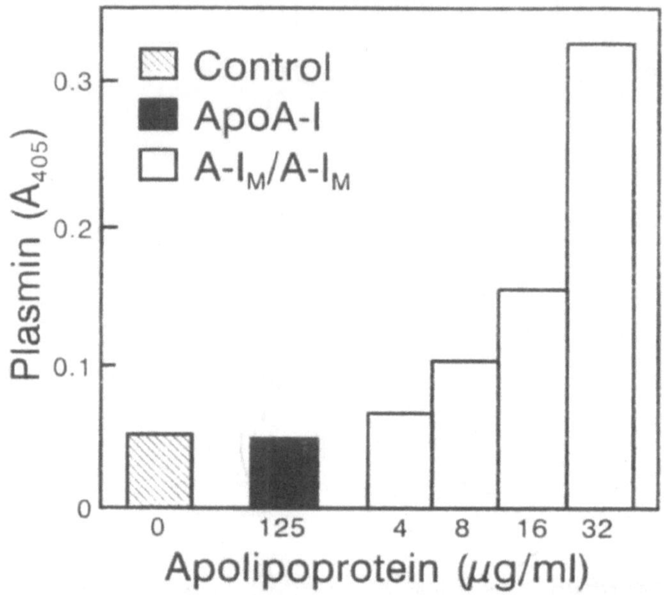

Figure 3. Effect of apoA-I and A-I_M/A-I_M on plasminogen activation. Glu-plasminogen was incubated with apoA-I or A-I_M/A-I_M and plasmin generation monitored with the S-2251 chromogenic substrate (courtesy of Dr. J. Chmielewska).

Since A-I_M/A-I_M was effective in inhibiting intimal thickening only when administered before lesion induction, additional preventive mechanisms on early events in lesion formation can be hypothesized. These would include: a) inhibition of the deposition of the complement membrane attack complex on endothelial cells [8]; b) direct effect on smooth muscle cell proliferation. Indeed, a reduced incorporation of a thymidine analogue into replicating DNA was observed in A-I_M/A-I_M treated rabbits [25].

Conclusions

Studies on the A-I_M mutation and the subsequent development of its potential use in therapy offer an interesting example of how the current rapid progress in recombinant DNA technology allows the direct evaluation of hypotheses raised from clinical observations. The case of recombinant apolipoproteins, in particular of A-I_M/A-I_M, is of special interest, because rapidly emerging clinical technologies permit a direct, noninvasive evaluation of arterial wall conditions [27]. When these techniques achieve world-wide application, the need for direct correction of initial or more advanced arterial lesions will prompt the use of recombinant proteins capable of promoting a rapid regression of atheromatous lesions. These 20 years of studies have, in any case, provided an exciting opportunity for establishing a direct link between a genetic observation, evaluation of the phenotypic expression and translation into a usable therapeutic tool.

References

1. Glomset JA. The plasma lecithin: Cholesterol acyltransferase reaction. J Lipid Res 1968;9:155-62.
2. Gordon DJ, Rifkind BM. High density lipoprotein: The clinical implications of recent studies. N Engl J Med 1989;321:1311-16.
3. Sorci Thomas M, Kearns MW, Lee JP. Apolipoprotein A-I domains involved in lecithin-cholesterol acyltransferase activation. Structure:function relationships. J Biol Chem 1993;268:21403-409.
4. Allan CM, Fidge NH, Morrison JR, Kanellos J. Monoclonal antibodies to human apolipoprotein AI: Probing the putative receptor binding domain of apolipoprotein AI. Biochem J 1993;290:449-55.
5. Rothblat GH, Mahlberg FH, Johnson WJ, Phillips MC. Apolipoproteins, membrane cholesterol domains, and the regulation of cholesterol efflux. J Lipid Res 1992; 33:1091-97.
6. Aoyama T, Yui Y, Morishita H, Kawai C. Prostaglandin I_2 half-life regulated by high density lipoprotein is decreased in acute myocardial infarction and unstable angina pectoris. Circulation 1990;81:1784-91.
7. Saku K, Ahmad M, Glass-Greenwalt P, Kashyap ML. Activation of fibrinolysis by apolipoproteins of high density lipoproteins in man. Thromb Res 1985;39:1-8.
8. Hamilton KK, Zhao J, Sims PJ. Interaction between apolipoproteins A-I and A-II and the membrane attack complex of complement. Affinity of the apoproteins for polymeric C9. J Biol Chem 1993;268:3632-38.
9. Badimon JJ, Badimon L, Galvez A, Dische R, Fuster V. High density lipoprotein plasma fractions inhibit aortic fatty streaks in cholesterol-fed rabbits. Lab Invest 1989;60:455-62.
10. Badimon JJ, Badimon L, Fuster V. Regression of atherosclerotic lesions by high density lipoprotein plasma fraction in the cholesterol-fed rabbit. J Clin Invest 1990; 85:1234-41.
11. Trachtenberg JD, Cochrane H, Sun S, et al. Apolipoprotein A-I inhibits atherosclerotic lesions progression. Circulation 1993;88:I-552.
12. Carlson LA. Effect of a single infusion of recombinant human proapolipoprotein A-I liposomes (synthetic HDL) on plasma lipoproteins in patients with low high density lipoprotein cholesterol. Nutr Metab Cardiovasc Dis 1995;5:85-91.
13. Yamada N, Inoue I, Kawamura M, et al. Apolipoprotein E prevents the progression of atherosclerosis in Watanabe heritable hyperlipidemic rabbits. J Clin Invest 1992; 89:706-11.
14. Franceschini G, Sirtori CR, Capurso A, Weisgraber KH, Mahley RW. A-I_{Milano} apoprotein. Decreased high density lipoprotein cholesterol levels with significant lipoprotein modifications and without clinical atherosclerosis in an Italian family. J Clin Invest 1980;66:892-900.
15. Gualandri V, Franceschini G, Sirtori CR, et al. A-I_{Milano} apoprotein. Identification of the complete kindred and evidence of a dominant genetic transmission. Am J Hum Genet 1985;37:1083-97.

16. Weisgraber KH, Rall SC, Bertsot TP, Mahley RW, Franceschini G, Sirtori CR. Apolipoprotein AI_{Milano}. Detection of normal AI in affected subjects and evidence for a cysteine for arginine substitution in the variant AI. J Biol Chem 1983;258:2508-13.
17. Segrest JP, Jones MK, De Loof H, Brouillette CG, Venkatachalapathi YV, Anantharamaiah GM. The amphipathic helix in the exchangeable apolipoproteins: a review of secondary structure and function. J Lipid Res 1992;33:141-66.
18. Franceschini G, Vecchio G, Gianfranceschi G, Magani D, Sirtori CR. Apolipoprotein $A\text{-}I_{Milano}$. Accelerated binding and dissociation from lipids of a human apolipoprotein variant. J Biol Chem 1985;260:16321-25.
19. Lins L, Brasseur R, De Pauw M, et al. Helix-helix interactions in reconstituted high-density lipoproteins. Biochim Biophys Acta 1995;1258:10-18.
20. Wilson C, Wardell MR, Weisgraber KH, Mahley RW, Agard DA. Three-dimensional structure of the LDL receptor-binding domain of human apolipoprotein E. Science 1991;252:1817-22.
21. Yi Y, Jonas A. Properties of an N-terminal proteolytic fragment of apolipoprotein AI in solution and in reconstituted high density lipoproteins. J Biol Chem 1995; 270:11290-97.
22. Schmidt HH, Remaley AT, Stonik JA, et al. Carboxyl-terminal domain truncation alters apolipoprotein A-I in vivo catabolism. J Biol Chem 1995;270:5469-75.
23. Roma P, Gregg RE, Meng MS, et al. In vivo metabolism of a mutant form of apolipoprotein A-I, apo $A\text{-}I_{Milano}$, associated with familial hypoalphalipoproteinemia. J Clin Invest 1993;91:1445-52.
24. Calabresi L, Vecchio G, Longhi R, et al. Molecular characterization of native and recombinant apolipoprotein $A\text{-}I_{Milano}$ dimer. The introduction of an interchain disulfide bridge remarkably alters the physicochemical properties of apolipoprotein A-I. J Biol Chem 1994;269:32168-74.
25. Soma MR, Donetti E, Parolini C, Sirtori CR, Fumagalli R, Franceschini G. Recombinant apolipoprotein $A\text{-}I_{Milano}$ dimer inhibits carotid intimal thickening induced by perivascular manipulation rabbits. Circ Res 1995;76:405-10.
26. Ameli S, Hultgardh Nilsson A, Cercek B, et al. Recombinant apolipoprotein $A\text{-}I_{Mileno}$ reduces intimal thickening after balloon injury in hypercholesterolemic rabbits. Circulation 1994;90:1935-41.
27. Pignoli P, Tremoli E, Poli A, Oreste P, Paoletti R. Intimal plus medial thickness of the arterial wall: A direct measurement with ultrasound imaging. Circulation 1986;74:1399-406.

ENVIRONMENT-BY-GENE INTERACTIONS: POLYMORPHISMS AT THE LIPOPROTEIN LIPASE (LPL) LOCUS

Quiping Zhang, Elisabeth Cavallero, Julian Cavanna, Andrea Kay, Aline Charles, Bernard Jacotot, and David J. Galton
Department of Human Metabolism and Genetics, St Bartholomew's Hospital, London EC1A 7BE, United Kingdom and Department of Internal Medicine, Hôpital Mondor, Creteil, France

Introduction

Untreated noninsulin-dependent diabetics have abnormal fasting lipid profiles with elevation of plasma triglycerides greater than 2.8 mmol/l and reduced HDL cholesterol to less than 0.9 mmol/l in more than 25% of cases [1]. Some factors responsible for this may be the increased flow of free fatty acids to the liver that augments hepatic synthesis and secretion of triglyceride (TG)-rich lipoprotein combined with a clearance defect of triglyceride-rich lipoproteins in the periphery by muscle and adipose tissue by impaired action of lipoprotein lipase. However, some noninsulin-dependent diabetics develop a severe lipemia with fasting plasma TG greater than 20 mmol/l suggesting that additional factors are operating.

Recently more than thirty mutations of lipoprotein lipase have been described including large insertions and deletions, frameshift mutations, splicing defects, and nonsense and missense mutations (for review see [2]). In the homozygous state these can impair the activity of the enzyme leading to a Type I chylomicronemia syndrome associated with eruptive xanthomata, episodes of acute pancreatitis, and lipemia rationales [3]. Heterozygotes for these mutations can also show abnormal lipid profiles on aging, or when factors such as obesity, pregnancy, or exposure to oral contraceptives are present. The possibility therefore arises that subjects with severe diabetic lipidemia are carriers for such mutants and the interaction of the metabolic state of diabetes in the presence of mutants of lipoprotein lipase predisposes to the lipemia. We have therefore examined 18 subjects with severe diabetic lipemia (plasma triglycerides ranging from 20 to 80 mmol/l) and have found 7 to possess mutations of lipoprotein lipase. Five of these mutants are previously reported in the literature whereas two are described here for the first time.

A. M. Gotto, Jr. et al. (eds.), Drugs Affecting Lipid Metabolism, 355–359.

Methods and Results

SUBJECTS

Eighteen subjects (Table 1) with known or recently diagnosed type II diabetes and severe hyperlipemia (fasting TG > 1000 mg/dl or 11.4 mmol/L), were referred for admission to the Endocrinology or Lipid Units of the H. Mondor Hospital between March 1993 and February 1994 and were included in this study. There were 15 men (mean age 45.6; range 39-72 years; mean BMI 31 kg/m^2; mean fasting blood glucose 15.2 mmol/l; and mean alcohol intake 191 gm/wk). The three women had a mean age of 43 years; mean BMI of 37 kg/m^2; mean fasting blood glucose 12.5 mmol/l; and mean alcohol intake of 13 gm/wk. Five patients had eruptive xanthomata and six had symptoms of pancreatitis. The other main clinical and metabolic features are outlined in Table 1.

Table 1. Clinical details of patients under study.

	Diabetic		Weight	Height	Plasma TG	Alcohol Intake	Therapy
	Yr	Sex	Kg	Cms	mmol/l		
G	29	M	80	170	24	Occasional	Glibenclamide
C	42	M	93	178	24	Abuse	Insulin pump
H	41	M	111	175	15	None	Diet alone
L	43	M	127	180	75	None	Insulin pump
H	45	M	77	171	40	Occasional	Insulin pump
H	36	M	85	162	13	Occasional	1000 Kcal diet
M	47	M	98	164	23	Abuse	Diet
C	44	M	103	158	19	None	Biguanide
C	60	M	130	180	35	Frequent	Insulin pump
D	74	M	83	173	20	None	Biguanide
A	58	M	88	178	29	Abuse	Biguanide
K	38	M	88	177	62	Abuse	Insulin pump
L	48	M	92	177	95	Abuse	Insulin pump

After 11.7 ± 3.6 (range 8-20) days in hospital 7 additional patients received treatment with fibrates for further improvement of lipid levels (gemfibrozil in 6 and fenofibrate in 1). The different treatments the patients thus received during hospitalization do not allow reliable conclusions about treatment responses.

METHODS

Total cholesterol, triglyceride and HDL-cholesterol (after precipitation of B-containing lipoproteins by phosphotungstic acid and magnesium chloride) were determined with an Abbot Diagnostics VP analyzer using enzymatic reagents (Boehringer Mannheim, Germany). Apolipoproteins A1 and apo-B were measured by immunoturbidometric methods using Daichi kits (Tokyo, Japan).

DNA METHODS

DNA extraction. DNA was prepared from peripheral leucocytes using a Nucleon II kit (Scotlabs Ltd, UK) and resuspended in TE buffer. DNA was quantified by spectrophotometry at 260 mM.

Amplification of LPL gene exons. Oligonucleotide primers were synthesized (IGI Ltd. UK) to allow the amplification of individual exons of the LPL gene. For each exon, flanking intronic DNA (sequence courtesy of K. Oka) was examined for potential PCR primer sites using PRIMER software and primer pairs identified. In each pair, one primer was biotinylated at the 5' end. Typical PCR reaction conditions were as follows: 50 → 100 ng DNA, 50 mM KCl, 10 mM Tris-HCl (pH 8.3), 2.0 mM $MgCl_2$ 0.001% (w/v) gelatin, 200 µM dNTPs, 100 mM each primer and 2 units *Taq* polymerase (Life Sciences, UK) in a 100µl. reaction. Amplification was achieved in a Perkin Elmer Cetus 480 thermal cycler using an initial denaturing step of 94° C for 1 minute and then 35 cycles of 94° C for 30 seconds, 60° C for 1 minute, 72° C for 1 minute, followed by a final elongation step of 72° C for 10 minutes. Small aliquot were removed to test the PCR reactions on 1.5% agarose gels.

Sequencing of PCR products. PCR products were sequenced using the dideoxy chain termination method. The PCR products were treated by one of two methods.

(1) PCR products were incubated with streptavidin-coated magnetic beads (Dynal Ltd. UK). After washing, the bound PCR product was denatured and the biotinylated strand recovered. The bound single stranded product was then sequenced using the Sequenase II kit (Amersham Life Sciences, UK) and the nonbiotinylated primer.

(2) The PCR product was sequenced directly after treatment with Exonuclease I and Shrimp Alkaline Phosphatase (Sequenase PCR product sequencing kit, Amersham Life Sciences, UK).

The reaction products from sequencing reactions were electrophoresed on 6% acrylamide-bisacrylamide (19:1), 7 M urea gels using a glycerol tolerant gel buffer. The gels were prewarmed and samples were electrophoresed at 50 V/cm. Subsequent to electrophoreses, the gels were fixed in 10% acetic acid and vacuum dried. Dry gels were autoradiographed for 18 → 72 hours with Hyperfilm Amersham Life Sciences, UK and the sequence read off the developed autoradiograph.

Results

The mutations in the lipoprotein lipase gene revealed by DNA sequence analysis are shown in Table 2, and eight of the eighteen subjects carried mutants in the heterozygous state. The silent codon mutation at threonine 361 would not be expected to have much functional effects on the activity of lipoprotein lipase but could act as a disease marker. No catalytic triad mutations were found (residues $Asp^{156} \rightarrow His^{214} \rightarrow Ser^{132}$) but exons 3 and 5 (where 2 of the mutations occurred) code for protein domains flanking the catalytic cleft of the enzyme. With regard to the most severely lipemic subjects at presentation (patients 16, 3, and 11, with plasma triglycerides of 79, 76, and 45 mmol/l respectively) no mutations were detected at the LPL locus. Possibly regulatory sequences of the LPL gene or other genetic loci may be involved. The mean plasma TG of the patients carrying the LPL mutants after treatment was 5.0 + 2.3 (n = 8) mmol/l compared to 7.9 + 5.5 (n = 10) mmol/l of the others. The numbers studied are probably too small to draw conclusions with regard to the impact of these mutants on effects of therapy.

Table 2. LPL gene mutations in diabetic lipemic subjects.

Exon/Intron	Nucleotide	$\alpha\alpha$ Residue	Individuals	Publication Information
3	G^{579}-A	Val^{108}- Val GTG⇒ GTA	17, 18	In literature
5	G^{818}-A	Gly^{188} - Glu GGG⇒ GAG	13, 17	In literature
	C^{829}-T	Arg^{192} - Ter CGA⇒ TGA	12	Unpublished
6	A^{1127} - G	Asn^{291} - Ser AAT⇒ AGT	6, 9	In literature
7	C^{1308} - G	Phe^{351} - Leu TTC⇒ TTG	8	Unpublished
8	C^{1338} - A	Thr^{361} - Thr ACE⇒ ACA	9, 14	Unpublished
9	C^{1595} - G	Ser^{447} - Ter TCA⇒ TGA	12, 13	In literature

Discussion

We have identified two new mutants of lipoprotein lipase by DNA analysis of 18 patients with marked diabetic lipemia. One of these in exon 5 terminates the enzyme protein at amino acid 192. This would be expected to abolish catalytic activity of the enzyme since it is known that carboxy terminal truncation at residue 381 reduces catalytic activity by about 85% [4]. The heterozygous state may be unaffected or show a mild lipemia; but when associated with diabetes m, a condition that predisposes to hypertriglyceridemia, a severe lipemia may develop. The other newly described variant ($Phe^{351} \rightarrow$ leu) may affect enzyme function due to steric differences between the 2 amino acids; however, this mutant will need further evaluation since both residues are hydrophobic. It is of interest however that the severity of the lipemia in this case (19 mmol/l at presentation) was similar to the lipemia with the truncated mutant (18.9 mmol/l). The severity of the diabetes at presentation was also similar (fasting blood glucoses of 13 mmol and 19.5 mmol/l, respectively) so this enzyme may be expected to show reduced activity.

Further work is in progress to determine the population frequencies of the newly described mutants ($Arg^{192} \rightarrow$ Ter and $Phe^{351} \rightarrow$ leu) and their effects on the catalytic activity of lipoprotein lipase.

Acknowledgements

This project is supported by Grant PL 931211 of the Commission of the European Communities and the Joint Research Board of St Bartholomew's Hospital.

References

1. Stern MP, Patterson JK, Haffner SM, Hasudu MP, Mitchell BD. Lack of awareness and treatment of hyperlipidaemia in type II diabetes in community surveys. JAMA 1989;56:360-64.
2. Hayden MR. Molecular genetics of human lipoprotein lipase deficiency. In: Bearn AG, editor. Genetics of coronary heart disease. Oslo: Institute of Medical Genetics, University of Oslo Press, 1992:112-15.
3. Galton DJ, Krone W. Hyperlipidaemia in practice. London: Gower Medical Publishing, 1991:27-37.
4. Kozaki K, Gotoda T, Kawamura M, et al. Mutational analysis of human lipoprotein lipase by carboxyterminal truncation. J Lipid Res 1993;34:1765-72.

RESPONSE TO INTERVENTION: APOLIPOPROTEIN E AS A PARADIGM

Eric Boerwinkle*
Human Genetics Center, University of Texas--Houston Health Science Center, PO Box 20334, Houston, Texas 77225, USA

Introduction

It is a developing paradigm in medical practice and biomedical research that both genetic and environmental factors are key contributors to disease etiology and pathophysiology. The age of molecular medicine, so often referred to as a futuristic ideal for which we are ill prepared, is here today. However, consideration of both genetic and environmental components is necessary for predicting those individuals at increased risk for disease and treating those already afflicted. However, simultaneous recognition of both is too often only rhetorical, with research efforts pursuing either genetic factors or environmental factors alone. Human geneticists stress the role of genes and familial factors influencing risk of disease, down-playing the role of environmental and stochastic elements. Epidemiologists and most medical practitioners, on the other hand, describe and manipulate environmental factors contributing to disease, ignoring the role of genetic contributors to disease etiology or response to treatment.

The chronic diseases of later life such as hypertension and coronary artery disease (CAD) are common in all Westernized countries. These diseases are the result of interactions among numerous environmental and genetic factors. Disease liability is not attributable to a single factor such as a solitary foodstuff or a single genetic alteration. As a result, the contribution to disease risk of any single gene or environmental factor is likely to be small when compared to all other risk factors combined. Also, the genes affecting disease risk do not act alone; they are constantly interacting with other genes and with environmental factors. Therefore, the effect of a gene measured in one environment may be very different than its effect in another.

The use of genetic information in predicting susceptibility to the common chronic diseases presents several unique problems and opportunities. Mankind is witnessing spectacular advances in the prevention and understanding of most single-gene disorders. These advances have revolutionized the detection and treatment of many of the rare inborn errors of metabolism. It is the great promise of molecular genetics and the human genome initiative that these advances will also impact on the common chronic diseases. There are many reasons why measures of DNA variation may improve the ability to predict

A. M. Gotto, Jr. et al. (eds.), Drugs Affecting Lipid Metabolism, 361–369.

interindividual differences in disease beyond that provided by established risk factors: 1) an individual's genotype does not change throughout life (barring somatic mutation), 2) the genotype is not influenced or changed by the disease process, 3) DNA variation can be measured more accurately than most intermediate predictor traits, 4) measurement of DNA variation is potentially less expensive, 5) measurement of DNA variation is required for assessing genotype-specific responses to environmental challenge (e.g. drug or dietary therapy), 6) the intermediate physiologic traits underlying disease may be unknown or inaccessible to measurement, and 7) the ability of other traits (e.g. weight) to predict disease may be genotype-dependent.

Once a genetic etiology has been assigned to a disease, however, there is a tendency to oversimplify the relationship between genotype and endpoint when making statements about risk or treatment. For example, sickle cell anemia is caused by a defect in a single gene; however there is considerable heterogeneity in the onset of disease and its severity. Interesting, the β-globin genes was the first human gene cloned and characterized and the sickle-cell mutation was the first such substitution described, but these early advances have done very little for treating the patient with sickle-cell anemia. Clearly, genetic defects may predispose a patient to coronary artery disease (CAD) (e.g. low density lipoprotein [LDL]-receptor mutations leading to familial hypercholesterolemia). However, the effects of such gene mutations are subject to modification and amelioration by other genetic and environmental factors.

The Role of Genes in Normal Lipid Variation

Two basic lines of evidence document the role of genes in affecting lipid levels. First, several inborn errors of lipid metabolism have been reported and characterized. For example, Brown and Goldstein [1] have described lesions in the low density lipoprotein LDL receptor gene that lead to elevated LDL levels and premature atherosclerosis. Similarly, an insertion in the gene encoding lipoprotein lipase (LPL) causes a deficiency in LPL activity resulting in familial combined hyperlipidemia [2]. The second line of evidence comes from quantitative genetic studies showing that a significant fraction of variability in lipid, lipoprotein, and apolipoprotein (apo) levels is attributable to polymorphic genetic variability. For example, Hamsten et al. [3] estimate that the proportion of population variability in high density lipoprotein-cholesterol (HDL-C) and apo B levels attributable to genetic factors is 0.42 and 0.51, respectively. This value is 0.53 for total serum cholesterol levels and 0.98 for plasma Lp(a) levels. Of particular interest in the biometrical genetic studies of coronary heart disease (CHD) risk factors has been the detection of statistical evidence for single unknown genes with large effects. Hasstedt et al. [4] report the characteristics of such a "major gene" with a large effect on HDL-C levels. Apo A-I is the major apolipoprotein in HDL, and Moll et al. [5] report evidence supporting the existence of a gene with a large effect on plasma apo A-I levels. Evidence supporting the role of a single locus with a large effect on plasma lipoprotein(a) [Lp(a)] levels is well established. Apolipoprotein(a), the unique protein component of Lp(a), is closely linked and homologous to the serum protease plasminogen [6]. Linkage analyses using a protein polymorphism in plasminogen have determined that the major gene contributing to Lp(a) levels is likely the apolipoprotein(a) [apo(a)] structural gene [7], and Boerwinkle et al. [8] estimate that 90% of the interindividual variation in plasma Lp(a) levels is attributable to length and sequence variation at the apo(a) gene.

Although traditional quantitative genetic studies indicate that genes are contributing, they do not yield information about the identity and role of specific gene loci. Knowledge concerning individual loci is necessary for determining which individuals carry specific mutations, and for studying the interaction between genes and environments. Advances in atherosclerosis research and molecular biology have identified numerous genes and gene products that may be contributing to cardiovascular disease. Plasma lipids do not circulate freely but rather are transported as lipoprotein particles containing specific proteins known as apolipoproteins. The lipoproteins, named by their density properties, are initially synthesized at the intestinal wall or by the liver. During circulation various enzymes alter the lipid and protein components of these particles. The lipoprotein particles may be taken up by cell surface receptors which recognize and bind the apo moieties. The genes encoding these apolipoproteins, enzymes, and receptors are candidates for those responsible for the underlying polygenetic and major gene effects discussed above.

The gene whose effects on normal lipid variation are best understood is apolipoprotein E. Apo E is a structural component of chylomicrons, very low density lipoproteins (VLDL) and a subset of HDL. Apo E plays a major role in lipid metabolism through cellular uptake of lipoprotein particles by apo E-specific and apo B/E receptors on the liver and other tissues [9]. Human apo E is polymorphic with three alleles, $\epsilon 2$, $\epsilon 3$, and $\epsilon 4$ coding for three isoforms E2, E3, and E4, respectively. In a sample of 223 unrelated individuals from Nancy, France, the relative frequencies of the $\epsilon 2$, $\epsilon 3$, and $\epsilon 4$ alleles were 0.13, 0.74, and 0.13, respectively [10].

E2-containing lipoproteins have lower affinity for hepatic lipoprotein receptors compared to lipoproteins containing E3 [11]. In addition, the conversion of VLDL to LDL in the plasma of patients with familial type III hyperlipoproteinemia is impeded by the apo E2 isoform but can be restored by addition of apo E3 [12], suggesting a role of apo E in the conversion of VLDL to LDL. Consistent with the function of the apo E2 isoform, studies have shown a reduction in the clearance of postprandial lipoproteins in subjects carrying an $\epsilon 2$ allele [13]. *In vitro*, the receptor binding affinity of E4-containing lipoproteins may be similar to those containing the common E3 isoform, but *in vivo* apo E4-containing lipoproteins are cleared more rapidly from circulation than those containing apo E3.

Numerous reports have indicated that the apo E polymorphism influences plasma lipid levels. Hallman et al. [14] studied the frequency and effects of the apo E polymorphisms among nine ethnically and geographically diverse populations. They concluded that although the frequencies of the apo E alleles are heterogeneous among populations the effects of this gene are relatively consistent: the average effect of the $\epsilon 2$ allele is to lower plasma cholesterol levels and the average effect of the $\epsilon 4$ allele is to raise plasma cholesterol levels. Using family data, Boerwinkle and Sing [15] directly estimated that the apo E polymorphism accounts for 12.5% of the overall polygenetic variance of total serum cholesterol levels. Boerwinkle and Utermann [16] investigated the effect of the apo E polymorphism on plasma apo E and total cholesterol levels in a sample of 563 blood bank donors from Marburg and Giessen, Germany. The average effects of the apo E alleles are shown in Table 1. The effects of the apo E polymorphism on plasma apo E levels were in the opposite direction from that for total cholesterol levels. Dallongeville et al. [17] concluded that the apo E polymorphism also influences fasting plasma triglyceride levels; compared to individuals with the ε3/3 genotype, ε3/4 subjects had higher fasting triglyceride levels. Based on the results of several epidemiologic studies, an association between apo E genotypes and prevalent CAD has been established [18-20]. The frequency of the ε2 allele is reduced among CAD patients, while the frequency of the ε4 allele is generally increased.

Table 1. Average effects of the apo E polymorphism[1].

Phenotype	ε2	ε3	ε4	Variance[2]
Apolipoprotein E (mg/dL)	0.95	-0.04	-0.19	20.2%
Total Cholesterol (mg/dL)	-14.2	-0.16	7.09	4.0%

[1]From Boerwinkle and Utermann (1988); [2]Percent of the total phenotypic variance attributable to the apo E polymorphism.

Genotype by Environment Interaction

The regulation of gene expression and the action of gene products are determined by the micro- and macro-environments of the organism and its cellular constituents. These environments are influenced by both the expression of other genes and by the ecology of the organism such as its diet. Much has been discussed about the potential for, and effects of, genotype by environment interaction, but only a few studies have attempted to quantitate the role of genotype by environment interaction in humans. Although biometrical genetic studies are important because they provide evidence supporting interaction, they are complicated and generally do not reveal the biological nature of any significant interactions. Genotype by environment and genotype by genotype interaction studies are greatly enhanced by incorporation of measured genotype information. One example of this approach is given by studies emplying the apo E polymorphism.

Nestruck et al. [21] reported significant interaction between the apo E polymorphism and the cholesterol-lowering drug probucol. Probucol has both antioxidant and lipid-lowering properties, and was previously shown to have a variable efficacy among patients [22]. Nestruck et al. [21] reported that probucol-treated type II hyper-cholesterolemic individuals with an ε4 allele showed a larger reduction in plasma cholesterol levels when compared with ε3/3 individuals. They hypothesize that the E4 isoform and probucol act synergistically to promote enhanced lipoprotein catabolism.

Gueguen et al. [23] investigated the interaction between the apo E polymorphism and longitudinal changes in several CHD risk factors in a sample of 158 nuclear families from Nancy, France. The estimated frequencies of apo ε2, ε3, and ε4 alleles in this sample were .120, .764, and .116, respectively. There was no significant evidence for an effect of the apo E polymorphism on the longitudinal profile of any of the variables considered. These result are consistent with other reports that have demonstrated consistency of apo E effects in both children and adults [15]. However, there was a significant interaction between apo E effects and weight change on the longitudinal change of serum triglyceride and β-lipoprotein levels. Accompanying weight gain, individuals with an ϵ4 allele showed a larger increase in triglyceride levels (0.15 ± .03 mmol/l/Kg) compared to individuals with no ϵ4 allele.

Tikkanen et al. [24] and Xu et al. [25] investigated the effects of the apolipoprotein E polymorphism in a sample of adults from Finland who switched from their normal diet to a diet low in total and saturated fat. The frequencies of the apo E alleles in this sample, and their effects on lipid levels when the subjects were on their normal diets were similar to those previously reported in other studies from Finland [26]. In contrast, when the subjects switched to a diet lower in total and saturated fat, average total serum cholesterol levels were not statistically significantly different among apo E genotypes. A direct test of whether dietary response differs among apo E genotypes, however, did not detect significant differences [25]. The decrease in total serum cholesterol levels on the low total and saturated fat diet was not significantly different among apo E types.

Because of its recognized importance in remnant clearance, the apolipoprotein [apo] E gene has been targeted for studying postprandial lipid response. It has been argued that prolonged postprandial lipemia is conducive to the development of atherosclerosis, and case-control studies have shown that late postprandial lipid levels are predictive of CAD, even when HDL is simultaneously considered [27]. To estimate the contribution of the apo E polymorphism to distinct metabolic aspects of postprandial lipoprotein metabolism, Boerwinkle et al. [28] measured multiple parameters of postprandial response in a biracial sample of 474 individuals taking part in the Atherosclerosis Risk in Communities (ARIC) Study. The profile of postprandial triglyceride and retinyl palmitate response for each of the common apo E genotypes is shown in Figure 1A and B, respectively. The profile of postprandial triglyceride levels was not different among the common apo E genotypes. Postprandial triglyceride concentrations increased from 128.6 (± 75.2) mg/dl at fasting to 270.8 (± 130.5) mg/dl at 3.5 hours followed by a decrease to 193.7 (± 137.1) mg/dl at 8 hours. The profile of postprandial retinyl palmitate was significantly different among apo E genotypes. The profile of response was very similar among apo E genotypes between fasting and 3.5 hours but diverged between 3.5 hours and 8 hours. Late postprandial retinyl palmitate levels were significantly higher in individuals with the ϵ2/3 genotype compared to the other apo E genotypes. For example, average late postprandial retinyl palmitate levels were 1462.9 (± 736.9) mg/dl in ϵ2/3 individuals compared to 1072.0 (± 604.2) mg/dl in the ϵ3/3s. More than 7% of the interindividual variation in postprandial retinyl palmitate response was attributable to the apo E polymorphism. As expected, the contribution of the apo E polymorphism to the other three response variables was less than that for retinyl palmitate. The contribution of the apo E polymorphism to the interindividual variation in response was less than 2% for total triglycerides. For comparative purposes, 4.1% of the variance in fasting LDL-cholesterol concentrations in this sample of Caucasians was attributable to the apo E polymorphism; a value similar to that reported previously in other populations [16]. Therefore, the proportional contribution of apo E to the interindividual variance in postprandial response as measured by retinyl palmitate is greater than that for fasting LDL-cholesterol.

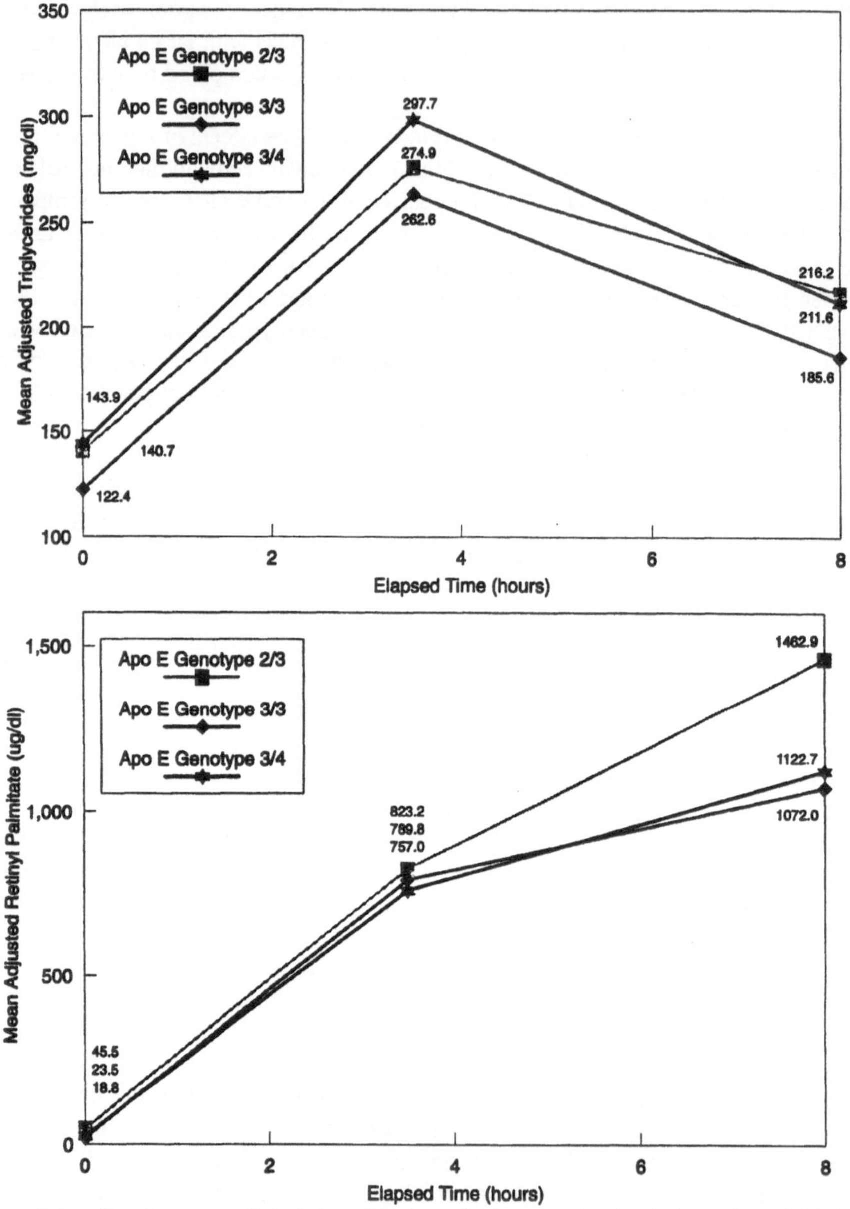

Figure 1. Profile of postprandial triglyceride (panel A) and retinyl palmitate (panel B) levels for each of the common apo E genotypes in 397 Caucasian subjects from the ARIC study.

Conclusion

The above discussion underscores the role of genotype-by-environment interaction in determining CHD risk factor variation. Knowledge of these interactions will impact the ability to implement the two basic objectives of this research--prediction and etiology. Genotype-by-environment interaction will confound the ability to use gene information to identify individuals at increased risk for disease without detailed consideration of environmental effects. However, if individuals with a genetic susceptibility can be identified early, they may be counseled toward alternative, more healthy, environments. By understanding more about these interactions, they can be exploited for the design and implementation of more efficacious intervention strategies. The light shed on chronic disease etiology by discovery of its genetic basis is likely to be of immediate value in suggesting effective interventions based on knowledge of genotype-by-environment interactions. Epidemiologists traditionally teach that the identification of a risk factor for a disease represents an opportunity for intervention and possibly prevention. For the foreseeable future, we will not be intervening or preventing disease by altering those genes influencing the common chronic diseases. The challenge for the future is to identify those genotypes that are susceptible to specific environmental influences, such as diet or drugs, so that appropriate action can be taken.

Acknowledgements

This work was supported by grants HL-40613, and contracts N01-HC55015, N01-HC55016, N01-HC55018, N01-HC55019, N01-HC55020, N01-HC55021, N01-HC55022 with the National Heart, Lung and Blood Institute. Eric Boerwinkle is an Established Investigator of the American Heart Association and the recipient of a Research Career Development Award from the National Institutes of Health (HL-02453).

References

1. Brown MS, Goldstein JL. Familial hypercholesterolemia. In: Scriver CR, Beaudet AL, Sly WS, Valle D, editors. The metabolic basis of inherited disease. New York: McGraw Hill, 1989:1215-50.
2. Langlios S, Deeb S, Brunzell JD, Kastelein JJ, Hayden MR. A major insertion accounts for a significant proportion of mutations underlying human lipoprotein lipase deficiency. Proc Natl Acad Sci USA 1989;86:948-52.
3. Hamsten A, Iselius L, Dahlen G, de Faire U. Genetic and cultural inheritance of serum lipids, low and high density lipoprotein cholesterol and serum apolipoproteins A-I, A-II, and B. Atherosclerosis 1986;40:199-208.
4. Hasstedt SJ, Ash KO, Williams RR. A reexamination of major locus hypotheses for high density lipoprotein cholesterol levels using 2170 persons screened in 55 Utah pedigrees. Am J Med Genet 1986;24:57-66.
5. Moll PP, Michels VV, Weidman WH, Kottke BA. Genetic determination of plasma apolipoprotein AI in a population-based sample. Am J Hum Genet 1989;44:124-39.

6. McLean JW, Tomlinson JE, Kuang W, et al. cDNA sequence of human apolipoprotein(a) is homologous to plasminogen. Nature 1987;330:132-37.
7. Drayna DT, Hegele RA, Hass PE, et al. Genetic linkage between lipoprotein(a) phenotype and a DNA polymorphism in the plasminogen gene. Genomics 1989;3:230-36.
8. Boerwinkle E, Leffert CC, Lin J-P, Lackner C, Chiesa G, Hobbs HH. Apolipoprotein(a) gene accounts for greater than 90% of the variation in plasma lipoprotein(a) concentrations. J Clin Invest 1992;90:52-60.
9. Mahley RW, Innerarity TL, Rall Jr SC, Weisgraber KH, Taylor JM. Apolipoprotein E: Genetic variants provide insights into its structure and function. Current Opinion in Lipidology 1990;1:87-95.
10. Boerwinkle E, Visvikis S, Welsh D, Steinmetz J, Hanash SM, Sing CF. The use of measured genotype information in the analysis of quantitative phenotypes in man. II. The role of the apolipoprotein E polymorphism in determining levels, variability, and covariability of cholesterol, betalipoprotein and triglycerides in a sample of unrelated individuals. Am J Med Genet 1987;27:567-82.
11. Weisgraber KH, Innerarity TL, Mahley RW. Abnormal lipoprotein receptor-binding activity of the human E apoprotein due to cystein-arginine interchange at a single site. J Biol Chem 1982;257:2518-21.
12. Ehnholm C, Mahley RW, Chappell DA, Weisgraber KH, Ludwig E, Witztum JL. Role of apolipoprotein E in lipolytic conversion of b-very low density lipoproteins to low density lipoprotein in type III hyperlipoproteinemia. Proc Natl Acad Sci USA 1984;81:5566-70.
13. Weintraub MS, Eisenberg S, Breslow JL. Dietary fat clearance in normal subjects is regulated by genetic variation in apolipoprotein E. J Clin Invest 1987;80:1471-77.
14. Hallman DM, Boerwinkle E, Saha N, et al. The apolipoprotein E polymorphism: A comparison of allele frequencies and effects in nine populations. Am J Hum Genet 1991;49: 338-49.
15. Boerwinkle E, Sing CF. The use of measured genotype information in the analysis of quantitative phenotypes in man. III. Simultaneous estimation of the frequencies and effects of the apolipoprotein E polymorphism and residual polygenetic effects on cholesterol, betalipoproteins and triglyceride levels. Ann Hum Genet 1987;51:211-26.
16. Boerwinkle E, Utermann G. Simultaneous effects of the apolipoprotein E polymorphism on apolipoprotein E, apolipoprotein B, and cholesterol metabolism. Am J Hum Genet 1988;42: 104-12.
17. Dallongeville J, Lussier-Cacan S, Davignon J. Modulation of plasma triglyceride levels by apo E phenotype: A meta-analysis. J Lipid Res 1992;33:447-54.
18. Menzel HJ, Kladetzky RG, Assman G. Apolipoprotein E polymorphism and coronary disease. Arteriosclerosis 1983;3:310-15.
19. Lenzen HJ, Assman G, Buchwalsky R, Schulte HS. Association of apolipoprotein E polymorphism, low-density lipoprotein cholesterol, and coronary artery disease. Clin Chem 1986;32:778-81.
20. Cumming AM, Roberts FW. Polymorphism at the apoprotein-E locus in relation to risk fo coronary disease. Clin Genet 1984;25:310-13.
21. Nestruck AC, Bouthillier D, Sing CF, Davignon J. Apolipoprotein E polymorphism and plasma cholesterol response to probucol. Metabolism 1987;36:743-47.
22. Cortese C, Marenah CB, Miller NE. The effects of probucol on plasma lipoproteins in polygenic and familial hypercholesterolemia. Atherosclerosis 1982;44:319-25.
23. Gueguen R, Visvikis S, Steinmetz J, Siest G, Boerwinkle E. An analysis of genotype effects

and their interactions by using the apolipoprotein E polymorphism and longitudinal data. Am J Hum Genet 1989;45:793-802.
24. Tikkanen MJ, Huttunen JK, Ehnholm C, Pietinen P. Apolipoprotein E_4 homozygosity predisposes to serum cholesterol elevation during a high-fat diet. Arteriosclerosis 1990;10: 285-88.
25. Xu C-F, Boerwinkle E, Tikkanen MJ, Huttunen JK, Humphries S, Talmud P. Genetic variation at the apolipoprotein gene loci contribute to response of plasma lipids to dietary change. Genet Epidemiol 1990;7:261-75.
26. Ehnholm C, Lukka T, Kuusi T, Nikkila E, Utermann G. Apolipoprotein E polymorphism in Finnish population: Gene frequencies and relation to lipid concentrations. J Lipid Res 1986; 27:227-35.
27. Patsch JR, Miesenbock G, Hopferwieser T, et al. Relation of triglyceride metabolism and coronary artery disease. Studies in the postprandial state. Arterio and Thromb 1992;12:1336-45.
28. Boerwinkle E, Brown S, Sharrett AR, Heiss G, Patsch W. Apolipoprotein E polymorphism influences postprandial retinyl palmitate but not triglyceride concentrations. Am J Hum Genet 1994;54:341-60.

MOLECULAR GENETICS OF CHOLESTEROL TRANSPORT AND CHOLESTEROL REVERSE TRANSPORT DISORDERS, AND CORONARY HEART DISEASE

Hiroshi Mabuchi, Kunimasa Yagi, Tatsuo Haraki, Toshinori Higashikata, Akihiro Inazu, Kouji Kajinami, and Junji Koizumi
The Second Department of Internal Medicine, Kanazawa University School of Medicine, Takara-machi 13-1, Kanazawa 920, Japan

Introduction

Cholesterol synthesized in the liver is secreted as very low density lipoprotein (VLDL), which is degraded by lipoprotein lipase and hepatic triglyceride (TG) lipase into intermediate density lipoprotein (IDL) and low density lipoprotein (LDL). LDL is taken up by the LDL receptor in the peripheral cells. Familial hypercholesterolemia (FH) is a disorder of LDL receptor abnormalities, and the resultant high-LDL-cholesterolemia produces atherosclerosis [1]. On the other hand, HDL_3 takes up cholesterol from the peripheral cells, and the cholesterol is esterified by LCAT, and the cholesteryl-ester in the HDL_2 with apoE is taken up by the liver, or it is transported into VLDL, IDL, or LDL by cholesteryl-ester transfer protein (CETP) [2].

First, we will describe LDL-receptor gene and apolipoprotein B-100 gene abnormalities, then CETP deficiencies, and finally the combination of these two metabolic abnormalities and coronary heart disease (CHD).

LDL-Receptor Abnormalities in Familial Hypercholesterolemia

We have collected 17 homozygotes and more than 1,400 heterozygotes of FH in the Hokuriku district of Japan. Six of the 17 homozygotes died during the past 20 years. Sudden cardiac death or heart failure was the cause of death in each of the 6 deceased homozygotes [3]. The average age of death was 26 years, and the average serum cholesterol level was 772 mg/dl.

One hundred heterozygotes died, and the causes of death are shown in Table 1. Forty-one patients died of myocardial infarction, 20 of sudden cardiac death, and 7 of heart failure or after CABG surgery. Thus, 68 of 100 patients (68%) died of coronary heart disease. The mean age of death in male heterozygotes was 58 years, which was significantly

A. M. Gotto, Jr. et al. (eds.), Drugs Affecting Lipid Metabolism, 371–377.

younger than 69 years in female heterozygotes. The mean serum cholesterol level was 357 mg/dl in the males and 344 mg/dl in the females.

Table 1. Causes of death in patients with heterozygous familial hypercholesterolemia.

Cause of Death	Number		Age		Cholesterol (mg/dl)		Triglyceride (mg/dl)	
	M	F	M	F	M	F	M	F
CHD	40	28	57 ± 13	70 ± 8	364 ± 67	344 ± 56	147 ± 52	157 ± 82
Stroke	3	5	63 ± 6	71± 5	379 ± 90	338 ± 90	157 ± 78	110 ± 12
Cancer	9	4	59 ± 9	61 ± 10	340 ± 73	339 ± 30	199 ± 107	159 ± 38
Others	7	4	64 ± 18	75 ± 13	315 ± 89	360 ± 44	132 ± 53	89 ± 36
Total	59	41	58 ± 13	69 ± 9	357 ± 71	344 ± 63	155 ± 66	146 ± 73

M, male; F, female. Data are mean ± SD.

More than 150 different mutations in the LDL receptor gene have been reported in the world [4]; thus, FH is a highly heterogeneous disease at the molecular level. Eight variants of the LDL receptor gene have been identified in our laboratory (Figure 1). Four mutants showed large deletions detected by Southern blot analysis, and four mutants were point mutations detected by SSCP analysis and direct sequencing of PCR products. These eight mutants of 86 patients from 33 families accounted for only 16.5% of FH. There seemed to be no founder gene effect in Japanese FH.

FH Tonami-1 [5], FH Tonami-2 [6], and FH Kanazawa-2 were most frequent mutants. FH Tonami-2 has a variant of LDL receptor gene with 10Kb deletion eliminating exons 2 and 3. This mutant gene deleted the first and second repeats of ligand binding domain of LDL receptor. The physiological activity of FH Tonami-2 receptor was 40% of that of the normal receptor, and the LDL receptor of the heterozygotes have 70% of normal activity. Mean serum cholesterol level of the four homozygotes of FH Tonami-2 was 587 mg/dl, and was significantly lower than those of classical FH homozygotes (713 mg/dl). All 4 true homozygotes with FH Tonami-2 are presently alive at ages 70, 59, 56, and 41, while six classical FH homozygotes died at an average of 26 years of age. The eldest two homozygotes have never been treated by LDL-apheresis, while the younger two patients have been treated by LDL-apheresis.

From these results we conclude that FH Tonami-2, caused by a partially impaired LDL receptor with small deletion in its binding domain, produces a mild type of FH, whereas other mutants produce severe type of FH. Serum lipoprotein cholesterol levels among the six mutants were compared. The mean LDL cholesterol level in the heterozygous FH Tonami-2 was 222 mg/dl, and was significantly lower than 272 mg/dl in the FH Tonami-1 heterozygotes. FH Tonami-2 heterozygotes have also survived longer than classical FH heterozygotes. Five out of 32 heterozygotes survived to reach eighty years of age. Several heterozygotes of FH Tonami-2 showed normocholesterolemia.

The mean HDL-cholesterol level in FH Kanazawa-2 was 34 mg/dl, and it was significantly lower than 46 mg/dl in FH Tonami-1. Thus, FH Kanazawa-2 produces a severe type of FH.

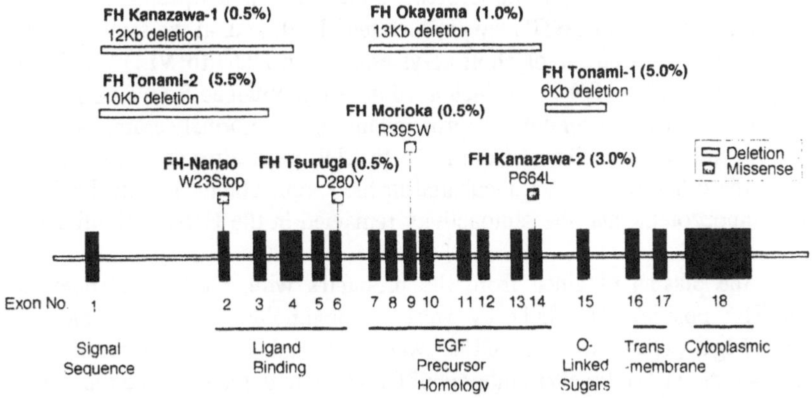

Figure 1. Location of familial hypercholesterolemia mutations in the low density lipoprotein (LDL) receptor gene. Eight mutants of the LDL receptor gene have been identified in our laboratory.

Absence of Familial Defective Apolipoprotein B-100 in Japanese FH Patients

Familial defective apolipoprotein B-100 (FDB) has been shown to be clinically indistinguishable from FH. To estimate the frequency of FDB in the Japanese population, we searched for this mutation among 385 patients clinically diagnosed as heterozygous FH from 350 unrelated families. No individuals with apo B 3500 mutation were detected. Although the apo B 3500 mutation has been frequently identified in many Caucasian populations [7], our results suggest that this mutant is a rare cause of genetic hypercholesterolemia in Japan [8].

Cholesteryl-Ester Transfer Protein (CETP) Deficiency in Familial Hyper-HDL-Cholesterolemia

Serum LDL is a positive coronary risk factor, and HDL above 60 mg/dl is a negative risk factor for coronary atherosclerosis [9]. Familial hyperalphalipoproteinemia has been known to be associated with low incidence of atherosclerosis. Recently, we found that this syndrome can be produced by CETP deficiency .

The proband, SY, is a 58-year-old Japanese man and was found to have hypercholesterolemia of 317 mg/dl and the HDL-cholesterol level was 247 mg/dl, about four times the normal HDL-cholesterol level [10]. Agarose gel electrophoresis of serum lipoprotein showed a pale β band of LDL and a dark α band of HDL. This serum lipoprotein pattern is similar to those found in rat serum, in which species CETP activity is deficient. Therefore, we studied CETP in this patient.

The plasma CETP is a hydrophobic glycoprotein and facilitates the transfer of cholesteryl-ester from HDL_2 to lipoproteins containing apolipoprotein B [2]. Thus, we thought that a deficiency of CETP may produce high HDL and, at the same time, low LDL levels. To study the transfer of cholesteryl ester from HDL to VLDL and LDL, [^{3}H] cholesteryl-ester labelled HDL_3 was incubated in serum obtained from a normal subject or from the patients with hyperalphalipoproteinemia. In the normal serum, radioactivity of cholesteryl-ester was transferred from HDL to LDL peak after an 8 hour incubation at 37°C. On the other hand, when incubated in the serum obtained from the patient with hyperalphalipoproteinemia, the radioactivity remained in the HDL peak after incubation [10].

In the plasma obtained from the proband's wife, CETP was detected at its characteristic position of 74KD by western immunoblot analysis using anti-CETP monoclonal IgG (TP2). However, CETP was undetectable in the plasma of the proband (SY) or his sister (KH). Smaller amounts of CETP were detected in the four children.

Human CETP gene located on the long arm of chromosome 16, and is comprised of 16 exons interrupted by 15 introns, and the gene spans 25 kb. Preliminary Southern blot analysis using the CETP cDNA revealed no major insertions or deletions of the CETP gene in the proband. The proband's genomic DNA was used as a substrate for amplification of the 16 exons and exon/intron junctions of the CETP gene by PCR. At the 5' splice donor of intron 14 (position +1) there was a G to A change altering the strictly conserved G-T intron splice donor to A-T (Int14 A)[11]. The proband (SY) and his sister (KH) showed the A at the first position of intron 14. The proband's wife is a normal subject, and showed the G at the position. Four children were heterozygotes with both A and G at this position of the splicing ladder.

The proband was born to a consanguineous marriage, and three homozygotes and 10 heterozygotes were confirmed in this family (Figure 2). As all the siblings are heterozygotes or homozygotes, either of the parents should be a homozygote.

Serum lipid and lipoprotein levels in 10 homozygotes and 20 heterozygotes were compared with those in 16 unaffected subjects [12]. Mean serum cholesterol level in the homozygotes was 271 mg/dl, and HDL-cholesterol level was markedly increased to 164 mg/dl, while the LDL-cholesterol level in the homozygotes decreased to 77 mg/dl, and was lower than 117 mg/dl of unaffected subjects. The heterozygotes showed intermediate values between the homozygotes and the unaffected subjects. HDL-cholesterol levels in family members showed a trimodal distribution, although the unaffected and the heterozygotes showed some overlapping. The cutting point of the heterozygotes and the homozygotes is approximately 100 mg/dl. Correlational analysis of lipoprotein and CETP levels using homozygotes, heterozygotes, and unaffected revealed a strong inverse relation between

CETP levels and the ratio of the HDL_2 levels to the sum of HDL_2 and HDL_3 levels, and the correlation coefficient was -0.790. A positive correlation was found between CETP and LDL-cholesterol levels (r = 0.517). The lipoprotein profile of persons with CETP deficiency, that is high-HDL and low LDL levels, is potentially antiatherogenic and may be associated with "longevity syndrome."

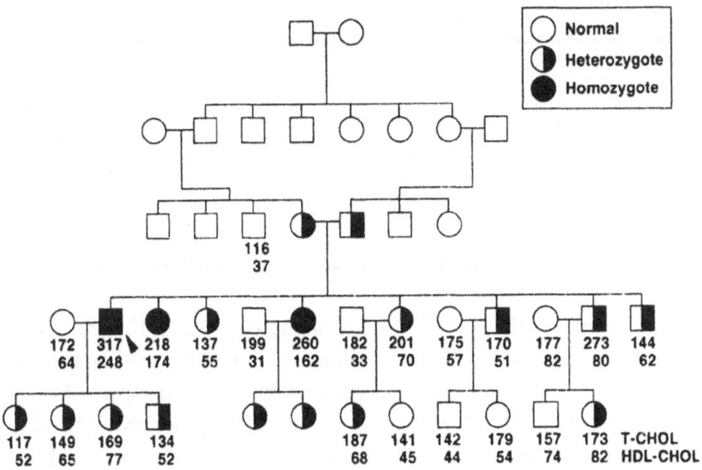

Figure 2. The pedigree of a family with CETP deficiency due to intron 14 G-A mutant. The proband is shown by the arrow.

Recently we found two novel mutants of CETP gene (Figure 3) and a total of four mutants have been identified in Japan [13]. One splice donor site mutant is a thymidine insertion in +3 position in intron 14, which will, again, result in splicing defect. Another new mutant is a missense mutation in exon 15, producing change of aspartic acid in 442 into glycine (D442G). As a whole, four mutants of CETP gene have been reported in Japan and other Asian countries, such as Korea and China.

Next, allele frequency of these mutant genes in the general Japanese subjects were studied. As a result, nine of 718 unrelated general subjects showed Int14 A mutation, and 59 were found to have the D442G mutation. Thus, the frequency of the two mutant allele in the general population in Japan was estimated to be about 1.3% in the Int14A mutant and 8.2% in D442G [13]. These two mutations accounted for about 10% of the total variance of HDL-C in the Japanese. Int14A and D442G are highly frequent, almost 1 in 10 general Japanese subjects. Thus, these two common mutants of CETP gene might raise the HDL-cholesterol levels and reduce coronary heart disease in the Japanese.

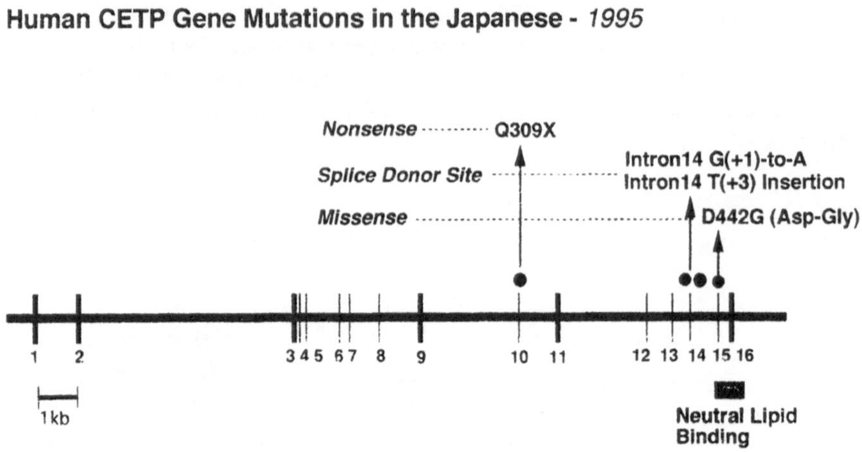

Figure 3. Location of four mutations in the CETP gene.

Double Heterozygotes of FH and CETP Deficiency, and Coronary Heart Disease

Finally, we found unique patients with double heterozygotes of FH and CETP deficiency [14]. The proband is 57 year-old man with angina pectoris. His brother died at 44 year-old of myocardial infarction. The proband received coronary angiographic study and the two-vessel disease was treated by PTCA. By screening CETP-gene mutant, the proband was proved to be a FH heterozygote combined with heterozygous CETP-deficiency, and his HDL-cholesterol level was 77 mg/dl. Thus, the combination of FH and CETP-deficiency produced severe coronary atherosclerosis in the proband and his younger brother.

We have screened CETP gene abnormalities in 288 unrelated Japanese FH patients, and found 22 double heterozygotes of FH and CETP gene and 1 heterozygous FH patient combined with homozygous CETP deficiency. These 22 double heterozygotes were often complicated by coronary heart disease, and 2 patients suffered myocardial infarction and 5 showed angina pectoris. Thus, 7 of the 22 patients showed definite coronary heart disease.

From these findings we suggest that atherogenicity of hyper-LDL-cholesterolemia in FH is more powerful than antiatherogenicity of hyper-HDL-cholesterolemia in CETP deficiency.

Conclusions

Several conclusions may be drawn: 1) LDL receptor gene abnormalities are highly heterogeneous in Japan, and the variation of LDL receptor mutant may determine the severity of hypercholesterolemia and coronary heart disease in FH; 2) no patients with apoB 3500 mutation were detected in Japanese FH patients; 3) two common mutants of CETP gene produce CETP deficiency and resultant antiatherogenic lipoprotein pattern (i.e. hyper-HDL-cholesterolemia and hypo-LDL-cholesterolemia), and the frequency of the mutant allele is about 1 in 10 subjects in Japan; and 4) double heterozygotes of FH and CETP deficiency produce premature coronary heart disease. Atherogenicity of hyper-LDL-cholesterolemia in FH is more powerful than antiatherogenicity of hyper-HDL-cholesterolemia in CETP deficiency.

References

1. Goldstein JL, Brown MS. Familial hypercholesterolemia. In: Scriver CR, Beaudet AL, Sly WS, Valle D, editors. The metabolic basis of inherited disease. 6th ed. . New York: McGraw-Hill Company, 1989:1215-50.
2. Tall AR. Plasma lipid transfer proteins. Annu Rev Biochem 1995;64:235-57.
3. Mabuchi H, Miyamoto S, Ueda K, et al. Causes of death in patients with familial hypercholesterolemia. Atherosclerosis 1986;61:1-6.
4. Hobbs HH, Brown MS, Goldstein JL. Molecular genetics of the LDL receptor gene in familial hypercholesterolemia. Hum Mut 1992;1:445-66.
5. Kajinami K, Mabuchi H, Itoh H, et al. New variant of low density lipoprotein receptor gene. FH-Tonami. Arteriosclerosis 1988;8:187-92.
6. Kajinami K, Fujita H, Koizumi J, Mabuchi H, Takeda R, Oota M. Genetically determined mild type of familial hypercholesterolemia including normo-cholesterolemic patients: FH-Tonami-2. Circulation 1989;80:II-278.
7. Myant NB. Familial defective apolipoprotein B-100: A review, including some comparisons with familial hypercholesterolemia. Atherosclerosis 1993;104:1-18.
8. Nohara A, Yagi K, Inazu A, Kajinami K, Koizumi J, Mabuchi H. Absence of familial defective apolipoprotein B-100 in Japanese patients with familial hypercholesterolemia. Lancet 1995;345:1438.
9. Expert Panel on Detection, Evaluation, and Treatment of High Blood Cholesterol in Adults. Summary of the second report of the National Cholesterol Education Program (NCEP) expert panel on detection, evaluation, and treatment of high blood cholesterol in adults (Adult Treatment Panel II). JAMA 1993;269:3015-23.
10. Koizumi J, Mabuchi H, Yoshimura A, et al. Deficiency of serum cholesteryl-ester transfer activity in patients with familial hyperalphalipoproteinemia. Atherosclerosis 1985;58:175-86.
11. Brown ML, Inazu A, Hesler CB, et al. Molecular basis of lipid transfer protein deficiency in a family with increased high-density lipoproteins. Nature 1989;342: 448-51.
12. Inazu A, Brown ML, Hesler CB, et al. Increased high-density lipoprotein levels caused by a common cholesteryl-ester transfer protein gene mutation. N Engl J Med 1990;323:1234-38.
13. Iazu A, Jiang X-C, Haraki T, et al. Genetic choleteryl ester transfer protein deficiency caused by two prevalent mutations as a major determinant of increased levels of high density lipoprotein cholesterol. J Clin Invest 1994;94:1872-82.
14. Haraki T, et al. Submitted for publication.

INSULIN RESISTANCE AND LIPID DISORDERS

R. Carmena, J.F. Ascaso, A. Merchante, and F.J. Ampudia
Department of Medicine, Endocrine Service, Hospital Clínico Universitario, 46010 Valencia, Spain

Introductory

Insulin resistance (IR) can be defined as a diminution of the biological response to a given concentration of insulin. Although the term IR was originally used to indicate impaired insulin action on glucose metabolism in liver, muscle, and adipose tissue, abnormal insulin activation of metabolic pathways involved in lipid metabolism, such as lipoprotein lipase (LPL) activity, free fatty acids (FFA) mobilization, and hepatic lipoprotein metabolism have also been reported. Insulin resistance was first described in diabetic patients and plays an important part in type I and type II diabetes mellitus and in the risk for the disease in nondiabetics [1]. Over the past decade, a more subtle and much more common form of IR has been observed in persons not treated with insulin and is characterized by hyperinsulinemia in the presence of normal or elevated plasma glucose levels [2]. This condition, which can be genetic and/or acquired, has a broad clinical spectrum that includes rare genetic syndromes, obesity, polycystic ovary syndrome, glucocorticoid or growth hormone excess, uremia, and glucose intolerance, among others [2,3]. Also in the last decade, the syndrome of IR has been recognized as an important factor predisposing to several chronic diseases, including hypertension, dyslipidemia, and atherosclerosis [2,4,5].

If the capacity of the pancreas to compensate is normal, resistance to the glucoregulatory actions of insulin leads to compensatory hyperinsulinemia and, as a consequence, IR individuals with normal glucose tolerance are hyperinsulinemic. The rationale for using plasma insulin concentration as a surrogate for IR, as in epidemiological studies in nondiabetic populations, has been that, provided the pancreatic insulin response is undiminished, insulin concentrations will rise to maintain normoglycemia, to a degree related to the severity of IR [6]. Accordingly, hyperinsulinemia in the presence of normal or elevated levels of blood glucose can be considered a marker of tissue IR. It should be emphasized that, in the context of enhanced risk for coronary heart disease, it is the IR syndrome, not hyperinsulinemia, that is considered the basic disturbance [7].

The different methods used to measure insulin action *in vivo* have been extensively reviewed [8]. Strictly speaking, it is insulin sensitivity, the inverse of IR, that is measured. All methods have their shortcomings and some of their main difficulties have been recently

A. M. Gotto, Jr. et al. (eds.), Drugs Affecting Lipid Metabolism, 379–388.

highlighted [8]. The insulin suppression test, the first to be introduced, and the euglycemic hyperinsulinemic clamp technique and its variations, considered by some as the reference method for measurement of IR, are rather laborious and complex and have been mainly used in small experimental studies [6,8]. The minimal model approach, introduced by Bergman et al. [9], avoids the procedural difficulties of the clamp by utilizing a computer program, and measures the dynamic insulin response to a glucose injection. It is now widely used in clinical research and, in well-defined groups of patients, is considered a valuable alternative to the glucose clamp for the assessment of insulin sensitivity [8,10,11].

One major difficulty in attempts to study IR is that there is not yet a quantitative definition available [6]. Numerous studies have shown that within an apparently healthy population, the range of insulin sensitivity is remarkably large, 3- to 7-fold variations having been reported. As much as 25% of the normal population is as insulin resistant as are subjects with impaired glucose tolerance or noninsulin-dependent diabetes mellitus (NIDDM) [2,12]. An ethnic difference in the role of the IR/hyperinsulinemia syndrome in determining blood pressure levels has been established and could possibly apply also to other manifestations of the syndrome such as lipid abnormalities [13,14]. More studies are needed to further evaluate this issue.

Insulin Resistance and Lipid Metabolism

CONSEQUENCES OF INSULIN RESISTANCE ON LIPID METABOLISM

Several well-characterized alterations of lipid metabolism are commonly associated with IR, although they are difficult to interpret in terms of cause and effect. As hypothesized by Frayn [15], the observed lipid changes could stem from disruption of the normal, precise co-ordination of postprandial lipid metabolism by insulin. One important consequence of IR is the loss of the suppressive effect of insulin on fat mobilization from adipose tissue. As a result, there is an increase in free fatty acids (FFA) flux owing to reduced suppression of lipolysis. The failure to suppress FFA release in the postprandial period may explain the increased hepatic very low density lipoprotein-triglyceride (VLDL-TG) secretion that has been described in IR subjects [16]. It has been shown that insulin acutely inhibits hepatic secretion of VLDL-TG and apoB-100, and in IR states, an increase in VLDL-TG and VLDL-apoB secretion is usually observed [17,18,19].

Insulin, by activation of the inactive, precursor form, exerts an important effect on LPL activity [20]. Consequently, in IR states there is impaired postprandial TG clearance and decreased transfer of cholesterol into high density lipoprotein (HDL) due to deficient LPL action combined with increased hepatic lipase activity. This complex of lipoprotein disturbances tends to increase the plasma concentrations of the small, dense LDL particles, the so-called "type B phenotype," which is considered atherogenic [21].

In summary (Table 1), in IR states the lipid abnormalities include elevated plasma VLDL-TG and VLDL-apoB concentrations, decreased HDL-cholesterol, elevation of plasma free fatty acids (FFA) (both fasting and postprandial), enhanced postprandial lipemia, and presence of small, dense low density lipoprotein (LDL) particles. These changes have been described as the "atherogenic lipoprotein phenotype" (ALP) [22].

Table 1. Alterations in lipid metabolism associated with IR.

• Elevation of plasma total and VLDL-TG, VLDL-apoB
• Lowering of HDL-cholesterol (HDL_2)
• Elevation of plasma FFA (impaired postprandial suppression)
• Enhanced postprandial lipemia
• Small, dense LDL particle distribution

PATHOPHYSIOLOGY

Although the association between hypertriglyceridemia and both glucose intolerance and hyperinsulinemia was described some decades ago [23,24], the elucidation of cause and effect remains a major challenge; i.e. are lipid changes secondary to IR or vice versa?

Several mechanisms must be considered in order to explain the association between IR and both glucose and lipoprotein abnormalities. As stated above, one implicit assumption has been that IR is the underlying factor and that the changes in lipid metabolism are secondary [15]. This assumption is based on much evidence suggesting that hypertriglyceridemia is a consequence of IR, irrespective of the glucose tolerance status [25], and on the recent demonstration, in two prospective studies [26,27], that fasting hyperinsulinemia precedes hypertriglyceridemia and low plasma HDL-cholesterol concentrations. Bjorntorp has hypothesized that the primary event could be IR initially localized only in adipose tissue [28]. This would result in an increased FFA efflux, with secondary effects causing or amplifying IR in muscle and liver. In fact, in visceral obesity, the elevated flux of FFA to the liver is associated with insulin resistance [28]. Most kinetic studies [29] have shown that IR induces overproduction of VLDL-TG rich particles by increasing the availability of FFA. In addition, increased synthesis and decreased removal rate may coexist, due to reduced adipose tissue LPL activity [20].

On the other hand, abnormal lipid and lipoprotein concentrations could induce an impairment in insulin action. There is evidence that hypertriglyceridemic NIDDM subjects, with plasma triglycerides levels between 260-1600 mg/dl (3-18 mmol/L) are more IR than matched NIDDM subjects without hypertriglyceridemia [30,31]. Since the report of Randle et al. [32], it is known that high plasma concentrations of FFA result in a decreased systemic glucose uptake in the muscle and liver and impaired insulin sensitivity. Steiner et al. have shown [33] that hypertriglyceridemia can lead to IR even without concomitant obesity or noninsulin dependent diabetes, and that high plasma VLDL concentrations downregulate insulin receptors. This IR may be the basis for the hyperinsulinemia response to a glucose challenge and in turn could further aggravate hypertriglyceridemia, perpetuating a vicious cycle. In a recent study, induction of acute hypertriglyceridemia by Intralipid® infusion in normal subjects caused a reduction in insulin sensitivity when the plasma triglyceride levels reached 6 mmol/L (530 mg/dl) [34]. The effects of triglyceride on glucose metabolism and insulin sensitivity were found to be independent of those due to circulating FFA. The triglyceride effect on carbohydrate and insulin metabolism was found to occur via triglyceride hydrolysis using the intracellular FFA pathway, without interference with the circulating FFA pool. From their own data and that in the literature the authors conclude that in normal subjects, plasma triglyceride levels influence glucose metabolism only above 5 mmol/L (440 mg/dl) [32].

Apolipoprotein E polymorphisms may influence the well-established relations of hyperinsulinemia to hypertriglyceridemia in insulin resistant/hyperinsulinemic conditions. It has recently been shown that in contrast to apoE2 and apoE3 carriers, who showed higher plasma triglyceride concentrations with fasting hyperinsulinemia, healthy premenopausal women with the apoE4 isoform had similar plasma triglyceride concentrations at high and low fasting insulin levels [35]. In another study, conducted in nondiabetic subjects from a biethnic population, the apoE 3/2 phenotype was associated with lower plasma levels of fasting and 2-hour post-prandial insulin [36]. It therefore seems possible that apoE polymorphism could explain some of the lipid variations observed in the IR syndrome in different populations.

Intervention studies might help to clarify the sequence of events. Steiner [37] has shown that reduction of plasma triglyceride concentrations with gemfibrozil in nondiabetic hypertriglyceridemic subjects resulted in reduction of the insulin response to a glucose load. On the other hand, in hypertriglyceridemic NIDDM subjects, 12 weeks of gemfibrozil therapy decreased triglyceride levels by 42% but did not improve insulin sensitivity, glucose levels, or glucose and FFA turnover and oxidation [38]. Along the same lines, treatment of nondiabetic men with combined hyperlipidemia (type IIb) with bezafibrate for 2 months caused a 42% reduction in mean plasma triglyceride concentrations with no significant influence on insulin sensitivity as measured by the euglycemic hyperinsulinemic clamp technique [39]. In a similar study, diabetic and nondiabetic hypertriglyceridemic subjects treated with bezafibrate for two months did not show significant changes in peripheral insulin sensitivity despite a 46% reduction in plasma VLDL-triglyceride concentrations [40]. It should be emphasized, however, that mean plasma triglyceride concentrations following bezafibrate remained at 260 ± 37 mg/dl (3.00 ± 0.42 mmol/L) and 312 ± 180 mg/dl (3.52 ± 2.03 mmol/L), respectively, in the last two studies, while in Steiner's study improvement was observed only in those subjects whose triglyceride decreased below 150 ± 42 mg/dl (1.70 ± 0.48 mmol/L). In conclusion, the studies reviewed above suggest that, in some cases, hypertriglyceridemia may cause, or at least aggravate, IR. The possibility of a hypothetical threshold value for plasma triglyceride to cause IR could be entertained, as has recently been hypothesized with the triglyceride/HDL relationship [41]. Further studies are needed in diabetic and nondiabetic subjects with hypertriglyceridemia to help clarify these complex interactions among which IR remains a central feature [2,13,15].

Factors Modulating the Effects of Insulin Resistance on Lipid Metabolism

An ethnic difference in the role of the IR/hyperinsulinemia syndrome in determining blood pressure levels has been well established [13,14] and could possibly apply also to other manifestations of the syndrome such as lipid abnormalities. Laws et al. [42] have reported that Asian-Indian men and women are more IR and have more severe dyslipidemia than control individuals from a European ancestry matched for age and BMI. More studies are needed to further evaluate this issue.

As recently reviewed by Taskinen [43], the association between insulin action and lipid metabolism could also be influenced by factors affecting both glucose and lipid metabolism, like obesity, abdominal distribution of fat, physical activity, diet, smoking habits, age, gender, etc. The amount of visceral fat is an important factor modulating the degree of insulin sensitivity and the lipid profile and may explain the major metabolic differences between men and women [43,44]. It seems unlikely, however, that a simple or "primary" change would account for all the interrelated disturbances associated with IR. Thus, although it is broadly accepted that IR and its manifestations are not dependent on obesity or a sedentary life style, they will be exacerbated if individuals become obese or less active.

Insulin Resistance in Hypercholesterolemia

Several studies have shown that hereditary and acquired hypercholesterolemia are associated neither with IR, as measured by the euglycemic clamp technique, nor with intracellular defects of glucose metabolism. Population based studies have shown a weak or no association between plasma total cholesterol concentrations and insulin levels [45,46], and in the San Antonio study there was no significant hyperinsulinemia associated with isolated hypercholesterolemia [13].

Karhapaa et al. [47], using the euglycemic hyperinsulinemic clamp technique, recently studied 13 adult FH and 25 non-FH hypercholesterolemic patients and control groups. Their results showed that glucose, insulin, and C-peptide responses in a oral glucose tolerance test were similar in all groups. During the euglycemic hyperglycemic clamp studies, FH and non-FH patients and control subjects displayed similar rates of whole-body glucose uptake. In addition, oxidative and nonoxidative glucose utilization, lipid oxidation, and suppression of plasma FFA levels by insulin were similar in the three groups. In another study, conducted in Taiwan in 15 thin, nondiabetic, men and women with type IIa hypercholesterolemia, no differences from controls were observed in plasma glucose and insulin responses to standard meals or during the insulin suppression test [48].

Thus, according to all available evidence, monogenic, polygenic, and environmental hypercholesterolemia are not associated with an impaired insulin action.

Insulin Resistance in Familial Combined Hyperlipidemia

Familial combined hyperlipidemia (FCHL) is a dyslipidemic syndrome, probably representing a mixture of various disease entities, that may result from the interaction of several metabolic and environmental factors. The prevalence of FCHL may be as high as 1% of the general population. It is the most common familial form of hyperlipidemia in young survivors of myocardial infarction, and may cause at least 10% of premature coronary heart disease [49,50]. Manifest hyperlipidemia before the age of 20 years is uncommon and no specific biological marker for FCHL has yet been found. Hepatic overproduction of VLDL apoB-100 has been demonstrated in FCHL subjects [51]. Diagnosis is generally based on family studies: occurrence of primary hyperlipidemia with varying phenotypic expression (types IIa, IIb, IV) in the proband and among his first degree relatives, elevated plasma apoB levels, and a positive history of premature cardiovascular disease indicate FCHL.

Several studies have described the presence of IR in FCHL subjects. In studies of familial dyslipidemic hypertension (FDH), Hunt et al. [52] found that about one third of the sibships with FDH met lipid criteria for FCHL. This subgroup displayed significantly higher plasma total and LDL-cholesterol, apoB, triglycerides, and (after adjusting for BMI) fasting insulin concentrations than did non-FCHL subjects. Mean plasma insulin concentrations were 22.1 and 16.2 mU/L in FCHL and non FCHL subjects, respectively ($p = 0.004$), with no difference in fasting plasma glucose levels between the two groups. Castro Cabezas et al. [53], in their study of 6 FCHL kindreds, found that plasma insulin concentrations were positively correlated with plasma apoB and triglyceride and inversely correlated with HDL-cholesterol concentrations. Since the body mass index (BMI) in these FCHL subjects was significantly lower than in Hunt's et al. [52], the authors concluded that obesity was not an obligatory feature of the IR syndrome in FCHL. On the other hand, fasting FFA were elevated in FCHL compared to normal controls or to patients with familial hypertriglyceridemia. Thus, the clustering of cardiovascular risk factors associated with IR in FCHL indicates a common metabolic basis for the FCHL phenotype and IR which is probably mediated by an impaired fatty acid metabolism. As discussed above, the presence of small, dense LDL particles (phenotype B) with increased atherogenic potential is an additional lipid anomaly that has been described in IR states and in FCHL subjects [21].

The effect of the 2 allele and IR on combined hyperlipidemia (type IIb) in a group of nonobese individuals has recently been estimated with measurements of fasting insulin [54]. Combined hyperlipidemic patients had higher fasting insulin concentrations compared with hypercholesterolemic patients with similar plasma glucose concentrations. There were significantly more smokers and carriers of the 2 allele among combined hyperlipidemics (type IIb) than in hypercholesterolemic (type IIa) individuals. Thus, the expression of the combined hyperlipidemic phenotype seems to be influenced by at least three independent factors: IR, 2 allele, and smoking.

We have compared 20 unrelated FCHL male subjects with 16 healthy, unrelated controls of similar age, gender, and BMI (R. Carmena, J.F. Ascaso, A. Merchante, F.J. Ampudia, unpublished data). All subjects were normotensive and diabetes was excluded by previous oral glucose tolerance test. Mean age and BMI were 45.6 ± 7 years and 27.8 ± 3 kg/m^2, respectively in patients and 42.9 ± 7 and 27.1 ± 3, respectively, in the controls. Insulin sensitivity was measured with a modified version of the minimal model technique in which a bolus of 300 mg/kg of glucose was administered at time 0, followed 20 minutes later by a bolus of 0.03 U/kg of regular insulin. Blood samples for glucose and insulin were obtained at 28 time intervals during three hours and the results were entered into computer program MINMOD. In nondiabetic populations, values obtained with this method have correlated significantly with clamp-derived measures of insulin sensitivity [6,11]. We found significantly lower insulin sensitivity (Si) values in the combined hyperlipidemia and hypertriglyceridemic subjects (types IIb and IV) than in controls or hypercholesterolemic (type IIa) subjects. Si values in FCHL subjects correlated significantly with fasting FFA plasma levels (r = -0.67), plasma insulin at 120 minute postglucose challenge (r = -0.62), BMI (r = - 0.60) and plasma triglyceride concentrations (r = -0.55). Table 2 contains a summary of a subset of our results.

Table 2. Summary of results obtained in 20 FCHL patients and 16 control subjects.

	IIa		IIb		IV		Controls	
N	5		8		7		16	
Age (years)	47	±7.5	46	±7.9	44.1	±6.0	42.6	±7.0
BMI kg/m^2	27.4	±1.9	27	±2.0	28.1	±2.8	27.1	±3.0
Waist/Hip Ratio	0.97	±0.05	0.99	±0.06	1.00	±0.05	0.96	±0.05
LDL-C mg/dL	195.7*	±33.1	205	±33.7*	125.1	±25.2	130.8	±27.8
HDL-C mg/dL	37.7	±3.4	37	±8.8	32.5	±8.2*	40.3	±7.4
Triglyc mg/dL	150.7	±28.4	313	±78.2*	401.5	±121.5*	158.3	±60.6
Fasting FFA mEq/L	299.8	±168.5	538	±184.6*	531.6	±93.4*	332.3	±125.6
Si min^{-1} µU^{-1} mL	1.89	±1.1	1.8	±0.7*	0.91	±0.8*	2.83	±1.3

* $p < 0.05$ versus control

According to our results and published data [47,48], IR occurs in hypertriglyceridemic FCHL subjects (types IIb and IV). We also found that FCHL subjects with decreased insulin sensitivity had hyperinsulinemia, elevated fasting FFA and apo B levels, and tended to have higher waist/hip ratio than the other groups. On the other hand, insulin sensitivity in hypercholesterolemic FCHL (type IIa) subjects did not differ from normal control subjects of similar BMI, gender, and age. Likewise, these latter two groups had similar fasting FFA plasma levels and insulin secretion (expressed as the area under the curve). Our results, obtained with a modified minimal model technique, are in agreement with published data in which insulin sensitivity was measured with other methods [47,48].

Conclusion

Insulin resistance is a common phenomenon, frequently associated with lipid disorders: increased FFA mobilization, hypertriglyceridemia, low plasma HDL-cholesterol concentrations, presence of small, dense LDL particles, and enhanced postprandial lipemia. Hypercholesterolemic subjects (type IIa) do not show impaired insulin action but subjects with combined hyperlipidemia (type IIb) or hypertriglyceridemia (type IV) have reduced insulin sensitivity. As discussed above, a cause-and-effect relation between IR and lipid abnormalities has yet to be established. Although arguments in favor of both hypotheses do exist, the driving force behind the chain of events associated with lipid disturbances is more likely to be IR. Intervention studies in nonobese FCHL types IIb and IV subjects, with correction of triglyceride values to below 150 mg/dl (1.70 mmol/L) may help to clarify this interesting issue.

References

1. Kahn, CR. Insulin resistance: A common feature of diabetes mellitus. N Engl J Med 1986;315:252-54.
2. Reaven GM. Pathophysiology of insulin resistance in human disease. Physiol Rev 1995;75:473-86.
3. Moller DE, Flier JS. Insulin resistance. Mechanisms, syndromes, and implications. N Engl J Med 1991;325:93848.
4. Reaven GM. The role of insulin resistance and hyperinsulinemia in coronary heart disease. Metabolism 1992;41(1):16-19.
5. Després JP, Maretter A. Relation of components of insulin resistance syndrome to coronary disease risk. Current Opin Lipidol 1994;5:274-89.
6. Godsland IF, Stevenson JC. Insulin resistance: Syndrome or tendency? Lancet 1995; 346:100-03.
7. Stern MP. The insulin resistance syndrome: The controversy is dead, long live the controversy! Diabetologia 1994;37:956-58.
8. Scheen AJ, Paquot N, Castillo MJ, Lefebvre PJ. How to measure insulin action in vivo. Diabet Metabol Rev 1994;10:151-88.
9. Bergman RN, Finegoog DT, Ader M. Assessment of insulin sensitivity in vivo. Endrocr Rev 1985;6:45-86.
10. Fulcher GR, Walker M, Alberti KGMM. The assessment of insulin action *in vivo*. In: Alberti KGMM, DeFronzo RA, Keen H, Zimmet P, editors International textbook of diabetes mellitus. Chichester: John Wiley, 1992:513-29.
11. Swan JW, Walton C, Godsland IF. Assessment of insulin sensitivity in man: A comparison of minimal model-and euglycemic clamp-derived measures in health and heart failure. Clin Sci 1994;86:317-22.
12. Williams B. Insulin resistance: The shape of things to come. Lancet 1994;344:521-24.
13. Ferrannini E, Haffner SM, Mitchell BD, Stern MP. Hyperinsulinemia: The key feature of a cardiovascular and metabolic syndrome. Diabetologia 1991;34:416-22.
14. Zimmet PZ, Collins VR, Dowse GK, et al. for the Mauritius Noncommunicable Disease Study: Is hyperinsulinemia a central characteristic of a chronic cardiovascular risk factor clustering syndrome? Mixed findings in Asian, Indian, Creole and Chinese Mauritians. Diabetic Med 1994;11:388-96.
15. Frayn KN. Insulin resistance and lipid metabolism. Curr Opin Lipidol 1993;4:197-204.
16. Coppack SW, Evans RD, Fisher RM, et al. Adipose tissue metabolism in obesity: lipase action in vivo before and after a mixed meal. Metabolism 1992;41:264-72.
17. Barlett SM, Gibbons GF. Short- and longer-term regulation of very low density lipoprotein secretion by insulin, dexamethasone and lipogenic substrates in cultured hepatocytes. A biphasic effect of insulin. Biochem J 1988;249:37-43.
18. Kwiterovich PO. Genetics and molecular biology of familial combined hyperlipidemia. Curr Opin Lipidol 1993;4:133-43.
19. Lewis GF, Uffelman KD, Szeto LW, Weller B, Steiner G. Interaction between free fatty acids and insulin in the acute control of very low density lipoprotein production in humans. J Clin Invest 1995;95:158-66.

20. Eckel RH. Lipoprotein lipase. A multifunctional enzyme relevant to common metabolic diseases. N Engl J Med 1989;320:1060-68.
21. Austin MA, Horowitz H, Wijsman E, Krauss RM, Brunzell J. Bimodality of plasma apolipoprotein B levels in familial combined hyperlipidemia. Atherosclerosis 1992; 92:67-77.
22. Austin MA, King MC, Vranizan KM, Krauss RM. Atherogenic lipoprotein phenotype. A proposed genetic marker for coronary heart disease. Circulation 1990; 82:495-506.
23. Farquhar JW, Frank JW, Gross RC, Reaven GM. Glucose, insulin and triglyceride responses to high and low carbohydrate diets in man. J Clin Invest 1966;45:1648-56.
24. Avogaro P, Crepaldi G, Enzi G. Association of hyperlipidemia, diabetes mellitus and mild obesity. Acta Diabetol Lat 1967;4:572-90.
25. Laakso M, Sarlund H, Mykkanen L. Insulin resistance is associated with lipid and lipoprotein abnormalities in subjects with varying degrees of glucose tolerance. Arteriosclerosis 1990;10:223-31.
26. Haffner SM, Valdez RA, Hazuda HP, Mitchell BD, Morales PA, Stern MP. Prospective analysis of the insulin-resistance syndrome (Syndrome X). Diabetes 1992;41:715-22.
27. Mykkanen L, Kuusito J, Haffner SM, Pyorala K, Laakso M. Hyperinsulinemia predicts multiple atherogenic changes in lipoproteins in elderly subjects. Arterioscler Thromb 1994;14:518-26.
28. Bjorntorp P. Fatty acids, hyperinsulinemia, and insulin resistance: Which comes first? Current Opin Lipidol 1994;5:166-74.
29. Tobey TA, Greenfield M, Kraemer F, Reaven GM. Relationship between insulin resistance, insulin secretion, very low density lipoprotein kinetics and plasma triglyceride levels in normotriglyceridemic man. Metabolism 1981;30:165-71.
30. Yki-Jarvinen H, Taskinen MR. Interrelationships among insulin's antilipolytic and glucoregulatory effects and plasma triglycerides in nondiabetic patients with endogenous hypertriglyceridemia. Diabetes 1988;37:1271-78.
31. Widen E, Ekstrand A, Salorante C, et al. Insulin resistance in type 2 (non-insulin-dependent) diabetic patients with hypertriglyceridemia. Diabetologia 1992;35:1140-45.
32. Randle PJ, Garland PB, Hales CN, Newsholme EA. The glucose fatty-acid cycle. Its role in insulin sensitivity and the metabolic disturbances of diabetes mellitus. Lancet 1963;i:785-89.
33. Steiner G, Vranic M. Hyperinsulinemia and hypertriglyceridemia, a vicious cycle with atherogenic potential. Int J Obesity 1982;6(1):117-24.
34. Piatti PM, Monti LD, Baruffaldi L, et al. Effects of an acute increase in plasma triglyceride levels on glucose metabolism in man. Metabolism 1995;44:883-89.
35. Despres JP, Verdon MF, Moorjani S, et al. Apolipoprotein E polymorphism modifies relation of hyperinsulinemia to hypertriglyceridemia. Diabetes 1993;42: 1474-81.
36. Valdez R, Stern MP, Howard BV, Haffner SM. Apolipoprotein E polymorphism and insulin levels in a biethnic population. Diabetes Care 1995;18:992-1000.
37. Steiner G. Altering triglyceride concentrations changes insulin-glucose relationships in hypertriglyceridemic patients. Double-blind study with gemfibrozil with implications for atherosclerosis. Diabetes Care 1991;14:1077-81.
38. Vuorinen-Markkola H, Yki-Jarvinen H, Taskinen MR. Lowering of triglyceride by gemfibrozil affects neither the glucoregulatory nor antilipolytic effect of insulin in type 2 (non-insulin-dependent) diabetes patients. Diabetologia 1993;36:161-69.
39. Karhapää P, Uusitupa M, Voutilainen E, Laakson M. Effects of bezafibrate on insulin sensitivity and glucose tolerance in subjects with combined hyperlipidemia. Clin Pharmacol Ther 1992;52:620-26.

40. Riccardi G, Genovese S, Saldalamacchia G, et al. Effects of bezafibrate on insulin secretion and peripheral insulin sensitivity in hyperlipidemic patients with and without diabetes. Atherosclerosis 1989;75:175-81.
41. Schaefer EJ, Lamon-Fava E, Ordovas JM, et al. Factors associated with low and elevated plasma high density lipoprotein cholesterol and apolipoprotein A-I levels in the Framingham offspring study. J Lipid Res 1994;35:871-82.
42. Laws A, Jeppesen JL, Maheux PC, Schaaf P, Ida Chen Y-D, Reaven GM. Resistance to insulin-stimulated glucose uptake and dyslipidemia in Asian Indians. Arterioscler Thromb 1994;14:917-22.
43. Taskinen M-R. Insulin resistance and lipoprotein metabolism. Current Opin Lipidol 1995;6:153-60.
44. Després JO. Dyslipidemia and obesity. Baillieres Clin Endocrinol Metab 1994;8:629-60.
45. Laakso M, Pyorala K, Voutilainen E, Marniemi J. Plasma insulin and serum lipids and lipoproteins in middle-aged non-insulin-dependent diabetic and non-diabetic subjects. Am J Epidemiol 1987;125:416-22.
46. Cambien F, Warner JM, Eschwege E, Jacqueson A, Richard JL, Rosselin G. Body mass index, blood pressure, glucose, and lipids: does plasma insulin explain their relationship? Arteriosclerosis 1987;7:197-202.
47. Karhapaa P, Voutilainen E, Kovanen PT, Laakso M. Insulin resistance in familial and nonfamilial hypercholesterolemia. Arterioscler Thromb 1993;13:41-47.
48. Sheu WH-H, Shieh S-M, Fuh MM-T, et al. Insulin resistance, glucose intolerance, and hyperinsulinemia. Hypertriglyceridemia versus hypercholesterolemia. Arteriosclerosis Thromb 1993;13:367-70.
49. Goldstein JL, Schrott HG, Hazzard R, Bierman EL, Motulsky AG. Hyperlipidemia in coronary heart disease. II. Genetic analysis in 176 families and delineation of a new inherited disorder, combined hyperlipidemia. J Clin Invest 1973;52:1544-68.
50. Grundy SM, Chait A, Brunzell JD. Familial combined hyperlipidemia workshop. Arteriosclerosis 1987;7:203-207.
51. Venkatesan S, Cullen P, Pacy P, Halliday D, Scott J. Stable isotopes show a direct relation between VLDL ApoB overproduction and serum triglyceride levels and indicate a metabolically and biochemically coherent basis for familial combined hyperlipidemia. Arterioscler Thromb 1993;13:1110-18.
52. Hunt SC, Wu LL, Hopkins PN, et al. Apolipoprotein, low density lipoprotein subfraction, and insulin associations with familial combined hyperlipidemia. Study of Utah patients with familial dyslipidemic hypertension.
53. Castro Cabezas M, de Bruin TWA, de Walk HW, Shoulders CC, Jansen H, Erkelens DW. Impaired fatty acid metabolism in familial combined hyperlipidemia. A mechanism associating hepatic apolipoprotein overproduction and insulin resistance. J Clin Invest 1993;92:160-168.
54. Sijbrands EJG, Westendorp RGJ, Höffer MJV, et al. Effect of insulin resistance, aspoE2 allele, and smoking on combined hyperlipidemia. Arterioscler Thromb 1994;14:1576-80.

INSULIN RESISTANCE AND LIPOPROTEINS IN HYPERTRIGLYCERIDEMIA: EFFECTS OF HYPOLIPIDEMIC DRUG TREATMENT

Finnbogi O. Karlsson and Alan J. Garber
Department of Medicine, Baylor College of Medicine, 6550 Fannin, Houston, Texas 77030, USA

Introduction

The dyslipidemia that is characterized by high serum triglycerides and low HDL (high density lipoprotein) cholesterol is a common metabolic disorder. It occurs primarily as hyperlipoproteinemia and secondarily as a consequence of other diseases affecting metabolism such as diabetes (type II or uncontrolled type I), hypothyroidism, obesity, and alcoholism [1]. Commonly, alteration of lipoprotein particle size or structure also coexist in the form of small dense low density lipoprotein (LDL) cholesterol as well as other modifications such as glycosylation, oxidation, and desialiation of lipoproteins [2-4]. The syndrome of insulin resistance and hyperinsulinemia are commonly seen in association with such dyslipidemia [5-6]. Whether the nature of this relationship is causal or associative is unclear however. It is possible, although less likely, that this relationship is a simple clustering of altered metabolic variables. Regardless, some evidence indicates that a failure of suppression of nonesterified fatty acids (NEFA) release and/or production from adipocytes by insulin is an important factor in the atherogenesis of this dyslipidemia and of the insulin resistance syndrome [7,8]. Epidemiological data indicate that this dyslipidemic, hyperinsulinemic metabolic profile is an important contributor to the etiology of atherosclerosis in nondiabetic and diabetic patients alike, and contributes in a major way to the risk of cardiovascular events in Western populations [9-13]. Elevated serum triglycerides alone have been found however to be less consistently significant in contributing to atherosclerosis in multivariate analyses. This may be related to the inability to isolate the individual metabolic importance of high triglycerides due to the concurrent defects associated with, rather than caused by, fasting high triglyceride levels, such as HDL cholesterol depletion and LDL cholesterol modifications as well as hyperinsulinemia *per se* [14].

Insulin itself has been implicated as a major factor in atherosclerotic plaque formation for over 4 decades [15,16]. A relationship between insulin resistance and alterations of lipoprotein composition or levels has been shown in subjects with "normal" glucose tolerance, with impaired glucose tolerance and in noninsulin dependent mellitus

A. M. Gotto, Jr. et al. (eds.), Drugs Affecting Lipid Metabolism, 389–396.

(NIDDM) [17-19]. Thus, it seems likely that the changes in lipoproteins and lipid levels are actually a causal pathogenic consequence of insulin resistance [20,21].

Pathophysiology and Biochemistry

The level of triglycerides in serum derives from both an exogenous component, i.e. dietary intake and absorption, as well as an endogenous component that includes both production of triglyceride-rich particles (first and foremost very low density lipoproteins [VLDL] in the liver) and the clearance of triglyceride-containing particles via lipolysis into various tissues for tissue specific roles. The exogenous component of hypertriglyceridemia is the result of intestinal absorption of cholesterol and triglycerides, the latter in the form of fatty acids in the proximal jejunum. These lipids are packaged into chylomicron particles by the intestinal mucosal cells and then travel through the intestinal lymphatic system into the systemic circulation. The chylomicron particle has a high triglyceride core that is hydrolyzed by lipoprotein lipase (LPL) of endothelial cells in peripheral tissues. This releases free fatty acids (FFA) that subsequently are used for aerobic energy production in muscle tissue and for storage as triglyceride fat in adipocytes. LPL activity is regulated by many components important in the insulin resistant state such as aerobic exercise and insulin itself. This association between insulin levels and LPL levels may however be tissue specific and less pronounced in muscle tissue than elsewhere. Fibric acid derivatives action to upregulate LPL enzymatic activity is thought to represent an important part of its hypolipidemic mechanism. The endproduct from LPL action upon chylomicrons is a smaller chylomicron remnant particle which has been implicated as having significant atherogenic characteristics [22]. This remnant, which is relatively cholesterol rich, is removed by the liver via a specific cell surface receptor. The liver is thus provided with cholesterol which leads to a reduction of LDL receptors, a reduction of LDL clearance by the liver, and therefore higher concentrations of LDL in the circulation, thus augmenting or accelerating atherosclerosis. This chylomicron remnant removal activity may be enhanced by the LPL, thus revealing a second important consequence of reduced LPL activity associated with insulin resistance and hypertriglyceridemia [23]. The hepatic lipase activity that is increased in hyperinsulinemic patients can possibly lead to lowering of the HDL cholesterol [24]. There is, however, controversy whether or not this enzyme may be insulin sensitive, or whether this defective enzyme activity is an independent alteration in low HDL cholesterol disease states.

An association between postprandial lipids and coronary artery disease (CAD) has been suggested for close to half a century but experimental evidence has been unpersuasive until the last decade [25].

The endogenous component of VLDL, which is synthesized and secreted by the liver, is also affected by LPL. VLDL is metabolized to intermediate density lipoprotein (IDL) which is subsequently converted primarily to LDL via hepatic lipase and/ or taken up by the liver by an LDL receptor-mediated process and to a lesser degree by peripheral tissues. HDL metabolism is intimately associated with the metabolism of triglyceride-rich lipoprotein particles described above. Nascent HDL is secreted by the intestine and the liver. It matures quickly by addition of surface components, acquired from triglyceride-rich lipoprotein particles during their catabolism. The mature HDL_3 particle is then esterified by LCAT. The particle becomes the larger HDL_2 particle which can carry more cholesterol and is closely associated with reverse cholesterol transport, i.e. returning cholesterol from peripheral tissues to the liver for excretion and catabolism. The cholesteryl esters of HDL can also be exchanged for triglycerides to triglyceride-rich lipoprotein particles. This is mediated by CETP, which is increased in insulin resistant states. A triglyceride-rich HDL_2 lipoprotein particle can then via hepatic lipase be converted back to HDL_3 by removal of the triglyceride core. If clearance of triglyceride-rich lipoprotein particle remnants is decreased, cholesteryl ester transfer increases thereby depleting HDL cholesterol and increasing the atherogenicity of triglyceride remnant particles [26].

Therapeutic Considerations

Treatment of these metabolic abnormalities by lifestyle maneuvers, such as diet and exercise as well as treatment of secondary causes of hyperlipidemia, is often only partially effective in correcting the lipid abnormalities. The addition of hypolipidemic agents is frequently necessary. The inadequate results with dietary and exercise interventions may well be due to lack of long-term patient compliance as seen with any long-term therapeutic interventions, but to a greater extent with these lifestyle maneuvers. The usual recommendations of a low fat diet may however also play a role as studies with high carbohydrate diets indicate that they lead to a deterioration of glycemic control, increased insulin resistance and accentuated postprandial lipemia. This occurs because of increased production of VLDL which is of a greater magnitude than the corresponding rise in hepatic lipoprotein lipase activity secondary to increased serum insulin concentration [27].

Lipoprotein lipase acts also upon VLDL particles in a manner similar to its action upon chylomicrons. However, the endproduct of VLDL hydrolysis is IDL cholesterol which is one of the most atherogenic lipoprotein particles [22]. Drug therapy for elevated VLDL triglyceride levels are fibric acid derivatives and/or nicotinic acid [28]. However, nicotinic acid has been relatively contraindicated in patients with diabetes because of its ability to cause worsening of blood sugar control. The extent to which this occurs has however not been well established and data to the contrary have been advanced [29,30]. Gemfibrozil however, in the Helsinki Heart Study appeared to benefit diabetic patients more than other patients in a subgroup analysis, in which it was very effective in reversing dyslipidemia and reducing coronary events. The latter was not statistically significant owing perhaps to the small number of patients studied [31,32]. Effects of gemfibrozil alterations of glycemic control have been reported in some but not all studies [33-35].

Fibric acid derivatives however, tend to raise LDL cholesterol only if VLDL triglycerides are elevated [36,37]. This increase is thought to be transient and represents a reverse cholesterol transport augmentation. Some data also exists that this LDL increase occurs with other therapies used to lower TG and that this rise is transient [38,39]. The fact that insulin itself may be a major driving force of LDL turnover via LDL receptor activity might also explain this rise in LDL as insulin levels have been shown to fall after treatment with these hypolipidemic agents. Another possible factor is that modified LDL particles such as small dense LDL may be less effective inhibiting cholesterol synthesis [40].

There are limited reports of improved glucose metabolism and decreased insulin resistance associated with the use of these hypolipidemic agents [41]. The effect of both fibrates and nicotinic acid upon carbohydrate metabolism has, however, not been studied in detail, although a recent study from Sane et al. looked at insulin sensitivity and antilipolytic efficacy of insulin before and after treatment of mild hypertriglyceridemia in nondiabetic patients [42]. A comparison of the effects of gemfibrozil and simvastatin was reported recently in NIDDM patients. Insulin sensitivity was found to decrease to a similar degree with either agent [43]. Gemfibrozil increased FFA levels in this study but simvastatin did not. The authors did not have a clear explanation for the apparent effect upon the insulin sensitivity.

Evidence exists that elevated serum fatty acids can inhibit cellular glucose metabolism both short and long term [44]. Experimental data has however been contradictory which may be related to the findings of Kleiber et al. which indicated that ambient plasma NEFA concentrations had no direct effect upon glucose metabolism but that antecedent elevations did [45]. Controversial findings with other fibrates have been reported, where CHO metabolism and insulin sensitivity have been shown to improve along with lowering of FFA levels. A comparison with pravastatin was performed where an alteration of these parameters was not found [46].

Most cases of clinical hypertriglyceridemia are thought to involve both overproduction of VLDL in the liver and reduced lipolysis in the periphery. The dyslipidemia is therefore due more to endogenous disturbance of lipid metabolism then simply to overingestion. This may in fact explain the inadequate response to excellent dietary adherence where both saturated fat intake and total caloric intake are reduced. Such overproduction has been found to occur in NIDDM, obesity, diet, and alcohol overuse, as well as in genetic dyslipidemias. Reduced lipolysis occurs with NIDDM. The pharmacological agents that have been used to treat those abnormalities of triglyceride metabolism are thought to work predominantly through enhanced LPL activity (fibrates) or decreased hepatic VLDL production (niacin). Associated increases in both hepatic lipase and cholesteryl-ester transfer protein activity have also been reported with fibrates [47]. HMG-CoA reductase inhibitors have not been widely used in the treatment of the high triglyceride/low HDL cholesterol dyslipidemia in the past as their effect upon these dyslipidemic components has been of much less magnitude then the effects of fibrates and niacin. The use of HMG-CoA reductase inhibitors however has been found to be safe and without major effects upon glucose metabolism by many investigators [48-50]. Adverse effects upon glucose tolerance have not been found significant, (but see [43]), although there is a trend toward increased serum insulin with a lowering trend in glucose in one study [51]. The use of HMG-CoA reductase inhibitors in combination with other agents has increased as experience has accumulated on the safety and efficacy of such combinations for severe cases of combined lipid disturbances [52-54].

Postprandial triglyceride concentrations have been indicated as the best predictor of severity of coronary disease. Accentuation of large, triglyceride-rich particles is a component of the insulin resistant state. This includes both the maximal triglyceride increase and the magnitude of postprandial lipemia (area under the triglyceride curve over 8 hours after the meal). Single triglyceride levels at 6 and 8 hours were shown to be both the most discriminatory and accurate variables in predicting presence or absence of coronary artery disease [55,56]. The reported superior improvement in postprandial lipoprotein clearance with gemfibrozil therapy over lovastatin is therefore of major importance with regards to therapeutic treatment decision making [57]. The change from small dense LDL to large LDL particles that has been reported with niacin if triglyceride levels can be reduced below 140 mg/dl is also of great importance because of the very high risk of CAD contributed to such particles [3,58].

Because of the somewhat unclear association of mildly high triglyceride levels to cardiovascular events and the potential long-term adverse effects of the classical pharmaceutical approach upon overall survival, several points need to be explicitly kept in mind when therapeutic considerations are made. It has been shown that in a healthy population, as triglyceride levels increase to 1.134 mmol/l, (100 mg/dl), small dense LDL particles appear in the plasma and circulating levels of normal, native, larger, less atherogenic (pattern A) LDL decline. When the triglyceride levels reach 1.70 mmol/l (150 mg/dl), normal pattern A LDL is eliminated and only the small dense LDL particles are seen. A similar cumulative distribution curve can be drawn using HDL levels. If HDL declines below 1.03 mmol/l (40 mg/dl) small dense LDL particles appear and the normal LDL particles disappear [59,60]. It is also important to keep in mind that not all triglyceride elevations accelerate atherosclerosis and the treatment approach should be tailored to the risk of pancreatic disease in some clinical situations (triglyceride elevation associated with vegetarian diet, or secondary to estrogens, fibrin drugs, and the use of alcohol) [61].

In patients with diabetes, dyslipidemia is the most accurate predictor of CAD mortality. Therapies which improve triglycerides but worsen LDL cholesterol may not produce an overall beneficial outcome. Further research is needed.

References

1. Taskinen MR. Quantitative and qualitative lipoprotein abnormalities in diabetes mellitus. Diabetes 1992;41:12-17.
2. Musliner TA, Krauss RM. Lipoprotein subspecies and risk of coronary disease. Clin Chemistry 1988;34:B78-B83.
3. Krauss RM. Low-density lipoprotein subclass and risk of coronary artery disease. Current Op Lipidology 1991;2:248-52.
4. Suehiro T, Ohguro T, Sumiyoshi R, et al. Relationship of low-density lipoprotein particle size to plasma lipoproteins, obesity and insulin resistance in Japanese men. Diabetes Care 1995; 18:333-38.
5. Byrne CD, Wareham NJ, Brown DC, et al. Hypertriglyceridemia in subjects with normal and abnormal glucose tolerance: Relative contributions of insulin secretion, insulin resistance and suppression of plasma non-esterified fatty acids. Diabetologia 1994;37:889-96.

6. Laws A, Reaven GM. Evidence for an independent relationship between insulin resistance and fasting plasma HDL-cholesterol, triglyceride and insulin concentrations. J Int Med 1992; 231:25-30.
7. Reaven GM. Role of insulin resistance in human disease. Diabetes 1988;37:1595-1607.
8. Byrne CD, Wareham NJ, Brown DC, et al. Hypertriglyceridemia in subjects with normal and abnormal glucose tolerance: Relative contributions of insulin secretion, insulin resistance and suppression of plasma non-esterified fatty acids. Diabetologia 1994;37:889-96.
9. Ebenbichler CF, Kirchmair R, Egger C, Patsch JR. Postprandial state and atherosclerosis. Curr Op Lipidol 1995;6:286-90.
10. Assmann G, Schulte H. Relation of high density lipoprotein cholesterol and triglycerides to incidence of atherosclerotic coronary heart disease. (The PROCAM experience). Am J Cardiol 1992;70:733-37.
11. Ducimetere P, Eschwege E, Papoz L, Richard J, Claude G, Rosselin G. Relationship of plasma insulin levels to the incidence of myocardial infarction and coronary heart disease mortality in a middle-aged population. Diabetologia. 1980;19:205-10.
12. Gotto AM. Hypertriglyceridemia: Risks and perspectives. Am J Cardiol 1992;70:19H-25H.
13. Stout RW. Insulin and atherosclerosis. In: Stout RW, editor. Diabetes and atherosclerosis. Kluwer Academic Publishers: Dordrecht, The Netherlands, 1992:165-202.
14. Stein Y, Gotto AM, Jr. A symposium: Triglycerides as a vascular risk factor: A global forum. Introduction. Am J Cardiol 1992;70:1H-2H.
15. Cruz AB, Amatuzio DS, Grande F, Hay LJ. Effect of intra-arterial insulin on tissue cholesterol and fatty acids in alloxan diabetic dogs. Circ Res 1961;9:39-43.
16. Tomkin GH, Owens D. Insulin and lipoprotein metabolism with special reference to the diabetic state. Diabetes/Metabolism Reviews 1994;10:225-52.
17. Garg A, Helderman JH, Koffler M, et al. Relationship between lipoprotein levels and in vivo action in normal young white men. Metabolism 1988;37:982-87.
18. Abbott WGH, Lillioja S, Young AA, et al. Relationship between plasma lipoprotein concentrations and insulin action in an obese hyperinsulinemic population. Diabetes 1987;36: 897-904.
19. Laakso M, Sarlund H, Mykkanen L. Insulin resistance is associated with lipid and lipoprotein abnormalities in subjects with varying degrees of glucose tolerance. Arteriosclerosis 1990;10: 223-31.
20. Garcia-Webb P, Bonser AM, Whiting D, Masarei JRL. Insulin resistance: A risk factor for coronary heart disease? Scand J Clin Lab Invest 1983;43:677-85.
21. Stout RW. Hyperinsulinemia, dyslipidemia and atherosclerosis. In: Moller DE, editor. Insulin resistance. Baffins Lane: Chichester, 1993:355-85.
22. Chung BH, Segrest JP. Cytotoxicity of remnants of triglyceride-rich lipoproteins: An atherogenic insult. Adv Exp Med Biol 1991;285:341-51.
23. Beisiegel U, Weber W, Bengtsson-Olivera G. Lipoprotein lipase enhances the binding of chylomicrons to low density lipoprotein receptor related protein. Proc Natl Acad Sci USA 1991;1(88):8342-46.
24. Baynes C, Henderson V, Anyaoku V, et al. The role of insulin insensitivity and hepatic lipase in the dyslipidemia of type 2 diabetes. Diabetic Med 1991;8:560-66.
25. Moreton JR. Chylomicronemia, fat tolerance and atherosclerosis. J Lab Clin Med 1950;35: 373-84.
26. Gotto AM. Hypertriglyceridemia: Risks and perspectives. Am J Cardiol 1992;70:19H-25H.

27. Chen YD, Coulston AM, Zhou MY, et al. Why do low-fat high-carbohydrate diets accentuate postprandial lipemia in patients with NIDDM? Diabetes Care 1995;18:10-16.
28. Grundy SM, Vega GL. Two different views of the relationship of hypertriglyceridemia to coronary heart disease. Implications for treatment. Arch Dear Dr. Van Berkel:Intern Med 1992;152:28-34.
29. Parson WB Jr. Studies of niacin use in hypercholesterolemia. Arch Int Med 1961;107:653-67.
30. Dunn FL. Treatment of lipid disorders in diabetes mellitus. Med Clin N America 1988;72: 1379-98.
31. Frick MH, Elo O, Haapa K, et al. Helsinki Heart Study: Primary-prevention trial with gemfibrozil in middle-aged men with dyslipidemia. Safety of treatment, changes in risk factors, and incidence of coronary heart disease. NEJM 1987;317:1237-15.
32. Manninen V, Tenkanen L, Koskinen P, et al. Joint effects of serum triglyceride and LDL and HDL cholesterol concentration on coronary heart disease in the Helsinki Heart Study. Circulation 1992;85:37-45.
33. Konttinen A, Kuisma I, Ralli R, et al. The effect of gemfibrozil on serum lipids in diabetic patients. Ann Clin Res 1979;11:240-45.
34. Goldberg R, Labelle P, Zupkis R, Ronca P. Comparison of the effects of lovastatin and gemfibrozil on lipids and glucose control in non-insulin-dependent diabetes mellitus. Am J Cardiol 1990;66:16B-21B.
35. Wong TK, Nagi L, Levin SR, Hershman JM. Comparison of lipid-lowering agents in glipizide treated non-insulin dependent diabetic patients. Diabetes 1991;40(1):395A.
36. Schwandt P, Richter WO, Weisweiler P, Neureuther G. Cholestyramine plus pectin in treatment of patients with familial hypercholesterolemia. Atherosclerosis 1982;44:379-83.
37. Kesaniemi YA, Grundy SM. Influence of gemfibrozil and clofibrate on metabolism of cholesterol and plasma triglycerides in man. JAMA 1984;251:2241-47.
38. Morgan WA, Rosenstock J, Raskin P. A comparison of fish oil or corn oil supplements in hyperlipidemic subjects with NIDDM. Diabetes Care 1995;18:83-86.
39. Axelrod L. Perspectives in Diabetes; Omega-3 fatty acids in diabetes mellitus. Gift from the sea? Diabetes 1989;38:539-43.
40. Owens D, Maher V, Collins P, et al. Cellular cholesterol regulation - a defect in the type 2 (non-insulin-dependent) diabetic in poor metabolic control. Diabetologia 1990;33:93-99.
41. Mikhailidis DP, Mathur S, Barradas MA, Dandona P. Bezafibrate retard in type II diabetic patients. Effects on hemostasis and glucose homeostasis. J Cardiovasc Pharmacol 1990;16(9): 26-29.
42. Sane T, Knudsen P, Vuorinen-Markkola H, et al. Decreasing triglyceride by gemfibrozil therapy does not affect the glucoregulatory or antilipolytic effect of insulin in nondiabetic subjects with mild hypertriglyceridemia. Metabolism: Clinical & Experimental 1995;44:589-96.
43. Ohrvall M, Lithell H, Johansson J, Vesby B. A comparison between the effects of gemfibrozil and simvastatin on insulin sensitivity in patients with non-insulin-dependent diabetes mellitus and hyperlipoproteinemia Metabolism: Clinical and Experimental 1995;44:212-17.
44. Randle PJ, Priestman DA, Mistry S, Halsall A. Mechanisms modifying glucose oxidation in diabetes mellitus. Diabetologia 1994;37(2):s155-s161.
45. Kleiber H, Munger R, Jallut D, et al. Interaction of lipid and carbohydrate metabolism after infusion of lipids or lipid lowering agents: Lack of direct relationship between free fatty acid concentration and glucose disposal. Diabetes Metabolism, 1992;18:84-90.

46. Inoue I, Takahashi K, Katayama S, et al. Improvement of glucose tolerance by bezafibrate in non-obese patients with hyperlipidemia and impaired glucose tolerance. Diabetes Research and Clinical Practice 1994;25:199-205.
47. Kahri J, Vuorinen-Markkola H, Tilly-Kiesi M, et al. Effect of gemfibrozil on high density lipoprotein subspecies in non-insulin dependent diabetes mellitus. Relations to lipolytic enzymes and to the cholesteryl ester transfer protein activity. Atherosclerosis 1993;102:79-89.
48. Garg A, Grundy SM. Management of dyslipidemia in NIDDM. Diabetes Care 1990;13:153-69.
49. Raskin P, Ganda OP, Schwartz S, et al. Efficacy and safety of pravastatin in the treatment of patients with type I or type II diabetes mellitus and hypercholesterolemia. Am J Med 1995;99: 362-69.
50. Behounek BD, McGovern ME, Kassler-Taub KB, et al. A multinational study of the effects of low-dose pravastatin in patients with non-insulin-dependent diabetes mellitus and hypercholesterolemia. Clin Cardiol 1994;17:558-62.
51. McCrea JB, Fruncillo RJ, Holland SD, et al. Lovastatin does not affect oral glucose tolerance in hypercholesterolemic patients. J Clin Pharmacol 1993;33:581-85.
52. Glueck CJ, Oabes N, Speirs J, Tracy T, Lang J. Gemfibrozil-lovastatin therapy for primary hyperlipidemias. Am J Cardiol 1992;70:1-9.
53. Wiklund O, Angelin B, Bergman M, et al. Pravastatin and gemfibrozil alone and in combination for the treatment of hypercholesterolemia. Am J Med 1993;94:13-20.
54. Davignon J, Roederer G, Montigny M, et al. Comparative efficacy and safety of pravastatin, nicotinic acid and the two combined in patients with hypercholesterolemia. Am J Cardiol 1994;73:339-45.
55. Patsch JR, Miesenbock G, Hopferwieser T, et al. Relationship of triglyceride metabolism and coronary artery disease: Studies in the postprandial state. Arteriosclerosis Thromb 1992;12: 1336-45.
56. Davidson MB. Clinical implications of insulin resistance syndromes. Am J Med. 1995;99: 420-26.
57. Simo IE, Yakichuk JA, Ooi TC. Effect of gemfibrozil and lovastatin on postprandial lipoprotein clearance in the hypoalphalipoproteinemia and hypertriglyceridemia syndrome. Atherosclerosis 1993;100:55-64.
58. Superko HR, Krauss RM. Differential effects of nicotinic acid in subjects with different LDL subclass patterns. Atherosclerosis 1992;95:69-76.
59. Austin MA, King MC, Vranizan KM, Krauss RM. Atherogenic lipoprotein phenotype: A proposed genetic marker for coronary heart disease. Circulation 1990;82:495-506.
60. Austin MA, Breslow JL, Hennekens CH, et al. Low density lipoprotein subclass patterns and the risk of myocardial infarction. JAMA 1988;260:1917-20.
61. Castelli WP. Epidemiology of triglycerides: A view from Framingham. Am J Cardiol 1992;70:3H-9H.

HYPERINSULINEMIA (INSULIN RESISTANCE), PLASMA LIPIDS AND CORONARY HEART DISEASE

Tsuguhiko Nakai and Ryuichi Fujiwara
Third Department of Internal Medicine, Fukui Medical School, Matsuoka-Cho, Fukui Prefecture, 910-11, Japan

Introduction

We showed that plasma levels of apolipoprotein (apo) A-I and apo B are powerful discriminators in normolipidemic patients with coronary heart disease (CHD) and that the hyperinsulinemic response may indicate an enhanced susceptibility to CHD [1]. Several studies indicate that hyperinsulinemia and insulin resistance are associated with unfavorable changes in plasma lipid and lipoprotein concentrations characterized by elevated total and very low density lipoprotein (VLDL), triglycerides, and decreased high density lipoprotein (HDL) cholesterol [2,3]. Insulin resistance and compensatory hyperinsulinemia are potential risk factors for CHD as well as central components of a cluster of metabolic abnormalities accelerating the atherosclerotic process. However, the relationship between hyperinsulinemia and CHD varies among differing ages and degrees of glucose tolerance. We studied lipid and apolipoprotein levels and their association with postglucose challenge measures of insulinemia in angiographically assessed CHD patients of middle-aged and elderly men with varying degrees of glucose tolerance [4].

Methods

A coronary angiogram was recorded in 127 male subjects, including 41 with normal glucose tolerance, 41 with impaired glucose tolerance (IGT), and 45 with noninsulin-dependent diabetes mellitus (NIDDM). We determined the presence and severity of coronary arterial stenosis in the 15 segments of the artery designated by the American Heart Association. CHD was considered to be present if ≥ 1 lesions narrowed the lumen of any of the 15 arterial segments by > 75%. Patients with such lesions were considered to have CHD, whereas those without narrowing or with < 25% narrowing of the lumen were considered to have normal coronary arteries. Patients were divided into 2 groups according to the results of coronary angiography: the group with normal coronary arteries (n = 33) and the group with CHD (n = 94). The severity of atherosclerotic changes was also assessed by grading the stenotic lesions as follows: 0 = luminal reduction < 25%; 1 = luminal reduction

A. M. Gotto, Jr. et al. (eds.), Drugs Affecting Lipid Metabolism, 397–403.

of 25% to 50%; 2 = luminal reduction of 50% to 75%; 3 = luminal reduction of 75% to 90%; 4 = luminal reduction of 90% to 95%; 5 = luminal reduction of 95% to 99%; and 6 = total occlusion. The points used to grade each branch of the coronary artery were added and the coronary score was obtained. The total coronary score was used to reflect the severity of CHD. The diagnosis of diabetes mellitus and IGT was confirmed by a 2-hour oral glucose tolerance test (75 g of glucose) according to the World Health Organization Expert Committee on Diabetes Mellitus. Only diabetic patients with NIDDM and those treated only with diet were included in the study. Venous blood samples were collected for determination of blood glucose and plasma insulin levels before, and 30, 60, and 120 minutes after glucose ingestion. The glucose and insulin response to the glucose load was calculated as the sum of glucose values and the sum of plasma insulin levels during the test, respectively. The early responses of glucose and insulin to a glucose load were calculated as the differences between 0 and 30 minutes of glucose values and plasma insulin levels, respectively. The ratios of the insulin release to the glucose values for the corresponding periods of time were also calculated. Plasma lipoproteins and apolipoproteins were determined using plasma samples drawn after a 14-hour overnight fast. Plasma cholesterol and triglyceride concentrations were measured enzymatically. For HDL cholesterol determination, VLDL was first removed by ultracentrifugation at a density of 1.006 g/ml. Cholesterol concentration was measured enzymatically in the supernatant after precipitation of low density lipoprotein with sodium heparin and manganese chloride using the VLDL-free fraction. Plasma apo A-I and apo B levels were determined by single radial immuno-diffusion. Data are presented as mean $\pm$ SEM. Data were stored in a Statistical Analysis System database. Distributions of categorical data were compared using the chi-square test with Yates' correction. Group differences for continuous variables were evaluated by 2-tailed t tests. Correlations were calculated with Pearson's correlation coefficients. Stepwise multiple regression analysis was performed to analyze the independent relation of the risk factors to the coronary score. A p level < 0.05 was considered statistically significant.

Results

Characteristics of the study population are summarized in Table 1 [4]. The cumulative lifetime consumption of tobacco was significantly higher in the CHD group. The coronary score of the CHD group averaged 13.1 $\pm$ 1.4. Total cholesterol and triglyceride levels were significantly higher in subjects with than without CHD. Plasma concentration of HDL cholesterol in the CHD group was significantly lower than that in the normal group. Plasma apo B levels were significantly higher in the CHD than in the normal group, and plasma apo A-I levels were significantly lower in the CHD group. A hyperinsulinemic response to an oral glucose load was observed in subjects with CHD. In subjects with normal glucose tolerance, no significant differences in total cholesterol and triglyceride levels were observed between the 2 groups; however, HDL cholesterol and plasma apo A-I levels were significantly lower in the CHD than in the normal group. The plasma apo B level was significantly higher in the CHD group. The elevation of plasma insulin concentrations during the test period and the early phase of the glucose challenge were significantly higher in the

Table 1. Biochemical features of subjects studied.

	Coronary Arteries		
	Normal (n = 33)	Narrowed (n = 94)	p Value
Age (year)	59.8 ± 1.7	58.9 ± 1.0	0.648
Total Cholesterol (mg/dl)	167 ± 5	186 ± 3	0.0006
Triglycerides (mg/dl)	100 ± 4	118 ± 3	0.0007
HDL Cholesterol (mg/dl)	47 ± 2	36 ± 1	0.0001
Apolipoproteins			
A-I (mg/dl)	114 ± 4	88 ± 2	0.0001
B (mg/dl)	89 ± 3	117 ± 2	0.0001
Basal Plasma Glucose (mg/dl)	96 ± 2	97 ± 1	0.629
Basal Plasma Insulin (μU/ml)	9.4 ± 0.6	9.5 ± 0.4	0.896
Sum of Glucose Values (mg/dl)	628 ± 17	632 ± 11	0.850
Sum of Plasma Insulin Values (μU/ml)	152 ± 13	229 ± 10	0.0001

Values are expressed as mean ± SEM. HDL = high density lipoprotein.

CHD than in the normal group. In subjects with IGT, total cholesterol and triglyceride levels were significantly higher in subjects with than without CHD. The plasma concentration of HDL cholesterol in the CHD group was significantly lower than that in the normal group. The level of plasma apo A-I was significantly lower in the CHD than in the normal group, whereas the plasma apo B level was significantly higher in the CHD group. A hyperinsulinemic response to an oral glucose load was observed in subjects with CHD. The clinical and metabolic characteristics of the subjects with NIDDM showed that total cholesterol and triglyceride levels were higher in subjects with than without CHD. There were significant differences in the levels of HDL cholesterol, plasma apo A-I, and plasma apo B between the 2 groups. The CHD group had significantly higher insulinemic measures during the glucose challenge. To investigate the possibility that the relation between hyperinsulinemia and clinical features, lipid concentrations, and apolipoprotein concentrations could be curvilinear, we calculated the clinical and metabolic data in the tertiles of the sum of plasma insulin values during the test period of the glucose challenge. Tertiles were based on the sum of plasma insulin levels during the glucose challenge in all subjects with normal glucose tolerance, IGT, and NIDDM. Increasing tertiles of the sum of postglucose insulin levels were also associated with increases in total cholesterol, triglycerides, and apo B, and with reductions in HDL cholesterol and apo A-I. The relation between the sum of plasma insulin levels during the glucose challenge and abnormal lipid and apolipoprotein levels was positive and linear with respect to total cholesterol, triglycerides, and apo B levels, and negative and linear with respect to HDL cholesterol and apo A-I levels. Stepwise multiple linear regression analyses were performed to assess the contribution of plasma lipid and apolipoprotein concentrations, body mass index, and the sum of postglucose insulin values to the variation in coronary score. The analyses indicated that plasma apo A-I and apo B concentrations were more accurate predictors of coronary score than the corresponding levels of plasma lipids in this group of subjects.

Table 2 shows the metabolic data of the elderly men aged 65 to 80 years (n = 42).

Table 2. Biochemical features of elderly men.

	Coronary Arteries		
	Normal (n = 19)	Narrowed (n = 23)	p Value
Age (year)	69.5 ± 1.5	71.9 ± 1.3	0.233
Total Cholesterol (mg/dl)	145 ± 2	178 ± 6	0.0001
Triglycerides (mg/dl)	100 ± 3	124 ± 2	0.0001
HDL Cholesterol (mg/dl)	42 ± 1	36 ± 1	0.0001
Apolipoproteins			
A-I (mg/dl)	108 ± 1	76 ± 4	0.0001
B (mg/dl)	89 ± 2	106 ± 3	0.0002
Basal Plasma Glucose (mg/dl)	92 ± 1	89 ± 2	0.258
Basal Plasma Insulin (μU/ml)	9.1 ± 0.8	9.4 ± 0.7	0.784
Sum of Glucose Values (mg/dl)	602 ± 49	594 ± 61	0.647
Sum of Plasma Insulin Values (μU/ml)	137 ± 6	212 ± 69	0.0001

Values are expressed as mean ± SEM. HDL = high density lipoprotein.

There were no differences in the mean age, body mass index, the cumulative life consumption of tobacco, and the prevalence of hypertension between the 2 groups. Total cholesterol, triglyceride, and apo B levels were higher in men with than without CHD. The levels of HDL cholesterol and plasma apo A-I were significantly lower in the elderly with

CHD. The CHD group had a significantly higher insulinemic measures during the glucose challenge. Metabolic characteristics of the elderly men with varying degrees of glucose tolerance were compared. In each of the men with normal, IGT, and NIDDM, there were no significant differences in the mean age, body mass index, and the prevalence of hypertension between the men with CHD and those without CHD. The men with CHD had a significantly lower plasma level of HDL cholesterol, and apo A-I and higher levels of apo B than the normal group with normal glucose tolerance. The men with CHD had a significantly lower plasma levels of HDL cholesterol and plasma apo A-I than the men without CHD in patients not only with IGT but also with NIDDM. Both plasma total cholesterol and triglycerides levels were higher in the CHD group with either IGT or NIDDM than in the CHD group with normal glucose tolerance. Graded reduction in plasma apo A-I and graded increase in plasma apo B were observed with the change of glucose tolerance for the worse. The elderly men with CHD were remarkably similar in hyperinsulinemia to the middle-aged men with CHD independent of the glucose tolerance status. Stepwise multiple linear regression analyses were performed to assess the contribution of plasma lipid and apolipoprotein concentrations, body mass index, and the sum of postglucose insulin values to the variation in coronary score. The elderly had similar results of the multiple regression analyses as in the middle-aged men, indicating the independent effect of plasma levels of apo A-I and apo B on the severity of CHD.

Discussion

In the present study, we showed that postglucose hyperinsulinemia was associated with higher plasma total cholesterol, triglycerides, and apo B levels, and with lower HDL cholesterol and apo A-I levels in CHD patients of middle-aged and elderly men with varying degrees of glucose tolerance. The elderly are in general prone to glucose intolerance and diabetes as well as to CHD. Therefore, the study of coronary metabolic risk factors in the elderly is particularly important. Although aging is associated with glucose intolerance, little information about the relation of insulin levels and CHD in the elderly has been reported. One prospective study suggests that hyperinsulinemia is a predictor of CHD independent of blood pressure and total cholesterol levels in the elderly [5]. The present study demonstrated that hyperinsulinemia was related to the risk of CHD in the elderly and middle-aged men. Hyperinsulinemia may be associated with the development of compositional changes in lipids as well as with changes in absolute levels of lipids and apolipoproteins that predisposed toward coronary atherosclerosis independent of the glucose tolerance status in both middle-aged and elderly men. Hyperinsulinemia may contribute to the development of atherosclerosis via a number of plausible mechanisms [6]. There is substantial evidence that insulin may regulate the various arterial cell functions. Insulin has been shown to stimulate the DNA synthesis of vascular smooth muscle cells [7], to enhance LDL receptor activity [8], to augment endogenous lipid synthesis by vascular cells [9,10], and to promote collagen formation. Several mechanisms have been proposed to explain how hyperinsulinemia affects the metabolism of lipids and apolipoproteins. It has been demonstrated that hyperinsulinemia can induce an overproduction of triglyceride-rich

VLDL in the liver by increasing the availability of free fatty acids as precursors of *de novo* triglyceride synthesis [11,12]. In addition to increased synthesis, the rate of VLDL removal by peripheral tissues from the circulation can be reduced in subjects with hyperinsulinemia. The association between higher levels of apo B and hyperinsulinemia may also be explained by an increased hepatic secretion of apo B in response to insulin resistance [13,14]. In the case of HDL, hyperinsulinemia correlates with an increase in the fractional catabolic rate of iodine-125 apo A-I/HDL and a reduction of plasma HDL cholesterol concentration [15]. In addition, the low concentration of HDL cholesterol in hyperinsulinemia may be linked to low lipoprotein lipase activity, which seems to characterize insulin-resistant states [16]. One must consider that abnormalities in lipid and apolipoprotein concentrations impair the action of insulin. High concentrations of VLDL lead to an impairment of insulin action [17].

Conclusion

In conclusion, insulin resistance and hyperinsulinemia play a central role in the development of risk factors associated with coronary heart disease in both middle-aged and elderly men. Hyperinsulinemia may be associated with the development of compositional changes in lipids as well as changes in the absolute levels of lipids and apolipoproteins that predispose to coronary atherosclerosis, independent of glucose tolerance status in both middle-aged and elderly men.

Acknowledgement

This work was supported by a Grant-in-Aid for Scientific Research from the Ministry of Education, Science, and Culture of Japan.

References

1. Fujiwara R, Kutsumi Y, Hayashi T, et al. Metabolic risk factors in the normolipidemic male patients with angiographically defined coronary artery disease. Jpn Circ J 1990;54:493-500.
2. Orchard TJ, Becker DJ, Bates M, Kuller LH, Drash AL. Plasma insulin and lipoprotein concentrations: An atherogenic association? Am J Epidemiol 1983;118:326-37.
3. Modan M, Halkin H, Lusky A, Segal P, Fuchs Z, Chetrit A. Hyperinsulinemia is characterized by jointly disturbed plasma VLDL, LDL, and HDL levels. A population-based study. Arteriosclerosis 1988;8:227-36.
4. Fujiwara R, Kutsumi Y, Hayashi T, et al. Relation of angiographically defined coronary artery disease and plasma concentrations on insulin, lipid, and apolipoprotein in normolipidemic subjects with varying degrees of glucose tolerance. Am J Cardiol 1995;75:122-26.
5. Welborn TA, Weame K. Coronary heart disease and cardiovascular mortality in Busselton with reference to glucose and insulin concentrations. Diabetes Care 1979;2:154-60.
6. Stout RW. Insulin and atheroma. 20-yr perspective. Diabetes Care 1990;13:631-59.
7. Fujiwara R, Hayashi T, Nakai T, Miyabo S. Diltiazem inhibits DNA synthesis and Ca^{2+} uptake induced by insulin, IGF-I, and PDGF in vascular smooth muscle cells. Cardiovasc Drugs Ther 1994;8:861-69.

8. Young IR, Stout RW. Effect of insulin and glucose on the cells of the arterial wall: interaction of insulin with dibutyryl cyclic AMP and low-density lipoprotein in arterial cells. Diabetes Metab 1987;13:301-306.
9. Stout RW. The effect of insulin and glucose on sterol synthesis in cultured rat arterial smooth muscle cells. Atherosclerosis 1977;27:271-78.
10. Fujiwara R, Shimada A, Tamai T, Nakai T, Miyabo S. Effects of insulin, insulin-like growth factor-I, and phorbol esters on neutral cholesteryl esterase activity in cultured rat vascular smooth muscle cells. J Lab Clin Med 1995;126:240-49.
11. Steiner G, Vranic M. Hyperinsulinemia and hypertriglyceridemia: A vicious cycle with atherogenic potential. Int J Obes 1982;6:117-24.
12. Tobey TA, Greenfield M. Kraemer F, Reaven GM. Relationship between insulin resistance, insulin secretion, very low density lipoprotein kinetics and plasma triglyceride levels in normotriglyceridemic man. Metabolism 1981;30:165-71.
13. Dashti N, Wolfbauer G. Secretion of lipids, apolipoproteins, and lipoproteins by human hepatoma cell line, HepG2: effects of oleic acid and insulin. J Lipid Res 1987;28:423-26.
14. Dashti N, Williams DL, Alaupovic P. Effects of oleate and insulin on the production and cellular mRNA concentrations of apolipoproteins in HepG2 cells. J Lipid Res 1989;30:1365-73.
15. Golay A, Zech L, Shi MZ, Jeng CY, Chiou Y-AM, Chen Y-DI. Role of insulin in regulation of high density lipoprotein metabolism. J Lipid Res 1987;28:10-18.
16. Oida K, Nakai T, Hayashi T, Miyabo S, Takeda R. Plasma lipoproteins of monosodium glutamate-induced obese rats. Int J Obes 1984;8:385-91.
17. Bieger WP, Michel G, Barwich D, Biehl K, Wirth A. Diminished insulin receptors on monocytes and erythrocytes in hypertriglyceridemia. Metabolism 1984;33:982-87.

DIABETES AND ATHEROSCLEROSIS: THE DIABETES ATHEROSCLEROSIS INTERVENTION STUDY (DAIS)

George Steiner
DAIS Project Office and WHO Collaborating Center for the Study of Athersclerosis in Diabetes, The Toronto Hospital (General Division) and the University of Toronto, Toronto, Canada M5G 2C4

Atherosclerosis in Diabetic Populations

Atherosclerosis has been called the major complication of diabetes [1]. In Caucasians it accounts for two-thirds to three-quarters of the deaths occurring in diabetes. This is two to three times the number in similar nondiabetic populations [2-4]. The prevalence of peripheral arterial disease in diabetes is increased even more than that of coronary disease [3]. In those populations with a low incidence of atherosclerosis the absolute magnitude of the problem may be less; however, the frequency of such vascular disease in those with diabetes is still nearly double that seen in those without diabetes [5-7]. Hence, the association of atherosclerosis with diabetes exists across all racial and national groups.

The increase in coronary disease occurs whether the patient population has insulin dependent diabetes (IDDM) or noninsulin dependent diabetes (NIDDM) [4,8-10]. Nearly 80% of those with diabetes have NIDDM. Furthermore, populations with NIDDM are older than those with IDDM [11]. Hence, the number of patients with coronary disease and NIDDM is much greater than the number with coronary disease and IDDM.

Anything that can be done to diminish coronary atherosclerosis in those with diabetes, particularly NIDDM, will have a major health impact.

Atherogenic Factors in Diabetes

In attempting to reduce atherosclerosis in diabetes one should understand the factors that have been associated with atherogenesis, particularly those may be influenced by diabetes. They have been the subject of several reviews [1,12] and cover virtually every aspect of atherogenesis. Diabetes has been suggested to influence elements of vascular biology such as endothelial cell function and proliferation; abnormalities in blood clotting, both in the soluble and in the cellular elements that are involved; and stresses on the vessel walls that might result from hypertension and altered rheology. The resistance to insulin and hyper-insulinemia found in many with diabetes have also been suggested to increase

A. M. Gotto, Jr. et al. (eds.), Drugs Affecting Lipid Metabolism, 405–411.

atheroslcerosis, either directly or indirectly. Epidemiologic evidence about the association of hyperglycemia and atheroslcerosis is conflicting. However, glycemia could increase atherogenisis through glycation of a variety of proteins and through advanced glycation endproducts. Smoking and nephropathy both increase the risk of macrovascular disease in diabetic populations. Finally both quantitative and qualitative changes in lipoproteins that could lead to atherosclerosis are found in diabetes.

This paper will focus on the dyslipoproteinemias associated with diabetes. This is not to suggest that these are the only, or even the most important atherogenic factors in diabetes. However, as will be noted later, epidemiologic studies indicate that they are associated with a significant increase in the risk of diabetic patients for macrovascular disease.

Dyslipoproteinemias in Diabetes

The most frequently observed lipid abnormality in diabetes is hypertriglyceridemia [13]. This is mainly due to an increase in the number of small, dense (Sf 12-60) triglyceride-rich lipoproteins in the plasma [13]. In those without diabetes, mild and moderate hypertriglyceridemia also reflects an increase in the numbers of Sf 12-60 lipoprotein particles [14]. Increased levels of such small triglyceride-rich lipoproteins are associated with increased angiographically demonstrated coronary artery disease [15].

Levels of plasma cholesterol and low density lipoproteins (LDL) are not very different in diabetic populations from those in general populations [13]. However, there are some suggestions that improvement of glycemic control in diabetes is accompanied by a reduction in LDL levels [16]. Even though there may not be important quantitative differences in LDL concentrations between those with diabetes and those without, there are important qualitative difference in the LDL of those with diabetes. These include an increase in the oxidation of LDL [17], an increase in the glycation of LDL [18], and the presence of small, dense LDL [19]. All of these changes can increase the atherogenicity of this lipoprotein.

A variety of high density lipoprotein (HDL) changes have been reported in diabetes [20]. These may well reflect the coexisting plasma triglyceride levels, coexisting obesity, and the use of insulin in the management of the hyperglycemia.

The presence of hypertriglyceridemia may even precede the development of overt diabetes [21]. Hypertriglyceridemia is often observed together with the insulin resistance and hyperinsulinemia that are seen in the syndrome of insulin resistance [22]. Chronic hyperinsulinemia has been found both in animals and in humans to increase the production of triglyceride-rich lipoproteins [23-25]. This is in contrast to the acute response to insulin. In the latter situation triglyceride-rich lipoprotein production decreases. In part the acute response to insulin is due to an insulin-induced decline in the plasma concentration of free fatty acids and, in part, it may reflect a direct effect of insulin on very low density lipoprotein (VLDL) production [26].

The coronary risk impact of hypertriglyceridemia in diabetes has been suggested by the WHO Multinational Study [27] and by the Paris Prospective Study [28]. The consequences of hypercholesterolemia in diabetic individuals was indicated by the Multiple Risk Factor Intervention Trial [2]. Although plasma cholesterol levels in people with diabetes are similar to those in people without, that study showed that increasing cholesterol levels were accompanied by an increase in the incidence of coronary artery disease. The shape of the incidence versus cholesterol curve in those with diabetes was similar to that seen in those without diabetes. However, for any given cholesterol level, those with diabetes had a three- to four-times higher incidence of coronary artery disease.

Recommendation for the Treatment of Dyslipoproteinemias in Diabetes

Several groups, such as the American Diabetes Association [29], have suggested desirable levels for plasma lipids in diabetic patients. These are based on pathophysiologic rationale and on extrapolation from lipid lowering studies conducted with nondiabetic populations. In the case of LDL, these include clinical event studies, such as the Lipid Research Clinics - Coronary Primary Prevention Trial [30] and the 4S Study [31], as well as angiographic studies [32-34]. In the case of HDL, the major trial evidence is found in the Helsinki Heart Study [35]. In the case of triglycerides, there are no primary prevention trials. The trial data comes from secondary intervention studies [36] and from post hoc subgroup analyses [37].

There have been two intervention studies which did not set out to examine the lipid hypothesis in diabetes. However, as they included some diabetic individuals post hoc analyses have been conducted on their diabetic subgroups. These are the Helsinki Heart Study [38] and the 4S Study [39]. In the former, treatment with gemfibrozil was found to reduce plasma triglyceride levels and to increase plasma HDL levels. These changes were found in those with diabetes as in those without. In the diabetic population, as in the general population, there were fewer fatal and nonfatal myocardial infarctions in those treated with active gemfibrozil than in those treated with placebo. However, the groups were too small to show statistical significance. In the 4S Study individuals were treated with simvastatin or placebo. Plasma cholesterol levels declined in those treated with the active drug whether or not they had diabetes. Those with diabetes had fewer total coronary events. However, in contrast to the population without diabetes, there was no difference in mortality in those diabetic people treated with simvastatin versus those treated with placebo. This probably again reflects small diabetic populations. Furthermore, both of these studies suffer the problems that occur in post hoc subgroup analyses. Thus, to date, no study has been completed that was specifically designed to examine the effect of correcting dyslipoproteinemias on coronary disease in a diabetic population. Until this is done, we will not know for certain whether the treatment targets are justified, not justified, or perhaps even too high.

The Diabetes Atherosclerosis Intervention Study (DAIS)

Against this background, the World Health Organization asked a group of experts from universities in a number of countries to develop a protocol to test the lipid hypothesis in individuals with noninsulin dependent diabetes. The protocol which emerged was one which involved a double-blind randomized controlled trial in which the effects of treating dyslipoproteinemias in diabetes on the angiographic progression and/or regression of coronary disease would be examined. The group decided to use a drug versus placebo design and selected to use the 200 mg micronized form of fenofibrate as the active test drug. Laboratoires Fournier agreed to supply the drug and to underwrite the study.

The details of the protocol are the subject of a separate publication [40]. In summary, the study is recruiting men and women between the ages of 45 and 65 years who have noninslin dependent diabetes, who may or may not have had a prior coronary event, who have at least moderately controled glycemia, and who have moderate hyperlipidemia. Sample size calculations predicted that the study will need 260 participants to have a 90% power to detect a 0.15 mm difference in average mean segment diameter of the coronary arteries and for a 2.5% one-sided test of the hypothesis that active treatment with fenofibrate will be beneficial in terms of coronary artery disease. Randomization will continue until the end of 1995. At the time of writing (October 1995), 332 have been randomized in the eleven centers located in Europe and Canada. Randomization occurs by center, gender, and prior coronary intervention. During a baseline, prerandomization period all participants will be on the study diet which approximates an AHA step I diet that is adapted to the needs of a population with NIDDM. During this baseline period they will have to have glycemic control comparable to that which might be found in community medical practices and lipoprotein levles that are comparable to those that are found most frequently in diabetic populations: plasma triglyceride concentrations between 1.7 to 5.2 mmol/l with LDL-cholesterol concentrations not exceeding 4.5 mmol/l, or LDL-cholesterol concentrations between 3.5 to 4.5 mmol/l with plasma triglyceride concentrations not exceeding 5.2 mmol/l, or both of the above, plus a plasma cholesterol/HDL-cholesterol ratio not lower than 4. Prior to randomization, all participants have a coronary angiogram performed according to standardized protocol which must show at least one 15% narrowing of a coronary artery. A repeat angiogram performed according to the same protocol will be conducted after at least three years of active or placebo treatment. The equipment in all angiography units is regularly monitored and all angiograms are read in a blinded fashion at the Core Angiography Lab in Toronto. The biochemical determinations for the European clinics are conducted in a core laboratory located in Helsinki. Those for the Canadian clinics are performed at a core laboratory located in Vancouver. Both laboratories are standardized to the Canadian Reference Foundation and, through it, the lipoprotein determinations are standardized against the Centers for Disease Control. The Project Office is located at the University of Toronto and the data management occurs at the University of North Carolina.

References

1. Steiner G. Atherosclerosis, the major complication of diabetes. In: Vranic M, Hollenberg CH, Steiner G, editors. Comparison of type I and type II diabetes. New York: Plenum Publishing Corp., 1985:277-97.
2. Stamler J, Vaccaro O, Neaton JD, Wentworth D. Diabetes, other risk factors, and 12-yr cardiovascular mortality for men screened in the Multiple Risk Factor Intervention Trial.

Diabetes Care 1993;16:434-44.
3. Wilson PF, Kannel WB. Epidemiology of hyperglycemia and atherosclerosis. In: Ruderman N, Williamson J, Brownlee M, editors. Hyperglycemia, Diabetes and Vascular Disease. Oxford: Oxford University Press, 1992:21-29.
4. Haffner SM, Stern MP, Rewers M. Diabetes and atherosclerosis: Epidemiological considerations. In: Draznin B, Eckel RH, editors. Diabetes and atherosclerosis. Amsterdam: Elsevier Science Publishers, 1993:229-54.
5. Diabetes Drafting Group. Prevalence of small vessel and large vessel disease in diabetic patients from 14 centres: The World Health Organization Multinational Study of Vascular Disease in Diabetics. Diabetologia 1985;28:615-40.
6. Nelson RG, Sievers ML, Knowler WC, et al. Low incidence of fatal coronary heart disease in Pima Indians despite high prevalence of non-insulin-dependent diabetes. Circulation 1990;81:987-95.
7. Montour LT, Macaulay AC, Adelson N. Diabetes mellitus in Mohawks of Kahnawake, PQ: A clinical and epidemiologic description. Can Med Assoc J 1989; 141:549-52.
8. Moss SE, Klein R, Klein BEK. Cause-specific mortality in a population-based study of diabetes. Am J Public Health 1991;81:1158-62.
9. Krolewski AS, Kosinski EJ, Warram JH, et al. Magnitude and determinants of coronary artery disease in juvenile-onset insulin-dependent diabetes mellitus. Am J Cardiol 1987;59:750-55.
10. Pyorala K, Laakso M, Uusitupa M. Daibetes and atherosclerosis: An epidemiologic view. Diabetes Metab Rev 1987;3:463-24.
11. Warram JH, Rich SS, Krolewski AS. Epidemiology and genetics of diabetes mellitus. In: Kahn CR, Weir GC, editors. Joslin's Diabetes Mellitus 13th Ed. Philadelphia: Lea & Febiger, 1994:201-215.
12. Chait A, Bierman EL. Pathogenesis of macrovascular disease in diabetes. In: Kahn CR, Weir GC, editors. Joslin's Diabetes Mellitus 13th Ed. Philadelphia: Lea & Febiger, 1994:648-64.
13. Steiner G. The dyslipoproteinemias of diabetes. Atherosclerosis 1994;110 (Suppl):S27-S33.
14. Poapst M, Reardon M, Steiner G. Relative contribution of triglyceride-rich lipoproteins particle size and number of plasma triglyceride concentration. Arterioscler 1985;5:381-90.
15. Steiner G, Schwartz L, Shumak S, Poapst M. The association of increased levels of intermediate-density lipoproteins with smoking and with coronary artery disease. Circulation 1987;75:124-30.
16. Pietri A, Dunn FL, Raskin P. The effect of improved diabetic controlon plasma lipid and lipoprotein levels. A comparison of conventional therapy and continuous subcutaneous insulin infusion. Diabetes 1980;29:1001-1005.
17. Morel DW, Chisholm GM. Antioxidant treatment of diabetic rats inhibits lipoprotein oxidation and sytotoxicity. J Lipid RE 1989;30:1827-34.
18. Steinbrecher UP, Witztum JL. Glucosylation of low-density lipoprotein to an extent comparable to that seen in diabetes slows their catabolism. Diabetes 1984;33:130-34.
19. Feingold KR, Grunfeld C, Pang M, et al. LDL subcalss phenotypes and tirlgyceride metabolism in non-insulin dependent diabetes. Arterisclerosis Thrombosis 1992; 12:1496-1502.
20. Nikkila EA. High density lipoproteins in diabetes. Diabetes 1981;30(2):82-87.
21. Haffner SM, Stern MP, Hazuda HP, et al. Cardiovascular risk factors in confirmed prediabetics: Does the clock for coronary heart disease start ticking before the onset of clinical diabetes? JAMA 1990;263:2893-98.
22. Lewis G, Steiner G. Hypertirlgyceridemia and its metabolic consequences as a risk factor for

atherosclerotic cardiovascular disease (ASCVD) in noninsulin dependent diabetes mellitus (NIDDM). Diabetes Metabolism Revs; in press.
23. Streja DA, Marliss EB, Steiner G. The effects of prolonged fasting on plasma triglyceride kinetics in man. Metabolism 1977;26:505-16.
24. Steiner G, Haynes FJ, Yoshino G, Vranic M. Hyperinsulinemia and in vivo very-low-density lipoprotein-triglyceride kinetics. Am J Physiol 1984;246:E187-92.
25. Steiner G, Vranic M. Hyperinsulinemia and hypertriglyceridemia, a vicious cycle with atherogenic potential. Int J Obesity 1982;6(1):117-24.
26. Lewis GF, Uffelman KD, Szeto LW, Weller B, Steiner G. Interaction between free fatty acids and insulin in the acute control of very low density lipoprotein production in humans. J Clin Invest 1995;95:158-66.
27. West KM, Ahuja MMS, Bennett PH, et al. The role of circulating glucose and triglyceride concnetrations and their interactions with other "risk factors" as deter minants of arterial disease in nine diabetic population samples from the WHO Multinational Study. Diabetes Care. 1983;6:361-69.
28. Fontbonne A, Eschwege E, Cambien F, et al. Hypertriglyceridemia as a risk factor for coronary heart disease mortality in subjects with impaired glucose tolerance or diabetes. Results from an 11-year follow-up of the Paris Prospective Study. Diabetologia 1989;32:300-304.
29. American Diabetes Association Consensus Statemnet. Detection and management of lipid disorders in diabetes. Diabetes Care 1993;16(2):106-112.
30. Anonymous. The Lipid Research Clinics Coronary Primary Prevention Trial results. II. The relationship of reduction in incidence of coronary heart disease to cholesterol lowering. JAMA 1984;251:365-74.
31. Scandinavian Simvastatin Survival Study Group. Randomized trial of cholesterol lowering in 4444 patients with coronary heart disease: The Scandinavian Simvastatin Survival Study (4S). Lancet 1994;344:1383-89.
32. Brown BG, Hillger L, Zhao XQ, Poulin D, Albers JJ. Types of changes in coronary stenosis severity and their relative importance in overall progression and regression of coronary disease. Observations from the FATS Trial. Familial Atherosclerosis Treatment Study. Ann NY Acad Sci 1995;748:407-17.
33. Watts GF, Lewis B, Brunt JNH, et al. Effects on coronary artery disease of lipid-lowering diet, or diet plus cholestyramine, in the St Thomas' Atherosclerosis Regression Study (STARS). Lancet 1992;339:563-69.
34. Waters D, Higginson L, Gladstone P, et al. Effects of monotherapy with an HMG-CoA reductase inhibitor on the progression of coronary atherosclerosis as assessed by serial quantitative arteriography. The Canadian Coronary Atherosclerosis Intervention Trial. Circulation 1994;89:959-68.
35. Huttunen JK, Manninen V, Manttari M, Koskinen P, Romo M, Tenkanen L, Heinonen OP, Frick MH. The Helsinki Heart Study: Central findings and clinical implications. Ann Med 1991;23:155-59.
36. Carlson LA, Rosenhamer G. Reduction of mortality in the Stockholm Ischaemic Heart Disease Secondary Prevention Study by combined treatment with clofibrate and nicotinic acid. Acta Med Scand 1988;223:405-18.
37. Tenkanen L, Pietila K, Manninen V, Manttari M. The triglyceride issue revisited. Findings from the Helsinki Heart Study. Arch Intern Med 1994;154:2714-20.
38. Koskinen P, Manttari M, Manninen V, et al. Coronary heart disease incidence in NIDDM

patients in the Helsinki Heart Study Joint effects of serum triglyceride and LDL cholesterol and HDL cholesterol concentrations on coronary heart disease risk in the Helsinki Heart Study. Implications for treatment. Diabetes Care 1992;85: 37-45.

39. Pyorala K, Pedersen TR, Kjekshus J. The effect of cholesterol lowering with simvastatin on coronary events in diabetic patients with coronary heart disease. Diabetes 1995;44(1):35A

40. Steiner G, for the DAIS Project Group. The Diabetes Atherosclerosis Intervention Study (DAIS). A Study Conducted in Cooperation with the World Health Organization. Diabetologia; in press.

WHAT ARE CRITERIA FOR TREATMENT OF DYSLIPIDEMIA IN WOMEN?

John C. LaRosa
Tulane University Medical Center, 1430 Tulane Avenue, New Orleans, Louisiana 70112, USA

Introduction

Dyslipoproteinemia is prevalent in women as well as in men. In both, its consequences of premature atherosclerosis and coronary artery disease (CAD) morbidity and mortality are common. In the United States, as many women (about 250,000) die each year of heart attacks as do men. In fact, atherosclerosis in women is responsible each year for more death and disability than all forms of cancer combined.

Lipoprotein Risk Factors in Women

Until about age 55 (that is, until the postmenopause), low density lipoprotein (LDL) cholesterol levels are lower in women than in men. After age 55, the relationship is reversed. From then onward, women have higher levels than do men of the same age. These differences in later life may, in part, be related to the higher coronary mortality in younger hypercholesterolemic men, leaving those men with lower cholesterol levels in the older age groups. Even so, the postmenopausal rise in LDL is confirmed in longitudinal follow-up [1].

Coronary risk rises with increases in LDL levels and falls with increases in high density lipoprotein (HDL) levels, in women as well as in men [2]. There are, however, some quantitative differences. In women, HDL levels are not only higher throughout the lifespan, but HDL is a more potent predictor of risk than LDL, suggesting that HDL may function differently in women [3,4].

LDL does not predict risk in women as strongly as in men [2]. Studies in female primates have demonstrated that the presence of circulating estrogen interferes with LDL uptake in the arterial wall [5]. This may be related to the antioxidant properties of estrogen [6]. At any given level, therefore, LDL is probably less atherogenic in women than in men.

Because HDL comprises a greater fraction of total cholesterol in women than in men and is more protective, and because LDL is less potent, total cholesterol is a less reliable predictor of CAD risk in women [7]. It is erroneous, however, to conclude from this that lipoproteins are unimportant as risk factors in women. As in men, long-term follow-up shows that total cholesterol is a predictor of both CAD and total mortality risk in women

A. M. Gotto, Jr. et al. (eds.), Drugs Affecting Lipid Metabolism, 413–423.

[8].

In younger women as in men, triglyceride levels are not a statistically independent predictor of coronary risk when HDL and LDL are considered in multivariate analysis [9]. This is not the case in older, postmenopausal women, however, in whom triglycerides are an independent predictor of coronary risk [10]. This may not be a direct effect of triglycerides. High triglyceride levels are associated with the appearance of a small, dense, more easily oxidized form of LDL [11]. This form of LDL is more prominent in older women [12].

In cross-sectional studies, lipoprotein(a) [Lp(a)] appears to be a cardiovascular risk factor in both men and women [13,14]. Levels of Lp(a) are higher in women than in men throughout most of the lifespan, particularly in the postmenopausal period [15].

Nonpharmacologic Modifiers of Lipoproteins in Women

DIET

Dietary recommendations assume that men and women have equivalent responses [16]. Such an assumption may not be appropriate. Small-scale studies, mostly in premenopausal women, have suggested that women experience less lowering of both LDL and HDL when adhering to a low-cholesterol, low saturated-fat diet compared with men of the same age [17-19]. Whereas these studies involved small numbers of subjects, a large-scale study of 2,000 postmenopausal women (compared with men of comparable age) demonstrated a greater decline in LDL and triglyceride levels in men than in women, and a greater decline in HDL levels in women than in men, when all subjects followed a very low-fat diet [20]. Thus, although low-fat diets do not appear to be harmful in women, their effect is less dramatic than in men of the same age.

WEIGHT AND BODY FAT DISTRIBUTION

As with those involving dietary compositional change, studies of weight loss suggest that weight loss in women may not necessarily be associated with favorable changes in circulating lipoproteins. Indeed, in one study, lowered HDL levels were observed in women with the same degree of weight loss that, in the men in the study, was associated with an increase in HDL levels [21].

It is tempting to speculate that these different responses in diet and weight loss between men and women may be related to differences in body fat distribution. In men, fat accumulates in the "android" pattern - around the trunk - thereby increasing the waist-to-hip ratio. In most women, however, body fat is more likely to accumulate in the buttocks and thighs, the "gynecoid" pattern. Truncal fat in both men and women is correlated with increases in LDL, decreases in HDL, and an increased risk of coronary disease and total mortality [22,23].

It is likely that, in men, these adverse changes in CAD risk are in part, mediated by an increased insulin resistance and hyperinsulinemia. Relationships between truncal fat and these factors are not as well demonstrated in women [24], despite the fact that women with a tendency to distribute fat in the android pattern have higher levels of circulating testosterone [25]. Nevertheless, in women, as in men, truncal obesity is a potent predictor of mortality [26].

Levels of other endogenous estrogens may also be of importance. Adipose tissue synthesis of estrogen from androstenedione can serve as a source of estrogen in postmenopausal women [27]. Thus, the benefits of weight reduction in older women may be offset by the loss of estrogen-producing adipose tissue. As a result, expected increases in HDL and declines in LDL may be less prominent than in men. The precise relationships between total body fat, body fat distribution, gender, and endogenous hormones remain to be delineated.

EXERCISE

As with low-fat diets and weight reduction, exercise also appears to be more effective in raising HDL and lowering LDL in men than in women [28]. In addition, premenopausal women respond to exercise with lipoprotein changes that are smaller than those in older, postmenopausal women [29]. This implies that the higher level of endogenous estrogen in premenopausal women may be a modulator of these physiologic responses. The relationships between exercise, changes in total body fat and body fat distribution, and changes in endogenous hormone levels are incompletely understood.

DIABETES

Until reaching their 60s and 70s, nondiabetic women have lower rates of CAD than do nondiabetic men.

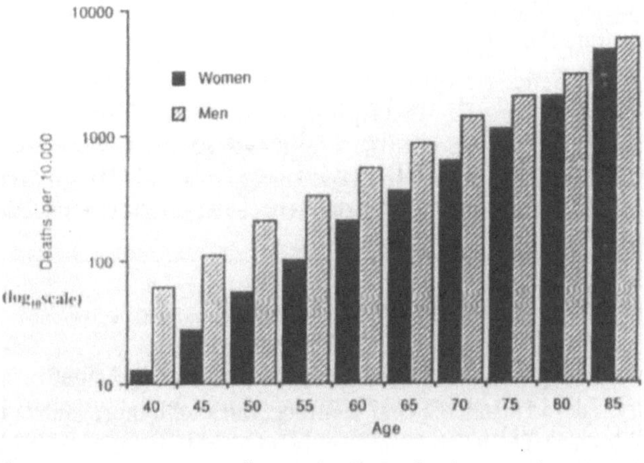

Figure l. Death due to coronary artery disease in the United States in 1986. (Reprinted with permission from [30]).

Diabetic men and women, however, have virtually the same rate of coronary disease.

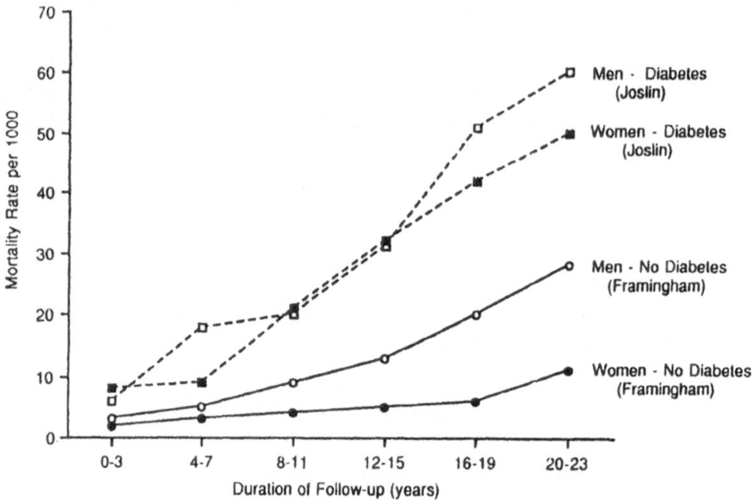

Figure 2. Coronary artery disease mortality and diabetes. (Reprinted with permission from *American Journal of Medicine Supplement* [31]).

One explanation for this adverse effect of diabetes in women is that diabetic women have greater and more adverse changes in their lipoprotein levels than do diabetic men. In some studies, LDL levels are higher in diabetic women than in diabetic men [31]. Other studies, however, demonstrate that diabetic women continue to have more favorable lipoprotein levels than do diabetic men [32]. In any case, the magnitude of the differences is insufficient to explain adequately the profound effect of diabetes in women. It appears, however, that circulating levels are not the whole explanation. Differences in coronary risk associated with declining levels of HDL and rising levels of LDL are greater in diabetic women than in diabetic men, again implying differences in lipoprotein functioning in women compared to men [33].

Oral Contraceptives, Lipoproteins, and CAD Risk

Studies of oral contraception have raised concern that their use might be associated with increased coronary risk [34]. Indeed, oral contraceptives with more androgenic progestins do raise LDL and lower HDL levels significantly, even in low dose forms [35,36]. Studies using those older contraceptives demonstrated greatly enhanced risk of myocardial infarction in women over 35 years of age, taking oral contraceptives, who also smoked [37].

Newer oral contraceptives, however, containing less androgenic progestins do not have these lipoprotein effects [38]. Follow-up studies for up to 12 years after cessation of oral contraceptive use (using older preparations) do not demonstrate increased risk of vascular disease [39]. Unless adverse effects take longer to be manifest, therefore, it seems unlikely that, in the absence of smoking, the effects of oral contraceptives on circulating lipoproteins have any long-term adverse effects on heart disease risk.

Postmenopausal Hormone Replacement, Lipoprotein, and CAD Risk

In numerous cohort studies of postmenopausal women, unopposed estrogen has been associated with a dramatically lowered risk of both CAD and all-cause mortality [40]. Unopposed estrogen has favorable effects on lipoproteins, lowering LDL and raising HDL. When progestins are added, the HDL-raising effect is lost with medroxyprogesterone, although not with micronized progesterone. LDL-lowering, however, is not affected [41]. In one cohort study, estrogen alone or combined with progestin was associated with a lower risk of nonfatal myocardial infarction [42,43].

Which of these beneficial effects are related to favorable lipoprotein changes is uncertain. Estrogen alone or in combination with progestin has other favorable effects. Both exogenous estrogen usage and estrogen/progestin combinations, as well as tamoxifen, have been shown to lower Lp(a) levels [44-46]. In addition, estrogen lowers fibrinogen levels [41], inhibits acetylcholine-induced vasospasm in the area of atheroma [47], interferes with platelet aggregation [48], and, as noted, interferes with LDL arterial wall uptake.

Treatment of Lipoprotein Disorders in Women

Evidence of Benefit in Women

As lipoprotein metabolism is not identical in women and men, it is not unreasonable to ask whether cholesterol lowering has the same importance in preventing CAD in women. Critics contend that there are insufficient clinical trial data to justify cholesterol-lowering interventions in women since most cholesterol-lowering studies were done with men. On the other hand, the available data indicate that cholesterol lowering is important in both women and men. In the Newcastle [49], Edinburgh [50], and Finnish [51] Mental Hospital studies, all of which were carried out in the 1960s and early 1970s, both men and women were included and the gender-specific data analyzed separately. A meta-analysis of these three studies [52] demonstrated that equivalent cholesterol-lowering in women and men was associated with equivalent reductions in coronary death rates. Aggressive LDL cholesterol lowering and HDL cholesterol raising in severely hypercholesterolemic men and women [53] has been shown to inhibit progression of CAD and induce regression of coronary disease in both sexes. Finally, in the recently completed Scandinavian Simvastatin Survival Study (4S), women had the same decline in overall coronary event rate as men with equivalent LDL cholesterol-lowering. There were insufficient women in the study to observe any effect on overall mortality rates, which declined significantly in men [54].

Current Guidelines for Treatment of Lipoprotein Disorders in Women

Guidelines for the detection, evaluation, and treatment of hypercholesterolemia and related disorders have been developed by the National Cholesterol Education Program (NCEP) [16]. These guidelines recommend that LDL be the primary target of intervention but that total and HDL cholesterol be the primary screening parameters. Table 1 lists the NCEP definitions of normal total and LDL cholesterol levels [16]. These were not considered to be different in women compared with men. However, HDL cholesterol is not considered a primary target for intervention. Individuals with low levels of HDL (defined in the guidelines as < 35 mg/dL [0.9 mEq/L]) are considered to have an additional risk factor.

Table 1. National Cholesterol Education Program categories for total and low-density lipoprotein (LDL) cholesterol.

	Total Cholesterol	LDL Cholesterol
Normal	< 200 mg/dL (5.2 mEq/L)	< 130 mg/dL (3.4 mEq/L)
Borderline	200-239 mg/dL (5.2-6.2 mEq/L)	130-159 mg/dL (3.4-4.1 mEq/L)
High	> 240 mg/dL (> 6.2 mEq/L)	> 160 mg/dL(> 4.1 mEq/L)

Drug Therapy Guidelines:

Those with LDL > 190 mg/dL (4.9 mEq/L) after trial of diet.
Those with LDL > 160 mg/dL (4.1 mEq/L) after trial of diet if CAD is present or in the presence of two (women) or one (men) other risk factor(s).

CAD = coronary artery disease; from Ref. 16.

Triglycerides are not addressed in depth in these guidelines. When triglyceride levels are > 200 mg/dL [2.3mEq/L], hygienic therapeutic intervention is recommended, including diet, weight loss, and exercise. Drugs to lower triglyceride levels are recommended only if other lipoprotein abnormalities are present; for example, if LDL levels are also high, if HDL is low, if triglycerides are very high (> 1,000 mg/dL [11.4 mEq/L]), or if there is a personal or family history of CAD or other manifestations of atherosclerosis.

Selection of both men and women for evaluation beyond total cholesterol and HDL measurement is limited to those with cholesterol levels > 240 mg/dL (6.2 mEq/L), or screening cholesterol levels of 200-239 mg/dL (5.2-6.2 mEq/L) and established coronary disease or other risk factors. Similarly, subjects with LDL levels > 190 mg/dL (4.9 mEq/L), or between 160 and 190 mg/dL (4.1-4.9 mEq/L), in the presence of established disease or other risk factors, are candidates for drug therapy.

Other risk factors indicating a requirement for full lipoprotein evaluation include age (men > 45, women > 55), gender, cigarette smoking, hypertension, diabetes, HDL < 35 mg/dL (0.9 mEq/L), or a family history of coronary disease.

The major difference when applying these guidelines to men compared with women is the awareness that men develop CAD at an earlier age and therefore should be considered candidates for more intensive interventions at age > 45, whereas in women, risk increases at age > 55. In this way, the guidelines account for the fact that the risk of coronary disease is lower in women than in men throughout most of their lifespan and that drug intervention in particular should be more limited in women than in men. In addition, the guidelines set higher LDL thresholds for drug intervention in premenopausal women (LDL > 220 mg/dL [5.7 mEq/L] than in postmenopausal women (LDL > 190 mg/dL [4.9 mEq/L]).

Table 2. Unique NCEP guidelines for women.

Screening	Total cholesterol and HDL > 20y/o
Age	> 55y/o a risk factor
LDL Cutpoint for Drugs	> 220 mg/dL (5.7 mEq/L) before menopause
	> 190 mg/dL (4.9 mEq/L) after menopause
Drugs	ERT as intermediate between diet and hypolipidemic drugs

ERT = estrogen replacement therapy; from Ref. 16.

Coronary disease is the most common form of death and disability in women as well as in men. No algorithm, however, can substitute for physician judgment. Diabetic women, for example, have the same risk of CAD as diabetic men and, therefore, it may be appropriate to initiate drug therapy in a premenopausal diabetic woman.

As already noted, there is reason to expect a lesser response to diet in women than in men. There is no reason, however, to expect that drug therapy will be less effective in women than in men. Indeed, in the regression study involving hypercholesterolemic men and women mentioned previously [53], and in the 4S [54], LDL decreases and HDL increases were virtually identical in woman compared with men.

A unique aspect of lipoprotein management in women, however, may be estrogen replacement therapy (ERT). ERT is viewed in the NCEP guidelines as an intermediate therapy between diet and lipid-lowering drugs for hypercholesterolemic, postmenopausal women, as estrogen tends to lower LDL and raise HDL levels. These recommendations are based on prospective population studies [40]. Clinical trials that clearly demonstrate the benefits (and perhaps the drawbacks) of ERT on coronary morbidity and mortality, and indicate the most beneficial hormone regimen(s), have not yet been done.

Summary

Lipoprotein disorders occur in women as well as in men. Moreover, they result in an increase in CAD risk in both sexes. There are differences, however. In women, HDL levels are a better predictor of coronary risk than in men, and triglyceride levels appear to be a better independent predictor of risk in postmenopausal women than in men of the same age. It appears, therefore, that LDL is a less important risk factor in women, perhaps because estrogen protects the arterial wall against LDL deposition. Clinical trial evidence of the benefit of cholesterol lowering in women is scarce. Available evidence, however, indicates that alterations in circulating lipoproteins are beneficial in preventing CAD in women as well as in men.

Postmenopausal hormone replacement therapy (HRT) has the potential to modify lipoprotein levels and, therefore, coronary risk, in women. Available cohort studies indicate that HRT lowers CAD risk.

Current guidelines for the detection and treatment of lipoprotein abnormalities set higher thresholds for lipoprotein evaluations in hypercholesterolemic women and higher thresholds for drug treatment of women who have raised levels of LDL. They do not, however, exclude women from cholesterol detection, evaluation, or treatment. For women as well as men, treatment of hypercholesterolemia is an important step in lowering the risk of CAD.

References

1. Matthews KA, Meilahn E, Kuller LH, Kelsey SF, Caggiula AW, Wing RR. Menopause and risk factors for coronary heart disease. N Engl J Med 1989;321: 641-46.
2. Eaker ED, Castelli WP. Coronary heart disease and its risk factors among women in the Framingham Study. In: Eaker ED, Packard B, Wenger N, et al, editors. Coronary Heart Disease in Women. New York: Haymarket Doyma, 1987:122-30.
3. Gordon DJ, Probstfield JL, Garrison RF, et al. High-density lipoprotein cholesterol and cardiovascular disease: Four prospective studies. Circulation 1989;79:8-15.
4. Bass KM, Newschaffer CJ, Klag MJ, Bush TL. Plasma lipoprotein levels as predictors of cardiovascular death in women. Arch Intern Med 1993;153:2209-16.
5. Wagner JD, Clarkson TB, St Clair RW, Schwenke DC, Adams MR. Estrogen replacement therapy (ERT) and coronary artery (CA) atherogenesis in surgically postmenopausal cynomolgus monkeys. (abstract) Circulation 1989;80(II):331.
6. Rifici VA, Khachadurian AK. The inhibition of low-density lipoprotein oxidation by 17-β estradiol. Metabolism 1992;41:1110-14.
7. Jacobs D, Blackburn H, Higgins M, et al. Report of the conference on low blood cholesterol: mortality associations. Circulation 1992;86:1046-60.
8. Knapp RG, Sutherland SE, Keil JE, Rust PF, Lackland DT. A comparison of the effects of cholesterol on CHD mortality in black and white women: Twenty-eight years of follow-up in the Charleston Heart Study. J Clin Epidemiol 1992;45:1119-29.
9. Austin MA. Epidemiologic associations between hypertriglyceridemia and coronary heart disease. Semin Thromb Hemost 1988;14:137-42.
10. Castelli WP. The triglyceride issue: a view from Framingham. Am Heart J 1986;112: 432-37.

11. de Graaf J, Hak-Lemmers HLM, Hectors MPC, et al. Enhanced susceptibility to in vitro oxidation of the dense low-density lipoprotein subfraction in healthy subjects. Arteriosclerosis 1991;11:298-306.
12. Campos H, McNamara JR, Wilson PWF, Ordovas JM, Schaefer EJ. Differences in low-density lipoprotein subfractions and apolipoproteins in premenopausal and postmenopausal women. J Clin Endocrinol Metab 1988;67:30-35.
13. Dahlen GH. Incidence of Lp(a) lipoprotein among populations. In: Scanu AM, editor. Lipoprotein(a). New York: Academic Press, 1990:151-73.
14. Sandkamp M, Assmann G. Lipoprotein(a) in PROCAM participants and young myocardial infarction survivors. In: Scanu AM, editor. Lipoprotein(a). New York: Academic Press, 1990:205-209.
15. Utermann G. The mysteries of lipoprotein(a). Science 1989;246:904-10.
16. Expert Panel on Detection, Evaluation, and Treatment of High Blood Cholesterol in Adults. Summary of the second report of the National Cholesterol Education Program (NCEP) expert panel on detection, evaluation, and treatment of high blood cholesterol in adults (Adult Treatment Panel II). JAMA 1993;269:3015-23.
17. Mensink RP, Katan MB. Effect of monounsaturated fatty acids versus complex carbohydrates on high-density lipoproteins in healthy men and women. Lancet 1987;1(8525):122-5.
18. Masarei JRL, Rouse IL, Lynch WJ, Robertson K, Vandongen R, Beilin LJ. Effects of a lacto-ovo vegetarian diet on serum concentration of cholesterol, triglyceride, HDL-C, HDL_2-C, HDL_3-C, apoprotein-B, and Lp(a). Am J Clin Nutr 1984;40:468-78.
19. Ernst N, Fisher M, Bowen P, Schaefer EJ, Levy RI. Changes in plasma lipids and lipoproteins after a modified fat diet. Lancet 1980;2(8186):111-3.
20. Barnard RF. Effects of life-style modification on serum lipids. Arch Intern Med 1991;151:1389-94.
21. Brownell KD. Differential changes in plasma high-density lipoprotein-cholesterol levels in obese men and women during weight reduction. Arch Intern Med 1981; 141:1142-6.
22. Soler JT, Folsom AR, Kushi LH, Prineas RJ, Seal US. Association of body fat distribution with plasma lipids, lipoproteins, apolipoproteins A-1 and B in postmenopausal women. J Clin Epidemiol 1988;41:1075-81.
23. Lapidus L, Bengtsson C, Larsson B, Pennert K, Rybo E, Sjostrom L. Distribution of adipose tissue and risk of cardiovascular disease and death: A 12-year follow-up of participants in the population study of women in Gothenburg, Sweden. BMJ 1984;289:1257-61.
24. Donahue RP, Orchard TJ, Becker DJ, Kuller LH, Drash AL. Physical activity, insulin sensitivity, and the lipoprotein profile in young adults: The Beaver County study. Am J Epidemiol 1988;127:95-103.
25. Hauner H, Ditschuneit HH, Pal SB, Moncayo R, Pfeiffer EF. Fat distribution, endocrine and metabolic profile in obese women with and without hirsutism. Metabolism 1988;37:281-86.
26. Folsom AR, Kaye SA, Sellers TA, et al. Body fat distribution and 5-year risk of death in older women. JAMA 1993;269:483-87.
27. Grodin JM, Siiteri PK, MacDonald PC. Source of estrogen production in postmenopausal women. J Clin Endocrinol Metab 1973;36:207-14.
28. Lokey EA, Tran ZV. Effects of exercise training on serum lipid and lipoprotein concentrations in women: A meta-analysis. Int J Sports Med 1989;10:424-29.
29. Hartung GH, Moore CE, Mitchell R, Kappus CM. Relationship to menopausal status and exercise levels to HDL cholesterol in women. Exp Aging Res 1984;10: 13-18.
30. Bush TL. The epidemiology of cardiovascular disease in postmenopausal women. Ann NY

Acad Sci 1990;592:263-71.
31. Krolewski AS, Warram JH, Valsania P, Martin BC, Laffel LMB, Christlieb AR. Evolving natural history of coronary artery disease in diabetes mellitus. Am J Med 1991;90(2A):56-61.
32. Ikeda T, Terasawa H, Ishimnyura M, et al. Sex differences in plasma cholesterol and apolipoprotein B levels in nonobese type 2 diabetic subjects. Diabete Metab 1992; 18:465-67.
33. Goldschmid MG, Barrett-Connor E, Edelstein SL, Wingard DL, Cohn BA, Herman WH. Dyslipidemia and ischemic heart disease mortality among men and women with diabetes. Circulation 1994;89:991-97.
34. Thorogood M. Oral contraceptives and cardiovascular disease: An epidemiologic review. Pharmacoepidemiol and Drug Saf 1993;2:3-16.
35. Lipson A, Stoy DB, LaRosa JC, et al. Progestins and oral contraceptive-induced lipoprotein changes: A prospective study. Contraception 1986;34:121-34.
36. Notelovitz M, Feldman EB, Gillespy M, Gudat J. Lipid and lipoprotein changes in women taking low-dose, triphasic oral contraceptives: a controlled, comparative, 12-month clinical trial. Am J Obstet Gynecol 1989;160:1269-80.
37. Rosenberg L, Kaufman DW, Helmrich SP, et al. Myocardial infarction and cigarette smoking in women younger than 50 years of age. JAMA 1985;253:2965-69.
38. Speroff L, DeCherney A, Burkman RT Jr, et al. Evaluation of a new generation of oral contraceptives. Obstet Gynecol 1993;81:1034-47.
39. Colditz GA for The Nurses' Health Study Research Group. Oral contraceptive use and mortality during 12 years of follow-up: The Nurses' Health Study. Ann Intern Med 1994;120:821-26.
40. Henderson BE, Paganini-Hill A, Ross RK. Risk factors for coronary artery disease. Arch Intern Med 1991;151:75-78.
41. The PEPI Investigators. Effects of estrogen or estrogen/progestin regimens on heart disease risk factors in postmenopausal women: The Postmenopausal Estrogen/ Progestin Interventions (PEPI) Trial. JAMA 1995;273:199-208.
42. Falkeborn M, Persson I, Adami H-O, et al. The risk of acute myocardial infarction after oestrogen and oestrogen-progestogen replacement. Br J Obstet Gynaecol 1992;99:821-28.
43. Psaty BM, Heckbert SR, Atkins D, et al. The risk of myocardial infarction associated with the combined use of estrogens and progestins in postmenopausal women. Arch Intern Med 1994;154:1333-39.
44. Kim CJ, Jang HC, Min YK. Hormone replacement therapy lowers the plasma concentration of lipoprotein(a) in postmenopausal women. (abstract) Circulation 1992;86(l):866.
45. Shewmon DA, Stock JL, Heiniluoma KM, Arpano M, Ukena TR, Weale VW. Tamoxifen lowers Lp(a) in males with heart disease. (abstract) Circulation 1992;86 (I):338.
46. Soma MR, Osnago-Gadda I, Paoletti R, et al. The lowering of lipoprotein(a) induced by estrogen plus progesterone replacement therapy in postmenopausal women. Arch Intern Med 1993;153:1462-68.
47. Lieberman EH, Gerhard M, Yeung AC, et al. Estrogen improves coronary vasomotor responses to acetylcholine in post menopausal women. (abstract) Circulation 1993;88:I-79.
48. Bar J, Tepper R, Fuchs J, Pardo Y, Goldberger S, Ovadia J. The effect of estrogen replacement therapy on platelet aggregation and adenosine triphosphate release in postmenopausal women. Obstet Gynecol 1993;81:261-64.
49. Group of physicians of the Newcastle-upon-Tyne region. Trial of clofibrate in the treatment of ischemic heart disease. BMJ 1971;4:767-75.
50. Research Committee of the Scottish Society of Physicians. Ischaemic heart disease: A

secondary prevention trial using clofibrate. BMJ 1971;4:775-84.
51. Miettinen M, Turpeinen O, Karvonen MJ, Elosuo R, Paavilainen E. Effect of cholesterol-lowering diet on mortality from coronary heart-disease and other causes. Lancet 1972;2:835-38.
52. Rossouw JF. International trials. Cholesterol and heart disease in older persons and in women. (abstract) National Heart, Lung, & Blood Institute, National Institutes of Health, Bethesda, MD:1990.
53. Kane JP, Malloy MJ, Ports TA, Phillips NR, Diehl JC, Havel RJ. Regression of coronary atherosclerosis during treatment of familial hypercholesterolemia with combined drug regimens. JAMA 1990;264:3007-12.
54. Scandinavian Simvastatin Survival Study Group. Randomised trial of cholesterol lowering in 4444 patients with coronary heart disease: The Scandinavian Simvastatin Survival Study (4S). Lancet 1994;344:1383-89.

TREATMENT OF HYPERLIPIDEMIA IN WOMEN

Nanette K. Wenger
Division of Cardiology, Department of Medicine, Emory University School of Medicine, 69 Butler Street, SE, Atlanta, Georgia 30303, USA

Coronary Heart Disease in Women: The Importance of Preventive Interventions

Coronary heart disease is the leading cause of mortality and disability in U.S. women as well as in men, although women develop clinical manifestations of coronary disease on average 10 years later [1]. In the U.S., more women than men currently die each year from coronary heart disease [2], and coronary heart disease is likely to engender greater morbidity and mortality in women as the U.S. population ages, owing to the female predominance at elderly age.

In addition to accounting for about 250,000 deaths annually in U.S. women, coronary heart disease in women entails a direct health care cost of $11 billion annually, and a total economic cost approximating $22 billion [3,4]. The substantial age dependency of the occurrence of coronary heart disease in women is evident in that 1 in 9 women aged 45 to 64 years has clinical manifestations of coronary heart disease, in contrast to 1 in 3 women older than 65 years of age. That coronary heart disease engenders substantial morbidity as well is emphasized by the identification that 36% of women in the 55- to 64-year age group with coronary disease are disabled by symptoms of their illness, with the percentage disabled rising to more than 55% in women older than 75 years of age.

Additionally, once clinical manifestations of coronary heart disease appear, the outcomes for women are less favorable than for their male counterparts. Based on data from the Myocardial Infarction Triage and Intervention (MITI) Registry [5], hospital mortality in women with myocardial infarction approximates 16%, as compared with 11% for men. Women also have a greater one-year mortality following myocardial infarction than do men, with an earlier and more frequent recurrence of infarction [6,7], and more postinfarction angina as well. Potential contributors [8] include the lesser utilization of thrombolytic therapy; suboptimal application of other medical therapies, in that many drugs traditionally used for women have not been appropriately evaluated in populations of women; lesser referral to cardiac rehabilitation services following a coronary event [9]; and, until recent years, lesser use of risk stratification procedures during the hospitalization for myocardial infarction and consequent lesser referral for myocardial revascularization when appropriate [10].

A. M. Gotto, Jr. et al. (eds.), Drugs Affecting Lipid Metabolism, 425–438.

Women who undergo coronary artery bypass graft surgery have twice the hospital mortality described for men [11]. Data from the MITI Registry document a 13% hospital mortality for women versus 6.5 % for men with coronary artery bypass surgery [5,12]. Further, they have lesser graft patency, less symptomatic relief, and more reoperation within the initial 5 years following coronary artery bypass graft surgery. However, for women who survive the hospital stay, their 5-, 10-, and now 15-year survival is comparable to that for men.

Contemporary percutaneous transluminal coronary angioplasty has comparable procedural success and safety for both genders [13]. However, women obtain less symptomatic relief and their long-term survival is less favorable, at least in part related to their older age. The newer transcatheter revascularization procedures have a lesser success rate for women and a higher complication rate, both potentially related to the larger size of these new devices relative to the smaller coronary artery size of women than of men [14].

It remains uncertain whether the less successful myocardial revascularization for women reflects their older age; their comorbidity, particularly diabetes and hypertension; or that more of these procedures are performed on an urgent or emergency basis for more severe and unstable angina [15]; or a combination of these factors.

The unfavorable clinical outcomes once coronary heart disease becomes manifest highlight the need for preventive interventions. Rather than, to paraphrase a Broadway musical, asking "Why can't a woman be more like a man?", the challenge is to identify the features unique to women and to explore how these unique features warrant unique interventions.

Hyperlipidemia in Women: Clinical Implications

Although hyperlipidemia is associated with premature atherosclerosis and increased coronary morbidity and mortality in women as in men, and cholesterol-lowering in women is associated with comparable benefits to those in men, a number of characteristics of lipoprotein risk factors are specific for women. Low levels of high density lipoprotein cholesterol (HLD-C) are more potent predictors of risk for women than for men [16], with elevated low density lipoprotein cholesterol (LDL-C) levels less so [17]. Because of the lesser predictive value of LDL cholesterol in women than in men, total cholesterol level also less reliably predicts coronary risk [18]. Nevertheless, total cholesterol levels predict both coronary and total mortality in both genders. Data regarding the association of triglycerides and coronary heart disease are inconsistent. Elevated triglyceride levels have been described as a significant independent predictor of coronary risk for postmenopausal women [19], although studies do not uniformly support this postulate [20]. However, the combination of hypertriglyceridemia and low levels of HDL cholesterol appear to impart greater risk for women than for men, with HDL cholesterol levels below 45 mg/dl being a high-risk characteristic for women. Low HDL cholesterol continues to predict mortality even at elderly age [21].

Women have higher HDL cholesterol levels than do men across the life span, with an only modest decrease in HDL levels at menopause. On the other hand, LDL cholesterol levels are lower in women than in men until the menopausal years but rise sharply thereafter at least to age 70 years, such that, at older age, women have higher levels of LDL cholesterol than do comparably aged men [22]. Reduced activity of LDL receptors has been postulated as a major explanation for the hypercholesterolemia of postmenopausal women [23]; thus agents that increase LDL receptor activity such as the HMG-CoA reductase inhibitors and possibly estrogen therapy may be preferable for women. Retrospective analysis of some studies suggested greater reductions in LDL-C in women than in men treated with HMG-CoA reductase inhibitors [24,25].

Although controversial, Lp(a) is suggested to predict cardiovascular risk; Lp(a) levels are higher in women than in men, particularly in the postmenopausal years. Lp(a) levels are reduced by estrogen therapy, without alteration of this reduction by concomitant progesterone administration. [26,27].

High levels of LDL cholesterol and low levels of HDL cholesterol continue to predict coronary heart disease well into the eighth decade [28]. Cholesterol lowering produces benefit in women [29-32], with a comparable reduction in coronary death rates related to cholesterol-lowering in both genders.

Coronary disease rates for diabetic women approach those for comparably aged diabetic men, potentially related, at least in part, to the more pronounced lipoprotein abnormalities in diabetic women than in diabetic men [33,34]. Based on follow-up data from NHANES I, diabetes imparts a greater relative risk for women, 2.4, as compared with 1.9 for men [35].

The proceedings of a National Heart, Lung, and Blood Institute (NHLBI) Workshop [28] reporting pooled data on 86,000 women based on 25 populations in 22 U.S. and international cohort studies, examined the association of hyperlipidemia and coronary risk in women, because most individual studies did not include sufficient numbers of women to allow reliable estimates of risk. Risk was estimated by comparing the upper two quintiles to the lower two quintiles of lipid levels. Data are provided for total cholesterol, HDL cholesterol, LDL cholesterol, and triglyceride relationships. The relative risk for mortality from coronary heart disease in women younger than age 65 with cholesterol levels ≥ 240 mg/dl as compared with those whose levels were < 200 mg/dl was 2.44 (95% confidence intervals 2.16, 2.75). For women older than 65 years of age, the relative risk for coronary mortality in the higher as compared with the lower total cholesterol level group was 1.12 (95% confidence intervals 1.01, 1.25). For women younger than 65 years of age with an LDL cholesterol level greater than 160 mg/dl, as compared with women with LDL cholesterol levels below 140 mg/dl, the relative risk of mortality from coronary heart disease was 3.27; the relative risk value for women older than 65 years was 1.13, a nonsignificant difference. As regards HDL cholesterol levels, women younger than age 65 with an HDL level below 50 mg/dl, compared with women whose HDL level was greater than 60 mg/dl, had a relative risk for coronary mortality of 2.13; the relative risk for women aged 65 years and older was 1.75. Women younger than age 65 with triglyceride levels below 100 mg/dl, as compared with levels greater than 130 mg/dl, had a relative risk of 1.98; the relative risk for women older than age 65 was 1.39. The dilemma offered by these data is that women younger than 65 years of age, whose absolute risk for coronary heart disease is relatively low, have a high relative risk associated with elevations of total and LDL cholesterol levels and triglyceride levels and lowered levels of HDL cholesterol. By contrast, for women older than 65 years of age who have a higher absolute risk of coronary disease, only low HDL levels appear to be associated with increased mortality from coronary heart disease.

A subsequent National Heart, Lung, and Blood Institute Conference, based on data from 124,000 women derived from 11 cohort studies, showed no association between total cholesterol levels and either all-cause mortality or total cardiovascular mortality for women [18]. However, women with cholesterol levels ≥ 240 mg/dl had a relative risk for coronary heart disease of 1.56 compared to women with cholesterol levels of 160-199 mg/dl. Data from both this and the prior NHLBI conference are limited in that confounding variables, particularly associated cardiovascular risk factors (including menopausal status and hormone use), are not addressed.

Cholesterol lowering with pharmacotherapy was associated with improved endothelium-mediated vasodilation in women and men with coronary artery disease [36].

Nonpharmacologic Therapy of Hyperlipidemia in Women

Women appear to have less lowering of cholesterol levels with dietary interventions than do men [37,38], although these studies involved predominantly premenopausal women. Substantial cholesterol-lowering occurred with dietary therapy and exercise in a study of postmenopausal women [39].

Weight loss in women is also less consistently associated with favorable lipid changes than in men [40], possibly related to patterns of body fat distribution [41,42]. The relationship to insulin resistance and hyperinsulinemia requires clarification. Of particular concern in women is the adipose tissue/estrogen relationship, in that, in postmenopausal women, estrogen is synthesized from androstenedione in adipose tissue [43], such that weight reduction may be associated with estrogen loss. Therefore, the favorable effects associated with weight loss in women may be less prominent than those in men.

Exercise is minimally effective in producing a favorable lipid profile in premenopausal women but has a markedly favorable effect in postmenopausal women [44].

A recent retrospective study suggests that women with coronary disease participating in long-term cardiac rehabilitation achieve greater lipid benefits than do men [45].

Randomized Controlled Trials of Lipid Lowering in Women

There is a gender gap in the evidence available from randomized controlled trials that relate to the efficacy of lipid-lowering in women as compared with men in the primary and secondary prevention of coronary heart disease. Importantly, because women have lower rates of CHD than do men of similar age, even comparable reduction in CHD risk in men and women related to cholesterol-lowering will result in less benefit for women.

PRIMARY PREVENTION STUDIES

No recent trials address the effect of cholesterol-lowering on the primary prevention of coronary heart disease in women. The few available trials were conducted almost two decades ago.

In the Finnish mental hospital study [31], more than 6,000 women patients were randomized to either a cholesterol-lowering or a control diet for 6 years, with subsequent reversal of dietary therapies for the next 6 years. Cholesterol-lowering dietary therapy resulted in a reduction in serum cholesterol levels of about 12%, without a statistically significant reduction in coronary mortality, cardiovascular mortality, or all-cause mortality.

A second trial of dietary therapy, the Minnesota Coronary Survey [46], randomized more than 4,500 women patients in state mental hospitals or nursing homes to a low saturated fat, high polyunsaturated fat, low cholesterol diet versus control status. Despite a serum cholesterol reduction of 14% related to dietary therapy, there was no significant reduction in coronary mortality, cardiovascular death, cardiovascular events, or total mortality. However, this diet was higher in total fat than that currently recommended by the National Cholesterol Education Program.

The only primary prevention trial of pharmacotherapy that included women [47], randomized 1,184 women with total cholesterol levels greater than 250 mg/dl to colestipol versus placebo therapy in a 3-year study; however, about 20% of women had preexisting coronary heart disease. Despite an almost 10% reduction in total cholesterol levels, neither coronary heart disease mortality nor total mortality in women differed between treatment and control groups, despite this benefit seen for men.

SECONDARY PREVENTION STUDIES

Women were included in several trials of lipid-lowering therapies that evaluated effects on the secondary prevention of coronary heart disease.

In the Stockholm Ischemic Heart Disease Secondary Prevention Study [48], 555 survivors of myocardial infarction, 103 of whom were women, were randomized to clofibrate and nicotinic acid therapy versus placebo for 5 years. Although outcomes in women were not analyzed separately, total mortality was decreased by 26% in the total study population and coronary heart disease mortality by 36% ($p < .05$). Benefit was most pronounced, 60%, in the patient subgroup whose serum triglyceride level was lowered 30% more ($p < .01$).

Patients with myocardial infarction or with angina and electrocardiographic evidence of myocardial ischemia were included in the 6-year Scottish Society of Physicians trial; 124 of the 717 participants were women [30]. Coronary heart disease death rates did not differ significantly between clofibrate-treated and control women, and total mortality was not assessed.

Comparable categories of patients were included in a study by Physicians of the Newcastle-upon-Tyne region; 497 participants, 97 of whom were women, were randomized to clofibrate versus placebo therapy [29]. As in the Scottish study, the mean cholesterol level of participants was elevated, and cholesterol levels fell on average 41 mg/dl in the treated women. Although the coronary death rate for women on clofibrate was 3.8% as compared with 13.3% in the placebo group, this difference did not reach statistical significance, likely owing to the small number of coronary deaths; total mortality was not assessed.

In the Program on the Surgical Control of the Hyperlipidemias (POSCH), an angiographic study of lipid-lowering in hypercholesterolemic survivors of myocardial infarction, 78 of the 838 participants were women. The study compared dietary control of hyperlipidemia with surgery [49]; women who underwent partial ileal bypass surgery had a 24% lower plasma cholesterol level than did women on dietary therapy after 5 years. Angiographic disease progression was significantly less in surgically treated women, despite no significant change in overall or coronary heart disease mortality. The findings in women were comparable to those of the total study population.

A second angiographic study involved 72 participants, 41 of whom were women, with heterozygous familial hypercholesterolemia [50]. Comparison between dietary counseling versus dietary counseling and aggressive combination drug therapy for lipid-lowering for 2 years showed that LDL cholesterol levels decreased significantly more in the drug-treated women than in the control population, 39.6% versus 12.7%. Quantitative coronary angiography showed the mean cross-sectional area of the coronary arteries to be reduced in the diet-treated women but increased in the drug-treated women, suggesting regression of atherosclerosis. Lowering of LDL cholesterol (38%) and raising of HDL cholesterol levels (27%) in these severely hypercholesterolemic women thus limited the angiographic progression of coronary disease and even induced regression [50].

Although data are limited, lipid-lowering with drug therapy has shown comparable benefit in women to that in men in lessening atherosclerosis and coronary events [51]. The Scandinavian Simvastatin Survival Study (4S) [52] was the first trial to document the benefit of cholesterol-lowering both for women and for patients older than age 60 years in the secondary prevention setting, i.e. a population with defined coronary disease and hypercholesterolemia, with most of the participants having had myocardial infarction. Nineteen percent of the study population were women; the relative risk of a major coronary event in the treated group was 0.66 for men and 0.65 for women during the 5.4 year median follow-up.

Postmenopausal Hormone Therapy: Lipid Effects

The interest in hormone replacement therapy as a coronary preventive intervention for women was stimulated by the predominance of coronary heart disease in postmenopausal women and has been reenforced by a number of biologically plausible potential benefits of estrogen use. To date, the best-documented of these benefits includes a favorable effect on lipoprotein metabolism, with estrogen raising HDL cholesterol and lowering LDL cholesterol values by 10-15%; the elevation of triglyceride levels is an unfavorable consequence. Further, for any level of circulating lipids, lipid deposition and accumulation in the vascular wall is decreased in the presence of estrogen. Thus, an added postulate is that estrogen may protect against LDL cholesterol deposition in the vascular wall [53] or, potentially, may reduce LDL oxidation [54]. However, these lipoprotein benefits appear to account for only about 25% to 50% of the reported favorable estrogen effects, engendering much interest in nonlipid mediated mechanisms of cardioprotection. Among these postulated effects are direct effects on vascular reactivity (vasodilator activity), decreased endothelin levels [55], increased prostacyclin production, potential calcium antagonist activity, sympathetic effects, favorable alterations in thrombotic mediators, favorable effect on atherosclerotic plaque, and antioxidant effects [54], among others.

A uniform finding in a number of observational studies has been the substantial decrease in risk for coronary heart disease [56-58] and decrease in all-cause mortality associated with unopposed oral estrogen use [59]. Data from these observational studies and meta-analysis of these studies [57] describe a 35-50% lowered risk of coronary events associated with such estrogen therapy. This benefit persisted even after adjustment for age, blood pressure, and cigarette smoking, based on data from the Lipid Research Clinics Follow-up Study. Striking cardioprotection has been described with long-term hormone use [59], with lower mortality among current uses than for women who used estrogen in the distant past. In women $\geq$ 65 years old in the Cardiovascular Health Study [60], postmenopausal estrogen use was associated with lower levels of LDL-C, fibrinogen, glucose, insulin, and obesity and higher levels of HDL-C and socioeconomic status; lower measures of subclinical cardiovascular disease were present as well. Benefit was comparable for women 65 to 74 and those older than 75 years of age, suggesting that postmenopausal estrogen use may decrease cardiovascular risk in women well into the eighth decade of life. An even more dramatic reduction in coronary risk is described with baseline coronary heart disease, with benefit greater in women with moderate or severe disease at coronary angiography, although these data are limited by very small numbers of women patients followed over the long term [61]. However, problems with observational studies, as a category, relate to selection bias artifact, in that a healthy cohort of women is typically prescribed estrogen. Further, there may be self-selection, in that women who continue to use estrogen beyond the duration of menopausal symptoms, exhibit a health-related behavior, compliance to medication-taking, which may be a surrogate for an otherwise healthy lifestyle. That compliance bias exists is demonstrated by reports from a number of randomized controlled trials of cardiac therapies where compliant patients in the placebo group had a 30-50% survival advantage over their noncompliant counterparts [62].

Estrogen replacement may be an appropriate lipid-altering therapy for postmenopausal women [59]. Orally administered estrogen can decrease LDL-C and increase HDL-C; of concern is the increase in serum triglyceride levels associated with estrogen use, which is particularly prominent in women with baseline elevation of triglyceride level. Estrogen is described as even more effective in decreasing coronary risk in women with established coronary heart disease than in healthy women [57,61,63]. Retrospective analysis of the EXCEL trial data showed that concomitant estrogen therapy had no effect on either the efficacy or the safety profile of lovastatin in women with moderate hypercholesterolemia [25].

Results of the Postmenopausal Estrogen/Progestin Intervention (PEPI) trial [64] have provided important new information about the metabolic effects of hormone therapies. The hypothesis underlying the study was that women taking estrogen have a lower risk of coronary heart disease and that estrogen prevents coronary heart disease by its favorable effect on coronary risk factors. The treatment arms of the PEPI trial, administered in 28-day cycles, included conjugated equine estrogen at 0.625 mg daily; this dose of estrogen with medroxyprogesterone acetate 10 mg on days 1-12; estrogen with medroxyprogesterone acetate 2.5 mg daily; and estrogen with micronized progestin 200 mg on days 1-12; as contrasted with placebo therapy. The study involved 875 women, aged 45-64 years at 7 PEPI clinical centers, women both with and without hysterectomy, but who had no known contraindications to hormone therapy.

The important differences in the primary trial endpoints were higher HDL levels in each active PEPI treatment group compared with placebo, with HDL levels highest with isolated conjugated equine estrogen or estrogen with micronized progestin, compared with conjugated estrogen with either cyclic or continuous medroxyprogesterone acetate. LDL cholesterol levels were lower in each active treatment group than in placebo, and triglyceride levels were higher in each active treatment group than in placebo. The most compelling PEPI regimen for favorably influencing coronary heart disease risk factors in women with a uterus was estrogen and micronized progestin, and in hysterectomized women unopposed estrogen; these judgments derive from the 33% three-year rate of adenomatous or atypical endometrial hyperplasia in women with a uterus in the unopposed estrogen group, identifying that unopposed estrogen is inappropriate for women who have not had hysterectomy.

Concern with the potential extent of use of estrogen as a lipid-lowering therapy, in addition to the persisting controversial risk for breast cancer [65,66], in particular with prolonged hormone use, derives from a random sample of premenopausal women in the Kaiser Permanente system [67]. Among women aged 40-55 years, based on 3-year follow-up data, 9% had absolute contraindications to hormone use, identified as breast or endometrial cancer; 40% had an absolute or relative contraindication, with the latter including liver disease, endometriosis, thromboembolic disease, uterine fibroids, migraine headaches, gallbladder disease, seizures, endometrial hyperplasia, fibrocystic breast disease, and the like.

Needed are prospective trials of hormone use with clinical endpoints. Fortunately, the relevant questions are being asked and fortunately two randomized controlled trials are currently underway to answer these critical questions; the Heart and Estrogen/Progestin Replacement Study (HERS) addresses hormone use in women with defined coronary disease, whereas the Women's Health Initiative of the U.S. National Institutes of Health involves a predominantly well population of women. Unfortunately, answers will not be available until the 21st century.

Current Guidelines for Management of Hyperlipidemia in Women: Are They Adequate?

Recommendations of the Adult Treatment Panel II of the National Cholesterol Education

Program [68] were the first to address items of specific relevance for women. Recommendations from NCEP II consider age greater than 55 years or premature menopause without estrogen replacement as a risk factor for women, comparable to that of male gender and male age greater than 45 years. Additionally, a history of coronary heart disease in a first-degree female relative younger than age 65 is a risk factor, compared with risk for a male family member with coronary disease at age younger than 55 years.

In the NCEP II Guideline, comparable HDL cholesterol levels are targeted for women as for men; since HDL cholesterol levels are higher in women than in men across the life span (and since low HDL cholesterol levels are stronger risk attributes for women than for men), should higher levels of HDL cholesterol be considered to place women at risk than is the case for men?

Using the NCEP II guideline and NHANES III data [69], between 11 and 26% of postmenopausal women in the United States are likely to be candidates for lipid-lowering therapy, even after an adequate trial of dietary treatment. With aging of the total U.S. population, more women survive to the postmenopausal years and have elevated levels of LDL cholesterol.

Since nonpharmacologic measures appear less effective in reducing cholesterol levels for women than for men, should lifestyle modifications be intensified for women or should earlier pharmacologic interventions be considered?

Current guidelines set higher thresholds for lipoprotein evaluations in hypercholesterolemic women and higher thresholds for drug treatment in women who have raised levels of LDL cholesterol, an LDL > 220 in premenopausal women and > 190 in postmenopausal women [68]. Should diabetic women of younger age be identified as at increased risk? Specifically, should premenopausal diabetic women have a lower threshold for initiation of pharmacologic treatment of raised LDL cholesterol levels, comparable to that for postmenopausal women? The presence of diabetes essentially nullifies the gender-protective effect, even for premenopausal women [70].

Additionally, since 60% of episodes of myocardial infarction and more than half of all coronary artery bypass graft surgery and percutaneous transluminal coronary angioplasty procedures in women are performed in those older than 65 years of age, it seems prudent and reasonable that more intensive lipid-lowering interventions [71,72] be undertaken in women with defined coronary disease, even at older age. Since women with coronary heart disease are at high risk of recurrent coronary events [73], benefit from cholesterol-lowering is likely to be greater than for healthy women.

Warranting evaluation are the differences in the cholesterol:coronary heart disease relationship between black and white women, in that this correlation is described as less prominent for black women [74,75]. The postmenopausal increase in total cholesterol levels is reported as far less pronounced among black than among white women. Finally, since most of the limited data available derive from studies of middle-aged, middle to upper socioeconomic class, white women, can or should this information be extrapolated to nonwhite women, to elderly women, and to those of lower socioeconomic status.

Both specific lipid-altering drugs and hormone replacement therapy can favorably influence lipid profiles for women. What are the benefit:risk ratios for each approach; and should combined therapy be considered? Clearly, the most effective lipid-altering therapy for women remains to be determined; the role of combinations of estrogen or estrogen/progestin and/or lipid-lowering drugs remains to be delineated [28].

Acknowledgements

With appreciation to Jeanette Zahler for help in preparation of the manuscript.

References

1. Lerner DJ, Kannel WB. Patterns of coronary heart disease morbidity and mortality in the sexes: A 26-year follow-up of the Framingham population. Am Heart J 1986;111:383-90.
2. Bush TL. The epidemiology of cardiovascular disease in postmenopausal women. Ann NY Acad Sci 1990;592:263-71.
3. Wenger NK, Speroff L, Packard B. Cardiovascular health and disease in women. N Engl J Med 1993;329:247-56.
4. Eaker ED, Chesebro JH, Sacks FM, Wenger NK, Whisnant JP, Winston M. Cardiovascular disease in women. Circulation 1993;88:1999-2009.
5. Maynard C, Litwin PE, Martin JS, Weaver WD. Gender differences in the treatment and outcome of acute myocardial infarction. Results from the Myocardial Infarction Triage and Intervention Registry. Arch Intern Med 1992;152:972-76.
6. Tofler GH, Stone PH, Muller JE, et al. and the MILIS Study Group. Effects of gender and race on prognosis after myocardial infarction: Adverse prognosis for women, particularly black women. J Am Coll Cardiol 1987;9:473-82.
7. Greenland P, Reicher-Reiss H, Goldbourt U, Behar S, and the Israeli SPRINT Investigators. In-hospital and 1-year mortality in 1,524 women after myocardial infarction. Comparison with 4,315 men. Circulation 1991;83:484-91.
8. Clarke KW, Gray D, Keating NA, Hampton JR. Do women with acute myocardial infarction receive the same treatment as men? BMJ 1994;309:563-66.
9. Lavie CJ, Milani RV. Effects of cardiac rehabilitation and exercise training on exercise capacity, coronary risk factors, behavioral characteristics, and quality of life in women. Am J Cardiol 1995;75:340-43.
10. Kostis JB, Wilson AC, O'Dowd K, et al., for the MIDAS Study Group. Sex differences in the management and long-term outcome of acute myocardial infarction. A statewide study. Circulation 1994;90:1715-30.
11. Khan SS, Nessim S, Gray R, Czer LS, Chaux A, Matloff J. Increased mortality of women in coronary artery bypass surgery: Evidence for referral bias. Ann Intern Med 1990;112:561-67.
12. Maynard C, Weaver WD. Treatment of women with acute MI: New findings from the MITI Registry. J Myocard Ischemia 1992;4:27-37.
13. Welty FK, Mittleman MA, Healy RW, Muller JE, Shubrooks SJ Jr. Similar results of percutaneous transluminal coronary angioplasty for women and men with postmyocardial infarction ischemia. J Am Coll Cardiol 1994;23:35-39.
14. Movsowitz HD, Emmi RP, Manginas A, et al. Directional coronary atherectomy in women compared with men. Clin Cardiol 1994;17:597-602.
15. Wenger NK. Gender, coronary artery disease, and coronary bypass surgery (editorial). Ann Intern Med 1990;112:557-58.

16. Gordon DJ, Probstfield JL, Garrison RJ, et al. High-density lipoprotein cholesterol and cardiovascular disease. Four prospective American studies. Circulation 1989;79:8-15.
17. Eaker ED, Castelli WP. Coronary heart disease and its risk factors among women in the Framingham Study. In: Eaker ED, Packard B, Wenger N, et al., editors. Coronary heart disease in women. New York: Haymarket Doyma, 1987: 122-30.
18. Jacobs D, Blackburn H, Higgins M, et al. Report of the conference on low blood cholesterol: Mortality associations. Circulation 1992;86:1046-60.
19. Castelli WP. The triglyceride issue: A view from Framingham. Am Heart J 1986; 112:432-37.
20. Criqui MH, Heiss G, Cohn R, et al. Plasma triglyceride level and mortality from coronary heart disease. N Engl J Med 1993;328:1220-25.
21. Corti M-C, Guralnik JM, Salive ME, et al. HDL cholesterol predicts coronary heart disease mortality in older persons. JAMA 1995;274:539-44.
22. Kannel WB. Nutrition and the occurrence and prevention of cardiovascular disease in the elderly. Nutr Rev 1988;46:68-78.
23. Arca M, Vega GL, Grundy SM. Hypercholesterolemia in postmenopausal women. Metabolic defects and response to low-dose lovastatin. JAMA 1994;271:453-59.
24. Shear CL, Franklin FA, Stinnett S, et al. Expanded Clinical Evaluation of Lovastatin (EXCEL) study results. Effect of patient characteristics on lovastatin-induced changes in plasma concentrations of lipids and lipoproteins. Circulation 1992; 85:1293-1303.
25. Bradford RH, Downton M, Chremos AN, et al. Efficacy and tolerability of lovastatin in 3390 women with moderate hypercholesterolemia. Ann Intern Med 1993;118:850-55.
26. Utermann G. The mysteries of lipoprotein(a). Science 1989;246:904-10.
27. Kim CJ, Jang HC, Min YK. Hormone replacement therapy lowers the plasma concentration of lipoprotein(a) in postmenopausal women (Abst). Circulation 1992;86(I):I-866.
28. Manolio TA, Pearson TA, Wenger NK, Barrett-Connor E, Payne GH, Harlan WR. Cholesterol and heart disease in older persons and women. Review of an NHLBI Workshop. Ann Epidemiol 1992;2:161-76.
29. Group of Physicians of the Newcastle-upon-Tyne region. Trial of clofibrate in the treatment of ischaemic heart disease. BMJ 1971;4:767-75.
30. Report by a Research Committee of the Scottish Society of Physicians. Ischaemic heart disease: A secondary prevention trial using clofibrate. BMJ 1971;4:775-84.
31. Miettinen M, Turpeinen O, Karvonen MJ, Elosuo R, Paavilainen E. Effect of cholesterol-lowering diet on mortality from coronary heart-disease and other causes. A twelve-year clinical trial in men and women. Lancet 1972;ii:835-38.
32. Rossouw JF. International trials. Presented at the Cholesterol and Heart Disease in Older Persons and in Women June 18-19, 1990. NHLBI, NIH, Bethesda, MD, Program and Abstracts Book p. 22.
33. Ikeda T, Terasawa H, Ishimura M, et al. Sex differences in plasma cholesterol and apolipoprotein B levels in non-obese type 2 diabetic subjects. Diabete Metab 1992; 18:465-67.
34. Goldschmid MG, Barrett-Connor E, Edelstein SL, Wingard DL, Cohn BA, Herman WH. Dyslipidemia and ischemic heart disease mortality among men and women with diabetes. Circulation 1994;89:991-97.
35. Centers for Disease Control. Coronary Heart Disease Incidence by Sex - United States, 1991-1987. In: CDC Surveillance Summaries, July 1992. MMWR 1992;41 (No. SS-2):526-29.
36. Treasure CB, Klein JL, Weintraub WS, et al. Beneficial effects of cholesterol-lowering therapy on the coronary endothelium in patients with coronary artery disease. N Engl J Med

1995;332:481-87.

37. Mensink RP, Katan MB. Effect of monounsaturated fatty acids versus complex carbohydrates on high-density lipoproteins in healthy men and women. Lancet 1987;i:122-25.

38. Masarei JRL, Rouse IL, Lynch WJ, Robertson K, Vandongen R, Beilin LJ. Effects of a lacto-ovo vegetarian diet on serum concentrations of cholesterol, triglyceride, HDL-C, HDL_2-C, HDL_3-C, apoprotein-B, and Lp(a). Am J Clin Nutr 1984;40:468-79.

39. Barnard RJ. Effects of life-style modification on serum lipids. Arch Intern Med 1991;151:1389-94.

40. Brownell KD, Stunkard AJ. Differential changes in plasma high-density lipoprotein-cholesterol levels in obese men and women during weight reduction. Arch Intern Med 1981;141:1142-46.

41. Soler JT, Folsom AR, Kushi LH, Prineas RJ, Seal US. Association of body fat distribution with plasma lipids, lipoproteins, apolipoproteins A1 and B in postmenopausal women. J Clin Epidemiol 1988;41:1075-81.

42. Lapidus L, Bengtsson C, Larsson B, Pennert K, Rybo E, Sjostrom L. Distribution of adipose tissue and risk of cardiovascular disease and death: A 12 year follow up of participants in the population study of women in Gothenburg, Sweden. BMJ 1984;289:1257-61.

43. Grodin JM, Siiteri PK, MacDonald PC. Source of estrogen production in postmenopausal women. J Clin Endocrinol Metab 1973;36:207-14.

44. Hartung GH, Moore CE, Mitchell R, Kappus CM. Relationship of menopausal status and exercise level to HDL cholesterol in women. Exp Aging Res 1984;10:13-18.

45. Warner JG, Brubaker PH, Zhu Y, et al. Long-term (5-year) changes in HDL cholesterol in cardiac rehabilitation patients. Do sex differences exist? Circulation 1995;92:773-77.

46. Frantz ID Jr, Dawson EA, Ashman PL, et al. Test of effect of lipid-lowering by diet on cardiovascular risk. The Minnesota Coronary Survey. Arteriosclerosis 1989;9:129-35.

47. Dorr AE, Gundersen K, Schneider JC Jr, Spencer TW, Martin WB. Colestipol hydrochloride in hypercholesterolemic patients - effect on serum cholesterol and mortality. J Chron Dis 1978;31:5-14.

48. Carlson LA, Rosenhamer G. Reduction of mortality in the Stockholm Ischaemic Heart Disease Secondary Prevention Study by combined treatment with clofibrate and nicotinic acid. Acta Med Scand 1988;223:405-18.

49. Buchwald H, Campos CT, Matts JP, Fitch LL, Long JM, Varco RL, and the POSCH Group. Women in the POSCH trial. Effects of aggressive cholesterol modification in women with coronary heart disease. Ann Surg 1992;216:389-400.

50. Kane JP, Malloy MJ, Ports TA, Phillips NR, Diehl JC, Havel RJ. Regression of coronary atherosclerosis during treatment of familial hypercholesterolemia with combined drug regimens. JAMA 1990;264:3007-12.

51. Haskell WL, Alderman EL, Fair JM, et al. Effects of intensive multiple risk factor reduction on coronary atherosclerosis and clinical cardiac events in men and women with coronary artery disease. The Stanford Coronary Risk Intervention Project (SCRIP). Circulation 1994;89:975-90.

52. Scandinavian Simvastatin Survival Study Group. Randomised trial of cholesterol lowering in 4444 patients with coronary heart disease: The Scandinavian Simvastatin Survival Study (4S). Lancet 1994;344:1383-89.

53. Wagner JD, Clarkson TB, St. Clair RW, Schwenke DC, Adams MR. Estrogen replacement therapy (ERT) and coronary artery (CA) atherogenesis in surgically postmenopausal cynomolgus monkeys (Abst). Circulation 1989;80(II):331.

54. Rifici VA, Khachadurian AK. The inhibition of low-density lipoprotein oxidation by 17-β estradiol. Metabolism 1992;41:1110-14.
55. Polderman KH, Stehouwer CDA, van Kamp GJ, Dekker GA, Verheugt FWA, Gooren LJG. Influence of sex hormones on plasma endothelin levels. Ann Intern Med 1993;118:429-32.
56. Stampfer MJ, Colditz GA, Willett WC, et al. Postmenopausal estrogen therapy and cardiovascular disease. Ten-year follow-up from the Nurses' Health Study. N Engl J Med 1991;325:756-62.
57. Grady D, Rubin SM, Petitti DB, et al. Hormone therapy to prevent disease and prolong life in postmenopausal women. Ann Intern Med 1992;117:1016-37.
58. Barrett-Connor E, Bush TL. Estrogen and coronary heart disease in women. JAMA 1991; 265:1861-67.
59. Henderson BE, Paganini-Hill A, Ross RK. Decreased mortality in users of estrogen replacement therapy. Arch Intern Med 1991;151:75-78.
60. Manolio TA, Furberg CD, Shemanski L, et al. for the CHS Collaborative Research Group. Associations of postmenopausal estrogen use with cardiovascular disease and its risk factors in older women. Circulation 1993;88 (part 1):2163-71.
61. Sullivan JM, Vander Zwaag R, Hughes JP, et al. Estrogen replacement and coronary artery disease. Effect on survival in postmenopausal women. Arch Intern Med 1990;150:2557-62.
62. Petitti DA. Coronary heart disease and estrogen replacement therapy. Can compliance bias explain the results of observational studies? Ann Epidemiol 1994; 4:115-18.
63. Gruchow HW, Anderson AJ, Barboriak JJ, Sobocinski KA. Postmenopausal use of estrogen and occlusion of coronary arteries. Am Heart J 1988;115:954-63.
64. The Writing Group for the PEPI Trial. Effects of estrogen or estrogen/progestin regimens on heart disease risk factors in postmenopausal women. The Postmenopausal Estrogen/Progestin Interventions (PEPI) Trial. JAMA 1995;273:199-208.
65. Colditz GA, Hankinson SE, Hunter DJ, et al. The use of estrogens and progestins and the risk of breast cancer in postmenopausal women. N Engl J Med 1995;332:1589-93.
66. Stanford JL, Weiss NS, Voigt LF, Daling JR, Habel LA, Rossing MA. Combined estrogen and progestin hormone replacement therapy in relation to risk of breast cancer in middle-aged women. JAMA 1995;274:137-42.
67. Whitlock EP, Valanis B, Ernst D, Smith L. Prevalence of contraindications to hormone replacement therapy in middle-aged women in a managed care setting. J Wom Health 1995; 4:293-302.
68. Expert Panel on Detection, Evaluation, and Treatment of High Blood Cholesterol in Adults. Summary of the Second Report of the National Cholesterol Education Program (NCEP) Expert Panel on Detection, Evaluation, and Treatment of High Blood Cholesterol in Adults (Adult Treatment Panel II). JAMA 1993;269:3015-23.
69. Sempos CT, Cleeman JI, Carroll MD, et al. Prevalence of high blood cholesterol among US adults. An update based on guidelines from the Second Report of the National Cholesterol Education Program Adult Treatment Panel. JAMA 1993;269:3009-14.
70. Manson JE, Colditz GA, Stampfer MJ, et al. A prospective study of maturity-onset diabetes mellitus and risk of coronary heart disease and stroke in women. Arch Intern Med 1991; 151:1141-47.
71. Pearson T, Rapaport E, Criqui M, et al. Optimal risk factor management in the patient after coronary revascularization. A Statement for Healthcare Professionals from an American Heart Association Writing Group. Circulation 1994;90:3125-33.
72. Smith SC Jr., Blair SN, Criqui MH, et al. Consensus Panel Statement. Preventing heart attack

and death in patients with coronary disease. Circulation 1995;92:2-4.
73. Walsh JME, Grady D. Treatment of hyperlipidemia in women. JAMA 1995;274: 1152-58.
74. Knapp RG, Sutherland SE, Keil JE, Rust PF, Lackland DT. A comparison of the effects of cholesterol on CHD mortality in black and white women: Twenty-eight years of follow-up in the Charleston Heart Study. J Clin Epidemiol 1992;45:1119-29.
75. Demirovic J, Sprafka JM, Folsom AR, Laitinen D, Blackburn H. Menopause and serum cholesterol: Differences between blacks and whites. The Minnesota Heart Survey. Am J Epidemiol 1992;136:155-64.

TREATMENT OF DYSLIPIDEMIAS IN WOMEN: NORMAL DEVELOPMENTAL CHANGES IN SERUM LIPIDS

Marianne J. Legato
Columbia University College of Physicians and Surgeons, 962 Park Avenue, New York, New York 10028, USA

Introduction

An understanding of what constitutes significant dyslipidemia begins with a review of the normal pattern of serum lipoproteins. It changes throughout the life cycle and, in the case of women, during the various phases of the reproductive cycle.

Childhood

In children 7-17 years of age, there are significant gender and racial differences in serum lipoprotein concentrations [1,2].

Girls, whether white or black, have higher high density lipoprotein (HDL) values than boys even before puberty [2]. White males begin to develop adverse profiles at puberty however; as testosterone levels rise, their HDL, and apo 1A levels drop and low density lipoprotein (LDL) concentration rises [1]. These data correlate with the observation of the Bogalusa Heart Study that children whose fathers had myocardial infarction tended to be white [1]. This early adverse trend in the developmental life of white males may help explain the earlier onset of coronary artery disease (CAD) in their lives as compared with that of white women. The gender specific changes I have described in HDL levels with the onset of puberty are not seen in blacks, who as a group and regardless of gender have significantly higher levels of HDL than their white counterparts throughout childhood and adolescence [2].

Knowing the absolute values of serum lipoprotein concentrations is not enough to predict disease. Neufeld and Newburger point out that the connection between childhood dyslipidemia and subsequent CAD is not incontrovertibly established and there are no data showing that reducing cholesterol in childhood will reduce cardiac mortality [3]. Furthermore, the biology of the relationship between dyslipidemia and CAD may vary significantly between racial groups. In people dying between 6 and 30 years of age, aortic fatty streaks were greater in black males and females at all ages than in whites in spite of blacks' relatively more favorable pattern of HDL concentrations [4]. This is the case even

A. M. Gotto, Jr. et al. (eds.), Drugs Affecting Lipid Metabolism, 439–445.

though pubescent black males do not demonstrate the inverse relationship between testosterone and DHEA levels and HDL concentrations seen in white boys [5]. In contrast to fatty streaks, however, raised lesions or plaque was more extensive in white than in black adults, indicating that the factors involving transition from fatty streak to plaque might differ between the races [6].

NCEP suggests treatment of drug therapy in children older than 10 years of age whose LDL levels are > 190 or for children with LDL over 160 who have two additional risk factors, which include smoking, obesity, diabetes, or physical inactivity [7]. Such children are less than 10% of the population and will usually have genetic dyslipidemia and a positive family history for early atherosclerosis. The vast majority of children with dyslipidemia can be managed by diet and lifestyle changes alone. Children of families with hyperlipidemia or early heart disease are at special risk and should be monitored from the time they are two years old. Pediatricians should update their patients' family histories every few years to pick up an occurrence of early CAD. Therapy of dyslipidemic children begins with a twelve-month trial of diet and exercise; bile resins and niacin are the drugs of choice in this population.

The NHLBI's Dietary Intervention Study in Children (DISC) showed that modest lowering of LDL levels in a group of approximately 600 children, half of whom were girls, over a 3-year period did not interfere with adequate growth, iron stores, or satisfactory nutrition during adolescence [8]. There were no adverse psychological effects on treated teens and in fact, such children had less depression than control groups, perhaps as a function of the support provided by their group sessions.

It is important to monitor risk factors in teens with elevated serum lipids. Cigarette smoking, obesity, birth control therapy, and other drugs should trigger particularly close surveillance. Oral contraceptives are not absolutely contraindicated in the dyslipidemic teen, but the physician should choose preparations with minimal androgenic activity in girls with low HDL levels and follow such patients closely. Postpubertal teens who have completed linear growth should be regarded and treated as adults. Lovastatin is absolutely contraindicated in pregnancy.

Changes in Women's Lipids During Reproductive Life

Changes During the Menstrual Cycle

Kim and Kalkhoff studied women's serum lipid profile changes during the menstrual cycle, and matched the values against males of similar age over the same time period studied [9]. As might be anticipated, men showed stable concentrations of lipids over a month's time, while those of women varied quite dramatically.

Triglyceride concentrations are highest in women at the time of ovulation and fall during the luteal phase. They are always higher than those of aged matched men. The same is true of HDL levels, which are also consistently higher than those of males, and which rise even further after ovulation. LDL, total cholesterol, and apo B levels, on the other hand, are significantly depressed during the luteal phase. All three values, furthermore, are significantly lower than those of men throughout the cycle. Thus, women who cycle normally have a relatively less atherogenic profile of serum lipids, which may explain in part the natural advantage young women enjoy in the timing of CAD relative to young men. It may also account in part for the vulnerability of women who suffer premature menopause to coronary artery disease. The fluctuating levels of serum lipoproteins in menstruating women dictate the need for correlating laboratory values with the phase of the patient's monthly cycle, particularly when following serial values in dyslipidemic patients.

CHANGES DURING PREGNANCY

One of the most interesting facts about normal pregnancy is that while estrogen increases 16-fold at a steady rate during gestation, HDL levels peak at midterm. With the rise in insulin production and the onset of insulin resistance that occur in midgestation, however, HDL levels decline and are only 15% above normal by parturition [10,11]. In contrast, total cholesterol and triglyceride levels rise steadily throughout pregnancy [12].

With parturition, triglyceride values return to normal within about a week. LDL levels, on the other hand, stay elevated for at least 8 weeks with or without lactation. Why the high estrogen concentration of pregnancy does not seem to prevent this increased LDL cholesterol is poorly understood; it may be that high levels of endogenous progesterone during pregnancy plays a role. Serum lipid values do not reliably reflect baseline levels until six months after delivery.

Because of the relatively atherogenic serum lipid profile of pregnancy, some investigators maintain that early pregnancy (before age 20)[13] and multiple pregnancies [14,15] are a risk for CAD, while other studies show no correlation between multiple pregnancies and vulnerability [15]. In any case, physicians should identify women in the 95th percentile for triglycerides and cholesterol during pregnancy, even if their values fall to normal after delivery. Such women often belong to hyperlipidemic families [16] and should be followed carefully to see if they develop hyperlipidemia themselves. In particular, their physicians should use particular caution in supervising the use of oral contraceptives and advise against cigarette smoking and excessive weight gain in such patients.

In spite of serum lipoprotein concentration changes during gestation, there are no studies supporting the notion that hypercholesterolemic women who do become pregnant increase their risk for CAD. On the other hand, lipid lowering drugs should be discontinued during pregnancy and women with cholesterol over 350 mg/dl should confine their childbearing to a minimum amount of years so they can resume drug therapy as quickly as possible [17].

Montelongo and colleagues studied plasma lipoproteins during pregnancy in pregestationally and in gestationally diabetic women [18]. Interestingly, diabetes, whether gestational or pre-existing, did not intensify or otherwise affect the normal changes of serum lipoproteins during pregnancy, at least in those patients in whom near normal glycocylated serum hemoglobin levels indicated good metabolic control. On the other hand, glucose, free fatty acids (FFA), and ketone body concentrations were higher in diabetic than in control women, indicating that adipose tissue lipolytic activity and liver consumption of released

FFA for ketogenesis were increased. The failure of these metabolic changes to drive serum lipoprotein values above those of normal women during pregnancy was attributed to relatively lower levels of sex hormones, (i.e. beta estradiol, progesterone, and prolactin) in these patients than in nondiabetic women.

Serum Lipoproteins and the Menopause

There is general agreement that premature menopause, whether it occurs spontaneously or is surgical, produces an enhanced risk for developing CAD. Women who suffer an earlier than normal menopause should receive hormonal replacement therapy. The consequences of natural and timely menopause *per se* are less clear. When corrected for age and smoking, menopause brings with it no accelerated increase in the incidence of coronary artery disease. Nevertheless, there is a change in serum lipoprotein concentration, and the change is atherogenic. Total cholesterol and LDL levels increase, and HDL levels either remain the same [19] or decrease very slightly [20].

Another factor in the increased risk of the menopause is the fact that premenopausal women have less dense and less atherogenic LDL particles than men. With menopause, however, they develop more of the smaller, denser LDL particles which are apo B-enriched and which correlate with increased triglyceride and decreased HDL levels, all changes which are considered atherogenic [21].

NCEP recommends estrogen replacement therapy for postmenopausal women who continue to have elevated LDL in spite of optimal life style corrections [22]. The positive effects of ERT in the postmenopausal women include not only their favorable impact on HDL and LDL, but on the vasculature and platelets as well, and there is now a very convincing body of evidence documenting a 40-50% lower incidence of CAD in estrogen users compared with nonusers.

Dyslipidemia in the Old Woman

There are important changes in the relationship between elevated levels of total cholesterol and LDL and lower than optimal levels of serum HDL to CAD in the elderly. They are somewhat different for women than for men.

Krumholz and his colleagues studied almost a thousand patients whose mean age was 79. In this study, neither hypercholesterolemia, low HDL levels, nor a high total serum cholesterol to HDL ratio predicted all cause or coronary heart disease mortality, nor were they associated with higher numbers of hospitalization for myocardial infarction (MI) or unstable angina compared with control groups [23]. Almost twice as many women than men were studied. Surprisingly, survival curves in women with total cholesterol levels greater than 240 mg/dl were the best in the group. The authors concluded that total cholesterol alone should not be considered an important risk factor for mortality for elderly women, but point out that Barrett-Connor and colleagues [24] and Aronow et al. [25] both found that high levels of total cholesterol were associated with increased coronary events in the very elderly, both males and females. The authors add the additional caveat that they could not say whether or not individuals who had sustained a previous myocardial infarction were unaffected by elevated levels of total cholesterol and LDL: their sample of almost 1,000 individuals did not include many patients with a recent MI.

Corti and her colleagues, on the other hand, showed that low HDL does predict CHD mortality and the occurrence of new CAD events in patients over 70. Their enormous prospective study extended to 4.4. years of follow-up and included 2,527 women and 1,377 men [26]. Risk was still significant at age 80. Moreover, total cholesterol over 240 mg/dl or higher was significantly associated with CAD death in women but not in men. Low HDL levels were a risk for both genders.

The data from Framingham confirm these, and showed that while total cholesterol values decline in patients after 70, the risk of coronary events continues to be related to total cholesterol/HDL ratio into the 90s, although in women, the effect diminishes progressively as age increases. In contrast, the risk in men decreases substantially after age 55, but then levels off [27]. With each increment of total cholesterol to HDL ratio, there is a steeper risk gradient for women and over a ratio of 7.5, women appear to lose their advantage over men in terms of a lower incidence of CAD [24]. Total cholesterol alone did not predict CHD in men, but did for women at levels at or above 240 mg/dl.

Summary

In summary, the normal physiologic events of menstruation, pregnancy, and aging are all accompanied by significant changes in serum lipoprotein levels. These should be taken into account when making therapeutic decisions for the female patient.

Isolated values for total cholesterol should not be used to predict risk, particularly for women. Complete serum lipid determinations, done more than once, are most useful in assessing risk for CAD, particularly in the female patient. The practicing physician should also be aware of the different criteria for the diagnosis of clinically significant dyslipidemia in men and women.

References

1. Berenson GS, Srinivasan SR, Attingney W, et al. Insight into a bad omen for white men: Coronary artery disease--the Bogalusa Heart Study. Am J Cardiol 1989:64:32C-39C.
2. Srinivasan SR, Freedman DS, Webber LS, Berenson GS. Black-white differences in cholesterol levels of serum high-density lipoprotein subclasses among children: The Bogalusa Heart Study. Circulation 1987;76:272-79.
3. Neufeld EJ, Newburger JW. How should children with hypercholesterolemia be managed? Choices in Cardiology. 1992;7:233-36.
4. Berenson GS, Wattigney WA, Tracy RE, et al. Atherosclerosis of the aorta and coronary arteries and cardiovascular risk factors in persons aged 6 to 30 years and studied at necropsy. Am J Cardiol 1992;70:851-58.
5. Srinivasan SR, Freedman DS, Sundara GS, et al. Racial (black-white) comparisons of the relationship of levels of endogenous sex hormones to serum lipoproteins during male adolescence: The Bogalusa Heart Study. Circulation 1986;74:1226-34.

6. Freedman DS, Newman WP 3rd, Tracy RE, et al. Black-white differences in aortic fatty streaks in adolescence and early adulthood: The Bogalusa Heart Study. Circulation 1988;77:856-64.
7. NCEP. Report of the expert panel on blood cholesterol levels in children and adolescents. Pediatrics 1992;89(suppl):525-584.
8. The Writing Group for the DISC Collaborative Research Groups. Efficacy and safety of lowering dietary intake of fat and cholesterol in children with elevated low-density lipoprotein cholesterol. JAMA 1995;273:1429-35.
9. Kim H, Kalkhoff RK. Changes in Lipoprotein composition during the menstrual cycle. Metabolism. ;28:663-68.
10. Desoye G, Schweditsch M, Pfieffer KP, et al. Correlations of hormones with lipid and lipoprotein levels during normal pregnancy and postpartum. J Clin Endocrinol Metabl 1987;64:704.
11. Fahraeus L, Larsson-Cohn U, Wallentin L. Plasma lipoproteins including high density lipoprotein subfractions during normal pregnancy. Obstet Gynecol 1985;66: 468.
12. Potter JM, Nestel PJ. The hyperlipidemia of pregnancy in normal and complicated pregnancies. Am J Obstet Gynecol 1979;133:165.
13. Rosenberg L, Miller DR, Kaufman DW, et al. Myocardial infarction in women under 50 years of age. JAMA 1983;250:2801.
14. Beard CM, Fuster V, Annegers JR. Reproductive history in women with coronary heart disease: A case-control study. Am J Epidemiol 1984;120:108.
15. Bengtsson C, Rybo G, Westerberg H. Number of pregnancies, use of oral contraceptives and menopausal age in women with ischemic heart disease, compared to a population sample of women . Acta Med Scan 1973;549:75.
16. Knopp RH, Bergelin RO, Wahl PW, et al. Population based lipoprotein lipid reference values for pregnant women compared to non-pregnant women classified by sex hormone usage. Am J Obstet Gynecol 1982;143:626.
17. Miller VT. Dyslipoproteinemia in women. Endocrinology and Metabl Clinics of North America 1990;19:381-98.
18. Montelongo A, Lasuncion MA, Pallardo LF, Herrera E. Longitudinal study of plasma lipoproteins and hormones during pregnancy in normal and diabetic women. Diabetes 1992; 41:1651-59.
19. Bush T, Cowan L, Heiss G, et al. Ovarian function and lipid/lipoprotein levels. Results from the Lipid Research Clinics (LRC) Program. Am J Epidemiol 1984; 120:489.
20. Meilahn EN, Kuller LH, Matthews KA, et al. Change in lipoprotein lipids and apoproteins during the perimenopause. 29th meeting of AHA Council on Epidemiology. Washington DC, June 18-22, 1989.
21. Campos H, McNamara JR, Wilson RWF, et al. Differences in low density lipoprotein subfraction and apolipoproteins in premenopausal and postmenopausal women (Framingham). J Clin Endocrinol Metab 1988;67:30.
22. Summary of the second report of the National Cholesterol Education Program (NCEP) expert panel on detection, evaluation, and treatment of high blood cholesterol in adults (Adult Treatment Panel II) JAMA 1993;269:3015-23.
23. Krumholz HM, Seeman TE, Merrill SS, et al. Lack of association between cholesterol and coronary heart disease mortality and morbidity and all-cause mortality in persons older than 70 years. JAMA 1994;272:1335-40.
24. Barrett-Connor E, Suarez L, Khaw K, et al. Ischemic heart disease risk factors after age 50.

J Chronic Dis 1984;37:903-908.
25. Aronow WS, Herzig Ah, Etinenne F, et al. 41 month follow-up of risk factors correlated with new coronary events in 708 elderly patients. J Am Geriatr Soc 1989; 37:501-506.
26. Corti MC, Gurainik JM, Salive ME et al. HDL cholesterol predicts coronary heart disease mortality in older persons. JAMA 1995;274:539-44.
27. Wilson PWF, Kannel WB. Hypercholesterolemia and coronary risk in the elderly: The Framingham Study. Hypercholesterolemia and coronary risk. American Journal of Geriatric Cardiology 1993;March/April:52-56.

HYPOLIPIDEMIC TREATMENTS IN THE ELDERLY: THE "BRISIGHELLA STUDY" EXPERIENCE

Antonio Gaddi, Caterina Galetti, Ada Dormi, Maria Carmela Grippo, Sergio D'Addato, Zina Sangiorgi, and Silvana Rimondi
Center for the Study of Atherosclerosis and Metabolic Diseases "Giancarlo Descovich," Policlinico S. Orsola-Malpighi, Via Massarenti 9, 40138 Bologna, Italy and the Department of Medical Clinic and Applied Biotechnology, University of Bologna, Bologna, Italy

Introduction

An editorial recently published by JAMA [1] suggests to physicians a careful use of hypolipidemic drugs in older people. One year earlier another editorial underlined that screening and treatment of high blood cholesterol is appropriate only for "younger elderly people" in secondary prevention or in those with high risk of coronary heart disease (CHD) [2]. It is suggested that people in their late 70s or older should not be screened or treated [2].

The National Cholesterol Education Program (NCEP) considers healthy elderly patients as possible "candidates for cholesterol lowering therapy" [3] and that they then should not be excluded *a priori* from preventive measures. The task force composed of members of the European Societies of Cardiology, Atherosclerosis, and Hypertension states, that true benefits of drug treatment in the elderly are unknown [4]. However they note that if CHD risk (projected around 60 years of age) increases, intensive advice is needed for all risk factors (RF). On the other hand, as age increases, the relative risk decreases but the attributable risk increases markedly [5].

It is almost impossible to mark a cut-off age over which preventive measures are no longer useful [1], even if different lipid trends [6] and relative high gender- and race-related variabilities are considered. Evaluation of life expectancy might help the general practitioner (GP) in identifying patients to be treated [1], but we have to ask ourselves if it is possible to apply a "demographic" index, which varies greatly from year to year and from country to country, to individual subjects.

Subjects to be treated should be chosen on the following bases: (a) current quality of life; (b) the presence of the main risk factors [1]; and (c) the patients' wishes or "desires" [1] and, we think, free will. However, these factors are valid in every preventive measure we adopt in the elderly (and in adults too), not only for choice of hypolipidemic drug

A. M. Gotto, Jr. et al. (eds.), Drugs Affecting Lipid Metabolism, 447–458.

therapy.

In our opinion, the choice of subjects for a preventive medicine scheme should be decided on the basis of the strength of the statistical association between RFs and pathology incidence, as well as the strength of the tests demonstrating the preventive efficacy of a given therapy. It also should depend on the comprehensive evaluation of both the clinical situation of the individual subject and the suitability of preventive measures for a large number of people. Benefits of CHD primary and/or secondary prevention in the elderly strongly depend upon physicians' and patients' acceptance of guideline indications and their compliance over a long period without excessive social costs. Without these characteristics, any type of prevention (hypotensive, hypolipidemic, etc.) is completely useless.

For these reasons, we utilized the Brisighella Study database to verify:

(a) What is the true suitability, in an elderly rural population, of hypolipidemic preventive measures (nutritional information and "chronic and correct" drug employment advice) and,

(b) Whether an effect on lipid risk profile is detectable after several years of follow-up without special measures.

Methods

The Brisighella Study is epidemiological research on chronic diseases of social impact started by Professor Giancarlo Descovich in 1972 [7] and continued by him and his coworkers over the last 25 years. In 1986 the Study became part of the WHO European Risk Factors Coordinated Analysis (ERICA) [8] and, since 1990, is part of Risk Factors and Life Expectancy (RIFLE) [9]. The study structure is complex [10] and includes different phases and subprojects: (a) the observational phase, from 1972 to 1986 (record of mortality and morbidity for all causes and survey of risk factor trends) and (b) the preventive intervention phase, started in 1986 and still in progress (check of efficacy, cost, and reliability of preventive programs). During this phase several projects were performed: high risk (HR) intervention, special projects for schoolboys, whole population nutritional education program, media utilization (newspapers and video networks), training of GP on therapeutic guidelines, etc..

The study design includes periodic controls (every 3 months) of causes of fatal and nonfatal new events (according to the International Classification of Disease) and checks the following points (every 4 years for the whole population, every 6-9 months for HR population):

(a) complete anamnesis (personal, remote and recent pathological, drug use, and life style changes, etc.);

(b) physical examination, blood pressure, body weight and height measurement, ECG recording; since 1984, liver/gallstone US scan has also been performed by MICOL project staff [11]; standardized questionnaires or "reading and recording" methods (i.e. the Minnesota code for ECG) were adopted (when available) for anamnesis and physical examination according to indications of the WHO [12]; more detailed information in quoted references [7-8,10,13-14];

(c) record of nutritional habits by dietitian inquiry plus the "seven-day questionnaire" [14]; and

(d) evaluation of metabolic RF and hematological parameters: total cholesterol (TC), triglycerides (TG), high density lipoprotein-cholesterol (HDL-C; only since 1976), fasting blood sugars, uric acid, apoprotein AI and B (since 1980), plasma and red blood cell fatty acid profile (since 1984), and Lp(a) (since 1988).

Thyroid hormones, lipoprotein UC fractions, apoproteins and other were evaluated on random samples. Lipid tests were performed according to the general guideline as in [15]; method and standardization procedure revision was performed according to indications advised by Italian Lipid Clinics [16]; quality control was performed for as long as possible (about 18 years), on the standard of the WHO Lipid Reference Center of Prague (precision and accuracy within 3% for TC, TG, and HDL-C). Low density lipoprotein cholesterol (LDL-C) was calculated for this report with the Friedewald formula.

The main database of the Brisighella Study is composed of 15 million records. Current processing is performed on a specific file containing the elderly population data (n = 441) collected in 1980, 1984, 1988, and 1992. For all the possible interyear comparisons (1980 versus 1984, 1980 versus 1988, etc.) and for all the continuous variables (TC, LDL-C, HDL-C, TG, fasting blood sugar (FBS), uric acid, systolic and diastolic blood pressure), intraindividual differences were reckoned. TG log transformation was performed on TG absolute values; no age adjustments were used. Diet, drug adherence, and smoking were codified as dichotomous variables (smoke: 0 = no, 1 = yes; hypolipidemic and other drugs: 0 = none, 1 = yes; drug type: one code level for each drug was considered in a separate field).

Table 1 summarizes the elderly group characteristics compared with the whole population screened during the Brisighella Study.

We selected all the subjects > 60 years old in 1992 who had been checked in all the controls (1980, 1984, 1988). We thus obtained a homogeneous sample of elderly subjects in whom intraindividual differences of lipids and other RF can be calculated. Sample age distribution relative frequencies are as follows (data in 1992): 60-65 = 0.20; 66-70 = 0.29; 71-75 = 0.23, 76-80 = 0.18; 81-85 = 0.09, > 85 = 0.01.

This sample represents 68-74% of the elderly people living in Brisighella from 1980 to 1992 included in the historical cohort. The remaining 26-34% should be considered "less compliant" because they participated only in 1/4 (few), 2/4 (the majority), or 3/4 controls. However, all people (even the adults) received the same input of the preventive medicine programs.

At the end of 1985 a Nutrition Information Center was opened in Brisighella, and in February 1986, four dietitians began working on a nutrition education program (NEP).

The center was opened 3 days a week with free access (no charge, nor were appointments necessary). All the families living in Brisighella were informed of the NEP by letter (3,016 letters were sent), containing brochures on nutrition guidelines [17-19]. We advertised the center on posters and through the media. Dietitians informed people of all ages how to reduce their daily intake of saturated fats and cholesterol, encouraging the consumption of olive oil (is a local product) and corn oil. Moreover, information was given

Table 1. General view of enrollment procedures and intervention types during the Brisighella Study. White areas refer to the observational prospective phase; gray areas to the intervention phase. The boxed data is currently being analyzed.

	1972	1976	1980	1984	1986	1988	1992	1996
Ther. Guidelines (GPs)	No	No	No	No	No	Yes/No	Yes/No	Yes
Nutrition Information	No	No	No	No	Yes	Yes	Yes	Yes
Personalized Diets	No	No	No	No	No	No	Yes/No	?
Hypolipidemic Drugs	No	No	No	No	No	Yes	Yes	Yes
Hypotensive Drugs	No	No	No	No	No	No	Yes	Yes
n (all screened)	2939	381	2175	2292	-	3663	2878	?
n (historical cohort)	2939	381	2175	1800	-	1756	1564	?
4-year control data available	Yes	Yes	Yes	Yes	No	Yes	Yes	No
" " used in this processing	No	No	Yes	Yes	No	Yes	Yes	No
Elderly living and screened at all four controls	-	-	all = 441 m = 231 f = 210	→ → →	- - -	→ → →	→ → →	

on excessive salt and dairy product (except milk) intakes, and on the differences between butter and soft margarine. Written information and booklets were given and periodically sent home to all citizens. Personalized diet "prescription" was avoided when possible.

A rapid cholesterol measurement method is available in the center (Reflotron, BBR; dry-chemistry method; data not used for this paper) [16]. Since 1986, approximately 2,200 citizens have come to the nutrition center, some more than once (especially women) (Table 2). We estimated that at least 0.7 person for every Brisighella family has participated in the NEP.

In 1988 after a general population control, the HR project started. It included the summoning of HR subjects for a medical check-up and was directed to all (young, adults, and elderly) HR citizens. A specialized staff again estimated personal risk profile and gave advice on life-hygiene (but seldom specific diets: see Table 2). The patient was sent to his GP who decided the pharmacological therapy when necessary; for hypolipidemic drugs, GPs adopted a protocol based on fibrates (Gemfibrozil, 600 mg bid or, then, 1200 and 900 mg in one dose) and/or on ion exchange resins (IER: cholestyramine or microporous cholestyramine) or on their association. The GPs explained to patients that the hypolipidemic therapy was chronic and they invited people to make a check-up every 6 months. Through letters and/or phone calls, people were reminded of the check-up date, but people were always free to continue/stop the therapy, to come/not come to controls. Drug prescriptions were in conformity with National Sanitary System (SSN) rules. Among the 441 selected subjects, 1/4 participated to HR program, at least once per year.

Table 2. Type of intervention programs started in 1986 and 1988. Approximate percentages of "free" participation of elderly analyzed in this study in the NEP are given. Since 1988, gemfibrozil has been taken by 22% of the elderly population, IER (ion exchange resins) by 1-2%, other hypolipidemic drugs less than 6%. Other comments, see text.

Period of Follow up	1980-1986	1986-1992	1988-1992
1. Personalized Diet	No	No/Yes	No/Yes
(% of Elderly)	(0.0)	(<0.5%)	(<1.5%)
2. Nutrition Information	No	Yes	Yes
(% of Elderly, M/F)	(0.0)	(25-55%)	(10-25%)
Type of Information	-	Booklets Similar to AHA-I	Booklets Similar to AHA-I
	-	Dialog with Dietitian	Dialog with Dietitian
3. Distribution of Diet Food	No	Yes	No
4. Hypolipidemic Drugs			
(% Of Elderly)	<5%	3-5%	29%
Chronic Therapy	No	No	Yes/No
Drug Type	Various	Various	Gemfibrozil (600x2) and/or IER

The aim of this statistical evaluation is to verify whether the effects of "free" participation in the NEP (and to dietary advice sent home) or to the HR program is detectable: a) in the entire elderly sample and/or, b) only in high risk or ill subjects. Statistics were performed by BMDP and by Statgraphic 6.1 packages. After descriptive statistics, intraindividual difference distributions were checked, using the hypothesis that if a random effect is present in the population, two-controls, paired, intraindividual differences are normally distributed with mean, median, and mode near 0; moreover, the 99% interval of confidence for means and t-test statistics were performed on the differences. Multiple regression (stepwise, forward selection, F to enter or remove variables into the model = 4) was used to verify (in the entire elderly sample divided by sex) whether any detectable effect of the therapy exists on 1992 lipid values or whether they can be forecasted by 1992 or by 1988, 1984 and 1980 levels of other risk factors. Multiple ANOVA, using year (1980, 1984, etc.) and sex as classification factors, was also performed. In the second analysis (b), we selected the subgroups of elderly that proved hypolipoproteinemic and/or HR (and/or with a previous CHD) before the start of preventive programs and analyzed the effect of drug prescriptions made by the GPs in these subgroups. Moreover statistical analysis was performed on data from all the elderly aged > 60 and > 65 at each control (1980 = 642, 1984 = 446, 1988 = 895, 1992 = 764). Data are not discussed in this paper.

Results

Figure 1 illustrates the frequency histograms of triglyceride differences (males and females: pooled data) 1980 versus 1984, 1988, and 1990. During the first 4- year period an evident shift to the right was observed, while in 1988 and in 1992 intraindividual TG difference distribution shifted markedly to the left. In 1992, 76% of Brisighella elderly had triglyceride values lower than during the previous periods.

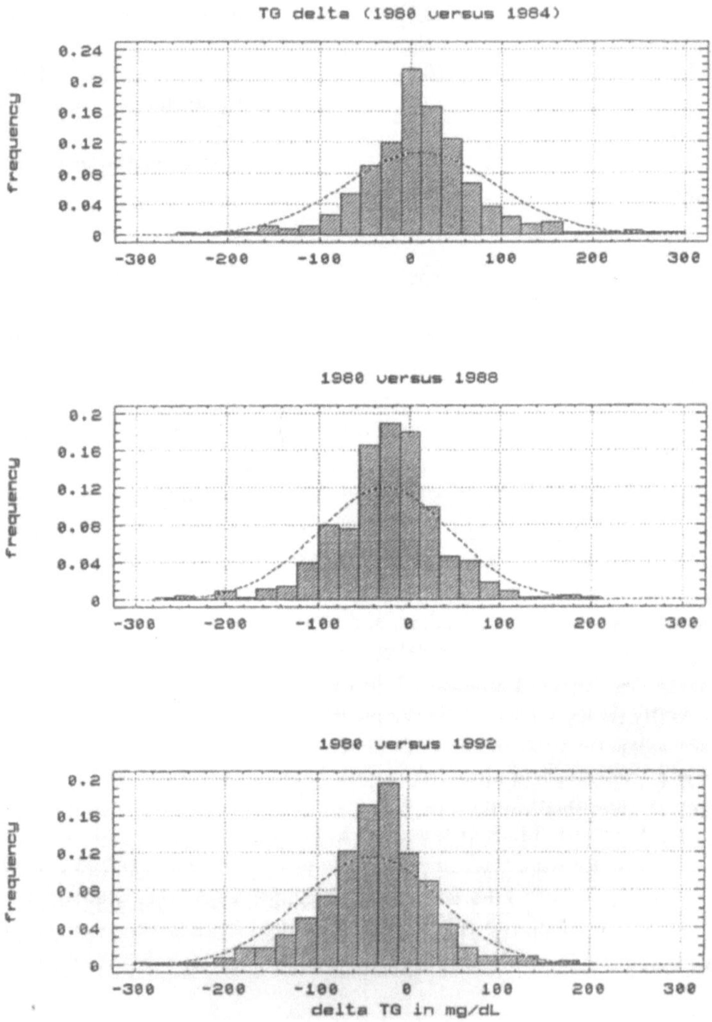

Figure 1. Distribution curves of TG differences in the elderly (males and females pooled data) between 1980 and 1984 (top), 1980 and 1988 (middle; NEP started in 1986), and 1980 versus 1992 (bottom; HR program started in 1988). See also Table 3.

The means of the differences, 99.0% confidence intervals for means, and t statistic, are reported in Table 3 for TG, LDL-C and HDL-C.

Table 3. Mean values and 99% confidence intervals for means and t statistics results for TG, LDL-C and HDL-C differences between 1980 and 1984, 1988, and 1992, in the entire elderly sample (m = 231, f = 210).

	Sex	Years	x	99% CI	t	p
TG	m	80-84	9.6	-5.9 25.3	1.60	0.109
	f	80-84	11.2	-1.9 24.3	2.21	0.027
	m	80-88	-22.4	-9.0 -35.7	-4.35	$1.9x10^{-5}$
	f	80-88	-32.0	-19.7 -44.3	-6.77	$2.7x10^{-8}$
	m	80-92	-44.2	-30.6 -57.8	-8.45	$1.2x10^{-14}$
	f	80-92	-37.0	-23.8 -50.2	-7.32	$1.2x10^{-8}$
LDL-C	m	80-84	8.97	1.8 16.1	3.27	0.001
	f	80-84	7.71	0.04 15.4	2.61	0.009
	m	80-88	-2.33	-8.2 3.6	-1.02	0.307
	f	80-88	-2.21	0.88 -10.9	-2.12	0.028
	m	80-92	-12.1	-5.7 -18.5	-4.09	$1.7x10^{-6}$
	f	80-92	-18.4	-11.2 -25.5	-6.68	$2.3x10^{-8}$
HDL-C	m	80-84	2.03	-0.1 4.2	2.51	0.012
	f	80-84	4.82	2.7 6.8	6.15	$1.1x10^{-8}$
	m	80-88	4.33	2.4 6.1	6.03	$6.3x10^{-9}$
	f	80-88	6.63	4.6 8.5	8.90	$3.8x10^{-8}$
	m	80-92	2.12	0.04 4.2	2.65	0.0083
	f	80-92	5.44	3.2 7.6	6.57	$1.9x10^{-8}$

Multiple ANOVA, performed on the absolute values at various controls, gave the same results (both for the 441 paired samples and for the entire elderly population; data not shown). The MANOVA solutions demonstrate effects for sex and for year, but not for their interaction. In short:

1) TG, higher in males, drops in both sexes after 1988 and 1992 controls; means (males and females; 1980, 1984, 1988, 1992, respectively): 161.3 mg/dL; 171.8 mg/dL; 134.2 mg/dL; and 120.7 mg/dL, respectively; MANOVA sex $F = 13.1$, $p = 0.0003$; year $F = 40.7$, $p < 0.0001$; interaction of sex by year $F = 0.89$, $p = 0.44$;
2) LDL-C, higher in females, drop in both sexes in 1992; means (as per TG): 163.1 mg/dL, 171.4 mg/dL, 159.4 mg/dL, 147.9 mg/dL, respectively; MANOVA sex $F = 76.6$, $p = 0.0001$; year $F = 25.3$, $p < 0.0001$, interaction $F = 0.483$, $p = 0.694$;
3) HDL-C, markedly higher in females, rising in both sexes at all controls; means (as per TG): 51.4, 54.9, 56.2, and 55.8, respectively; MANOVA sex $F = 113.6$, $p < 0.0001$; years F= 14.3, sex = 0.23; interaction $F = 1.43$, $p = 0.23$ (tables of means,

SEM and 95% CI subdivided by year, age-class, and sex are available on request).

The multiple regression analysis was performed by stepwise forward selection procedure on 1992 values of LDL-C, TG and HDL-C (dependent variables). This procedure demonstrates that in the entire elderly population, some predictors of lipid values in 1992 were found (Table 4).

Table 4. Multiple regression analysis on 1992 lipids in the entire elderly sample. The determination coefficient (R^2), the standard error of estimate (SEE) for full regression are given; (neg.)= negative coefficient. Single coeff., p, conditional sum of squares relative to single predictors are not shown; for the listed independent variables (predictors) p is always $< 3x10^{-4}$.

Dependent Variables	Males			Females		
	R^2	SEE	Predictors	R^2	SEE	Predictors
LDL-C (1992)	0.43	28.3	1988-LDL-C 1984-LDL-C 1992-FBS	0.35	29.0	1988-LDL-C 1984-LDL-C 1992-HDL-C (neg.)
TG (1992)	0.52	48.2	1988-TG 1980-TG 1988-HDL-C (neg.) 1980-HDL-C	0.47	43.4	1988-TG 1984-TG 1988-HDL-C (neg.) 1992-hypol. drug
HDL-C (1992)	0.57	8.3	1988-HDL-C 1984-HDL-C 1992-TG (neg.)	0.57	9.2	1988-HDL-C 1980-HDL-C 1992-TG (neg.) 1992-hypol. drug (neg) 1992-drug type (neg)

The main predictors for all the parameters, obviously, are the values of the same parameters as the previous controls (tracking). Drug therapy seems to influence TG and HDL-C only in 1992 (females) while hypolipidemic therapies given in the 1980-88 period do not show any significant effect on lipids. Other possible predictors with very low p values and that have a very slight effect on determination coefficient for full regression (not shown in Table 4) are: age and TG (1988 or 1992 values) for LDL-C values, age and LDL-C for TG, and LDL-C (1992) for HDL-C.

The analysis of lipid risk factors in high risk elderly subjects was performed on all the "every-4-year" differences (1980 versus 1984, 1984 versus 1988, etc.) in both: (a) hyperlipidemic subjects (TG > 200 and/or LDL-C >160 or > 190 mg/dL, evaluated at each control), and (b) in patients probably classified "at high risk" by the GP and that are treated by antihypertensive, hypolipidemic, and/or other cardiovascular drugs.

Eighty-five to 168 patients at each control are classified as per (a) or as per (b). In this subgroup analysis, we found several minor variations of lipids during the 1980-1984 period, although during the 1988-1992 phase more marked differences become visible. In particular, we recognize that:

1) the absolute number of hypolipidemic drug-treated patients, constant from 1980 to 1988 (around 2.5-5%), markedly increases in 1992 (to 29%). The number of well-treated subjects (evaluated on the basis of post-therapy lipid values) also increases: in 1992, mean TG values in 1988 hypertriglyceridemic elderly, treated by drugs from 1988-1992, is 126.5 mg/dL (SEM = 8.2) In this group, < 15% of the elderly showed slightly increased TG values.

2) the mean values of LDL-C decrease markedly and significantly from 1988 to 1992 in hypercholesterolemics (all phenotypes): from 193.5 mg/dL (SEM = 2.14) to 164.6 mg/dL (SEM = 3.22). In the same way, a marked increase of HDL-C from 1988 to 1992 was found both in elderly in the lowest HDL-C tertile (in 1988) and in the hypertriglyceridemics.

Preliminary Conclusions

At present, total and CHD mortality is decreasing in the Brisighella population. The database should be completed and reliable statistical analysis available by 1997-1998. It is obvious that only after this analysis can conclusions (efficacy yes/no/not ascertainable) be drawn. Thus, the conclusions now concern the suitability of nonexpensive preventive measures in a free-living elderly rural population.

In a previous published analysis of lipid trends in the entire elderly population of Brisighella [20] (1972, 1980, and 1984 data, analysis in 5-year age classes from the age of 60 to 80 years), an increase of TC and TG (HDL-C was not measured in 1972) was observed in both males and females. A slight decrease of TC was evident in the 80-85 age class. This study demonstrates that 1972-TC measurements are predictive for CHD mortality (code 410-414 of WHO-ICD 8th revision) in the subsequent 12 years of follow-up in males, 60-75 years old in 1972 (females = fewer events to perform multiple logistic function) [20]. The same conclusions on lipid trends are obtained utilizing data from 1980 to 1984 in 441 "paired" elderly. After the start of the NEP in the entire population, a marked decrease of triglycerides in the whole sample of elderly was observed; perhaps the age-increasing LDL-C trend previously observed [20] may be contrasted (Table 3). The multiple regression analysis suggests that in the entire female population a detectable effect of hypolipidemic drugs on TG and HDL-C is evident only in 1992. In 1992, after the NEP and the HR program, a marked reduction in LDL-C and in TG was also observed in high risk and hyperlipidemic elderly subjects.

Thus, nonguided therapies and/or life style spontaneous changes have no or little effects, while correct nutritional information and application of therapeutic guidelines seem to achieve evident results even in the elderly.

The cost/benefit ratio is low, taking into account that the majority of "preventive actions" were made by GPs, local authorities, and the people themselves. The only additional cost needed was for efficacy measurement and adherence methods already foreseen by the research protocol (for example, the plasma and RBC fatty acid profile).

Moreover, we demonstrated that the GPs' training and some specialized support (activities possible in Brisighella, where 6 GPs work, with one specialist one morning 3-times monthly) makes it possible to raise the benefit (in terms of lipid risk profile improvement) of pharmacological therapy in the population. Other benefits achieved with this preventive strategy, not discussed here, include the identification of familial hyperlipidemic subjects, new cases of diabetes and hypertension, some subjects with asymptomatic CHD and gallstones, etc. Future plans foresee the study of selective hypodysnutritional conditions and early diagnosis of atheromatic lesions, and treatment of identified "ill" people, without relevant additional resources and costs.

It can therefore be concluded that integrated prevention, including the most common chronic diseases and coordinated with early diagnosis, is not an unreachable goal but a question which depends on rationalization of medical resources and better health education and self-control among the population.

References

1. Denke MA, Winker MA. Cholesterol and coronary heart disease in older adults. No easy answer. JAMA 1955;274:575-79.
2. Hulley SB, Newman TB. Cholesterol in the elderly. Is it important? JAMA 1994;272: 1372-73.
3. Expert panel on the detection, evaluation and treatment of high blood cholesterol in adults (adults treatment panel II). Summary of second report of expert panel on the detection, evaluation and treatment of high blood cholesterol in adults. Circulation 1994;89:1329-45.
4. Piörälä K, De Backer G, Graham I, Poole-Wilson P, Wood D, on behalf of the task force of European Society of Cardiology, European Atherosclerosis Society and European Society of Hypertension. Prevention of CHD in clinical practice. Europ Heart J 1994;15:1300-31 and Atherosclerosis 1994;110:121-61.
5. Bilheimer DW. Clinical considerations regarding treatment of hypercholesterolemia in the elderly. Atherosclerosis 1991;91:s35-s57.
6. Miller NE, Nanjee MN. Hyperlipidemia in the elderly: Metabolic changes underlying the increases in plasma cholesterol and triglycerides during aging. Cardiovasc Risk Factors 1992;2:158-169.
7. Descovich GC, Mannino G, Lenzi S. Relationships between ischaemic heart disease, diet and lipid spectrum in a group of homogeneous population in Emilia Romagna. Gior It Cardiol 1974;4:373-81.
8. ERICA Research Group. The CHD risk map of Europe. The 1st report of the WHO-ERICA Project. Europ Heart J 1988;9:1-35.
9. Menotti A, Farchi G, Seccareccia F and the RIFLE Research Group. The prediction of coronary heart disease mortality as a function of major risk factors in over 30,000 men in the Italian RIFLE pooling project (risk factors and life expectancy). A comparison with the MRFIT primary screenes. J Cardiov 1994;1:263-70.
10. Descovich GC, D'Addato S, Dormi A, et al. The Brisighella heart study report from 1984 to 1989. In: Descovich GC, Gaddi A, Magri GL, Lenzi S, editors. Atherosclerosis and cardiovascular diseases. Dordrecht, The Netherlands: Kluwer Academic Publishers, 1990:622-31.
11. Attili AF, Carulli N, Roda E, et al. Epidemiology of gallstone disease in Italy: prevalence data

of the Multicenter Italian Study of Cholelithiasis (MICOL). Am J Epidem, 1995:141:158-65.
12. Rose GA, Blackburn H. Cardiovascular survey methods. World Health Organization. Geneva, 1969.
13. Descovich GC, Gaddi A, Minardi A, et al. The Brisighella Heart Project. In: Lenfant C, Albertini A, Paoletti R, Catapano AL, editors. Biotechnology of dyslipo-proteinemias. Application in diagnosis and control. New York: Raven Press, 1990: 311-17.
14. Gaddi A, Ciarrocchi A, Matteucci A, et al. Dietary treatment for familial hypercholesterolemia: Differential effects of dietary soy protein according to the apolipoprotein E phenotypes Am J Clin Nutr 1990;53:1191-96.
15. Manual of laboratory operations. Lipid Research Clinic Program: Lipid and lipoprotein analysis. DHEW Publicat., no (NHI) 75, 1974.
16. Sprovieri G, Lippi U, Graziani MS, Catapano A, Gaddi A, Manzato E, (Commissione Nazionale Congiunta AIPAC, SIBIoC, SIMEL, CISMEL, ASFA e Gruppo di Studio delle Malattie Dismetaboliche e dell'Aterosclerosi). Linee guida per la diagnostica di laboratorio delle dislipidemie. Biochim Clin 1995;19:198-205, and Patol Clin 1995; 1:42-48.
17. Descovich GC, Menotti A, on behalf of Italian Group of Epidemiology and Prevention. Rapporto Rimini 84: Prevenzione primaria della cardiopatia coronarica. Giorn It Arter, 1986;3:249-58.
18. Italian Consensus Conference. Lower cholesterol to prevent coronary heart disease. Finalized Project of Preventive and Rehabilitative Medicine. Rome, National Research Council Ed., 1986.
19. Italian National Nutrition Institute. Guide lines for healthy nutrition. Booklet printed by INN, Rome, 1985.
20. Descovich GC, Ceredi C, De Simone G, et al. The Brisighella Study: plasma lipid trend in the elderly observed over a twelve year period. In: Descovich GC, Gaddi A, Magri GL, Lenzi S, editors. Atherosclerosis and cardiovascular diseases. Dordrecht, The Netherlands: Kluwer Academic Publishers, 1990:38-48.

Addendum

BRISIGHELLA STUDY STAFF

Founder	Prof. G. C. Descovich (deceased 1993)
Mayor of Brisighella	T. Samore'
Scientific Coordinator	Prof. A. Gaddi, MD, PhD
Brisighella Coordinator	E. Pelliconi
Bologna Biomedical Staff	B. Descovich MD, C. Descovich MD, S. Fedeli MD, N. Scoz MD
-ECG	S. D'Addato MD
-Ecographic	D. Pomata MD
-ECG Reading/Coding	L. Finazzo MD, C. Mussoni MD, S. Rimondi MD
-Brisighella GP	L. Bagnaresi MD, J. Drei MD, I. Gamberi MD, A. Naldi MD, C. Samore', MD, P. Viozzi MD
Bologna Laboratory Staff	Z. Sangiorgi BD, G. La Regina BD, G. Copparoni, R. Mambelli
Bologna Nutritional Staff	C. Alberghini Diet., L. Lolli Diet.

Bologna Biometrics	A. Dormi MathD, Y. Piazzi Diet.
General Secretary	M. Nanni
Brisighella Anagraphic Staff	L. Sbarzaglia, L. Masi

CONTRIBUTORS LIST

1. Antonio Gaddi, MD, PhD, Atherosclerosis Center "Giancarlo Descovich," Dept. of Medical Clinic and Applied Biotechnology, University of Bologna
2. Caterina Galetti, MD., Atherosclerosis Center "Giancarlo Descovich," Dept. of Medical Clinic and Applied Biotechnology, University of Bologna
3. Ada Dormi, MathD., Atherosclerosis Center "Giancarlo Descovich," Dept. of Medical Clinic and Applied Biotechnology, University of Bologna
4. Maria Carmela Grippo, MD, Atherosclerosis Center "Giancarlo Descovich," Dept. of Medical Clinic and Applied Biotechnology, University of Bologna
5. Sergio D'Addato, MD, Atherosclerosis Center "Giancarlo Descovich," Dept. of Medical Clinic and Applied Biotechnology, University of Bologna
6. Silvana Rimondi, MD, Atherosclerosis Center "Giancarlo Descovich," Dept. of Medical Clinic and Applied Biotechnology, University of Bologna
7. Zina Sangiorgi, BD, Atherosclerosis Center "Giancarlo Descovich," Dept. of Medical Clinic and Applied Biotechnology, University of Bologna

DRUG TREATMENT OF HYPERLIPIDEMIA IN THE ELDERLY: HMG-CoA REDUCTASE INHIBITORS AND FIBRIC ACID DERIVATIVES

Alberto Zambon, Giovannella Baggio[1], and Gaetano Crepaldi[2]
University of Washington, Endocrinology/Metabolism, Box 356426, Seattle, Washington 98195-6426, USA, [1]University of Sassari, Viale S. Pietro, 8, 07100 Sassari, Italy, and [2]Institute of Internal Medicine, University of Padua, Via Giustiniani, 2, 35128 Padua, Italy

Introduction

The elderly are among the fastest growing segment of the population in the US and in most westernized countries. In 1990, those over the age 65 represented about 4% of the US population; now they constitute 13% of the US population and by the year 2030 they will constitute 20% according to the estimates of the U.S. Census Bureau. Similar estimates are available for most of western European countries, including Italy [1]. This phenomenon presents a challenge for the health care system in industrialized countries since chronic diseases are common in the elderly causing several degrees of disability. Therapy of chronic conditions may not cause a significant prolongation of life, however a valid therapeutic end-point in the elderly would be compression of morbidity in the time before death, such as an independent life being maintained for a significantly longer period before death [2].

Atherosclerosis is strongly associated with aging [3] and several risk factors assume increased importance in the elderly such as hypertension, diabetes mellitus, and cigarette smoking, setting this group of patients in a high-risk category for CHD. Treatment of the large number of older patients with elevated serum cholesterol levels is often advocated to prevent coronary heart disease (CHD) [4] which is clearly the most common cause of death in old age. The vast majority (up to 80%) of deaths from CHD occurs beyond age 65 in both genders [5].

Yet in spite of remarkable evidence that hypercholesterolemia is associated with increased risk for CHD in young and middle-aged individuals [6], the importance of hypercholesterolemia as a risk factor for cardiovascular disease in persons older than 65 remains controversial. Studies of older populations, including the Framingham Heart Study, have reported conflicting results [7-9]. A recent report from the Established Populations for Epidemiologic Studies of the Elderly (EPESE) suggested that low high density lipoprotein cholesterol (HDL-C) predicts CHD mortality and occurrence of new CHD events in persons older than 70 years, while elevated total cholesterol was not found to be associated with

A. M. Gotto, Jr. et al. (eds.), Drugs Affecting Lipid Metabolism, 459–464.

CHD mortality in men [10]. The same study showed that in older women elevated total cholesterol may be a risk factor for CHD. Although the total cholesterol appears to lose power as a risk predictor in the elderly, lipoprotein subclasses, specifically HDL, may retain this power and thereby implicate dyslipidemia in the atherogenic process. Unfortunately primary prevention clinical trials have included relatively few elderly patients, and the question can be raised of whether results carried out in middle-aged patients can be extrapolated to the elderly.

Recently a secondary prevention, randomized trial among persons aged 35 through 70 years with CHD reported that lowering total and low density lipoprotein cholesterol with simvastatin, an inhibitor of hydroxymethylglutaryl coenzyme A (HMG-CoA) reductase, decreased all-cause and CHD mortality, as well as major coronary events, even in the subgroup of older patients (age 60-69) [11]. Because most patients with established CHD are aged 60 or more, the issue of secondary prevention becomes of great importance in the elderly population. Given the available data [11-14] it is reasonable to suggest that cholesterol lowering regimens have similar effects on the secondary prevention of CHD in middle-aged and elderly people making drug therapy for secondary prevention attractive in the elderly.

There are limited data presently available regarding the efficacy and safety of the hypolipidemic therapy in the elderly.

Hydroxymethylglutaryl Coenzyme A (HMG-CoA) Reductase Inhibitors

The HMG-CoA reductase inhibitors are suitable alternatives to other hypolipidemic therapies for the management of hypercholesterolemia in the elderly. Members of this drug class effectively lower the low density lipoprotein (LDL)-cholesterol level, and also, to a lesser extent, lower plasma triglycerides (TG) and increase HDL-cholesterol. Drugs in this class currently include lovastatin, simvastatin, pravastatin, and fluvastatin. These compounds inhibit the activity of the HMG-CoA reductase, the major rate-limiting enzyme in the cholesterol biosynthesis. When intracellular cholesterol synthesis is inhibited, human cells express more LDL receptors to obtain the cholesterol they require from LDL in the plasma [15]. LDL receptor synthesis is particularly stimulated in the liver. Side effects of these drugs include gastrointestinal distress, raised hepatic transaminases (1.3%), and myopathy (0.5%). Studies in the elderly with HMG-CoA reductase inhibitors have shown that these drugs are usually well tolerated and highly effective in a dose-dependent manner, reducing total cholesterol up to 35% and LDL-cholesterol up to 49% in patients ranging in age from 60 to 82 years [11, 16].

These results were confirmed in a large, multicenter study performed in Italy where the effect of 20 mg/day of pravastatin on 338 patients, aged 60-70 years, with diagnosis of primary hypercholesterolemia, was evaluated. More women participated in the study representing 74% of the subjects studied (Table 1). Age, BMI (Kg/m^2), and baseline levels of total cholesterol (TC), LDL-C, HDL-C, and TG are shown in Table 1.

Table 1. Anthropometric features and basal lipid values.

		Pravastatin	Bezafibrate
Age (yrs.)		67 ± 0.4	67 ± 0.3
BMI (Kg/h2)		25.6 ± 0.25	25.3 ± 0.4
Gender	M	87	36
	F	251	112
Cholesterol (mg/dl)		289 ± 1.7	291 ± 2.5
LDL-C		207 ± 1.7	210 ± 2.5
HDL-C		53 ± 0.7	52 ± 1.1
Triglycerides		144 ± 2.5	140 ± 4.3

Values are expressed as mean±SEM

After 24 weeks of treatment with pravastatin TC decreased by 19%, LDL-C by 27%, TG by 4%, and HDL-C increased by 7% (Figure1).

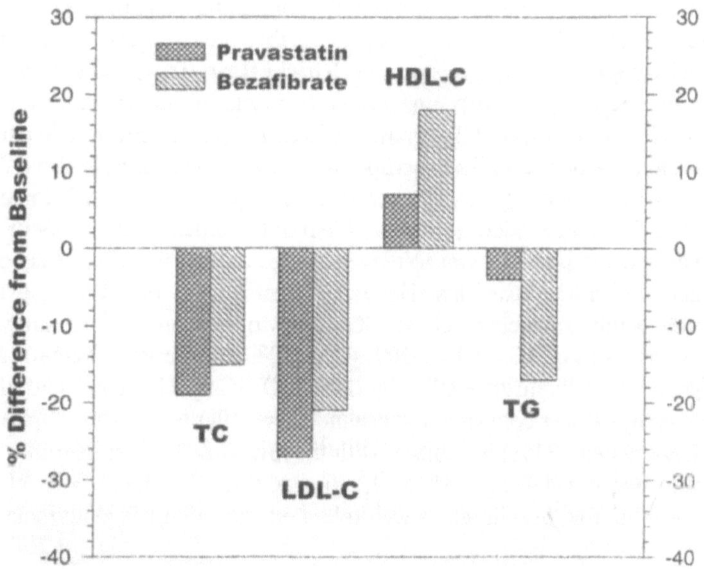

Figure 1. Effects of pravastatin and bezafribrate on plasma lipids. Values are expressed as % change from the baseline. TC, plasma cholesterol; LDL-C, low density lipoprotein cholesterol; HDL-C, high density lipoprotein cholesterol; TG, plasma triglycerides.

It is interestingly, however, to notice that when the subjects were stratified into four subgroups according to their baseline HDL-C levels (HDL-C ≤ 40 mg/dl; 41-50 mg/dl; 51-60 mg/dl; > 60 mg/dl), pravastatin increased HDL-C levels in subjects of the lowest quartile by 25%, whereas an increase by 9% was observed in subjects with baseline HDL-C between 41-50 mg/dl and no changes were observed in subjects with HDL-C greater than 51 mg/dl.

During the trial the number of drop-out patients was 56 out of 338 subjects (16.6%). The large majority of drop-outs were for reasons unrelated to the drug therapy and only one patient quit the study due to an increase in transaminase levels. These results confirm that the efficacy and safety of pravastatin were remarkable in elderly as well as in younger subjects.

FIBRIC ACID DERIVATIVES

Several fibric acid derivatives are available world-wide. This drug class includes clofibrate, gemfibrozil, bezafibrate, and fenofibrate. All of these agents effectively lower plasma triglycerides but they vary in their effect on the cholesterol level. Gemfibrozil was thoroughly evaluated in the Helsinki Heart Trial [17]. It is generally well tolerated. Side effects include epigastric distress, diarrhea, myalgias, abnormal liver function, anemia and lithogenic bile. The association of gemfibrozil and HMG-CoA reductase inhibitors increase the incidence of myositis (up to 5%). In some hypertriglyceridemic patients, gemfibrozil may cause the LDL-C to rise. The mechanism of action of gemfibrozil and the other fibrates is not completely defined although there is evidence that they stimulate lipoprotein lipase activity and inhibit triglyceride synthesis. In the Helsinki Heart Trial, gemfibrozil was found to reduce cardiovascular morbidity and mortality primarily in patients with combined hyperlipidemia (elevated TG and TC) and low HDL-C. It was less effective in patients with hypercholesterolemia alone (type 2a hyperlipoproteinemia). This drug is also indicated for use in patients with severe hypertriglyceridemia, especially those at risk for developing pancreatitis. Very few studies addressed the problem of the efficacy and safety of fibric acid derivatives in the elderly. Data are available from a large trial performed in Italy on 148 old subjects (Table 1) with primary hyperlipidemia treated with bezafibrate, a fibric acid derivative. In this study, subjects received 400 mg/day of bezafibrate for a study period of 24 weeks. Baseline levels of TC, LDL-C, HDL-C, and TG are shown in Table 1. At the end of the study period, bezafibrate lowered TC by 15%, LDL-C by 21% and TG by 17% while HDL-C increased by 18% as compared to baseline values (Figure 1). Bezafibrate increased HDL-C to a larger extent (31%) in subjects with the lowest HDL-C at baseline. The LDL-C/HDL-C ratio decreased from 4.18 to 2.9 ($p < 0.001$). No major side effects were observed, suggesting that bezafibrate is well tolerated and safe for aged population.

Conclusions

Management of elevated cholesterol in the elderly is controversial because few data are available evaluating efficacy/benefits of cholesterol-lowering drug therapy in old subjects. Some of the results presented are from the Italian Pravastatin and Bezafibrate Study, one of the largest, multicenter, randomized, double-blind studies comparing the efficacy, tolerability, and safety of pravastatin (an HMG-CoA reductase inhibitor) and bezafibrate (a fibric acid derivative) in elderly patients with primary hypercholesterolemia*. The results suggest that in the elderly the efficacy and safety of pravastatin and bezafibrate are comparable to those observed in younger subjects. Pravastatin is more effective in reducing total and LDL-C (19% and 27%, respectively) than bezafibrate (15% and 21%, respectively). Bezafibrate is more active in lowering plasma TG and increasing HDL-C (18%) as compared to pravastatin (7%) possibly through its specific effect on very low density lipoproteins (VLDL). Both drugs were well tolerated and safe for aged population. Of particular interest is the effect of pravastatin and bezafibrate on the HDL-C in the light of a recent report [10] suggesting that low HDL-C but not total cholesterol predicts CHD mortality and occurrence of new CHD events in persons older than 70 years.

Nevertheless, if drug therapy is warranted, a clear distinction should be made between drug therapy in the elderly for primary prevention of CHD compared with secondary prevention. For primary prevention, more patients would be exposed to drug therapy for the benefit of a few, and although this in itself may not contraindicate drug therapy in an old subject, lipid-lowering treatments in the elderly must withstand a cost-effectiveness analysis [18]. Therefore, because of the increased potential for adverse events, more stringent criteria should be used for patient selection of primary prevention than secondary prevention. Specifically subjects with chronic illness (cancer, dementia, etc.), or a limited life expectancy are not good candidates for drug therapy as treatment would be less likely to have benefits and more potential to cause harm. On the other hand, both the greater expected benefit and shorter duration of therapy needed to realize it, make drug therapy for secondary prevention attractive in the elderly. If this is the case pravastatin and bezafibrate appear to be safe and effective for treating hypercholesterolemia in the elderly.

References

1. Golini A, Lori A. Aging of the population: Demographic and social changes. Aging-Milano 1990;2:319-36.
2. Fries JF, Green LW, Levine S. Health promotion and the compression of morbidity. Lancet 1989;i:481.
3. Hazzard WR. Aging and atherosclerosis: Teasing out the contributions of time, secondary aging, and primary aging. Clin Geriatr Med 1985;1:251.
4. Kafonek S, Kwiterovich P. Treatment of hypercholesterolemia in the elderly. Ann Intern Med 1990;112:723-25.
5. National Center for Health Statistics. Vital statistics of the United States, 1988. Vol.II, Mortality, Part A. Washington DC: US Department of Health and Human Services, Public Health Service 1991:44-46. DHHS publication (PHS) 91-1101.
6. Castelli WP. Epidemiology of coronary artery disease. Am J Med 1984;76:4-12.
7. Shurtleff D. Some characteristics related to the incidence of cardiovascular disease and death using pooled repeated biennial measurements. In: Framingham Heart Study: An epidemiologic investigation of cardiovascular disease. Washington, DC: US Dept of Health, Education, and Welfare; 1974: section 30, table 1-3. DHEW publication NIH 74-599.

8. Kronmal RA, Cain KC, Ye Z, Omenn GS. Total serum cholesterol levels and mortality risk as a function of age: A report based on the Framingham data. Arch Int Med 1993;153:1065-73.
9. Reed D, Benfante R. Lipid and lipoprotein predictors of coronary heart disease in elderly men in the Honolulu Heart Program. Ann Epidemiol 1992;2:29-34.
10. Corti MC, Guralnik JM, Salive ME, et al. HDL cholesterol predicts coronary artery mortality in older persons. JAMA 1995;274:539-44.
11. Scandinavian Simvastatin Survival Study Group. Randomized trial of cholesterol lowering in 4444 patients with coronary artery disease: The Scandinavian Simvastatin Survival Study (4S). Lancet 1994;344:1383-89.
12. Shepherd J, Cobbe SM, Ford I, et al. Prevention of coronary heart disease with pravastatin in men with hypercholesterolemia. N Engl J Med 1995;333:1301-1307.
13. Goldman L, Weinstein MC, Goldman PA, Williams LW. Cost-effectiveness of HMG-CoA reductase inhibition for primary and secondary prevention of coronary heart disease. JAMA 1991;265:1145-51.
14. Denke M. Drug treatment of Hyperlipidemia in elderly patients. Curr Opin Lipidol 1993;4:56-62.
15. Brown MS, Goldstein JL. A receptor-mediated pathway for cholesterol homeostasis. Science 1986;232:34.
16. Kuhn P, Darioli R, Bovet P, Bercher L, Bruuner HR. Dose-dependent lipid-lowering effect of simvastatin (MK-733) in the elderly. Curr Therap Res 1989; 46:381.
17. Frick MH, Elo O, Haapa K, et al. Helsinki Heart Study: Primary-prevention trial with gemfibrozil in middle-aged men with dyslipidemia. Safety of treatment, changes in risk factors, and incidence of coronary artery disease. N Engl J Med 1987;317: 1237.
18. Avorn J. Benefit and cost analysis in geriatric care. N Engl J Med 1984;310:1294-1301.

Addendum

The Italian Pravastatin and Bezafibrate Study was coordinated by:

G. Crepaldi (Institute of Internal Medicine, University of Padua)
G.Baggio (Department of Geriatrics, University of Sassari)
S. Ventura (Institute of Internal Medicine, University of Perugia)
T. Segato (Institute of Ophthalmology, University of Padua)

PARTECIPATING GERIATRIC CENTERS

R. Balestrieri, S. Bertolini (University of Genoa), A. Capurso (University of Bari), P.U. Carbonin, A. Cocchi (Catholic University of Rome), D. Ceruso (University of Messina), D. Cucinotta (City Hospital Forli'), A. D'Alessandro (University of Florence), O. DeCandia (City Hospital of Padua), G. Descovich† (University of Bologna), F. Fabris (University of Turin), F.S. Feruglio (University of Trieste), S. Forconi (University of Siena), P. Forte (City Hospital of Rovigo), P. Fratino (University of Pavia), F. Mello (City Hospital of Venice), L. Motta (University of Catania), R. Navalesi (University of Pisa), A. Notarbartolo (University of Palermo), E. Paciaroni (I.N.R.C.A. Ancona), M. Passeri (University of Parma), M. Peruzza (City Hospital of Venice), A. Rappelli (University of Ancona), F. Rengo (University of Naples), U. Senin (University of Perugia), G. Valenti (University of Parma), C. Vergani (University of Milan), A.M. Zerman (City Hospital of Verona).

DRUG STRATEGIES FOR TREATMENT OF ACUTE AND POST-MI PATIENTS

Charles H. Hennekens
Harvard Medical School and Division of Preventive Medicine, Brigham and Women's Hospital, 900 Commonwealth Avenue East, Boston, Massachusetts 02215, USA

Introduction

Despite a dramatic decline in coronary heart disease (CHD) mortality over the past several decades, acute myocardial infarction (MI) remains the leading cause of death in the United States as well as in most developed countries, responsible for approximately one of every four fatalities or roughly 500,000 deaths each year [1]. Almost half of the deaths attributable to MI occur before the victims reach the hospital. Of those admitted to hospitals for MI, about 7-12% die during the course of their hospitalization, and an additional 10% die over the next several years [2-3].

An impressive decline in CHD mortality of approximately 2-3% per year has occurred over the past 30 years in the United States. CHD mortality rates have decreased among both men and women as well as among blacks and whites. Primary prevention measures, such as avoidance and cessation of cigarettes, lowering blood cholesterol, and increased diagnosis and treatment of hypertension, have played significant roles in the secular decline in CHD deaths. However, improvements in the treatment of MI patients, both in the peri-infarct period and in long-term management over the ensuing years, have also contributed importantly to the decline in CHD death rates. For example, 30-day mortality rates have declined during this time period from 20-30% to 5-10%.

Antithrombotic Therapy

Antithrombotic therapy with aspirin confers clear net benefits in the treatment of acute MI as well as in long-term secondary prevention following infarction. In acute MI, aspirin therapy confers unequivocal benefits in and should be administered to virtually all patients presenting with symptoms suggestive of infarction. Aspirin therapy in acute MI was evaluated in the Second International Study of Infarct Survival (ISIS-2), which randomized 17,187 patients presenting within 24 hours of the onset of symptoms [4]. Utilizing a 2 x 2 factorial design, the trial tested simultaneously the effects of intravenous streptokinase (1.5 million units) and oral aspirin (162 mg daily for 30 days, with the first tablet crushed or

A. M. Gotto, Jr. et al. (eds.), Drugs Affecting Lipid Metabolism, 465–471.

chewed to achieve a rapid clinical antithrombotic effect). At five weeks, those allocated to aspirin had experienced a statistically significant 23% reduction in vascular mortality (804 events versus 1,016; $p < 0.00001$). This benefit of approximately 23 lives per 1,000 patients treated was present regardless of the interval between onset of symptoms and treatment. There was only a small excess of minor bleeds, no excess of major bleeds, and, most importantly, no increase in hemorrhagic stroke associated with aspirin.

In long-term secondary prevention following MI, aspirin also confers a clear net benefit, which is additive to that of treatment during acute MI. In the Antiplatelet Trialists' Collaboration overview, among approximately 20,000 patients from 10 trials of patients with prior MI, allocation to antiplatelet therapy (principally with aspirin) yielded a statistically significant 15% reduction in two-year vascular mortality ($p < 0.005$) [5].

Heparin is also widely used as an antithrombotic therapy for acute MI. An overview of randomized trials of heparin in acute MI conducted prior to the use of aspirin suggested that its use is associated with a 16% mortality reduction, but also a two- to four-fold increase in bleeding rates [6-7].

Two large trials have assessed the clinical benefit of adding delayed subcutaneous heparin to a regimen of thrombolysis and aspirin: the Gruppo Italiano per lo Studio della Sopravvivenza nell'Infarto Miocardico (GISSI-2) and its international extension [8-9] and the Third International Study of Infarct Survival (ISIS-3) [10]. In these two trials, which randomized a total of more than 62,000 acute MI patients, there was no significant mortality benefit associated the addition of delayed subcutaneous heparin to a regimen of thrombolysis and adequate dose aspirin (325 mg in GISSI-2; 162 mg in ISIS-3). Heparin-treated patients in both trials experienced significant excesses in bleeding. In GISSI-2, there was a significant excess of noncerebral bleeding requiring transfusion, while in ISIS-3 heparin-treated patients experienced a significant excess of definite or probable cerebral hemorrhage as well as noncerebral bleeding requiring transfusion.

It had been suggested that the optimal benefit-to-risk profile for heparin requires immediate intravenous administration (within 4 hours of the start of thrombolytic therapy), and at doses sufficient to achieve consistent elevations of the activated partial thromboplastin time. This approach was tested in the Global Utilization of Streptokinase and Tissue Plasminogen Activator to Treat Occluded Arteries (GUSTO-1) trial, which directly compared immediate IV heparin with delayed subcutaneous heparin among patients treated with aspirin and streptokinase [11]. There was no significant mortality benefit of immediate IV heparin (7.4%) compared with delayed subcutaneous heparin (7.2%). Hemorrhagic stroke rates in the two groups were similar.

Thus, after the randomization of more than 62,000 patients in GISSI-2 and ISIS-3, there was no clear evidence that delayed subcutaneous heparin adds to the mortality benefit attainable with aspirin alone in patients receiving thrombolysis, regardless of the agent. Further, data from more than 20,000 patients in GUSTO-1 reveal no clear benefit of immediate IV heparin compared with delayed subcutaneous heparin in patients treated with aspirin and streptokinase. Newer antithrombotic agents are now undergoing evaluation in randomized trials.

Thrombolytic Therapy

Thrombolytic therapy confers a clear net benefit on in-hospital mortality rates among acute MI patients. A comprehensive overview of all trials of thrombolytic therapy enrolling more than 1,000 patients indicates that, in those with ST elevation or bundle branch block who are treated within 12 hours of symptom onset, this therapy saves 20-30 lives per 1,000 patients [12]. Benefits are greater for those treated within 6 hours, but are still substantial for those treated up to 12 hours after symptom onset.

Although the benefits of thrombolysis are clear, there has been controversy over which of the principal thrombolytic agents has the optimal benefit-to-risk ratio. GISSI-2, which directly compared streptokinase and tissue plasminogen activator (tPA), found no mortality difference between the treatments, but a significant excess among tPA-treated patients of total stroke (4 per 1,000, $p < 0.008$) and a nonsignificant excess of cerebral hemorrhage (3 per 1,000, $p = 0.10$) [8-9]. ISIS-3, which compared streptokinase, tPA, and anisoylated plasminogen streptokinase activator complex (APSAC), also found no mortality difference, but a significant excess with tPA of total stroke (4 per 1,000, $p < 0.001$) and cerebral hemorrhage (3 per 1 000, $p < 0.001$) [10]. GUSTO-1 found a 9 per 1,000 mortality benefit with accelerated tPA and IV heparin, but a significant excess of total stroke (3 per 1,000, $p < 0.05$) and cerebral hemorrhage (2 per 1,000, $p < 0.03$) in comparison to streptokinase with delayed subcutaneous heparin [11].

Thus, the totality of evidence indicates any overall differences in efficacy, safety or ease of administration of streptokinase, tPA, or APSAC are small in relation to the substantial benefits that would result from the wider use and earlier administration of any thrombolytic therapy.

Beta-Blockers

Beta-blockers are effective anti-ischemic, antiarrhythmic, and hypotensive agents, which reduce myocardial wall stress and infarct size when used in acute MI. Beta-blocker therapy has been demonstrated to confer significant mortality benefits in acute MI. The First International Study of Infarct Survival (ISIS-1), which randomized over 16,000 acute MI patients worldwide, demonstrated a significant 15% reduction in 7-day vascular mortality among those receiving atenolol versus placebo ($p < 0.04$) [13], and an overview of beta-blocker trials in acute MI demonstrated a significant mortality benefit of 13 lives per 1,000 patients treated [14].

Net mortality benefits of beta-blocker therapy were clear prior to the widespread use of more recent acute MI therapies. No large-scale randomized trials have been conducted, however, to assess the effects of beta-blockers in conjunction with aspirin, thrombolysis, or angiotensin converting-inhibitors. In long-term therapy, an overview of several randomized trials beta-blocker therapy has demonstrated clear benefits of prolonged administration on vascular mortality, sudden death and reinfarction [14].

Beta-blockers, therefore, should be considered for all acute MI patients without clear contraindications, such as severe congestive heart failure, asthma, or hypotension, and treatment should be continued for at least two years.

Angiotensin Converting Enzyme Inhibitors

Several randomized trials have demonstrated significant benefits on mortality as well as reductions in reinfarction and ventricular arrhythmias from the use of angiotensin converting enzyme (ACE) inhibitors in acute MI [15-19]. GISSI-3 and ISIS-4 randomized a total of more than 70,000 patients within 24 hours of the onset of acute MI symptoms to ACE inhibitor therapy (lisinopril in GISSI-3; captopril in ISIS-4) or placebo [18-19]. The two trials demonstrated a 35-day mortality benefit of about 5 lives per 1,000 patients treated.

In long-term treatment of post-MI patients with left ventricular dysfunction, ACE inhibitors also confer small, but significant, mortality benefits. In the Acute Infarction Ramipril Efficacy (AIRE) Study, after an average treatment duration of 15 months, patients randomized to ramipril experienced a 27% mortality reduction ($p = 0.002$) [16], while the Survival and Ventricular Enlargement (SAVE) Trial demonstrated a 19% mortality reduction with captopril after 42 months of treatment ($p = 0.014$) [17].

Thus, ACE inhibitor therapy should be considered for all eligible patients within 24 hours of the onset of acute MI symptoms, and should be continued long-term in those with left ventricular dysfunction. Whether long-term benefits accrue to all post-MI patients requires further investigation.

Calcium Channel Blockers, Magnesium, and Nitrates

Calcium channel blockers. Calcium channel blockers have been evaluated in randomized trials and found to confer no net mortality benefit. In the Nifedipine and Angina Myocardial Infarction Study (NAMIS), short-term mortality was, in fact, higher among those receiving nifedipine than placebo ($p = 0.018$) [20]. By six months, however, there was no significant mortality difference. Similar results have been found in the Secondary Prevention Re-infarction Israeli Nifedipine Trial (SPRINT II) [21] and the Trial of Early Nifedipine in Acute Myocardial Infarction [22]. Thus, calcium channel blockers do not appear to reduce mortality in acute MI. Subgroup analyses from some trials have raised the possibility of benefits of calcium antagonists with negative chronotropic effects in preventing reinfarction, angina, and death in patients with normal ventricular function, but this hypothesis requires testing randomized trials.

Magnesium. As regards the use of intravenous magnesium in acute MI, the Second Leicester Intravenous Magnesium Intervention Trial (LIMIT-2), which randomized 2,316 patients with suspected acute MI, demonstrated a 24% mortality reduction associated with magnesium ($p = 0.04$) [23]. A mortality benefit was also observed in a meta-analysis that included LIMIT-2 and several earlier, small trials [24]. However, ISIS-4, which tested magnesium in over 58,000 patients with suspected acute MI, found no evidence of any mortality benefit overall or among subgroups of those treated within 6 hours, those who received magnesium soon after thrombolytic therapy, or those not receiving thrombolysis

[19]. Thus, current evidence does not support the use of magnesium as therapy in acute MI.

Nitrates. With respect to nitrates, based on their clear benefits in reducing ischemic chest pain, and on basic and clinical research findings demonstrating an ability to limit infarct size and improve left ventricular function, randomized trials have evaluated their possible mortality benefit in acute MI. While a meta-analysis of several trials of small sample size demonstrated a large and significant mortality benefit (12% versus 20.5%, $p < 0.001$) [25], the results of GISSI-3 [18] and ISIS-4 [19] in over 70,000 patients indicate no mortality benefit of nitrates in acute MI. Both trials, however, did find nitrate therapy to be effective and safe for the control of ischemic chest pain.

Conclusion

There are clear and substantial mortality benefits in acute MI from the use of aspirin as well as thrombolytics, alone as well as in combination with one another and with beta-blockers and ACE inhibitors. Data from randomized trials do not provide support for net mortality benefits of calcium antagonists, magnesium or nitrates in acute MI, although nitrates are effective and safe for relief of ischemic chest pain. The estimated short-term benefit of aspirin in acute MI is 23 lives per 1,000 patients treated within 24 hours, and for thrombolytic therapy, 20-30 lives per 1,000 patients treated within 12 hours. For beta-blockers this benefit is 13 lives per 1,000, and for ACE inhibitors it is 5 lives per 1,000 patients treated.

Long-term therapy following MI with aspirin, beta-blockers, and ACE inhibitors will save additional lives. However, it is important to bear in mind that so, too, will other risk reductions measures that are effective in both primary and secondary prevention, including smoking cessation, cholesterol lowering, control of elevated blood pressure, and avoidance or management of obesity [3]. Despite impressive gains over that past three decades, acute MI remains the leading cause of death in the U.S. The greater utilization during and after MI of therapies with proven net benefits will contribute further to reductions in the public health burden of MI.

References

1. American Heart Association. Heart and stroke facts: 1995 statistical supplement. Dallas, Texas:American Heart Association, 1994.
2. Moss AJ, Benhorin J. Prognosis and management after a first myocardial infarction. N Engl J Med 1990;322:743-53.
3. Manson JE, Tosteson H, Ridker PM, et al. The primary prevention of myocardial infarction. N Engl J Med 1992;326:1406-16.
4. ISIS-2 (Second International Study of Infarct Survival) Collaborative Group. Randomized trial of intravenous streptokinase, oral aspirin, both or neither among 17,187 cases of suspected acute myocardial infarction. Lancet 1988;ii:349-60.
5. Antiplatelet Trialists' Collaboration. Collaborative overview of randomized trials of antiplatelet treatment. Part I: Prevention of vascular death, myocardial infarction and stroke

by prolonged antiplatelet therapy in different categories of patients. Br Med J 1994; 308:81-106.

6. MacMahon S, Collins R, Knight C, Yusuf S, Peto R. Reduction in major morbidity and mortality by heparin in acute myocardial infarction (abstract). Circulation 1988;78(II):98.
7. O'Donnell CJ, Ridker PM, Hebert PR, Hennekens CH. Antithrombotic therapy of acute myocardial infarction. J Am Coll Cardiol 1993;25:23S-29S.
8. Gruppo Italiano per lo Studio della Sopravvivenza Nell'Infarto Miocardico. GISSI-2: A factorial randomized trial of alteplase versus streptokinase and heparin versus no heparin among 12,490 patients with acute myocardial infarction. Lancet 1990;336:65-71.
9. The International Study Group (ISG). In-hospital mortality and clinical course of 20,891 patients with suspected acute myocardial infarction randomized between alteplase and streptokinase with or without heparin. Lancet 1990;336:71-75.
10. ISIS-3 (Third International Study of Infarct Survival) Collaborative Group. ISIS-3: A Randomized Trial Comparing SK vs tPA vs APSAC and comparing aspirin plus heparin vs aspirin alone among 41,299 suspected acute myocardial infarction. Lancet 1992;339:1-18.
11. The GUSTO Investigators. An international randomized trial comparing four thrombolytic strategies for acute myocardial infarction. N Engl J Med 1993;329:673-82.
12. Fibrinolytic Therapies Trialists' (FTT) Collaborative Group. Indications for fibrinolytic therapy in suspected acute myocardial infarction: Collaborative overview of mortality and major morbidity results from all randomized trials of more than 1000 patients. Lancet 1994; 343:311-22.
13. ISIS-1 Collaborative Group. Randomized trial of intravenous atenolol among 16,027 cases of suspected acute myocardial infarction: ISIS-1. Lancet 1986;ii:57-66.
14. Yusuf S, Peto R, Lewis J, Collins R, Sleight P. Beta-blockade during and after myocardial infarction. An overview of the randomized trials. Prog Cardiovasc Dis 1985;27:335-71.
15. Kingma JH, van Gilst WH, Peels CH, Dambrink J-HE, Verheught FWA, Wielenga RP, for the CATS investigators. Acute intervention with captopril during thrombolysis in patients with first anterior myocardial infarction. Results from the Captopril and Thrombolysis Study (CATS). Eur Heart J 1994;15:898-907.
16. The Acute Infarction Ramipril Efficacy (AIRE) Study Investigators. Effect of ramipril on mortality and morbidity of survivors of acute myocardial infarction with clinical evidence of heart failure. Lancet 1993;342:821-28.
17. Pfeffer MA, Braunwald E, Moy LA, et al. Effect of captopril on mortality and morbidity in patients with left ventricular dysfunction after myocardial infarction. N Engl J Med 1992; 327:669-77.
18. Gruppo Italiano per lo Studio della Sopravvivenza Nell'Infarto Miocardico. GISSI-3. Effects of lisinopril and transdermal glyceryl trinitrate singly and together on 6-week mortality and ventricular function after acute myocardial infarction. Lancet 1994;343:1115-22.
19. ISIS-4 (Fourth International Study of Infarct Survival) Collaborative Group. ISIS-4: A randomized factorial trial assessing early oral captopril, oral mononitrate and intravenous magnesium sulphate in 58,050 patients with suspected acute myocardial infarction. Lancet 1995;345:669-85.
20. Muller JE, Morrison J, Stone PH, et al. Nifedipine therapy for patients with threatened and acute myocardial infarction: A randomized, double-blind, placebo-controlled comparison. Circulation 1984;69:740-47.
21. Sprint Study Group. The Secondary Prevention Re-Infarction Israeli Nifedipine Trial (SPRINT) II: Design and methods, results (abstract). Eur Heart J 1988;9(1):1914,1914A.

22. Wilcox RG, Hampton JR, Banks DC, et al. Trial of early nifedipine in acute myocardial infarction: The TRENT Study. Br Med J 1986;293:1204-1208.
23. Woods KL, Fletcher S, Roffe C, Haider Y. Intravenous magnesium sulphate in suspected acute myocardial infarction: Results of the second Leicester Intravenous Magnesium Intervention Trial (LIMIT-2). Lancet 1992;339:1553-58.
24. Teo KK, Yusuf S. Role of magnesium in reducing mortality in acute myocardial infarction: A review of the evidence. Drugs 1993;46:347-59.
25. Yusuf S, Collins R, MacMahon S, Peto R. Effect of intravenous nitrates on mortality in acute myocardial infarction: An overview of the randomized trials. Lancet 1988;1:1088-92.

NONCHOLESTEROL SERUM STEROLS IN SCANDINAVIAN SIMVASTATIN SURVIVAL STUDY

Tatu A. Miettinen, Timo Strandberg, Hannu T. Vanhanen, and Helena Gylling, for the 4S Group
Division of Internal Medicine, University of Helsinki, 00290 Helsinki, Finland

Introduction

A large placebo-controlled randomized multicenter Scandinavian Study, 4S, showed that in 4,444 patients with coronary heart disease a 25% decrease in serum cholesterol was recorded by an over-five-year simvastatin treatment (2,223 subjects), while the respective change in the placebo group (2,221 subjects) was 1% [1]. A highly significant decrease was observed in total (-30%) and coronary mortality (-42%). Simvastatin, like other statins, lowers serum cholesterol by inhibiting cholesterol synthesis [2]. This is associated with a significant fall in serum triglycerides and an increase in high density lipoprotein (HDL) cholesterol, two findings observed also in 4S. Statins can decrease cholesterol turnover and reduce biliary cholesterol secretion [3]. Cholesterol absorption efficiency is decreased in familial hypercholesterolemia (FH) but not in non-FH [3-5]. In the present subgroup study of 4S we evaluated some baseline factors regulating cholesterol synthesis and absorption, and tried to figure out effects of simvastatin on cholesterol metabolism by determining noncholesterol sterols in serum by gas liquid chromatograpy, expressing the values in terms of mmol/mol of total cholesterol. Cholesterol precursor sterols, Δ^8-cholestenol, desmosterol, and lathosterol are known to reflect cholesterol synthesis [6], while cholestanol and plant sterols (campesterol and sitosterol) are associated with cholesterol absorption, but they are also related to cholesterol turnover [6-7]. The study population included 434 coronary patients in the simvastatin group and 433 patients in the placebo group, and the measurements were performed at baseline, and 6 weeks, 12 months, and 66 months after randomization.

The higher the basal cholesterol concentration, the lower was the respective precursor sterol proportion ($r = -0.140$ for lathosterol; $n = 867$), suggesting that cholesterol synthesis is low at high cholesterol concentrations and high at low respective levels. Despite similar basal cholesterol values, the proportions of cholestanol and plant sterols were lower and those of the precursor sterols higher in obese (body mass index > 26) than lean subjects, findings shown earlier also in noncoronary subjects [8]. Simvastatin reduced, correspondingly, more the precursor sterol proportions (e.g. lathosterol -35 versus -32%;

A. M. Gotto, Jr. et al. (eds.), Drugs Affecting Lipid Metabolism, 473–476.

$p < 0.01$) and increased less plant sterol (e.g. campesterol +24 versus 27%; $p < 0.01$) in obese than in lean subjects. A higher basal cholesterol concentration in females than in males was associated with only inconsistent respective differences in noncholesterol sterols or their responses to simvastatin, even though the increase of the sitostanol proportion was 29% in females and 23% in males ($p < 0.001$). Figure 1 shows that simvastatin lowered serum cholesterol by 39% and 33% at 6 weeks and 66 months, respectively, with virtually no change in the placebo group. A marked-up to 36% decrease was observed in the

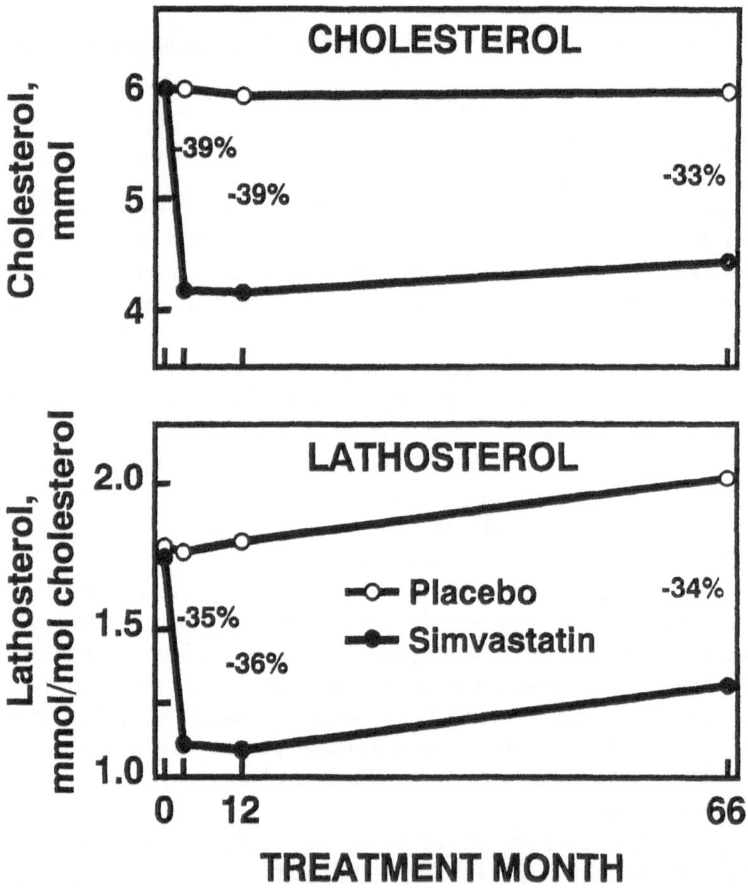

Figure 1. Cholesterol and lathosterol lowering by simvastatin.

lathosterol ratio by simvastatin as compared to the placebo treatment. Comparable changes were observed in Δ^8-cholestenol and desmosterol. In addition, the decrease in total (or low density lipoprotein [LDL]) cholesterol was positively associated with the decrease in the precursor sterol proportions (e.g. r = 0.138 for lathosterol; n = 422), suggesting that the higher the inhibition of cholesterol synthesis, the higher was the decrease in serum cholesterol. The decreases in cholesterol and the precursor sterol proportions caused by simvastatin were negatively related to their baseline values (r-values ranged from -0.398 to -0.892) and the higher the basal cholesterol level, the lower was the decrease in cholesterol synthesis (r = 0.131 for Δ^8-cholestenol change).

Cholestanol and Plant Sterols

The baseline proportions of cholestanol and plant sterols were only weakly, but positively, related to the baseline cholesterol levels, suggesting that increased cholesterol absorption contributed weakly to serum cholesterol. Figure 2 demonstrates that simvastatin increased the proportions of cholestanol and the two plant sterols (campesterol, sitosterol) to cholesterol by 12% to 36% as compared to placebo. Thus, the serum concentrations of

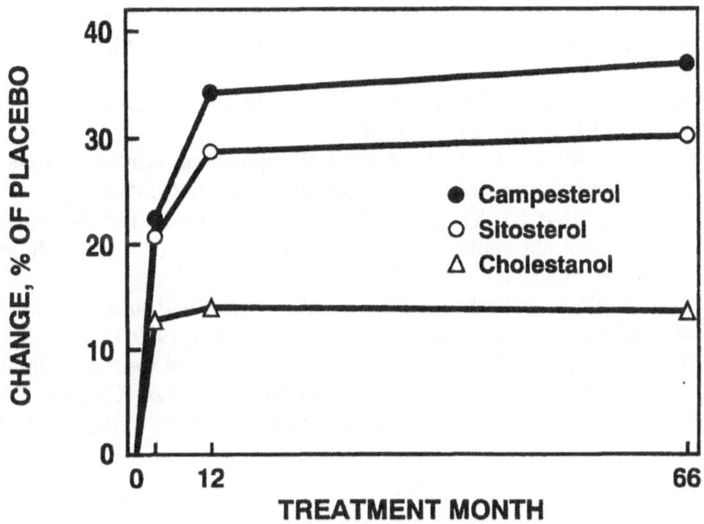

Figure 2. Relative increase of campesterol, sitosterol, and cholestanol by simvastatin.

these sterols were actually decreased, especially during the early phase of the treatment. Since simvastatin inhibits effectively cholesterol synthesis, it reduces also biliary secretion of cholesterol, resulting in reduced turnover of cholesterol [3]. This most likely also reduces turnover of cholestanol and plant sterols, resulting in their increased proportion to cholesterol at somewhat reduced serum concentrations. Simvastatin increased unlikely absorption of plant sterols, even though at reduced intestinal cholesterol pool a slight increase in their absorption was not excluded.

The higher the baseline proportions of cholestanol and plant sterols, the higher were their increases. In general, the proportions and the simvastatin-induced changes in proportions of cholestanol and plant sterols were negatively related to those of cholesterol precursors and opposite to respective correlations what the precursor sterol proportions had. Preliminary analyses suggested that the higher the baseline quartile of these sterols, the lower was the rate of simvastatin-induced decrease in major coronary events. This would mean that subjects with the high baseline proportions of these sterols are nonresponders to simvastatin-induced decrease in coronary events. No such association was observed for serum total baseline cholesterol in this subgroup.

References

1. The Scandinavian Simvastatin Survival Study Group. Randomized trial of cholesterol lowering in 4444 patients with coronary heart disease: The Scandinavian Simvastatin Survival Study Group (4S). Lancet 1994;344:1383-89.
2. Grundy SM. HMG-CoA reductase inhibitors for treatment of hypercholesterolemia. N Engl J Med 1988;319:24-33.
3. Vanhanen H, Kesäniemi YA, Miettinen TA. Pravastatin lowers cholesterol, cholesterol-precursor sterols, fecal steroids, and cholesterol absorption in man. Metabolism 1992;41:588-95.
4. Miettinen TA. Inhibition of cholesterol absorption by HMG-CoA reductase inhibitor. Eur J Clin Pharmacol 1991;40:Suppl 1:S19-S21.
5. Vanhanen HT, Miettinen TA. Cholesterol absorption and synthesis during pravastatin, gemfibrozil and their combination. Atherosclerosis 1995;115:135-46.
6. Miettinen TA, Tilvis RS, Kesäniemi YA. Serum plant sterols and cholesterol precursors reflect cholesterol absorption and synthesis in volunteers of a randomly selected male population. Am J Epidemiol 1990;131:20-31.
7. Miettinen TA, Tilvis RS, Kesäniemi YA. Serum cholestanol and plant sterol levels in relation to cholesterol metabolism in middle-aged men. Metabolism 1989;38: 136-40.
8. Miettinen TA. Regulation of serum cholesterol by cholesterol absorption. In: Parnham MJ, Niemann R, editors. Agents and action supplements AAS26. Cologne Atherosclerosis Conference No. 4: Cholesterol-Homeostasis. Basel: Birkhäuser Verlag, 1988:53-65.

MEDICAL MANAGEMENT OF POSTMYOCARDIAL INFARCTION PATIENTS

Haruo Nakamura and Toshio Shibuya
National Defense Medical College, Department of Medicine, 3-2 Namiki, Tokorozawa, Saitama 359, Japan

Introduction

The consensus panel statement of the American Heart Association [1] on preventing heart attack and death in patients with coronary disease recently indicates that comprehensive risk factor intervention extends overall survival, improves the quality of life, decreases the need for interventional procedures such as angioplasty and bypass grafting, and reduces the incidence of subsequent myocardial infarction (MI).

Specifically, many clinical sequelae may occur following myocardial infarction, which may determine the prognosis of the patient. Ventricular remodelling or dilation is one of the important events, leading to an increased risk of heart failure, cardiac rupture, arrhythmia, and death. Thromboembolic events due to increased hemostatic factors and the dysfunction of endothelium of the coronary artery caused by hyperlipidemia could result in a recurrence of myocardial infarction.

CURRENT DRUGS PRESCRIBED IN THE POST-MI PATIENTS

Based on the above points, administration of such drugs as β-blockers, angiotensin-converting enzyme (ACE) inhibitors, nitrates, thrombolytic agents, aspirin, and lipid lowering agents, is frequently recommended.

Analysis of drugs received by post-MI patients in our department between March 1995 and September 1995 showed that 80% of the subjects were taking aspirin, 64% β-blockers, 96% nitrates, 28% ACE inhibitors, and 36% lipid lowering agents. There is an increasing number of reports on the use of each drug. Examination on the effect of use of aspirin on mortality and morbidity rates in a subset of the control group of the program on the surgical control of the hyperlipidemia (POSCH) [2] was performed by the stratification of cigarette smoking status in hyperlipidemic post-MI patients. In current cigarette smokers at baseline with a mean follow-up of 8.3 years, the overall mortality rate was 45.2% in patients with no aspirin use and 10.4% in patients who reported even infrequent aspirin use. The overall mortality rate in former cigarette smokers was lower in patients with or without aspirin than that in current cigarette smokers. The relative risk of overall mortality in this

A. M. Gotto, Jr. et al. (eds.), Drugs Affecting Lipid Metabolism, 477–482.

group of aspirin users appeared to be smaller compared to nonaspirin users. Although the effect of in-trial aspirin use on former cigarette smokers did not reach statistical significance, the trends were similar to those observed in the current smokers.

The benefits of aspirin were also reported in animal experiments [3]. It was shown that of the rats that underwent left coronary artery occlusion, aspirin-treated rats had a less expanded infarct area than control rats, related to increased patency of the microvessels in the infarcted area.

We also have to consider other hemostatic factor antigens and tissue plasminogen activator antigens as a means of diminishing subsequent acute coronary syndromes.

Since 1972, many randomized, controlled trials of long-term β-adrenergic blocking therapy have been conducted in more than 18,000 survivors of acute myocardial infraction. These studies have shown convincingly the therapeutic benefit of initiating treatment for the typical trial patients. Analysis of data from Beta-Blocker in Heart Attack Trial (BHAT), a randomized, double-blind placebo-controlled trial, indicated that in patients who survived to one year with low-to-moderate risk, the clinical course using β-blocker therapy (propranolol) did not have a long-term beneficial effect and in contrast, among patients who had a high-risk clinical course such as worsening ischemia, heart failure, and arrhythmia, β-blockers significantly reduced mortality in the follow-up period [4].

The use of angiotensin-converting enzyme (ACE) inhibitors has also been reported to be beneficial in patients after acute myocardial infarction and the benefit seems to be greatest in patients with congestive heart failure or asymptomatic ventricular dysfunction which is an important prognostic indicator, possibly due to the process of ventricular remodeling.

The survival of myocardial infarction long-term evaluation trial was conducted to test the hypothesis that oral administration of an ACE inhibitor, zofenopril, to patients with acute anterior myocardial infarction who were not undergoing thrombolysis would improve their clinical outcome by reducing the incidence of major cardiovascular events [5].

During the six weeks of treatment, death or severe congestive heart failure occurred in 10.6% in the placebo group and in 7.1% in the zofenopril group. Examining the cumulative incidence of death from all causes regardless of whether there was prior congestive failure, it was found that there were 65 deaths in the placebo group (8.3%) as compared with 50 in the zofenopril group (6.5%). The reduction in the risk of death from all causes during the six-week treatment period was 22% and was almost entirely due to the reduction in cardiovascular mortality in zofenopril group.

Patients who received zofenopril for six weeks were significantly more likely to survive than patients who were given placebo. The difference in survival cannot be explained by the concomitant pharmacologic or surgical treatment.

The Fourth International Study of Infarct Survival (ISIS-4) [6] has also assessed the effect on mortality and major morbidity of the addition of each of three widely practicable treatment: one month of oral ACE inhibitor, one month of oral nitrates, and 24 hours of intravenous magnesium to the patients with definite or suspected acute myocardial infarction.

There was a significant 7% proportional reduction in 5-week mortality which corresponds to an absolute difference of 4.9 fewer deaths per 10,000 patients treated by ACE inhibitors for a month. They also pointed out that the absolute benefits appeared to be larger in certain higher risk groups, such as those presenting with a history of previous MI or with heart failure. In contrast, there were no significant reductions in 5-week mortality in mononitrate or magnesium treatments.

There is no longer any doubt about the benefit and safety of treating hypercholesterolemia in patients who have had a myocardial infarction. The placebo-controlled, multinational study was conducted to evaluate the use of pravastatin in 1,062 patients with hypercholesterolemia (200 to 300 mg/dl) and 2 or more additional risk factors for coronary artery disease [7].

At week 13, patients treated with pravastatin had significant reductions in low density lipoprotein cholesterol (LDL-C) (26%), total cholesterol (19%), and triglyceride (12%), and significant elevations in high density lipoprotein lipoprotein cholesterol (HDL-C) (7%). At that time 66% of the subjects taking pravastatin had achieved the target cholesterol goal (namely below 200 mg/dl) versus 7% of the patients taking placebo. Efficacy was maintained at 26 weeks. Serious adverse events were reported significantly more often in patients receiving placebo. Six of these events occurred in the pravastatin-treated group and 26 occurred in placebo-treated patients. Serious adverse cardiovascular events were reported in 1 pravastatin-treated patient and in 13 placebo-treated patients. There were no significant differences in noncardiocerebrovascular events.

The largest secondary prevention trial, the Scandinavian Simvastatin Survival Study (4S) [8] studied 4,444 patients with coronary heart disease and showed that after 5.4 years a 25%reduction in plasma cholesterol concentrations initially between 5.5 and 8.0 mmol/l resulted in 30% fewer deaths and 42% fewer coronary deaths.

Dosage of simvastatin was adjusted in order to reduce serum total cholesterol to 3.0-5.2 mmol/L. The primary endpoint was total mortality. During the study period 438 patients died, 256 in the placebo group and 182 in the simvastatin group. The relative risk was 0.70 with simvastatin. There were 189 coronary deaths in the placebo group compared with 111 in the simvastatin group. The relative risk of coronary death was 0.58 with simvastatin. There was no statistically significant difference between the two groups in the number of deaths from noncardiovascular causes.

The Kaplan-Meier 6-year probability of escaping major coronary events was 70.5% in the placebo group and 79.6% in the simvastatin group. The probability of escaping any coronary events was 56.7% in the placebo group and 66.6% in the simvastatin group. Simvastatin also reduced any atherosclerotic events and the patients risk of undergoing coronary artery bypass surgery or angioplasty. This study shows that long-term treatment of cholesterol lowering with simvastatin is safe and improves survival in coronary heart disease patients.

TREATMENT GOAL OF PLASMA LIPIDS

Trial evidence shows clear benefits from secondary prevention by reducing patient cholesterol level. However, a small double-blind trial, the Harvard Atherosclerosis

Regression Project [9], added some additional perspective by suggesting that patients with more normal cholesterol concentrations (between 4.5 and 6.0 mmol/L) might not benefit from statin treatment at least within three years.

Since Japanese patients with MI generally have mildly elevated or almost normal cholesterol levels, we treated those subjects with statins in order to obtain whether cholesterol-lowering treatment benefits the patients and to find out the target levels of plasma total cholesterol, triglyceride, HDL-cholesterol, and LDL-cholesterol to inhibit the progressive change of coronary atherosclerosis.

Ninety subjects (73 male and 17 female) were enrolled and received repeated quantitative coronary angiography during the interval of 3 years. Fifteen percent changes in stenosis were classified as either progression or regression. All quantitative aspects of the angiographic analysis were blinded as to patient's identity and the film sequence.

We found 34 patients experienced definite progression and 56 patients nonprogression. Table 1 shows baseline risk factors for the patient with or without progression. There were no significant differences in risk factors such as age, gender, incidence of hypertension, diabetes mellitus, and smoking habits.

Table 1. Baseline characteristics of patients.

	Progression		P	Odds Ratio
	(+)	(-)		
N	34	56		
Age (y/o)	56.3 ± 9.3	56.7 ± 8.7	0.85	
Gender (M/F)	31/3	42/14	0.1	3.4
Hypertension(+/-)	21/13	34/22	0.92	1.0
DM (+/-)	13/21	20/36	0.81	1.1
Smoking (+/-)	29/5	43/13	0.48	1.8

The mean total cholesterol at baseline was 202 mg/dl for nonprogression patients and was 219.7 mg/dl for progression patients. The difference was statistically significant. It fell 3% and 4% in the subjects with nonprogression and the subjects with progression respectively after the treatment. The subjects with progression have still relatively high cholesterol level, namely more than 200mg/dl. The changes in LDL-cholesterol in the patients with or without progression is shown in Figure 1. The mean LDL-cholesterol at baseline was 131.5 mg/dl for nonprogression patients and was 151.5 mg/dl for progression patients. This difference was again significant. It fell 6% in the nonprogression group and 4% in the progression group, respectively. LDL-cholesterol levels in the subjects with progression were significantly higher compared with those of nonprogression group, and remained more than 130 mg/dl.

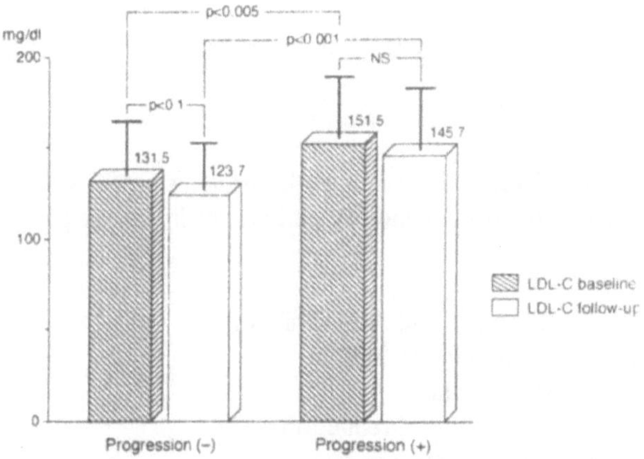

Figure 1. LDL-cholesterol levels for progression and nonprogression group

The mean triglyceride level at baseline was comparable in both groups. In the subjects without progression, it decreased by 11%, while in the subjects with progression, it remained at the baseline level.

The baseline HDL-cholesterol level averaged 41 mg/dl for the patients without progression. As shown in Figure 2, it rose 12% in the nonprogression group and fell 3% in the progression group, remaining below 40 mg/dl.

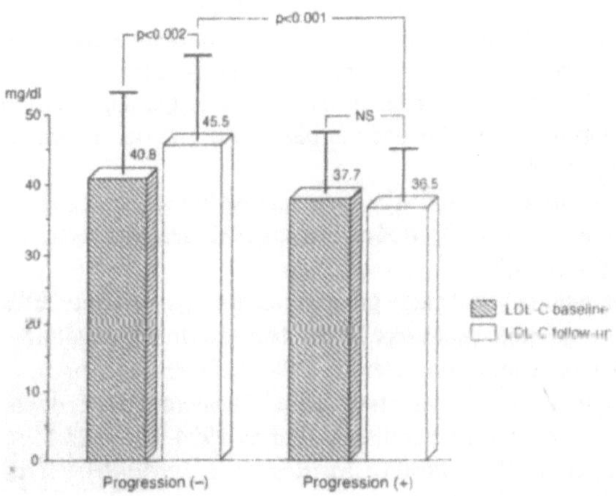

Figure 2. HDL-cholesterol levels for progression and nonprogression group

This trial has shown the benefits to the ischemic subjects with normal or mildly elevated blood cholesterol levels by reducing total cholesterol below 200 mg/dl, LDL-cholesterol below 130 mg/dl, triglyceride below 150 mg/dl, and by increasing HDL-cholesterol more than 40 mg/dl.

Thus, we speculate these figures will be the treatment goal for ischemic patients.

Conclusion

Considering the many factors determining the prognosis of post-MI patients such as ventricular dysfunction, hemostatic factors, and plasma lipids, we propose the term 2A'S-BCDE.

2A	stands for Aspirin and ACE inhibitor
S	stands for Smoking cessation
B	stands for β-blockers
C	stands for Cholesterol reduction
D	stands for Diet against obesity
E	stands for Exercise

References

1. Smith SC, Blair SN, Criqui MH, et al. Preventing heart attack and death in patients with coronary disease. Circulation 1995;92:2-4.
2. Fitch LL, Buchwald H, Matts JO, Johnson JW, Campos CT, Long JM. Effect of aspirin use on death and recurrent myocardial infarction in current and former cigarette smokers. Amer Heart J 1995;129:656-62.
3. Alhaddad IA, Tkaczerski L, Siddiqui F, Mir R, Brown EJ. Aspirin enhance the benefits of late reperfusion on infarct shape. Circulation 1995;91:2819-23.
4. Viscoli CM, Horwitz RI, Singer BH. Beta-blockers after myocardial infarction; Influence of first-year clinical course on long-term effectiveness. Ann Int Med 1993; 118:99-105.
5. Anbrosioni E, Borghi C, Magnani B. The effect of the angiotensin-converting- enzyme inhibitor zofenopril on mortality and morbidity after anterior myocardial infarction. N Engl J Med 1995;332:80-85.
6. ISIS-4. A randomised factorial trial assessing early oral captopril, oral mononitrate, and intravenous magnesium sulphate in 58650 patients with suspected acute myocardial infarction. Lancet 1995;345:669-85.
7. The pravastatin multinational study group for cardiac risk patients: Effects of pravastatin in patients with serum total cholesterol levels from 5.2 to 7.8 mmol/liter plus two additional atherosclerotic risk factors. Am J Cardiol 1993;72:1031-37.
8. Scandinavian Simvastatin Survival Study Group. Randomised trial of cholesterol lowering in 4444 patients with coronary heart disease. Lancet 1994;344:1383-89.
9. Sacks FM, Pasternak RC, Gibson CM, Rosner B, Stone PH. Harvard Athero-sclerosis Reversibility Project (HARP). Effect on coronary atherosclerosis of decrease in plasma cholesterol concentrations in normocholesterolaemic patients. Lancet 1994;344:1182-86.

EXPERIENCE IN CLINICAL USE OF NEW CHOLESTEROL LOWERING DRUGS

N. Nakaya
Tokai University Tokyo Hospital, 1-2-5 Yoyogi Shibuya-ku, 151 Tokyo, Japan

Introduction

Several powerful antihyperlipidemic drugs are now available. The most potent cholesterol-lowering drug is the HMG-CoA reductase inhibitor and the average reduction rate of LDL-cholesterol is 25-35%. If it is used in combination rate with an anion-exchange resin, the reduction rate will be increased to 35-45%. However, we need more powerful agents for the treatment of familial hypercholesterolemia or severe nonfamilial hypercholesterolemia. We have two candidates: one is CI-981(atorvastatin) and the other is NK-104.

A New HMG-CoA Reductase Inhibitor NK-104

The chemical structure of NK-104 is shown in Figure 1. This compound was synthesized by the Nissan Chemical Industry and the Phase II study is going on in Japan. In the Phase I 4-week study, daily doses of 1mg, 2mg, and 4mg of NK-104 and placebo were given to 35 hypercholesterolemic volunteers.

LDL-cholesterol decreased from around 150mg/dl to less than 90mg/dl in higher dose groups. The decreasing rates were 32% with 1mg, 37% with 2mg and 43% with 4mg. If we compare the reduction rate between once daily administration and twice daily administration, the latter was slightly more effective (Figure 2).

The reduction of serum triglyceride was also observed in higher dose groups and the maximum reduction was 28% in the 4-mg group. HDL-cholesterol increased in all groups and the maximum increase was observed in 4-mg group.

Apo A-I also increased in all groups except the placebo group, but a dose-dependent increase was not obtained in this study. Apo B decreased in all groups and dose dependently. The decreasing patterns were well matched to those of LDL-cholesterol. Apo E decreased significantly in all treated groups and decreasing rates were 20-30%.

In this study, NK-104 was given to mild hypercholesterolemic volunteers. Therefore, if it is given to much severe hypercholesterolemic patients, the greater reduction of LDL-cholesterol must be obtained. It is suggested in the Phase I study.

No clinically significant adverse events or abnormal changes in laboratory tests were

A. M. Gotto, Jr. et al. (eds.), Drugs Affecting Lipid Metabolism, 483–488.

observed except slight increase in GOT and GPT in a few cases.

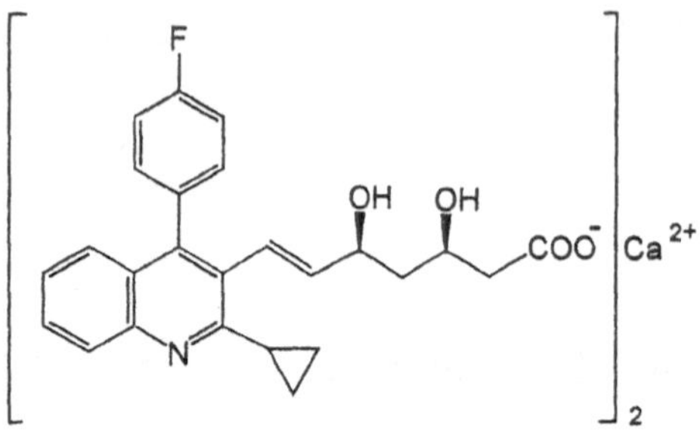

NK-104 $(C_{25}H_{23}FNO_4)_2Ca$ MW 881.0

Monocalcium bis[(3R,5S,6E)-7-[2-cyclopropyl-4-(4-fluorophenyl)-3-quinolyl]-3,5-dihydroxy-6-heptenoate

Figure 1. Chemical structure of NK-104.

A New Anion Exchange Resin MCI-196

Anion exchange resin is an ideal drug in the mode of action. Two drugs, cholestyramine and colestipol, are now available, but are not used frequently because of poor compliance. We are developing a new anion exchange resin, MCI-196, which has about 4 times stronger activity than cholestyramine has. The chemical structure of MCI-196 is shown in Figure 3.

The cholesterol-lowering effect was compared in cholesterol-fed rabbits between cholestyramine and MCI-196. The increase of serum cholesterol was dose-dependently inhibited by both drugs. However, the dose of MCI-196 was one-fourth of cholestyramine (Figure 4).

The cholesterol-lowering effect of MCI-196 was examined in the 4-week study of Phase I. Three grams of MCI-196 were administered to 18 hypercholesterolemic volunteers in three different ways: 1.5 g twice a day before morning and evening meals, 1.5 g twice a day after morning and evening meals, and 3g once a day before the evening meal. The biggest reduction (35.5%) was observed in the group receiving 1.5 g twice a day before meals (Figure 5).

Serum triglyceride and HDL-cholesterol did not change significantly. Gastrointestinal symptoms were observed in some subjects, but the incidence was less than those reported in cholestyramine treatment.

In the Phase II study, daily doses provided were between 2.5 g and 4.0 g; there was no difference in LDL-cholesterol reduction between daily doses of 3.0 g and 4.0 g (Figure

6). Therefore, 1.5 g twice a day before morning and evening meals was chosen for the Phase III study. These two drugs will be very helpful for the treatment of hypercholesterolemia.

Mean concentration of serum LDL-cholesterol

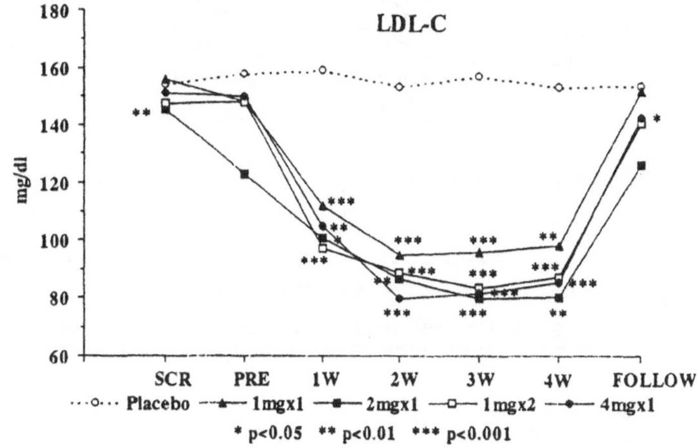

Mean change rate of serum LDL-cholesterol

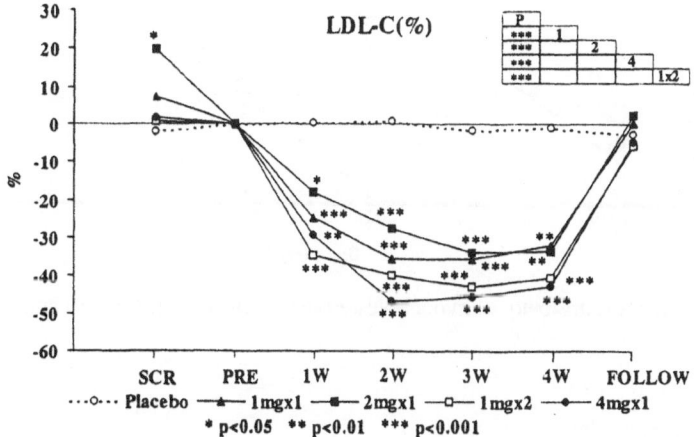

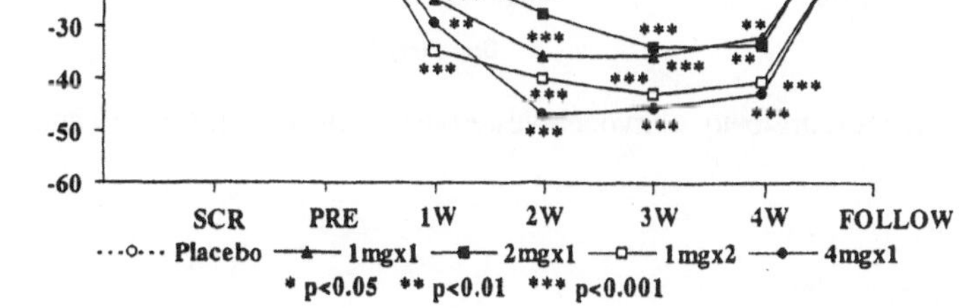

Figure 2. Mean concentration and mean percent change of serum LDL-cholesterol after administration of NK-104. ○, placebo; ▲, 1 mg x1; ■, 2 mg x1; □, 1mg x2; ●, 4mg x1; *, $p < 0.05$; **, p , 0.01; ***, p , 0.001.

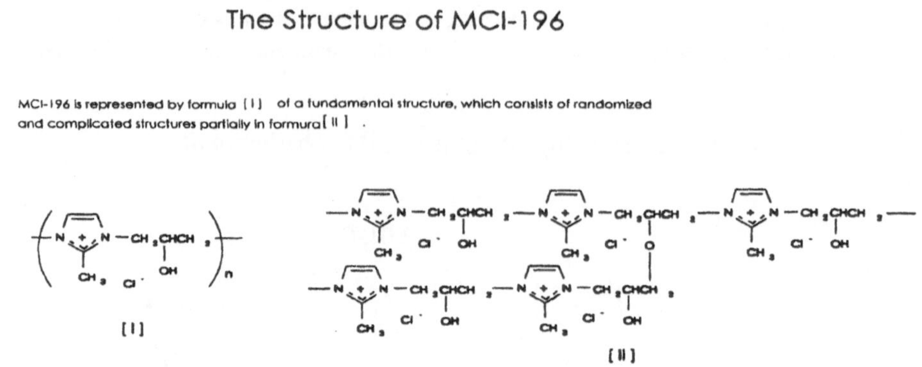

The Structure of MCI-196
MCI-196 is represented by formula [I] of a fundamental structure, which consists of randomized and complicated structures partially in formura[II] .
[I]
[II]

Figure 3. Chemical structure of MCI-196.

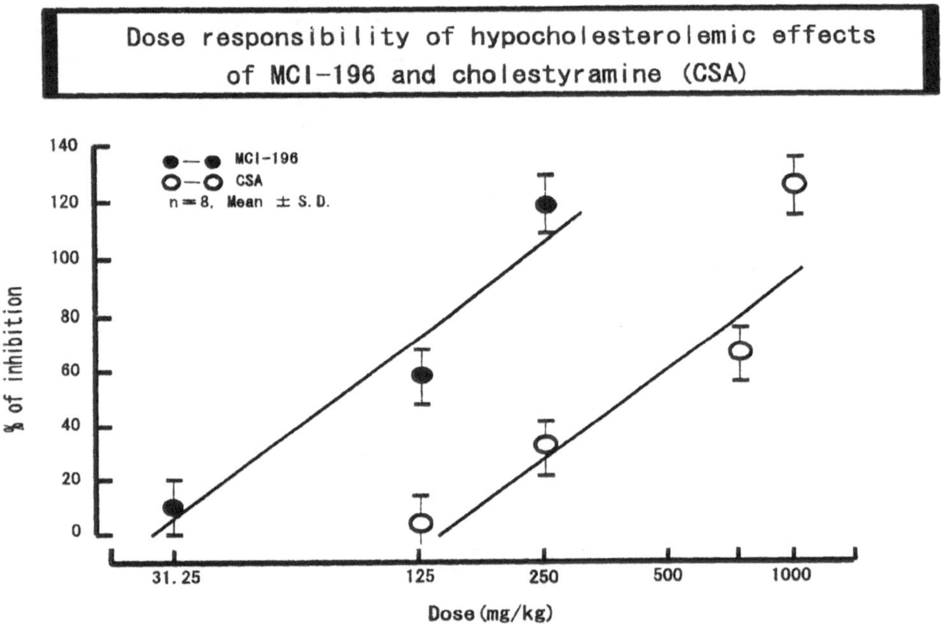

Figure 4. Dose responsibility of hypocholesterolemic effects of MCI-196 and cholestyramine (CSA).

LDL-c (No.2)

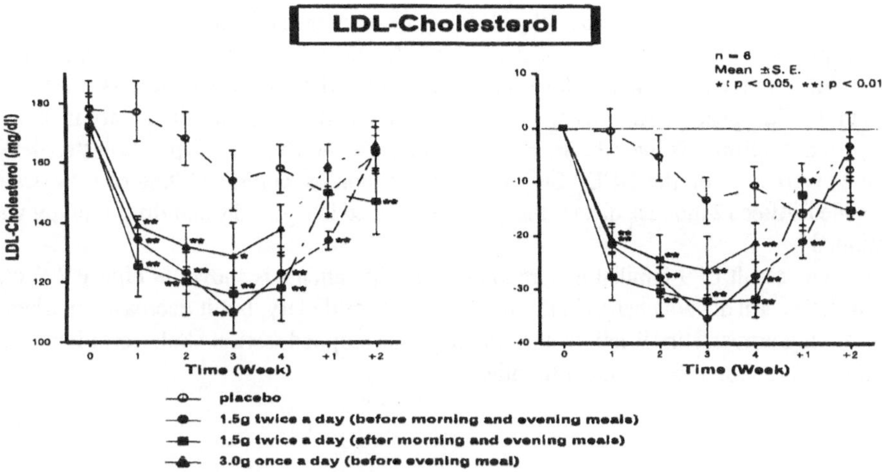

Figure 5. Mean concentration and mean percent change of serum LDL-cholesterol after administration of MCI-196. ○, placebo; ●, 1.5 g twice a day (before morning and evening meals); ■, 1.5 g twice a day (after morning and evening meals); ▲, 3.0g once a day (before evening meal).

LDL-c (No.1)

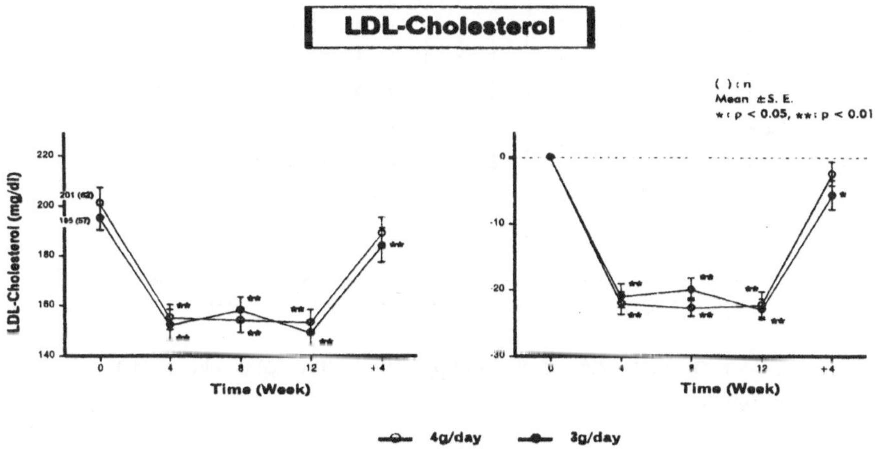

Figure 6. Mean concentration and mean percent change of serum LDL-cholesterol after administration of MCI-196. ○, 4 g/day; ●, 3 g/day.

Effect of Diet on Drug Therapy

Cholesterol-lowering drugs, especially HMG-CoA reductase inhibitors are more effective in the Japanese than in Europeans or Americans. A half-dose of pravastatin or simvastatin brings almost the same reduction of serum cholesterol in the Japanese patient as does a full dose in the European or American. The reason must be the difference in dietary habits.

To confirm this hypothesis, an experiment was performed. Hypercholesterolemic patients were kept on the NCEP Step II diet for 2 months, and then 20mg of pravastatin was added. After 12 months, dietary therapy was stopped intentionally and drug therapy was continued.

The result of 9 familial hypercholesterolemic patients is shown in Figure 7. Total serum cholesterol did not change in the first 2 months of dietary, but it decreased markedly after adding pravastatin. When dietary therapy was stopped, serum cholesterol increased significantly, about 10%, within 3 months.

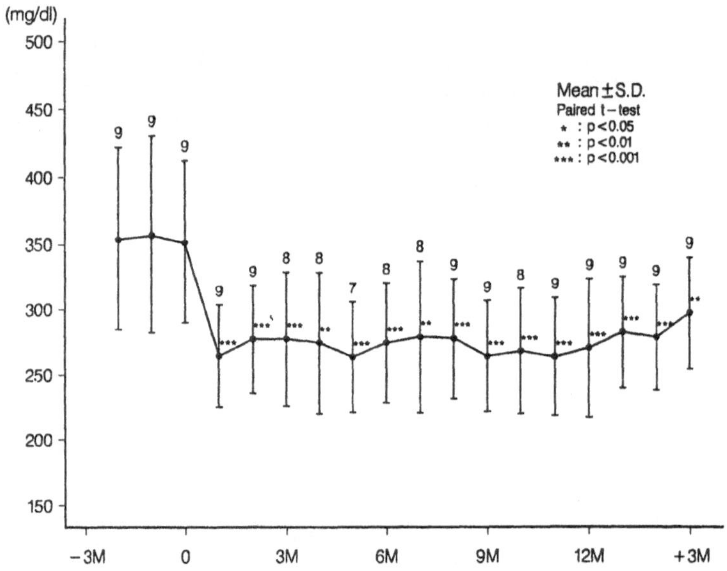

Figure 7. Effect of diet and drug therapy on serum total cholesterol in familial hypercholesterolemia.

This cholesterol changing pattern clearly shows that the dietary therapy can strengthen the effect of drug therapy, even when the dietary therapy alone has no effect on serum cholesterol level.

BUILDING BETTER COMPLIANCE: FACTORS AND METHODS COMMON TO ACHIEVING HEALTHY LIFESTYLE

John P. Foreyt and Walker S.C. Poston II
Behavioral Medicine Research Center, Baylor College of Medicine, One Baylor Plaza, Houston, Texas 77030, USA

Introduction

The treatment of obesity, hypercholesteremia, and cardiovascular disease is fraught with difficulty, since these disorders are chronic and often require the patient to make substantial lifestyle changes. Successful treatment is associated with dietary change, increasing physical activity, and when necessary, appropriate use of medications [1].

Unfortunately, the most common problems discussed in the literature are usually noncompliance with drugs, diet, and/or exercise [2-10]. For example, it has been estimated that only one-third of all patients follow a physician's or other health care provider's directions [2]. With regard to medication compliance, some researchers estimate that medication noncompliance (e.g. improper use or dosing or premature discontinuation) is responsible for up to 10% of all hospital admissions, increased mortality, and increased treatment costs [3]. In addition, it has been estimated that 30-50% of all prescriptions fail to produce the desired treatment effect because of noncompliance [4]. The total cost of medication noncompliance, which includes hospital admissions, lost productivity, excess premature mortality, increased ambulatory treatment costs, and nursing home admissions, has been estimated to exceed 100 billion dollars [4].

Dietary noncompliance is as least as frequent as medication noncompliance [5]. Dietary compliance is thought to be difficult because it is usually restrictive, diets are employed as methods of disease control rather than cure, and the dietary regimens must be employed indefinitely [5]. In fact, Ghali and colleagues [6] found that noncompliance to dietary changes as a precipitating cause accounted for 22% of the decompensated heart failure in their sample, while medication noncompliance alone only accounted for 6%. The combination of drug and dietary noncompliance accounted for 37%.

The picture for exercise compliance does not appear any better. Only 8.1 % of males and 7.0% of females in the U.S. are regularly active and engage in activity at the appropriate level of intensity to provide cardiovascular benefit [7]. In addition, 50% of individuals who start an aerobic exercise program stop within 6 months [8]. This is a particularly important problem, since men and women with low levels of fitness have

A. M. Gotto, Jr. et al. (eds.), Drugs Affecting Lipid Metabolism, 489–496.

significantly greater risk for morbidity and have higher all-cause and disease-specific mortality rates than more fit individuals [9].

Overall, patients who comply tend to have better medical outcomes than those who do not [10]. So why don't patients comply with treatment when it is obvious that by doing so they would live longer and lead healthier lives?

PREDICTORS OF COMPLIANCE

Numerous investigators have reviewed and cataloged research on predictors of compliance and/or noncompliance [3-5,8,11-17]. These factors have been grouped in various and overlapping ways and include patient factors, biological factors, social/environmental factors, disease-related factors, treatment factors, and relationship (patient-health care provider) interaction factors. Table 1 provides a summary of these different factors.

Table 1. Predictors of noncompliance.

Patient Factors: -Type and severity of the medical problem -Type and severity of any psychological disturbance -Lack of understanding -Conflicting health beliefs -Dissatisfaction -Lack of social support -Conflicting treatment expectations	Disease-Related Factors: -Chronicity and severity of condition -Presence or absence of symptoms -Stability of symptoms
Relationship Factors: -Poor rapport and communication -Failure to elicit negative feedback -Patient dissatisfaction -Negative beliefs about patient	Treatment Factors: -Characteristics of the treatment setting -Lack of cohesiveness of the treatment delivery system -Inconvenience and expense -Complexity -Side effects -Degree of behavioral change
Social/Environmental Factors: -Lack of economic resources -Family instability -Unemployment -Lack of social support -Societal and economic endorsement of unhealthy behaviors -Social stigma associated with treatment -Peer pressure	Biological Factors: -Sensory or cognitive disability -Disease instability -Unpleasant drug side effects -Unpleasant nondrug regimens -Interference of health behaviors with enjoyable behaviors -Misinterpretation of biological cues

The table is not exhaustive and the categories are not mutually exclusive (e.g. the biological factors can easily fit in another category). It is notable that no single factor is a primary predictor of compliance and/or noncompliance.

This complexity in predicting noncompliance is interesting given that some health care providers appear to believe that patient characteristics, specifically personality and demographic characteristics, are the best predictors of noncompliance [11]. In reality, there is little support for patient personality traits or demographic variables as predictors of compliance [3-5,11-17].

The best predictors of noncompliance tend to be factors that physicians and other health care providers can play a role in modifying. These factors include the relationship, patient beliefs and expectations, treatment, and social/environmental factors (e.g. poor patient-provider communication and rapport, failure to elicit negative feedback, patient dissatisfaction, negative beliefs about patients, patients' expectations about treatment and health beliefs, treatment complexity and duration, treatment side effects, degree of behavioral change required, inconvenience and expense, lack of family and other social support, and peer pressure).

Managing Noncompliance

Attitude Change

Health care providers can improve compliance by changing the way they think about the problem. Compliance/noncompliance is not a dichotomous issue or behavior. Individuals comply along a continuum and their compliance can vary over time and from treatment to treatment. One hundred percent compliance is often not necessary for the desired health outcome [3].

Noncompliance is not a disorder or a internal defect of the patient. The fact that noncompliance is so ubiquitous in medical treatment suggests that it is often the norm and not the exception. Noncompliance is "...the unavoidable byproduct of collisions between the clinical world and other competing worlds of work, play, friendship, and family life" [18] (p. 1305). Health care providers also have difficulty with compliance (e.g. health behaviors, professional behaviors) [19]. Noncompliance is normative, sometimes rational, and should be expected since change is difficult for most individuals and treatment often interferes with or changes important aspects of a patient's lifestyle [20].

Enhancing the Patient-Provider Relationship

The next group of interventions are broadly focused on enhancing the patient-provider relationship. Miller and Rollnick [21] provide evidence from the area of addictions that basic counseling and listening skills can enhance the patient-provider alliance and reduce resistance to change. They suggest that health care providers focus on 1) expressing empathy (e.g. communicating acceptance with skillful listening and accepting that ambivalence about change is normal); 2) developing discrepancies between the patient's current behavior and the desired health outcomes (e.g. make the patient aware of the consequences of not changing, outline the discrepancy between the patient goals and behavior, and have the patient present reasons for change); 3) avoiding arguing (arguments are counterproductive and increase a patient's defensiveness; instead, use resistance as a signal to change strategies); 4) rolling with the patient's resistance (involve the patient as a resource for problem-solving solutions, and offer new perspectives rather than imposing them); and 5) supporting self-efficacy (the physician's belief in the possibility of change is a motivator; remember that the patient is ultimately responsible for behavior change, and support and reinforce all efforts on the patient's part to change).

In addition, there are many simple interventions that can help to improve the patient-provider alliance. Patient education has been found to be an important part of most compliance interventions and works to address many of the patient and relationship predictors of noncompliance [22-24]. Examples of educating or providing information include ensuring that the patient understands the treatment instructions by writing them down, providing clear information about the diagnosis, discussing patient's beliefs about the illness and treatment, and assessing the patient's treatment expectations. Patient-provider alliance building is a very effective method of improving treatment compliance [25]. Utilizing many of the above mentioned strategies has been associated with decreased patient dropout rates and increased objectively-measured medication compliance (> 85%) in multi-year clinical trials [25].

Modifying or Enhancing the Treatment Regimen

Many empirically-validated and simple interventions include reducing the treatment complexity, improving the management of side effects, addressing office-oriented factors that affect satisfaction, predicting setbacks and problem-solving ways to manage them, making behavior changes in small increments, reducing inconvenience associated with treatment, providing ways for patients to get feedback about their progress, developing reasonable and varied treatment goals, and involving patients in assessment and treatment goal planning. For example, to improve medication compliance, a physician can simplify treatment complexity by reducing the number of medications or by reducing the number of doses by using longer acting medications [26].

Giving feedback about treatment progress and providing a way for patients to monitor their progress through self-monitoring can be very effective for both exercise and dietary adherence [1,12,27-28]. Providing prompts or reminders also can be very effective. For example, simple telephone reminders and memory devices have been found to improve medication compliance [3,26] and prompting patients to exercise through weekly phone calls has been found to significantly enhance compliance to a walking program [29].

Finally, modifying the goals of treatment and involving the patient in the goal-setting process can be very effective [12]. For example, exercise compliance has been a problem because patients often try to start exercising according to the American College of Sports Medicine (ACSM) guidelines [30], which most individuals in the US do not currently meet.

Instead, patient's can be encouraged to set more realistic goals and gradually build up to intense exercises over time, since there is evidence that even light-to-moderate physical activity (e.g. walking, gardening, etc) can provide important health benefits and reduce risk for mortality [8,9,26].

ENVIRONMENTAL AND SOCIAL FACTORS

A final group of interventions focus on modifying the patient's environment and support system. A primary intervention in this area is to involve family members in the treatment process. This can include having them attend special educational/informational sessions with the patient, having them present for appointments, and encouraging them to participate in appropriate components of the treatment program (e.g. dietary modification and exercise/physical activity). The beneficial effect of social support has been demonstrated for exercise, dietary change, and the treatment of obesity [1,12]. Enlisting social support does not have to be time consuming for the physician. For example, Fishman [31] described a novel intervention called the "90 Second Intervention" currently undergoing evaluation that involves having the patient call a family member or other individual from the physician's office to recruit their support for a low-intensity exercise program. The patient contracts with these supporters to be "health partners" in the exercise program. This intervention, minimal in terms of cost and time, may yield tangible improvements in exercise compliance.

Finally, while health care providers cannot resolve all of the potential environmental barriers to compliance (e.g. unemployment and social stigma), they can work with patients to problem-solve some of these environmental and support issues to make them more manageable. For example, if patients have difficulty enlisting family members as supporters in dietary change, the physician can keep referral lists of local community support programs that the patient could attend. In addition, the physician could provide periodic, brief booster sessions to check on the patient's progress and provide support [1].

SPECIAL POPULATIONS

Patients from different cultural/ethnic groups, older patients, and children may have unique needs with regard to complying to lifestyle change interventions. Several recent reviews [32-35] provide information about modifying some of the discussed methods to make them more applicable for special populations. For example, with some minority patients, special emphasis should be placed on including the family in treatment and assessing the patient's health beliefs and expectations for treatment [32]. In addition, assessing cognitive functioning and the impact of medical problems on the patient and family may be particularly important for improving compliance with older individuals [34]. Approaching each patient as an individual and utilizing the principles discussed in the section on enhancing the patient-provider relationship will provide physicians with much of the information they need to work with different populations.

Conclusion

Factors associated with the successful treatment of obesity apply equally to the treatment of cardiovascular diseases [1]. Programs should gradually reduce fat and increase physical activity (reducing the inconvenience of the treatment and the degree of behavioral change and complexity), utilize methods that provide the patient with feedback (providing information and including the patient in the treatment process), reduce environmental barriers, and improve social support. All of these methods have been found to be effective in improving compliance with medication, dietary change, and exercise. Most of them are fairly simple to implement and the physician's health care staff can be trained to deliver many of them.

Perhaps the most difficult area for some health care providers will be to allow that patients are ultimately their own change agents and that we need to enlist them as members of the treatment team if we are going to be successful in the long-term management of chronic health problems. This philosophy may require health care providers to change their attitudes about the issue of compliance and patients that do not appear to be cooperating with the treatment protocol. It may also encourage some physicians to pay greater attention to factors that are often labeled as "nonspecific," to alter the unequal nature of the patient-provider relationship, and to look at treatment from the perspective of the patient [18,20].

Acknowledgments

The authors wish to acknowledge that this work was partially supported by a Minority Scientist Development Award to Dr. Poston from the American Heart Association and with funds contributed by the AHA, Puerto Rico Affiliate and a grant from the National Heart, Lung, and Blood Institute, HL47052.

References

1. Foreyt JP, Goodrick GK. Factors common to successful therapy for the obese patient. Medicine and Science in Sports and Exercise 1991;23:292-97.
2. Becker MH. Patient adherence to prescribed therapies. Medical Care 1985;23:539-55.
3. Morris LS, Schulz RM. Patient compliance--an overview. Journal of Clinical Pharmacy and Therapeutics 1992;17:283-95.
4. Berg JS, Dischler J, Wagner DJ, Raia JJ, Palmer-Shevlin N. Medication compliance: A healthcare problem. The Annals of Pharmacotherapy 1993;27(Suppl):S1-S19.
5. Glanz K. Compliance with dietary regimens: Its magnitude, measurement, and determinants. Preventive Medicine 1980;9:787-804.
6. Ghali JK, Kadakia S, Cooper R, Ferlinz, J. Precipitating factors leading to decompensation of heart failure: Traits among urban blacks. Arch Intern Med 1988; 148:2013-16.
7. Casperson CJ, Christenson GM, Pollard RA. Status of the 1990 physical fitness and exercise objectives--Evidence from NHIS 1985. Public Health Reports 1986;101: 587-92.
8. Robinson JI, Rogers MA. Adherence to exercise programmes: Recommendations. Sports Med 1994;17:39-52.

9. Blair SN, Kohl HW, Paffenbarger RS, Clark DG, Cooper KH, Gibbons LW. Physical fitness and all-cause mortality: A prospective study of healthy men and women. JAMA 1989;262:2395-2401.
10. Horwitz RI, Horwitz SM. Adherence to treatment and health outcomes. Arch Intern Med 1993;153:1863-68.
11. Meichenbaum D, Turk DC. Facilitating treatment adherence: A practitioners guidebook. New York:Plenum Press, 1987:41-68.
12. Burke LE, Dunbar-Jacob J. Adherence to medication, diet, and activity recommendations: From assessment to maintenance. J Cardiovasc Nurs 1995;9:62-79.
13. Grunberg NE, Lord D. Biological barriers to adoption and maintenance of health-promoting behaviors. In: Shumaker R, Schron EB, Ockene, JK, Parker CT, Probsfield JL, Wolle JM, editors. The handbook of health behavior change. New York:Springer Publishing Company, 1990:221-30.
14. Dunbar J. Predictors of patient adherence: Patient characteristics. In: Shumaker R, Schron EB, Ockene, JK, Parker, CT, Probsfield, JL, Wolle, JM, editors. The handbook of health behavior change. New York:Springer Publishing Company, 1990:348-60.
15. Altman, DG. The social context and health behavior: The case of tobacco. In: Shumaker R, Schron EB, Ockene JK, Parker CT, Probsfield JL, Wolle JM, editors. The handbook of health behavior change. New York:Springer Publishing Company, 1990:241-69.
16. Friedman HS, DiMatteo MR. Patient-physician interactions. In: Shumaker R, Schron EB, Ockene JK, Parker CT, Probsfield JL, Wolle JM, editors. The handbook of health behavior change. New York:Springer Publishing Company, 1990:84-101.
17. Sherbourne CD, Hays RD, Ordway L, DiMatteo MR, Kravitz RL. Antecedents of adherence to medical recommendations: Results from the medical outcomes study. Journal of Behavioral Medicine 1992;15:447-68.
18. Trostle JA. Medical compliance as an ideology. Soc Sci Med 1988;27:1299-1308.
19. Ellrodt AG, Conner L, Riedinger M, Weingarten S. Measuring and improving physician compliance with clinical practice guidelines: A controlled intervention trial. Annals of Internal Medicine 1995;122:277-82.
20. Morris LS, Schulz RM. Medication compliance: The patient's perspective. Clinical Therapeutics 1993;15:593-606.
21. Miller WR, Rollnick S. Motivational interviewing: Preparing people to change addictive behavior. New York:The Guilford Press, 1991:51-63.
22. Becker MH. Theoretical models of adherence and strategies for improving adherence. In: Shumaker R, Schron EB, Ockene JK, Parker CT, Probsfield JL, Wolle JM, editors. The handbook of health behavior change. New York:Springer Publishing Company, 1990:5-43.
23. Smith TW, Leon AS. Coronary heart disease: A behavioral perspective. Champaign, IL: Research Press, 1992: 67-95.
24. Cramer JA. Optimizing long-term patient compliance. Neurology 1995;45(1):S25-S28.
25. Frank E, Kupfer DJ, Siegel LR. Alliance not compliance: A philosophy of outpatient care. J Clin Psychiatry 1995;56(1):11-17.
26. King AC. Community and public health approaches to the promotion of physical activity. Medicine and Science in Sports and Exercise 1994;26:1405-12.
27. Brownell KD, Cohen LR. Adherence to dietary regimens 2: Components of effective interventions. Behavioral Medicine 1995;20:155-64.
28. Barnard ND, Akhtar A, Nicholson A. Factors that facilitate compliance to lower fat intake. Arch Fam Med 1995;4:15358.

29. Lombard DN, Lombard TN, Winett RA. Walking to meet health guidelines: The effect of prompting frequency and prompt structure. Health Psychology 1995;14: 164-70.
30. American College of Sports Medicine. Position stand: The recommended quantity and quality of exercise for developing and maintaining cardiorespiratory and muscular fitness in healthy adults. Medicine and Science in Sports and Exercise 1990;22:265-74.
31. Fishman T. The 90-second intervention: A patient compliance mediated technique to improve and control hypertension. Public Health Reports 1995;110:173-78.
32. Lewis D, Belgrave FZ, Scott RB. Patient adherence in minority populations. In: Shumaker R, Schron EB, Ockene JK, Parker CT, Probsfield JL, Wolle JM, editors. The handbook of health behavior change. New York:Springer Publishing Company, 1990:277-92.
33. Aledort LM, Weiss H, Parker CT, Levi JR, Simon R. Life-style interventions in the young. In: Shumaker R, Schron EB, Ockene JK, Parker CT, Probsfield JL, Wolle JM, editors. The handbook of health behavior change. New York:Springer Publishing Company, 1990:293-314.
34. Roth HP. Problems with adherence in the elderly. In: Shumaker R, Schron EB, Ockene JK, Parker CT, Probsfield JL, Wolle JM, editors. The handbook of health behavior change. New York:Springer Publishing Company, 1990:315-26.

MANAGEMENT OF PRIMARY HYPERLIPIDEMIA WITH COMBINATION THERAPY

Haruo Nakamura
National Defense Medical College, Department of Medicine, 3-2 Namiki, Tokorozawa, Saitama 359, Japan

Introduction

Since epidemiologic, clinical, and genetic studies have clearly established the primary role of lipoproteins in atherogenesis, measures to lower plasma cholesterol have become fundamental to the practice of preventive cardiology [1].

The NCEP (National Cholesterol Education Program) panel recommended that drug therapy be initiated in patients with coronary heart disease who have plasma LDL cholesterol concentrations greater than 130 mg/dl with a goal of reducing them to less than 100 mg/dl or less than 130 mg/dl of non-HDL cholesterol [2]. Secondary prevention trials, especially those that measured results by angiography, suggest that optimal benefit is obtained at these concentrations. Meeting secondary prevention targets will require greater use of combined drug treatment.

Treatment Goal

Combined drug treatment is often applied if monotherapy does not reach the target goal of treatment, and also if adverse reactions of monotherapy can not be compensated.

Regarding the target goal of plasma lipids among Japanese with coronary artery disease, we repeated quantitative coronary angiography during the interval of 3 years. Ninety subjects were enrolled in this study and their plasma cholesterol levels had been treated mostly by statins prior to the first quantitative coronary angiography. The progressive changes were defined as having more than 15% stenotic alterations. After examination of the follow-up study, 34 cases were judged to be subjects with progression; it was also found that their LDL cholesterol levels were significantly higher than those of the subjects without progression. Also their HDL cholesterol levels were significantly lower than those of the subjects without progression.

We therefore considered that the target levels of plasma lipids were less than 200 mg/dl in total cholesterol, or less than 130 mg/dl in LDL cholesterol, less than 150 mg/dl in triglyceride, and greater than 40 mg/dl in HDL cholesterol.

To achieve these target goals, many subjects with hyperlipidemias are required to

A. M. Gotto, Jr. et al. (eds.), Drugs Affecting Lipid Metabolism, 497–504.

receive combined drug treatment. To examine whether a small dose of bile acid sequestrant used in combination with statin is more effective in reducing serum and LDL cholesterol levels than inhibitor use alone, a randomized double-blind study was conducted in subjects with severe hypercholesterolemia with serum cholesterol levels of 7.0 mmol/L (270 mg/dl) or more [3].

Subjects were randomly assigned to receive either colestipol 5g or 10g or placebo each morning in fixed dosage for 18 weeks. They simultaneously received incremental doses of simvastatin, starting placebo for 6 weeks and then 20 mg/night for another 6 weeks. For the final 6 weeks, the dose was increased to 40 mg/night. Respective maximum reductions in serum cholesterol, LDL cholesterol, and apolipoproteins B values in subjects taking combination therapy were 41%, 50%, and 43%, respectively, compared with lesser reductions of 32%, 38%, and 37%, respectively, in those taking simvastatin monotherapy. Combined treatment thus achieved the target goal of total cholesterol approximately 200 mg/dl. Low dose colestipol combined with simvastatin produced superior LDL cholesterol lowering compared with simvastatin alone. There was little difference in efficacy between 5 g/day and 10 g/day of colestipol or between 20 mg/day and 40 mg/day of simvastatin.

A randomized, placebo-controlled trial with a 24-week double-blind period was also conducted to compare LDL cholesterol-lowering efficacy of low dose combinations of cholestyramine and fluvastatin [4]. The 10 mg and 20 mg fluvastatin monotherapy groups showed moderate reductions in LDL cholesterol, -16% and -19% respectively. Reductions in LDL cholesterol that resulted from the addition of cholestyramine 8 g/day, to 10 mg and 20 mg of fluvastatin were greater than those observed with monotherapy, 26% and 31%, respectively. LDL cholesterol reductions of about 25% to 30% can be achieved with a low-dose combination therapy with fluvastatin and cholestyramine. This trial also showed the achievement of the target goal of LDL cholesterol level, about 130 mg/dl, by using combination therapy.

Another study was designed to determine the lowest effective doses of a bile acid sequestrant and a statin [5]. The efficacy of three drug regimens (cholestyramine resin 8 g/day, cholestyramine resin 8 g/day plus lovastatin 5 mg/day, and lovastatin 20 mg/day) was tested in 26 men with moderate hypercholesterolemia after a step-one cholesterol lowering diet. Each drug period was 3 months in duration, interspersed by a 1-month period of the step-one diet only. Cholestyramine resin therapy achieved significant reduction in LDL cholesterol levels from 173 mg/dl to 151 mg/dl. The addition of 5 mg of lovastatin to cholestyramine therapy achieved even lower levels, averaging 131 mg/dl. Lovastatin therapy at 20 mg/day produced a lowering of LDL cholesterol levels similar to that of the low-dose combination.

In the majority of familial hypercholesterolemia (FH), plasma LDL cholesterol levels are not normalized with a single drug regimen and thus combination therapy is usually required. A short-term, double-blind study was conducted to compare the efficacy and safety of fluvastatin when combined with cholestyramine (Group 1) or with bezafibrate (Group 2) in 38 heterozygous FH patients [6]. After 6 weeks of combination treatment, the combination of 40 mg/day of fluvastatin with 400 mg/day of bezafibrate in Group 2 reduced plasma LDL cholesterol levels by 35%, as compared with 32% in Group 1. Plasma triglyceride reduction and HDL cholesterol elevation of Group 2 were also significant. The combination was well tolerated and no notable abnormalities in aspartate aminotransferase (AST), alanine aminotransferase (ALT), and creatine kinase (CK) levels occurred. This trial indicated that fluvastatin-bezafibrate combination is superior to fluvastatin-cholestyramine combination for management of FH.

We conducted the comparative study to assess the efficacy of pravastatin (10 mg/day) (Group 1) and pravastatin with clinofibrate (600 mg/day) (Group 2) in mildly elevated hypercholesterolemic subjects [7]. Both groups showed similar reductions of total and LDL cholesterol levels. However, Group 2 showed more efficiently reduced triglyceride levels and significantly increased HDL-cholesterol levels than seen in Group 1. Both drugs were well tolerated without any serious adverse events.

Double-blind and placebo-controlled trial in Sweden and Finland was conducted to compare the efficacy and safety of pravastatin, gemfibrozil, combined therapy, and placebo in the treatment of 290 ambulatory patients with hypercholesterolemia [8].

Pravastatin reduced total cholesterol, LDL cholesterol, and apoprotein B by 26.3%, 33.5%, and 28.8%, respectively, which was more marked than gemfibrozil (15.2%, 16.8% and 15.3%, respectively). Gemfibrozil reduced VLDL cholesterol and triglyceride by 49.1% and 42.2%, respectively. It also increased HDL cholesterol by 15.2%. The combination of both drugs significantly reduced total cholesterol by 29.0%, LDL-cholesterol by 37.1%, and increased HDL cholesterol by 16.8%. Adverse events and clinical laboratory abnormalities were generally mild and transient in all groups. Although the combination may be useful in selected cases of combined hyperlipidemia, caution should be paid not to develop severe clinical side effects.

Gemfibrozil lowers only modestly serum cholesterol which in some cases may even be elevated as a response to triglyceride lowering. Since gemfibrozil treatment is known to be associated with reduced absorption of cholesterol and increased synthesis of cholesterol [9]. The agents of choice for the combination therapy should act by complementary mechanisms to diminish LDL cholesterol, be well tolerated by the patients, and not achieve efficacy at the expense of clinically significant additive side effects.

Complementary Actions

LDL comprises several distinct subclasses with differing physical, chemical, and metabolic properties. The profile characterized by a predominance of LDL-III, small dense LDL was originally identified and has been designated LDL subclass pattern B [10]. The evidence that individuals with small, dense LDL have a number of interrelated metabolic features associated with increased risk of coronary artery disease led to this designation.

The hyperlipidemia in familial combined hyperlipidemic (FCH) patients is characterized by elevation of both VLDL and LDL, whereas HDL, and particularly HDL_2 levels in plasma are often reduced. Another striking feature of this syndrome is the presence of small and dense LDL. The clinical trial was conducted to investigate the ability of pravastatin to favorably correct plasma lipid and lipoprotein levels and LDL structure in 12 FCH patients [11]. Pravastatin significantly lowered plasma total and LDL cholesterol levels by 21% and 32%, respectively. Triglyceride levels did not change, and apo B concentrations decreased by 9%, HDL cholesterol increased by 6% because of a significant 73% rise of HDL_2 cholesterol. The electrophoresis profiles at baseline showed the presence of a single major subpopulation of relatively small size (24.5 ± 0.5 nm); pravastatin decreased the mean diameter to 23.8 ± 0.6 nm. An LDL subclass pattern B persisted after treatment in the patients. These results were contradictory to the early study using simvastatin in type IIb patients, indicating LDL particle size increased significantly [12]. The difference in the results can be explained by the different response of triglyceride reductions to the agents. It seems necessary to reduce triglyceride significantly in order to obtain the alteration of LDL size.

The effect of ciprofibrate treatment on the atherogenic profile of LDL subspecies in combined hyperlipidemia was investigated in 6 patients. Analysis of 5 LDL subclasses separated by isopycric density gradient ultracentrifugation showed a predominance of dense LDL subspecies. Ciprofibrate (100 mg/day for 1 month) treatment effected marked reductions in both total plasma LDL and apo B levels. Triglyceride levels also decreased from 233 mg/dl to 156 mg/dl, or by 33%. The plasma profile of LDL subspecies was normalized to a significant degree as a result of preferential reduction in the elevated levels of both dense subspecies (LDL-4, LDL-5). Plasma levels of both apo B and triglyceride were significantly and positively correlated with those of LDL-4 and LDL-5, suggesting not only that the degree of triglyceride elevation is intimately linked to the extent of shift in LDL subclass profile towards denser subspecies, but also that triglyceride reduction upon treatment strongly influences LDL-4 and LDL-5 [13].

The effect of gemfibrozil or simvastatin on apo B -containing lipoproteins, and LDL subfraction profile was evaluated in a double-blind placebo-controlled, randomized trial of 45 patients with FCH [14]. Gemfibrozil reduced total cholesterol and triglyceride by 13% and 48,% respectively, whereas simvastatin reduced total cholesterol and triglyceride by 22% and 16%, respectively. LDL cholesterol was reduced with simvastatin. This decrease was due to a reduction in all isolated LDL subfractions except LDL-2, Gemfibrozil increased LDL-1 and LDL-2 cholesterol and reduced LDL-4 cholesterol resulting in a more buoyant LDL subfraction profile. In both groups, a predominance of small dense LDL remained despite therapy.

Another characteristic feature of the metabolic disturbances in FCH is considered to be overproduction of hepatic apolipoprotein B of VLDL. In addition, decreased lipoprotein lipase (LPL) activity has been shown in some cases [15]. Twenty-seven patients with FCH were divided into 2 groups, one with normal postheparin lipoprotein lipase (PHLPL) mass, the other with reduced PHLPL mass. Major plasma lipids are not statistically different at baseline in 2 groups. We started to treat both groups with pravastatin (10 mg/dl) for 8 weeks. Elevated triglycerides and reduced HDL cholesterol still remained in spite of treatment in low PHLPL mass group. Pravastatin in combination with bezafibrate (400 mg/day) treatment started and continued for another 8 weeks. As seen in Table 2, triglycerides decreased and HDL cholesterol increased significantly in the patients with low PHLPL mass. This study indicates that patients with FCH are heterogenous regarding LPL and that the combination treatment with statin with fibrate is preferable to improve lipid with profiles in the subjects with low LPL mass.

Table 1. Efficacy of combined treatment of type IIb with pravastatin and bezafibrate.

PHLPL Mass (mg/dl)		Baseline	Pravastatin (8W) (10 mg/day)	Pravastatin (10 mg/day) Bezafibrate(400 mg/day)
	TC	275	226**	214**
254	TG	254	186**	142**
(N = 12)	HDL-C	37	42*	44**
	LDL-C	187	139**	127**
	ApoB	154	130*	124**
	TC	284	235**	213**
132	TG	271	233*	154**
(N = 5)	HDL-C	36	38	43**
	LDL-C	194	150*	140**
	ApoB	150	136	125**

(mg/dl) *P < 0.05 **P < 0.01 (versus Baseline)

LDL Oxidizability

A large body of experimental data support the hypothesis that peroxidative processes play a role in atherogenesis. Additionally, there is accumulating epidemiological evidence of an association between antioxidant vitamin intake and reduced risk of coronary heart disease.

In a subgroup analysis using the extensive dietary and nutritional supplement database collected in the Cholesterol Lowering Atherosclerosis Study (CLAS), analysis was made to explore the association of supplementary and dietary vitamin E and C intake with the progression of coronary artery disease [16]. Analysis of variance revealed significantly less coronary lesion progression due to treatment with drug and supplementary vitamin E intake of 100 IU per day or greater. Within the drug group, benefit of supplementary vitamin E intake was found for all lesions, especially mild/moderate lesions. Although verification from carefully designed, randomized, serial arterial imaging end-point trials is needed, administration of antioxidants would be beneficial.

Probucol is not only a plasma lipid lowering drug, but also has antioxidant properties. We evaluated the angiographic changes in 12 hypercholesterolemic subjects with probucol 750 mg/day for 1 year. Fifteen percent stenotic change was classified as eitherprogression or regression.

The subjects with progression have slightly higher total cholesterol levels at baseline. No differences were observed in total cholesterol levels after 1 year of treatment in the subjects with or without progression. LDL cholesterol levels were elevated in the subjects with progression at baseline and treatment after 1 year showed still slightly elevated, greater than 150 mg/dl. LDL cholesterol in the subjects with regression was lower at baseline and remained lower than other subjects after 1 year probucol treatment.

Figure 1 shows that HDL cholesterol in the subjects with progression was lower at baseline and was further decreased after the treatment. Marked decrease of HDL cholesterol with the treatment of probucol such as below 30 mg/dl might adversely affect atherosclerosis development.

According to the results of Probucol Quantitative Regression Swedish Trial (PQRST) [17], the failure of probucol to affect femoral atherosclerosis was also considered partly due to the reduction of HDL2b. Dosage of probucol in the trial was 1000 mg per day and it reduced HDL cholesterol 56 mg/dl at baseline to 37.5 mg/dl after the treatment.

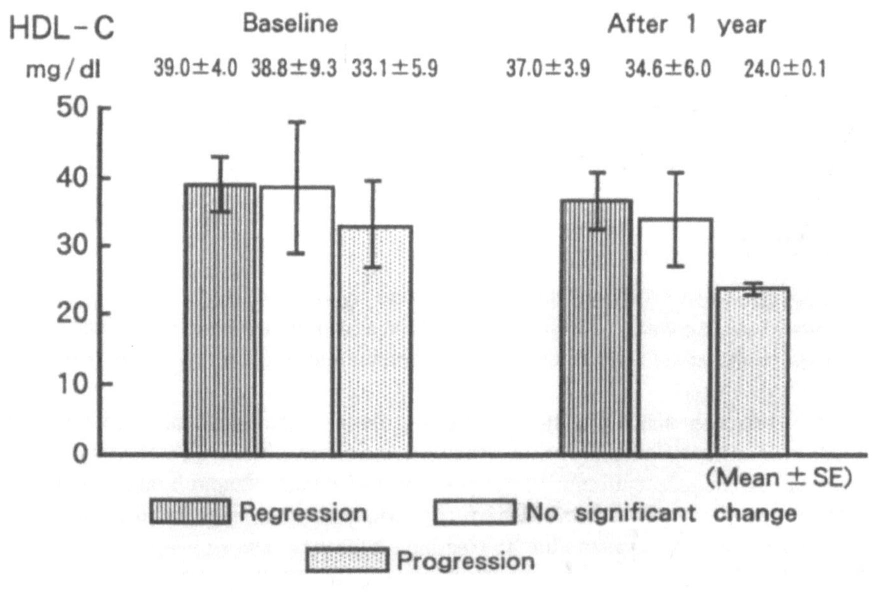

Figure 1. Changes in HDL C by probucol and angiographic changes (N = 12).

We have compared the effects of two dosage regimens of probucol on the plasma lipids and the lag time of LDL oxidizability. Probucol 750 mg/day administration significantly reduced total cholesterol, LDL cholesterol, and HDL cholesterol. Lag time was significantly lengthened by 750 mg/day probucol. The parameter changed similarly by the treatment of 500 mg/day probucol but to a lesser extent.

It might be preferable to combine other hypolipidemic agents with probucol of small dosage in order to protect against LDL oxidation and not to decrease HDL cholesterol markedly.

Conclusion

Combined treatment of hypolipidemic drugs should be consideredas a treatment option, based on the treatment goal of plasma lipids, complementary actions by drugs, and the possible contribution of antioxidants with cholesterol-lowering drugs to the retardation of atherosclerotic changes.

References

1. Havel RJ, Rapaport E. Management of primary hyperlipidemia. N Engl J Med 1995; 332:1491-98.
2. Adult Treatment Panel II, National Cholesterol Education Program Second Report of the Expert Panel on Detection, Evaluation and Treatment of High Blood Cholesterol in Adults. Circulation 1994;89:1333-1445.
3. Simons LA, Simons J, Parfitt A. Successful management of primary hypercholesterolemia with simvastatin and low-dose colestipol. Med J Australia 1992;157:455-59.
4. Sprecher DL, Abrams J, Allen JW, et al. Low-dose combined therapy with fluvastatin and cholestyramine in hyperlipidemic patients. Ann Int Med 1994;120: 537-43.
5. Denke MA, Grundy SM. Efficacy of low-dose cholesterol-lowering drug therapy in men with moderate hypercholesterolemia. Arch Int Med 1995;155:393-99.
6. Leitersdorf E, Muratti EN, Eliav D, et al. Efficacy and safety of a combination fluvastatin-bezafibrate treatment for familial hypercholesterolemia; Comparative analysis with a fluvastatin-cholestyramine combination. Am J Med 1994;96:401-407.
7. Saitama Mevalotin Study Group. Efficacy of combined treatment of pravastatin and clinofibrate. Progress in Medicine 1994;14:2182-89. (in Japanese)
8. Wiklund O, Angelin B, Bergman M, et al. Pravastatin and gemfibrozil alone and combination for the treatment of hypercholesterolemia. Am J Med 1993;94:13-20.
9. Vanhanen HT, Miettinen TA. Cholesterol absorption and synthesis during pravastatin, Gemfibrozil and their combination. Atherosclerosis 1995;115:135-46.
10. Austin MA, King MC, Vranizan KM, Krauss RM. Atherogenic lipoprotein phenotype; a proposed genetic marker for coronary heart disease risk. Circulation 1990;82:495-506.
11. Franceschini G, Cassionotti M, Vecchio G, et al. Pravastatin effectively lowers LDL cholesterol in familial combined hyperlipidemia without changing LDL subclass pattern. Arterioscler Thromb 1994;14:1569-75.
12. Zhao SP, Hollaar L, van't Hooft FM, Smelt AHM, Lenven JAG, van Laarse A. Effect of simvastatin on the apparent size of LDL particles in patients with type IIb hyperlipoproteinemia. Clin Chim Acta 1991;203:109-18.
13. Bruckert E, Dejazer S, Chapman MJ. Ciprofibrate therapy normalize the atherogenic low-density lipoprotein subspecies profile towards denser subspecies. Atherosclerosis

1993;100:91-102.

14. Bredie SJH, be Bruin TWA, Demacker PMN, Kastelein JJP, Stalenhoet AFH. Comparison of gemfibrozil versus simvastatin in familial combined hyperlipidemia and effects on apolipoprotein-B-containing lipoproteins, low density lipoprotein subfraction profile, and low density lipoprotein oxidizability. Am J Cardiol 1995;75:348-53.
15. Babirak SP, Brown BG, Brunzell JD. Familial combined hyperlipidemia and abnormal lipoprotein lipase. Arterioscler Thromb 1992;12:1176-83.
16. Hodis HN, Mack WJ, LaBree L, et al. Serial coronary angiographic evidence that antioxidant vitamin intake reduces progression of coronary artery atherosclerosis. JAMA 1995;273:1849-54.
17. Johnsson J, Olsson AG, Bergstrand L, et al. Lowering of HDL2b by probucol partly explains the failure of the drug to affect femoral atherosclerosis in subjects with hypercholesterolemia. Atheroscler Thromb Vasc Biol 1995;15:1049-1056.

DRUG COMBINATIONS IN THE PRACTICE OF A LIPID CLINIC

Massimo Liguori, Cecilia Sapio, Paolo Pauciullo, and Mario Mancini
Institute of Internal Medicine Medical School, University Federico II of Naples, via Pansini 5, 80131 Naples, Italy

Introduction

In the last few years the interest in the development of optimal strategies for the prevention of coronary disease in Western societies has been increasing. Particular attention has been, and will be given to the treatment of hyperlipidemia, one of the most important risk factors of coronary heart disease (CHD) [1]. The European Atherosclerosis Society stated that in patients at high risk intensive lipid lowering treatment should be considered [2,3], including multiple drug regimens when diet alone or single drug treatment proved insufficient. Combination drug therapy has been suggested in resistant hyperlipidemia such as some cases of familial combined hyperlipidemia (FCH) [4,5] and heterozygous familial hypercholesterolemia (FH) [6,7].

Safety and efficacy of bile acid sequestrants plus HMG-CoA reductase inhibitors [8-10] or bile acid sequestrants plus fibrates [4,5] have been demonstrated in controlled studies. The association of HMG-CoA reductase inhibitors and fibrates was found to be effective [11-13], but muscle damage in some patients has been reported [14,15].

In addition to these data on serum lipid levels and safety parameters, there is important experimental evidence confirming the impact of these intensive interventions on human clinical atherosclerosis. In the Stockholm Ischemic Heart Disease Secondary Prevention Study [16], the five-year effects of a combined treatment with clofibrate and nicotinic acid were observed in survivors of myocardial infarction (MI). The five-year incidence of both total and CHD mortality was significantly lower in the treated patients compared to a control untreated group of MI survivors. In the Cholesterol-Lowering Atherosclerosis Study [17], the Familial Atherosclerosis Treatment Study [18], and in the Atherosclerosis Specialized Center of Research Intervention Trial [19] significant delay of progression or regression of coronary atherosclerosis was achieved by treatments with colestipol plus lovastatin, or ternary drug combination.

The present study retrospectively evaluates the impact of some of above mentioned combined drug regimens in the clinical practice of an outpatient lipid clinic.

A. M. Gotto, Jr. et al. (eds.), Drugs Affecting Lipid Metabolism, 505–511.

Table 1. Stockholm Heart Study, 5-Year Mortality.

Group	Total	CHD
Control	82	73
Treatment	61*	47**

* $p<0.05$; ** $p<0.01$

Patient and Methods

In 1994, 704 (55% men) patients with primary hyperlipidemia were seen in the Outpatient Lipid Clinic of the Medical School of the University Federico II of Naples. Polygenic hypercholesterolemia was found in 18% of cases, FH in 40%, FCH in 35%, familial hypertriglyceridemia (FHTG) in 6%, and remnant disease (Type III) in 1% of cases. Patients were usually seen every 3 months. All patients were put on a lipid lowering diet with the following composition: carbohydrates 56%, fat 27% (cholesterol 200 mg, saturated fatty acid 5%, monounsaturated fatty acid 16%, P/S 1.14), and proteins 17%.

After 3 months of diet alone, patients who failed to achieve the serum lipids target levels recommended in EAS guidelines [3] were prescribed a drug treatment. During drug regimens diet prescription was always reinforced. If an at least 3-month lipid lowering treatment with one drug proved insufficient according to the above mentioned EAS Guidelines, a second drug was introduced.

Table 2. EAS 1993 Guidelines. Target cholesterol levels according to CHD risk.

	Mild	Moderate	High
Total (mg/dl)	195-230	195	175-195
LDL (mg/dl)	155-175	135-155	115-135

Seventy-seven patients (10.9% of the total, males = 41, females = 36), who were on lipid lowering combined drug regimen, were included in the present study. The mean age was 51 years and the types of hyperlipidemia were FH in 32 cases and FCH in 45 cases. Patient follow-up after the first drug occurred at 3 months and at 12 months after the second drug.

Serum and high density lipoprotein (HDL) cholesterol and serum triglycerides were

Serum and high density lipoprotein (HDL) cholesterol and serum triglycerides were determined by enzymatic method (Trinder, Boehringer, Mannheim-Germany) on COBAS instrument. HDL cholesterol was obtained after precipitation from total serum of apolipoprotein B containing particles by Na-phosphotungstate/magnesium chloride. Quality control of lipid analysis was performed by the WHO Reference Center. Coefficients of variation were: cholesterol 1.9%; triglycerides 0.9%; and HDL-cholesterol 1.4% [20]. Low density lipoprotein (LDL) cholesterol concentrations were calculated according to Friedewald whenever possible (total serum triglyceride concentrations lower than 400 mg/dl). In hypertriglyceridemic subjects serum was centrifuged at 40,000 rpm for 16 hours at a density of 1.019 kg/l of NaBr. At the end of the run, the supernatant, containing very low density lipoprotein (VLDL) and intermediate density lipoprotein (IDL), was analyzed for its cholesterol content. LDL cholesterol concentration was calculated as the difference between total serum cholesterol concentration and the sum of cholesterol concentrations in VLDL, IDL, and HDL.

Safety controls before and at least every 3 months in the first year of drug treatment included physical examination, serum alanine aminnotransferase (ALT), aspartate aminotransferase (AST), creatine phosphokinase (CPK), gamma glutamyl transpeptidase (GT), and alkaline phospatase (AP) determination. Statistical analysis were performed by two-tailed ANOVA.

Results

Average lipid lowering effects of dietary treatment alone on total cholesterol, LDL cholesterol, and triglycerides of our 77 patients were respectively 8.1%, 3%, and 15.1%. Table 3 shows the effects of bile acid sequestrants alone (8-16 g/day on average) and in combination with HMG-CoA reductase inhibitors (15-20 mg/day on average) in 46 patients (32 with FH, mean age 37 years, range 17-49; 14 with FCH, mean age 53 years, range 39-57). Total serum and LDL cholesterol dropped by 41% and 48%, respectively ($p < 0.001$), serum triglycerides were not significantly affected. HDL cholesterol rose by 19% ($p < 0.05$). Gastric discomfort was reported in 3 cases. Mild ALT (54 u/l) increase in one case and transitory myalgia were also observed. In no cases did side effects induce withdrawal from therapy.

Table 4 shows the effects of gemfibrozil alone (1200 mg/day on average) and in combination with bile acid sequestrants (8 g/day on average) in 24 patients with FCH, mean age 52 years, range 37-61. Total serum and LDL cholesterol fell by 24% and 21%, respectively ($p < 0.01$), serum triglycerides by 58% ($p < 0.001$). HDL cholesterol was increased by 27% ($p < 0.05$). No side effects were reported.

Table 5 shows the effects of at least one year of combined treatment with gemfibrozil (1200 mg/day) plus HMG-CoA reductase inhibitors (15-20 mg/day on average) in 7 patients with FCH, mean age 51 years, range 42-61. Total serum and LDL cholesterol were reduced by 35% and 36%, respectively ($p < 0.001$), and serum triglycerides by 61% ($p<0.001$). HDL cholesterol rose by 35% ($p < 0.05$). No side effects occurred after one year of treatment.

Table 3. Lipid lowering effect of cholestyramine alone (8-16 g per day) and in combination with HMG-CoA reductase inhibitors (15-20 mg per day). 46 patients; mg/dl (% changes versus baseline); FH=32; FCH=14.

	Baseline	First Drug 3 Months	Combination 12 Months
Total Serum Cholesterol	393	290 (-26)	232 (-41)***
LDL Cholesterol	301	218 (-30)	158 (-48)***
Serum Triglyceride	142	154 (+8)	130 (-8)
HDL Cholesterol	42	40 (-5)	50 (+19)*

*$p < 0.05$; ***$p < 0.001$ ANOVA

Table 4. Lipid lowering effect of gemfibrozil alone (1.2 g per day) and in combination with cholestyramine (8 g per day). 24 patients; mg/dl (% changes versus baseline); FCH.

	Baseline	First Drug 3 months	Combination 12 months
Total Serum Cholesterol	304	258 (-15)	232 (-24)**
LDL Cholesterol	207	191 (-8)	163 (-21)**
Serum Triglyceride	322	110 (-66)	135 (-58)***
HDL Cholesterol	33	45 (+36)	42 (+27)*

*$p < 0.05$; **$p < 0.01$; ***$p < 0.001$ ANOVA

Discussion

The aim of the present retrospective study was to assess the impact in the clinical practice of prescribing lipid lowering combined drug regimens in hyperlipidemic patients at high risk for CHD.

The distribution of various forms of hyperlipidemia in the patients attending the outpatient lipid clinic of the University of Naples is by no means representative of the distribution in the general population. Most cases of polygenic hypercholesterolemia and some cases of hypertriglyceridemia are in fact treated by general practitioners. This can explain the overrepresentation of FH and FCH among our patients.

All our patients assigned to a lipid lowering combined drug regimen qualified for FH or FCH, which both carry an increased risk of developing CHD, or had family or personal history of early CHD.

Table 5. Lipid lowering effect of gemfibrozil alone (1.2 g per day) and in combination with HMGCoA reductase inhibitors (15-20 mg per day). 7 patients; mg/dl (% changes versus baseline); FCH.

	Baseline	First Drug 3 months	Combination 12 months
Total Serum Cholesterol	344	289 (-16)	224 (-35)**
LDL Cholesterol	236	217 (-8)	150 (-36)**
Serum Triglyceride	363	135 (-63)	142 (-61)**
HDL Cholesterol	34	45 (+33)	46 (+35)*

*$p < 0.05$; **$p < 0.001$

Patients with FH were the majority in the group treated with bile acid sequestrants and HMG-CoA reductase inhibitors. The rationale for this association is based on:

1) Mode of action of the two drugs. They both decrease serum cholesterol by increasing LDL receptor activity in the liver. This activity is reduced in FH patients. Bile acid sequestrants increase cholesterol synthesis in the liver, an adverse effect which can be blocked by HMG-CoA reductase inhibitors.

2) Reduction of doses. Eight to sixteen grams of cholestyramine can be tolerated well, and a low-moderate dose of statins is a safety precaution in young patients (60% under age 40) who are expected to have a long exposure to drug therapy.

In spite of low doses of the drugs, with only mild side effects, a consistent total and LDL cholesterol reduction was obtained in our Lipid Clinic with this drug association, and most of the patients achieved a serum cholesterol level under the threshold of the "high risk" [21]. A lipid lowering effect of this size is associated with significant reductions of CHD morbidity and mortality in various clinical trials. Halted progression and even regression of atheroma was observed in some cases [18].

FCH was always the diagnosis in the patients treated with the association of gemfibrozil with either bile acid sequestrants or HMG-CoA reductase inhibitors. Gemfibrozil speeds up the catabolism of VLDL, which are synthesized in excess in FCH. The association of gemfibrozil with bile acid sequestrants or HMG-CoA reductase inhibitors, which enhance LDL receptor activity, counteracts the excess of circulating LDL, often present in FCH patients. In addition, this association can prevent the LDL cholesterol increase that has been observed following treatment with fibrates alone. Both associations proved effective, though HMG-CoA reductase inhibitors induced a more pronounced reduction of total and LDL cholesterol and total triglycerides.

Both associations significantly increase HDL cholesterol levels. The dose of gemfibrozil was the usual one of 1200 mg/day, but cholestyramine and statins were given at low-moderate doses (8 g/day and 15-20 mg/day, respectively). This might have contributed to treatment safety. In particular, no case of myopathy was observed in patients treated with fibrates and statins after one year of treatment.

The lipid lowering drugs associations mentioned above proved effective in reducing CHD events and halting the progression of atherosclerosis [16-19]. Moreover recently published data indicate that the association of a powerful antioxidant drug like probucol with a statin was able to reduce the vascular tone of coronary artery, an important determinant of coronary blood flow [22].

In conclusion, our data suggest that lipid lowering combined drug regimens are not common (about 10% of cases) in the practice of our outpatient Lipid Clinic. Patients with either FH or FCH, the most CHD-related forms of hyperlipidemia, are the usual candidates for this multiple drug therapy. Results in terms of serum lipid changes can be rewarding. However, low-moderate drug doses and careful safety monitoring are mandatory.

References

1. Mancini M, Pauciullo P. Clinical Relevance of Hyperlipidemia. Cardiovascular Drugs and Therapy 1990;4:1385-88.
2. Study Group of European Atherosclerosis Society. The recognition and management of hyperlipidemia in adults: A policy statement of the European Atherosclerosis Society. Eur Heart J 1988;9:571-600.
3. Prevention of coronary heart disease, scientific background and new clinical guidelines. International Task Force/EAS. Nutr Metab Cardiovasc Dis 1992;2: 113-56.
4. East C, Grundy SM. Single and combination lipid-lowering drug therapy for familial combined hyperlipidemia. Card Board Rev 1989;6:49-66.
5. East C, Bilheimer DW, Grundy SM. Combination drug therapy for familial combined hyperlipidemia. Ann Int Med 1988;115:25-32.
6. Gaddi A, Ciarrocchi A, Barozzi G, et al. Cholestyramine, gemfibrozil or their combination in the treatment of patients with familial hypercholesterolemia: A retrospective study. Adv Ther 1991;8:176-89.
7. Weisweiler P, Merk W, Jacob B, Schwandt P. Fenofibrate and colestipol: Effects on serum and lipoprotein lipids and apolipoproteins in familial hypercholesterolemia. Eur J Clin Pharm 1986;30:191-94.
8. Erkelens DW. Combination drug therapy with HMG-CoA Reductase Inhibitors and Bile Acid Sequestrants for Hypercholesterolemia. Cardiology 1990;77(4):3-38.
9. Emmerich J, Aubert I, Bauduceau B, et al. Efficacy and safety of simvastatin (alone or in association with cholestyramine). A 1- year study in 66 patients with type II hyperlipoproteinemia. Eur Heart J 1990;11:149-55.
10. Weisweiler P. Simvastatin plus low dose colestipol in the treatment of severe familial hypercholesterolemia. Curr Ther Res 1988;44:802-806.
11. Tilly-Kiesi M, Tikkanen MJ. Low density lipoprotein density and composition in hypercholesterolemic men treated with HMG-CoA reductase inhibitors and gemfibrozil. J Int Med 1991;229:427-34.
12. Glueck C, Speirs J, Tracy T. Safety and efficacy of combined gemfibrozil-lovastatin therapy for primary dyslipoproteinemias. J Lab Clin Med 1990;109:603-609.
13. Garg A, Grundy SM. Gemfibrozil alone and in combination with lovastatin for treatment of hypertriglyceridemia in NIDDM. Diabetes 1989;38:364-72.

14. Ross Pierce L, Wysowsky DK, Gross T. Myopathy and rhabdomyolysis associated with lovastatin-gemfibrozil combination therapy. JAMA 1990;264:71-75.
15. Illingworth DR, Bacon S. Influence of lovastatin plus gemfibrozil on plasma lipids and lipoproteins in patients with heterozygous familial hypercholesterolemia. Circulation 1989;79:590-96.
16. Carlson LA, Rosenhamer G. Reduction of mortality in the Stockholm Ischemic Heart Disease Secondary Prevention Study by combined treatment with clofibrate and nicotinic acid. Acta Med Scand 1988;223:405-18.
17. Cashin Hemphill L, Mack S, Pogoda JM, Sanmarco E, Azen SP, Blankenorhorn DM. Beneficial effects of colestipol-niacin on coronary atherosclerosis. A 4- year follow up. JAMA 1990;264:3013-17.
18. Brown G, Albers JJ, Fisher LD, et al. Regression of coronary artery disease as a result of intensive lipid-lowering therapy in men with high levels of apolipoprotein B. N Engl J Med 1990;323:1289-98.
19. Kane JP, Malloy MJ, Ports TA, Phillips NR, Diehl JC, Havel RJ. Regression of coronary atherosclerosis during treatment of familial hypercholesterolemia with combined drug regimens. JAMA 1990;264:3007-12.
20. Grafnetter D. World Health Organization (WHO) coordinated quality control in the lipid laboratory. Giorn Arteriosel 1977;2:113-28.
21. Holme I. An analysis of randomized trials evaluating the effect of cholesterol reduction on mortality and coronary heart disease incidence. Circulation 1990;82: 1916-24.
22. Anderson TJ, Meredith IT, Yeung AC, Frei B, Selwyn AP, Ganz P. The effect of cholesterol lowering and anti-oxidant therapy on endothelium-dependent coronary vasomotion. N Engl J Med 1995;332:488-93.

LONG-TERM EFFECT OF LDL-APHERESIS ON CORONARY HEART DISEASE

Peter Schwandt, Markus G. Donner, and Werner O. Richter
Medical Department II, Klinikum Grosshadern, Ludwig-Maximilians University Munich, D-81377 Munich

Introduction

Several intervention studies have shown that vigorous drug treatment of LDL-hypercholesterolemia can reduce the incidence of cardiovascular events in patients with coronary heart disease [1-3]. Today LDL-cholesterol levels of 100-120 mg/dl are generally accepted for preventing the progression of coronary atherosclerotic lesions [1-5]. LDL-apheresis is regarded as a potent means of treatment for patients with severe hereditary forms of LDL-hypercholesterolemia, who do not respond sufficiently to dietary and drug treatment. In Germany patients with angiographically proven coronary heart disease presenting with LDL-cholesterol concentrations > 130 mg/dl, despite maximal dietary and combined hypolipidemic drug treatment, are considered candidates for this procedure. The techniques most widely applied today are immunoadsorption [6,7], heparin-induced extracorporeal LDL precipitation (HELP) [8,9], and dextran sulfate adsorption [10,11]. In this presentation the long-term lipoprotein changes and the long-term results of coronary angiographies in 33 patients with heterozygous familial hypercholesterolemia treated with 3 different forms of LDL-apheresis are discussed.

Patients

A total of 33 patients (21 men, 12 women, mean age 47 $\pm$ 9 years) were regularly treated with LDL-apheresis. Eighteen patients underwent immunoadsorption, 8 were treated with HELP apheresis, and 7 with dextran sulfate adsorption. All patients suffered from heterozygous familial hypercholesterolemia (familial defective apolipoprotein B was excluded) and severe coronary heart disease documented by coronary angiography. In addition to a specific cholesterol-lowering diet all patients had been treated with various lipid-lowering agents such as anion-exchange resins, fibrates, nicotinic acid, probucol, and HMG-CoA reductase inhibitors. In all instances LDL-cholesterol exceeded 30% of the generally accepted goal for patients with coronary heart disease (i. e. 100 mg/dl). Therefore LDL-apheresis was initiated.

A. M. Gotto, Jr. et al. (eds.), Drugs Affecting Lipid Metabolism, 513–519.

During the study the patients further adhered to a lipid-lowering diet (300 mg cholesterol/day, 30% of daily energy intake as fat, 10% of saturated, monounsaturated, and polyunsaturated fatty acids each). In addition 19 patients were treated with simvastatin 40 mg/day, 1 patient with 30 mg/day, and 7 patients with 20 mg/day. Six patients did not take an HMG-CoA reductase inhibitor due to severe side effects. Patients also had to refrain from smoking. Treatments were scheduled weekly, although fortnightly in four patients. The patients were permitted to miss four treatments per year.

Procedures

The patients were connected to the systems via 2 venous accesses in the antecubital veins of both arms using 17 gauge needles.

Immunoadsorption

For LDL immunoadsorption blood was withdrawn at a flow rate of 50-60 ml/min. Blood cells and plasma were separated by a continuous blood flow cell separator (Celltrifuge II, Baxter Fenwal, Deerfield, Illinois, USA). Citrate dextrose solution (2.5-3.0 ml/min, ACD Formula B, Baxter Fenwal, Deerfield, Illinois, USA) and heparin (B. Braun, Melsungen, Germany (2,500 IU as a bolus and 2,500 to 3,500 IU/h as a continuous infusion) were used for anticoagulation. The plasma was alternately pumped into 2 columns containing polyclonal antihuman apolipoprotein B-100 antibodies coupled to sepharose 4B gel (LDL-Therasorb, Baxter Deutschland, Munich, Germany). After passage through the column the LDL-poor plasma was returned to the patient together with the previously separated blood cells by the second venous access in the opposite arm. Generally, each of the two columns was loaded twice (1,200 - 1,600 ml each cycle) during one treatment session. One column was loaded while the other one was being regenerated. The amount of plasma treated was increased when after two consecutive treatments the previously achieved post-treatment LDL-cholesterol levels could not be obtained. The regenerative process was initiated with glycine buffer (pH 2.8), followed by a phosphate buffered saline solution (PBS) and a 0.9 g/l sodium chloride solution using an automated adsorption-desorption device (ADA-System, Medicap, Ulrichstein, Germany). Treatment time was 3 to 4 hours. The maximum volume of 4-6 l of plasma treated was dependent on the duration of treatment (maximum 4 hours), the volume of the citrate-dextrose solution used (maximum of 700 ml), and the intended cholesterol level after treatment. Every patient had a set of two columns, which were regenerated after every loading and could be re-used for 40 to 50 treatments. After treatment the columns were rinsed with a phosphate-buffered saline solution containing 0.1 g/l sodium azide and stored in a refrigerator (4° C). Forty-eight hours before the next treatment the columns were rinsed with 1 l of sodium chloride (9 g/l) and a sample from this solution was taken for bacterial analysis. This was done for safety reasons, although in no case was bacterial growth in samples of the column fluid demonstrated. Before therapy the columns were again rinsed with 5 l of sodium chloride (9 g/l) to remove sodium azide. As tested on several occasions, after 1.2 l of rinsing no sodium azide was detectable in the eluate.

HELP

Blood was withdrawn at a flow rate of 50-60 ml/min. Heparin (2,500-3,500 IU as a bolus and 2,500 IU/h as a continuous infusion) was used for anticoagulation. Blood cells and plasma were separated by a 0.2 μm polypropylene membrane filter (Haemoselect, B. Braun, Melsungen, Germany). The blood cells were immediately given back to the patient. LDL was precipitated at a pH of 5.12 by adding an equal volume of an acetic acid buffer solution containing 100 IU heparin/ml to the plasma. The precipitated LDL was retained by a 0.4 μm polycarbonate membrane precipitation filter (B. Braun, Melsungen, Germany). The excess heparin in plasma was removed by an anion-exchange filter (two heparin-adsorber cartridges with DEAE-cellulose as an active ingredient, B. Braun, Melsungen, Germany). Finally, bicarbonate dialysis and ultrafiltration using a Cuprophane membrane filter with an effective surface area of 1.7 m^2 (B. Braun, Melsungen, Germany) was applied to remove the excess buffer volume and to restore the plasma to physiological pH. The plasma was then returned to the patient. During one treatment 2,500-3,000 ml of plasma were processed. The treatment time was dependent on the saturation of the precipitate removing filter and on post-treatment fibrinogen concentration, which was not to fall below 0.6 g/l. The procedure was performed using an automated system that regulates flows and monitors pressures (Plasmat-secura, B. Braun, Melsungen, Germany). The treatment time ranged between 2-3 hours and was primarily dependent on the plasma flow.

Dextran Sulfate Adsorption

Treatments were performed with the LDL apheresis system MA 01 (Kaneka Corporation, Osaka, Japan). Heparin was given for anticoagulation (2,000-2,500 IE as an initial injection, 0-2,000 IE/h continuously). Blood flow was set to 60-90 ml/min. Plasma was obtained by filtration (Plasmaflux P2S, Fresenius, Oberursel, Germany) at a rate of 30-40% of blood flow and alternately pumped into 2 columns (Liposorber LA-15, Kanegafuchi, Chemical Industry Corporation, Osaka, Japan) containing 150 ml cellulose-bound dextran sulfate, which adsorbs apo-B containing lipoproteins. The columns are designed for single use, the installation of 2 liposorbers, however, permits regeneration of one column while the other is being loaded. Thus, within one treatment one column can be used several times. The first column is loaded with 500 ml, the subsequent columns with 600 ml of plasma. Regeneration is performed with 105 ml of 41 g/l saline (Kaneka Corporation, Osaka, Japan). Before the next loading the columns are rinsed with 355 ml of Hartmann's solution (Fresenius, Bad Homburg, Germany).

The mean treatment period with LDL-apheresis was 4.4 $\pm$ 2.6 years. Twenty-three patients were treated longer than 2 years. Coronary angiography was performed every 2 years. The global change score of coronary arteries comparing angiograms at baseline and after every two years was estimated by a panel of expert angiographers. The interpretation of the global score, as reported before [1], is shown in Table 1.

Table 1. Assessment of coronary angiographies.

Global Score
-3 = Extreme Regression
-2 = Intermediate Regression
-1 = Definitely Discernible Regression
0 = No Demonstrable Change
1 = Definitely Discernible Progression
2 = Intermediate Progression
3 = Extreme Progression

Effects on Plasma Lipoproteins

Regular LDL-apheresis yielded a long-term decrease of total and LDL-cholesterol as well as of lipoprotein (a), while HDL-cholesterol increased. The long-term changes of these parameters are summarized in Table 2. Looking at the LDL-cholesterol concentrations we found that 11 patients still had a mean concentration (mean between the post-treatment value and the next pretreatment value) higher than 130 mg/dl, 4 were between 120-130 mg/dl, 7 between 110 and 120 mg/dl, 8 between 100 and 110 mg/dl, and three below 100 mg/dl.

Coronary Angiographies

The follow up of the global coronary score of native coronary vessels is listed in Table 3. In four patients a regression of coronary atherosclerosis was observed, in all other cases there was a stop in progression of coronary lesions (0 = no change). Eight patients had already undergone coronary bypass surgery, in two patients (+1, +3) a progression was found in the bypass vessels. No occlusion of native coronary stenoses was observed. Angiographically controlled regression studies in patients with familial hypercholesterolemia on LDL-apheresis have reported results for 2-3 year periods [12-15]. This presentation provides data on coronary angiographies for the course of up to 8.4 years LDL-apheresis treatment in several patients.

Table 2. Long-term effects of regular LDL-apheresis on serum lipoproteins (mg/dl). n = 33.

	Before First Apheresis under Diet + Lipid-Lowering Drugs	Mean Level of Last 5 Treatments of the Observation Period of Every Patient
Total Cholesterol	312 ± 105	198 ± 35
HDL-Cholesterol	40 ± 10	49 ± 9
LDL-Cholesterol	258 ± 62	127 ± 24
Lipoprotein(a)*	58 ± 48	25 ± 34
Ratio: LDL/HDL-Cholesterol	6.45	2.59

* median ± SD

Table 3. Global change score of native coronary arteries under LDL-apheresis.

Patient	Sex	Age (yr.)	Duration of Treatment (yr.)	Global Change Score	Patient	Sex	Age (yr.)	Duration of Treatment (yr.)	Global Change Score
LH	f	44	8.4	0	SJ	m	52	4.0	0
BF	m	38	8.3	0	ZA	m	62	3.1	0
KK	f	43	8.2	0	HE	f	52	3.0	0
RC	f	44	8.1	0	BA	m	49	3.0	0
SJ	m	47	8.1	-2	SH	f	50	3.0	0
RD	m	29	8	-1	KE	m	54	2.9	0
SB	f	43	7.3	0	SM	m	45	2.4	0
WF	m	37	7.3	-1	WK	m	49	2.4	0
SP	m	46	7.1	0	SK	f	60	2.3	0
MA	f	58	6.2	0	SB	f	49	2.3	0
LB	f	56	5.2	-1	RW	m	50	2.0	0
TW	m	33	5.1	0					

Side Effects

We did not observe any long-term clinically relevant side effects with any of the three procedures applied.

Conclusion

We conclude that in the long term LDL-apheresis, preferably in combination with an HMG-CoA reductase inhibitor, can improve the poor prognosis of patients with severe heterozygous familial hypercholesterolemia.

References

1. Blankenhorn DH, Nessim SA, Johnson RL, et al. Beneficial effects of combined colestipol-niacin therapy on coronary atherosclerosis and coronary venous bypass grafts. JAMA 1987; 257:3233-40.
2. Brown G, Albers JJ, Fisher LD, et al. Regression of coronary artery disease as a result of intensive lipid-lowering therapy in men with high levels of apolipoprotein B. N Engl J Med 1990;323:1289-98.
3. Scandinavian Simvastatin Survival Study Group. Randomized trial of cholesterol lowering in 4444 patients with coronary heart disease: The Scandinavian Simvastatin Survival Study (4S). Lancet 1994;344:1383-89.
4. MAAS Investigators. Effect of simvastatin on coronary atheroma: The Multicentre Anti-Atheroma Study (MAAS). Lancet 1994;344:633-38.
5. Watts GB, Lewis B, Brunt JNH, et al. Effects on coronary artery disease of lipid lowering diet, or diet plus cholestyramine, in the St. Thomas' Atherosclerosis Regression Study (STARS). Lancet 1992;339:563-69.
6. Stoffel W, Greve V, Borberg H. Application of specific extracorporeal removal of low density lipoprotein in familial hypercholesterolemia. Lancet 1981;II:1005-1007.
7. Richter WO, Jacob BG, Ritter MM, et al. 3-year treatment of familial heterozygous hypercholesterolemia by extracorporeal LDL-immunoadsorption with polyclonal apolipoprotein B antibodies. Metabolism 1993;42:888-94.
8. Eisenhauer T, Armstrong VW, Wieland H, et al. Selective removal of low density lipoproteins (LDL) by precipitation at low pH: First clinical application of the HELP system. Klin Wochenschr 1987;65:161-68.
9. Seidel D, Armstrong VW, Schuff-Werner P, for the HELP Study Group. The HELP-LDL-Apheresis Multicenter Study, an angiographically assessed trial on the role of LDL-apheresis in the secondary prevention of coronary heart disease. I. Evaluation of safety and cholesterol-lowering effects during the first 12 months. Eur J Clin Invest 1991;21:375-83.
10. Mabuchi H, Michishita I, Takeda M, et al. A new low density lipoprotein apheresis system using two dextran sulfate cellulose columns in an automated column regenerating unit (LDL-continuous apheresis). Atherosclerosis 1987;68:19-25.
11. Homma Y, Mikami Y, Tamachi H, et al. Comparison of selectivity of LDL removal by double filtration an dextran-sulfate cellulose column plasmapheresis. Atherosclerosis 1986;60:23-27.

12. Tatami R, Inoue N, Itho H, et al. Regression of coronary atherosclerosis by combined LDL-apheresis and lipid-lowering drug therapy in patients with familial hypercholesterolemia: A multicenter study. Atherosclerosis 1992;95:1-13.
13. Schuff-Werner P, Gohlke H, Bartmann U, et al. The HELP-LDL-apheresis multicenter study, an angiographically assessed trial on the role of LDL-apheresis in the secondary prevention of coronary heart disease. II. Final evaluation of the effect of regular treatment on LDL-cholesterol plasma concentrations and the course of coronary heart disease. Eur J Clin Invest 1994;24:724-32.
14. Borberg H, Oette K. Experience with and conclusions from three different trials on low density lipoprotein apheresis. In: Agishi T, Kawamura A, Mineshima M, editors. Therapeutic plasmapheresis (XII). Utrecht, The Netherlands: VSP, 1993:25-28.
15. Thompson GR, Maher VM, Matthews S, et al. Familial Hypercholesterolaemia Regression Study: A randomized trial of low-density-lipoprotein apheresis. Lancet 1995;345:811-16.

The H.E.L.P. System: Clinical Experience of 10 Years

Joachim Thiery and Dietrich Seidel
Institute of Clinical Chemistry, University Hospital Großhadern, Marchioninistraße 15, D-81366 Munich, Germany

Introduction

Premature coronary heart disease (CHD) and early death from cardiac consequences are the frequent outcomes of severe hypercholesterolemia in patients with elevated plasma levels of low density lipoproteins (LDL). In many patients suffering from CHD, high plasma concentrations of lipoprotein(a) (Lp(a)) and fibrinogen may potentiate the cardiovascular risk. Today, there is experimental and clinical evidence that plasma LDL-cholesterol (LDL-C) levels below 100 mg/dl diminish the risk of recurrent coronary events, reduce mortality, and can induce regression of vessel wall lesions in CHD-patients [1-4]. However, in some cases of severe hypercholesterolemia with plasma LDL-C concentrations above 240 mg/dl, LDL cannot sufficiently be decreased by maximal dietary and pharmacological therapy alone. Today, this group of high risk CHD patients can also be treated with an extracorporeal procedure to eliminate LDL, Lp(a), and fibrinogen from plasma circulation: the H.E.L.P.-LDL-apheresis system (heparin-mediated extracorporeal LDL:fibrinogen precipitation). For the last decade, we have investigated the clinical efficiency and safety of this selective plasma therapy in the treatment of CHD-patients with severe hypercholesterolemia.

The H.E.L.P. Apheresis System

The system has been developed and is manufactured by B. Braun Melsungen, Melsungen, Germany. The method is based on an increase of the positive charges on LDL and Lp(a) particles at low pH, allowing them to specifically form a network with heparin and fibrinogen in the absence of divalent cations [5]. Only a limited number of other heparin-binding plasma proteins are coprecipitated by heparin at low pH. Other proteins, such as apo A1, apo A2, albumin, or immunoglobulins, do not bind to heparin and are not affected [6,7].

The H.E.L.P. system has unique features:

1. it removes LDL, Lp(a), and fibrinogen with high efficiency;
2. it increases HDL on long-term treatment;
3. it does not alter or modify plasma lipoproteins;

A. M. Gotto, Jr. et al. (eds.), Drugs Affecting Lipid Metabolism, 521–529.

4. it does not change plasma concentrations of cell mediators;
5. it avoids the use of compounds with immunogenic or immunostimulatory activity;
6. it uses only disposable material and avoids regeneration of any of the used elements;
7. it is a technically safe and well-standardized procedure;
8. in short- and long-term treatment, tolerance and clinical benefits are excellent; and
9. its clinical utility has been established by the outcome of controlled clinical trials.

The major characteristics of the H.E.L.P. system are illustrated in Figure 1.

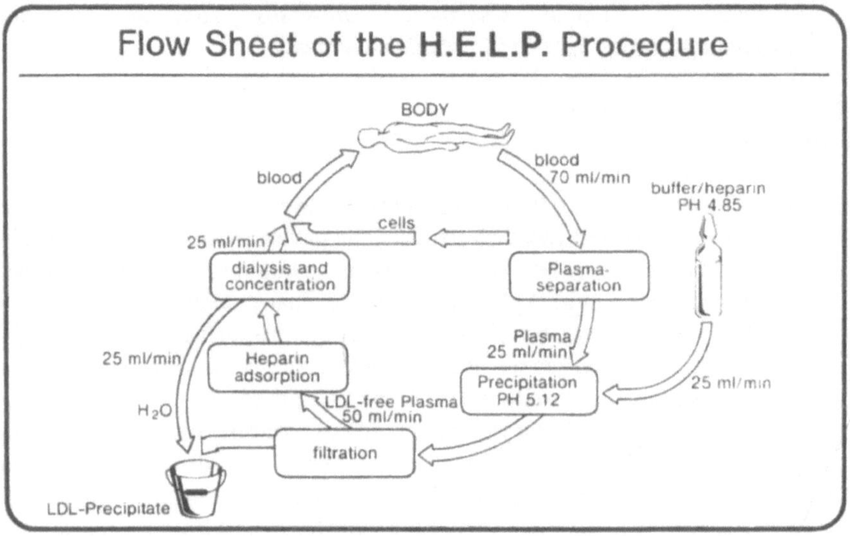

Figure 1. Flow sheet of the H.E.L.P. procedure.

In the first step, plasma is obtained by filtration of whole blood through a plasma separator. This is then mixed continuously with a 0.3 M acetate buffer of pH 4.85 containing 100 IU heparin/ml. A sudden precipitation occurs at a pH of 5.12, and the suspension is circulated through a 0.4 μm polycarbonate filter to remove the precipitated LDL, Lp(a), and fibrinogen. Excess heparin is absorbed by passage through an anion exchange column which binds only heparin at the given pH. The plasma buffer mixture is finally subjected to a bicarbonate dialysis and ultrafiltration to remove excess fluid and to restore the physiological pH, before the plasma is mixed with the blood cells and returned to the patient. All filter and tubings required for the treatment are sterile, disposable, and are intended for single use only. This makes it easy and reliable to work with the system and guarantees a steady quality for each treatment, independent of the clinic performing the procedure. Safety is assured by a visual display and two microprocessors operating in parallel. Due to the excellent tolerance of the procedure the patients leave the hospital shortly after the end of the treatment.

Clinical Experience With the H.E.L.P. System in CHD Patients with Severe Hypercholesterolemia

The clinical experience with the H.E.L.P. system goes back to 1984. Since then and up to 1995, approximately 500 patients were treated in almost 100,000 single treatments. Some patients have been treated for more than 10 years. Currently, the system operates in approximately 75 centers in Germany, Austria, Italy, Ireland, Hungary, Brazil, and in the US.

The efficiency of the system is 100% for the elimination of LDL, Lp(a), and fibrinogen. Per single treatment (lasting 1.5 to 2 hours), 2.8 to 3 liters of plasma are treated, causing an actual reduction of approximately 65-70% of these three compounds in plasma of the treated patients.

The rates of return to pre-apheresis concentrations for LDL differ between normocholesterolemics and heterozygous as well as homozygous familial hypercholesterolemic (FH) patients. In biweekly treatment intervals, the pretreatment values usually reach a new steady state after 4 to 8 treatments. Long-term effects of the H.E.L.P. treatment based on interval concentrations between two treatments (c after H.E.L.P. + c before H.E.L.P.:2) and expressed as percentage of plasma levels at the start are shown in Table 1.

Table 1. Long-term effects of the H.E.L.P. treatment based on interval concentrations between two treatments and expressed as percentage of plasma levels at the start.

Long-Term Effects of the H.E.L.P. Treatment Mean Interval Values of Approximately 6,000 Treatments			
LDL-Cholesterol	-51%	±	14
Lp(a)	-45%	±	5
Fibrinogen	-46%	±	15
Apoprotein B100	-45%	±	10
HDL-Cholesterol	+12%	±	2
Apoprotein A1	+9%	±	2

Of particular clinical relevance is the considerable effect that H.E.L.P. treatment has on blood rheological parameters, which are especially important in coronary heart disease. H.E.L.P. treatment reduces plasma viscosity by 15% and erythrocyte aggregation by 50%, while erythrocyte filtrability rises by 15% and tissue partial pressure of oxygen by 20-30%. It has been shown that the changes in plasma viscosity and erythrocyte aggregation are brought about by the reduction of both plasma fibrinogen and LDL [8].

Changes in blood viscosity lead to improvement equivalent to 8% reduction of the hematocrit, of course without changing the latter. It seems likely that the rapid improvement in clinical symptoms associated with coronary heart disease in treated patients, shown by a decrease in angina attacks and improvement in myocardial stress ability, is primarily related to improved rheology and in addition, possibly to a positive influence on endothelium function.

Clinical Utility of the H.E.L.P. Treatment

The first coronary angiograms two years after H.E.L.P. treatment in over 50 patients of the H.E.L.P. multicenter study [9] lend support to the hope that the regression of coronary heart disease is possible in humans. In this study, angiograms obtained before and after two years of regular treatment were quantitatively evaluated by an independent and blind evaluator [10]. The rate of regression was 1.8 times the rate of progression for the period of two years. This factor is independent of the cut-off value used to define significance of changes. In the H.E.L.P. multicenter study, only 15% of the coronary lesions progressed on the basis of an 8% detection limit for the significance to estimate the change.

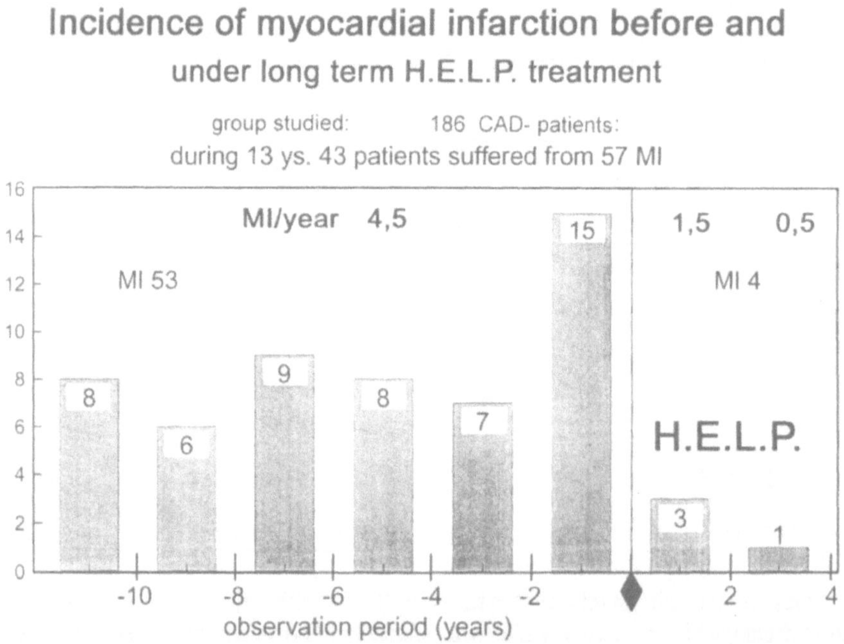

Figure 2. Effect of long-term H.E.L.P. treatment on the incidence of myocardial infarction. There is a significant reduction from 4.5 myocardial infarctions/year preceding the H.E.L.P. therapy to 1.5/year after 2 years, and to 0.5/year after 4 years of continuous H.E.L.P. therapy.

Figure 2 indicates the myocardial infarction incidence in a high risk coronary heart disease patient group (n = 186) which was followed by history for 10 years before undergoing H.E.L.P. therapy. On average, 4.5 myocardial infarctions (MI) per year and 16 in the preceding 2 years before the H.E.L.P. treatment were recorded. Immediately after the start of the H.E.L.P. treatment, the MI-incidence fell to 3 and to 1.5 per 2 years for the following 4 years after start of treatment. The prompt reduction of MI incidence of high risk patients following H.E.L.P. therapy may result from transforming unstable plaques into stable plaques and substantially testifies to the clinical efficiency of this treatment. Our results clearly demonstrate that regular H.E.L.P. treatment favorably influences the progression of coronary artery disease, decreases the incidence of coronary events, and enhances survival time of CHD patients.

Experience With a Combined H.E.L.P. and HMG-CoA Reductase Inhibitor Therapy

In cases with plasma cholesterol levels exceeding 300 mg/dl, the use of specified diets and drugs may not be sufficient if LDL concentrations < 100 mg/dl and regression of CHD is to be approached as a means of secondary intervention. We have therefore investigated the efficacy of a combined therapy, using HMG-CoA reductase inhibitors (lovastatin, pravastatin, simvastatin) in combination with the H.E.L.P. apheresis. These compounds significantly decrease the rate of return after H.E.L.P. apheresis by approximately 20% in both, heterozygous and homozygous FH patients [11,12].

When the two treatments are combined, a reduction of the interval LDL-C level of 70-80% may be achieved while Lp(a) and fibrinogen are not further affected (over the H.E.L.P. treatment alone, 45%). In the combined form, therapy intervals between the H.E.L.P. treatments may in many cases be stretched from 7 to 14 days, depending on the synthetic rates for LDL or upon the severity of CHD.

Typical Case Reports

CASE 1: PREMATURE CORONARY HEART DISEASE, STRONGLY ELEVATED LDL-, AND LP(A)-PLASMA CONCENTRATIONS

A typical follow-up kinetic for LDL and lipoprotein(a) under H.E.L.P. treatment of a patient with severe progressive coronary heart disease is shown in Figure 3. At the start of our therapeutic intervention, the 33-year-old MI patient had a history of coronary bypass and percutaneous transluminal coronary angioplasty (PTCA) treatment. He showed LDL cholesterol levels of 350 mg/dl and marked elevation of Lp(a) of 165 mg/dl.

LDL cholesterol could be lowered with an HMG-CoA reductase inhibitor (simvastatin) by about 48% to 170 mg/dl, but no effect on lipoprotein(a) levels was observed. However, in combination with regular H.E.L.P. treatment, we were able to maintain LDL-concentrations at an interval value of about 100 mg/dl. In addition, H.E.L.P. treatment brought about a marked decrease of post-apheresis lipoprotein(a) concentrations.

The interval Lp(a) levels maintained at about 60 mg/dl. Fibrinogen was lowered from a baseline value of 317 mg/dl to a H.E.L.P. interval value of 177 mg/dl, which is equivalent to a 44% reduction. A control angiography after 3 and 5 years revealed that the combined treatment did stop the very progressive coronary heart disease, which was developing in the patient prior to treatment. In addition, PTCA results before H.E.L.P. therapy were well maintained after 5 years of treatment.

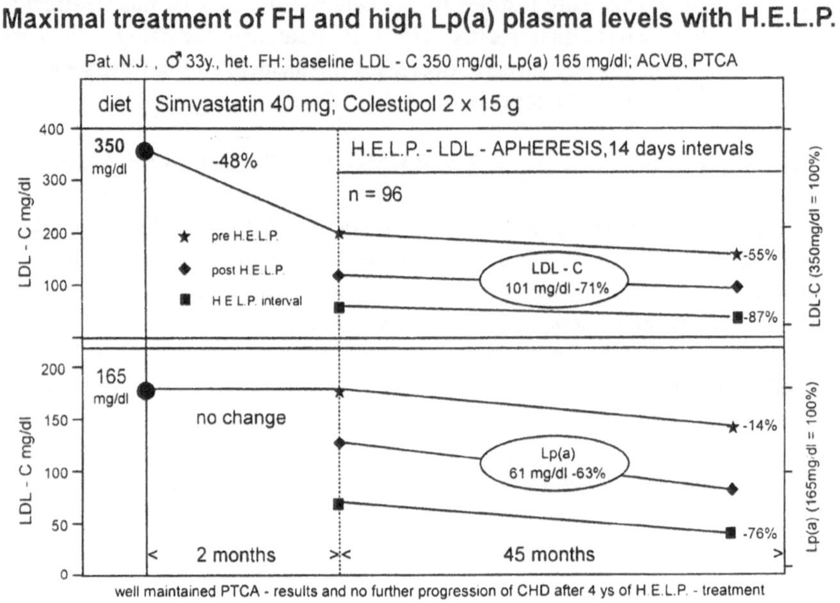

Figure 3. Effects of H.E.L.P. treatment in combination with simvastatin and colestipol on plasma LDL-cholesterol and Lp(a) concentrations in a CHD patient with heterozygous familial hypercholesterolemia and high Lp(a) levels. H.E.L.P. treatment started two months after conventional lipid lowering therapy. Values represent the mean of pre-, post-, and interval-H.E.L.P.-LDL, respectively. Lp(a) concentrations represent 45 months of combined plasma therapy.

CASE 2: HOMOZYGOUS FORM OF HYPERCHOLESTEROLEMIA

Early death from cardiac consequences of premature coronary sclerosis and aortic stenoses is the usual outcome of homozygous familial hypercholesterolemia [13]. Inherited as an autosomal dominant defect of the LDL receptor gene, this disease is characterized by very high plasma LDL cholesterol concentrations (between 600 and 1,000 mg/dl) and the development of severe cutaneous and tendon xanthomata in childhood. All conventional lipid lowering treatments with diet and medication are completely insufficient.

Since 1985, we have been following and treating a familial homozygous hypercholesterolemic (FHH) patient, born in 1979, with the H.E.L.P. apheresis procedure [12]. LDL cholesterol concentrations before the start of treatment exceeded 800 mg/dl. The follow-up of LDL concentrations under the H.E.L.P. treatment alone and in combination with lovastatin and regular cholestyramine is shown in Figure 4.

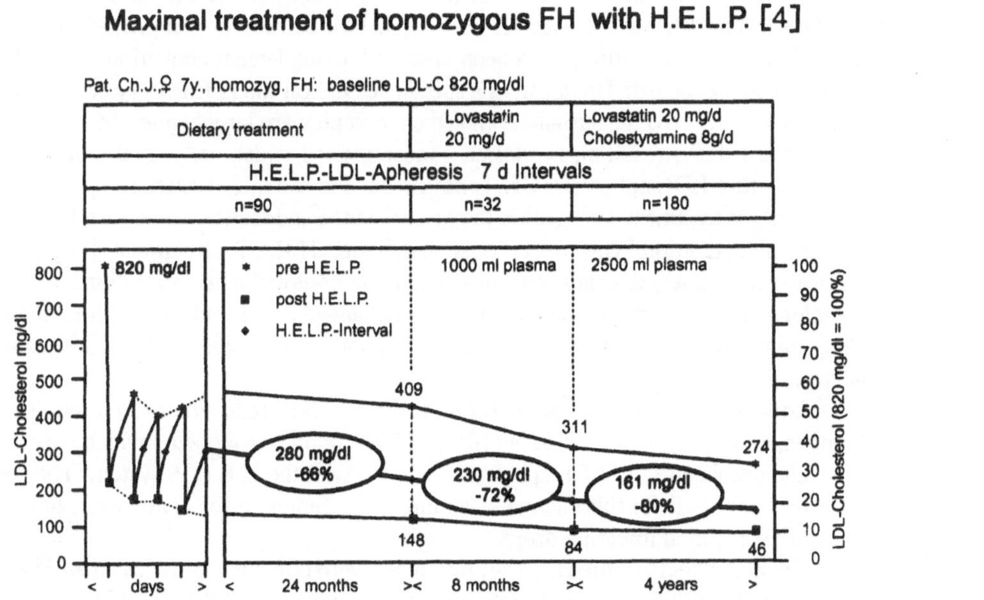

Figure 4. Effect of H.E.L.P. treatment in a child with homozygous familial hypercholesterolemia. Values represent the mean of pre-, post-, and weekly H.E.L.P. intervals. LDL-concentrations of H.E.L.P. treatment alone and in combination with lovastatin and cholestyramine.

The girl was treated for two years by weekly H.E.L.P. apheresis. Under this procedure the LDL-C interval levels were maintained below 280 mg/dl. At this time a rapid regression of existing multiple xanthomata could be observed. With additional medication of lovastatin and cholestyramine a further LDL decrease to 180 mg/dl could be achieved. The treated plasma volume recently could be enhanced from 1.5 to 2.5 liters. This resulted in a mean LDL cholesterol level of 160 mg/dl, which is equivalent to a decrease of 80% as compared to pretreatment values. The therapy is excellently tolerated. The girl is well and shows normal growth and age adequate development. No signs of cardiovascular symptoms have been noted as yet.

Treatment Tolerance and Safety of the H.E.L.P. System

At the end of the H.E.L.P. therapy, plasma concentrations of proteins that are not selectively precipitated by heparin at low pH were generally in the range of 80-90% of the initial values and returned to their original level no later than 24 hours after the end of the treatment [6,13]. Substitution of any kind has not been necessary in the years of clinical experience with the H.E.L.P. system. The H.E.L.P. procedure does not alter the physicochemical characteristics of LDL, nor does it alter the ligand quality of LDL for lipoprotein receptors. Special attention has been focused in all clinical trials on the effect of H.E.L.P. on hemostasis. All post-treatment controls were typical for extracorporeal procedures, and no critical bleeding complications have been observed. Complement activation is found in all extracorporeal procedures. However, as a specific feature on the H.E.L.P. system, activated complement C3, C4 and the terminal complement complex are largely adsorbed to the filter system of H.E.L.P., resulting in plasma concentrations which are actually below those measured before LDL apheresis. C5a is not retained in the filter system but plasma levels at the end of the treatment were within the normal range and leukocytopenia, a hallmark of complement activation, was never observed under H.E.L.P. treatment [14]. Plasma electrolytes, hormones, vitamins, enzymes, and immunoglobulin concentrations, as well as hematological parameters, remained virtually unchanged at the end of each treatment and on long-term application of H.E.L.P., alone and in combination with HMG-CoA reductase inhibitors.

Long-term observations show that besides the marked reduction of LDL cholesterol, fibrinogen, and Lp(a), some increase (10%) of HDL cholesterol occurs which may add to the antiatherogenic effect of LDL apheresis treatment with the H.E.L.P. system. The reason and the metabolic basis of this change is yet unknown. Similar effects, however, have been found with some lipid lowering drugs.

Adverse effects of the H.E.L.P. treatment were documented in less than 3% of all treatments and could be managed without any major problem [7,9,11,14,15].

Indication for the H.E.L.P. Therapy

Based on the experience of many centers, a German consensus panel has published differentiated guide lines as to when LDL apheresis should be applied [16].

LDL apheresis treatment is recommended in any of the following circumstances: 1) the presence of homozygous FH; 2) for primary prevention of CHD in young patients with severe hypercholesterolemia and a strong family history of CHD, provided LDL-C cannot be decreased below 200 mg/dl by a hyperlipidemic diet and maximal drug therapy; or 3) for secondary prevention of CHD in patients with severe CHD (stage III-IV) and marked hypercholesterolemia, provided LDL-cholesterol cannot be decreased below 135 mg/dl by maximal dietary and drug therapy.

Diet and drug therapy should be continued while the patients are on H.E.L.P.-LDL-apheresis treatment. The therapeutic goal in secondary prevention for LDL is 100 mg/dl.

References

1. Blankenhorn DH, Hodis HN. Arterial imaging and atherosclerosis reversal. Arteriosclerosis

and Thrombosis 1994;14:177-92.

2. Brown BG, Albers JJ, Fisher LD, et al. Regression of coronary artery disease as a result of intensive lipid-lowering therapy in men with high levels of apolipoprotein B. N Engl J Med 1990;323:1289-98.
3. The Scandinavian Simvastatin Survival Study Group. Randomized trial of cholesterol lowering in 4444 patients with coronary heart disease: Scandinavian Simvastatin Survival Study (4S). Lancet 1994;8934:1383-89.
4. Shepherd J, Cobbe SM, Ford I, et al. for the West of Scotland Coronary Prevention Study Group. Prevention of coronary heart disease with pravastatin in men with hypercholesterolemia. N Engl J Med 1995;333(29):1301-1307.
5. Seidel D, Wieland H. Ein neues Verfahren zur selektiven Messung und extrakorporalen Elimination von low-density lipoproteinen. J Clin Chem Clin Biochem 1982;20:684-85.
6. Eisenhauer T, Armstrong VW, Wieland H, Fuchs C, Scheler F, Seidel D. Selective removal of low density lipoproteins (LDL) by precipitation at low pH: First clinical application of the H.E.L.P. system. Klin Wschr 1987;65:161-68.
7. Seidel D, Armstrong VW, Schuff-Werner P, for the H.E.L.P. Study Group. The H.E.L.P.-LDL-apheresis multicenter study, an angiographically assessed trial on the role of LDL-apheresis in the secondary prevention of coronary heart disease. I. Evaluation of safety and cholesterol-lowering effects during the first 12 months. Eur J Clin Invest 1991;21:375-83.
8. Schuff-Werner P, Schütz E, Seyde WC, et al. Improved hemorheology associated with a reduction in plasma fibrinogen and LDL in patients being treated by heparin-induced extracorporeal LDL-precipitation (H.E.L.P.). Eur J Clin Invest 1989;19:30-37.
9. Schuff-Werner P, Gohlke H, Bartmann U, et al. and the H.E.L.P. Study Group. The H.E.L.P.-LDL-Apheresis Multicenter Study, an angiographically assessed trial on the role of LDL-apheresis in the secondary prevention of coronary heart disease. II. Final evaluation of the effect of regular treatment on LDL-cholesterol plasma concentrations and the course of coronary heart disease. Eur J Clin Invest 1994;24:724-32.
10. Reiber JHC. Morphologic and densitometric analysis of coronary arteries. In: Heintzen PH, Bürsch JH, editors. Progress in cardiovascular angiocardiography. Dordrecht, The Netherlands: Kluwer Academic Publishers, 1988:137-58.
11. Thiery J, Seidel D. LDL-apheresis: Clinical experience and indications in the treatment of severe hypercholesterolemia. Transfusion Science 1993;14:249-59.
12. Thiery J, Walli AK, Janning G, Seidel D. Low density lipoprotein plasmapheresis with and without lovastatin in the treatment of the homozygous form of familial hypercholesterolemia. Eur J Pediatric 1990;149:716-21.
13. Armstrong VW, Schleef J, Thiery J, et al. Effect of H.E.L.P.-LDL apheresis on serum concentrations of human lipoprotein(a): Kinetic analysis of the post-treatment return to baseline levels. Eur J Clin Invest 1989;19:235-40.
14. Würzner R, Schuff-Werner P, Franzke A, et al. Complement activation and depletion during LDL-apheresis by heparin-induced extracorporeal LDL-precipitation (H.E.L.P.). Eur J Clin Invest 1991;21:288-94.
15. Schultis H-W, von Bayer H, Neitzel H, Riedel E. Functional characteristics of LDL particles derived from various LDL-apheresis techniques regarding LDL-drug-complex preparation. J Lipid Res 1990;31:2277-84.
16. Greten H, Bleifeld W, Beil FU, et al. LDL-apherese. Ein therapeutisches Verfahren bei schwerer Hypercholesterinämie. Deutsches Ärzteblatt 1992;89:48-49.

LOWERING OF SERUM CHOLESTEROL LEVELS BY A CHOLESTEROL DERIVATIVE OF A NEW TRIANTENNARY CLUSTER GALACTOSIDE

Theo J.C. Van Berkel, Helene Vietsch, and Erik A.L. Biessen
Division of Biopharmaceutics, Leiden-Amsterdam Center for Drug Research, Sylvius Laboratory, University of Leiden, PO Box 9503, 2300 RA Leiden, The Netherlands

Introduction

Previous studies have demonstrated that cholesterol-derivatized galactosides exert an hypocholesterolemic effect by inducing hepatic uptake of (atherogenic) lipoproteins via galactose-recognizing receptors in the liver [1-3]. However, a prolonged infusion with high concentrations of these compounds was required, which may be caused by the low affinity for the galactose-recognizing asialoglycoprotein receptor on the parenchymal liver cell [4]. Both the low level of lipid-lowering activity and the lack of specificity for targeting lipoproteins to the asialoglycoprotein receptor was caused by the moderate affinity and specificity of the cholesterol-derivatized cluster galactoside for this receptor.

In the present study we show that both the affinity and specificity of a triantennary cluster galactoside for the asialoglycoprotein receptor could be significantly improved by elongation of the spacer that connects the terminal galactose moieties of a cluster galactoside with the branching point of the dendrite from 4Å to 20Å. In view of its high affinity, the most selective compound (TG(20Å)) may offer a new tool for the development of a more potent hypocholesterolemic therapeutic. Therefore, we synthesized the cholesterol derivative of this cluster galactoside (TG(20Å)C) and tested its cholesterol-lowering activity as well as its effect on the biliary secretion of bile-acids.

Results

Affinity and Specificity of Galactose-Terminated Triantennary Cluster Galactosides for the Hepatic Asialoglycoprotein Receptor

The affinity of the synthesized cluster galactosides (for structures see Figure 1A) for the hepatic asialoglycoprotein receptor was determined using competition studies of ^{125}I-ASOR binding to parenchymal liver cells. The affinity of the cluster galactoside for the asialoglycoprotein receptor increased dramatically with elongation of the spacer connecting

A. M. Gotto, Jr. et al. (eds.), Drugs Affecting Lipid Metabolism, 531–539.

1A

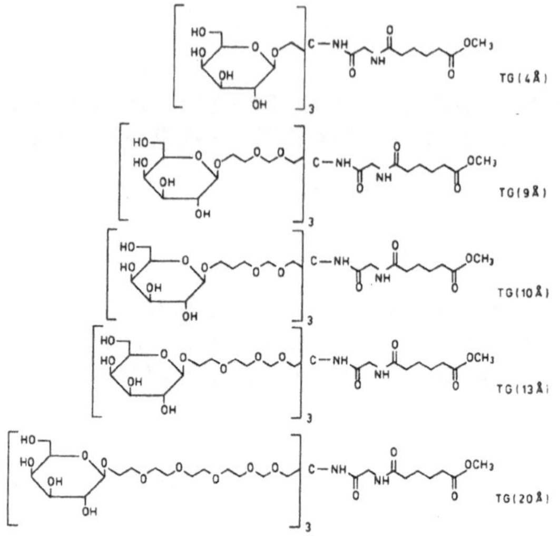

1B

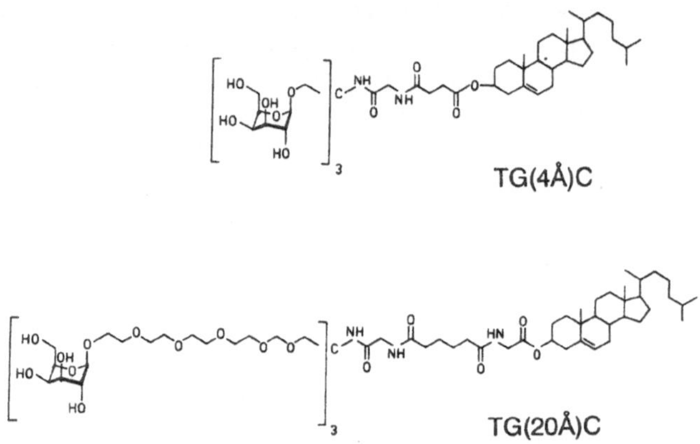

Figure 1. Chemical structures of the tested cluster galactosides.
1A: *N*-[Tris-*O*-(ß-D-galactopyranosyl)methyl]methyl-N^{α}-[1-(6-methyl)adipyl]glycinamide [TG(4Å)];*N*-[Tris-*O*-(ethyl-ß-D-galactopyranosyl)methoxymethyl]methyl-N^{α}-[1-(6-methyl)adipyl]glycinamide [TG(9Å)], *N*-[Tris-*O*-(propyl-ß-D-galactopyranosyl)methoxymethyl]methyl-N^{α}-[1-(6-methyl)adipyl]glycinamide [TG(10Å)]; *N*-[Tris-*O*-(3-oxapentanyl-ß-D-galactopyranosyl)methoxymethyl]methyl-N^{α}-[1-(6-methyl)adipyl]glycinamide [TG(13Å)]; *N*-[Tris-*O*-(3,6,9-trioxaundecanyl-ß-D-galactopyranosyl)methoxymethyl]methyl-N^{α}-[1-(6-methyl)adipyl]glycinamide [TG(20Å)].
1B: chemical structures of *N*-[Tris-*O*-(3,6,9-trioxaundecanyl-ß-D-galactopyranosyl)methyl]methyl-N^{α}-[1-(6-(5-cholesten-3ß-yloxy)glycyl)adipyl]glycinamide, TG(20Å)C], *N*-[Tris-*O*-(ß-D-galactopyranosyl)methyl]methyl-N^{α}-[(5-cholesten-3ß-yloxy)succinyl]glycinamide [TG(4Å)C].

the terminal galactosyls with the branching point of the dendrite (Figure 2). TG(20Å), provided with a 20 Å spacer, displayed a K_i of 190 nM while TG(4Å), having a 4Å spacer, was only marginally capable of inhibiting ^{125}I-ASOR binding (K_i = 390 μM). The cluster galactosides with intermediate spacer length, TG(9Å), TG(10Å) and TG(13Å), exhibited intermediate affinities (K_i = 1.2 μM, 19 μM, and 10 μM, respectively) for the asialoglycoprotein receptor. As a control, competition studies of ^{125}I-ASOR binding by unlabeled ASOR were performed. In agreement with previous studies, the affinity of ASOR for the ASGPr was in the low nanomolar range with an K_i of 6.46 ± 1.75 nM [5,6].

In addition to the asialoglycoprotein receptor on the parenchymal liver cell, the liver contains a second galactose recognizing receptor: the galactose/fucose receptor on the Kupffer cell [7-9]. To assess the cellular specificity of the synthesized cluster galactosides, we have determined the affinity of the galactosides for the competing galactose/fucose receptor on Kupffer cells using competition studies of ^{125}I-lactosylated LDL (Lac-LDL) binding to this receptor. Lac-LDL has been established to be specifically recognized by the fucose/galactose receptor on Kupffer cells [9]. ^{125}I-Lac-LDL binding to Kupffer cells could

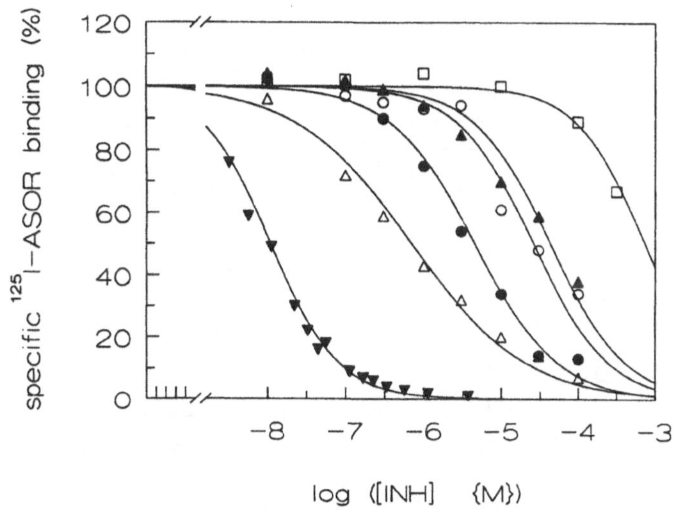

Figure 2. Displacement of ^{125}I-ASOR binding to the parenchymal liver cell by galactose-terminated cluster galactosides. Competition experiments of ^{125}I-ASOR binding to parenchymal liver cells were performed as follows. Rat parenchymal liver cells were incubated for 2 hours at 4° with a fixed concentration of 5 nM ^{125}I-ASOR in the absence or presence of unlabeled ASOR (▼) or one of the following cluster galactosides: TG(4Å) (☐), TG(9Å) (●), TG(10Å) (▲), TG(13Å) (○) and TG(20Å) (△). Binding is expressed as % of the specific binding, which is defined as the difference between total binding (absence of displacer) and nonspecific binding (100 mM N-acetyl galactosamine). The inhibition curves were fitted according to a single site competition binding equation using a computerized nonlinear regression procedure (Graph-Pad).

be inhibited for 78 % by excess unlabelled Lac-LDL at an K_i of 1.15 ± 0.30 nM (data not shown). By contrast, none of the compounds was capable of displacing ^{125}I-Lac-LDL binding from Kupffer cells at concentrations of up to 400 μM.

EFFECT OF TG(20Å)C ON THE CHOLESTEROL CONCENTRATION OF RAT SERUM

The galactoside with the highest affinity for the asialoglycoprotein receptor, TG(20Å), has been derivatized with a cholesterol moiety, yielding TG(20Å)C (Figure 1B) [10] and the biological activity of the compound has been evaluated in the rat. Although the rat is not the most appropriate model for evaluating the hypocholesterolemic activity of TG(20Å)C in terms of serum lipoprotein profile and cholesterol metabolism, utilization of the rat enables a direct comparison with earlier studies on the hypocholesterolemic activity of TG(4Å)C and mono-gal-chol [1-4,11,12]. The effect of an intravenous bolus injection of TG(20Å)C on the total serum cholesterol content in rats is shown in Figure 3. A dose-dependent decrease of cholesterol level was observed following injection of TG(20Å)C. Even at a dose of 56

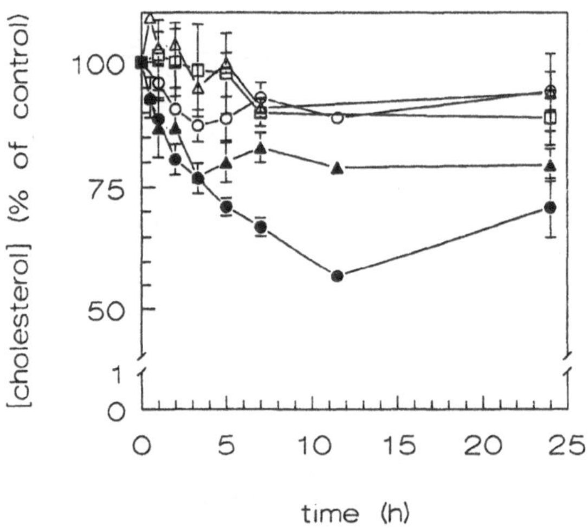

Figure 3. Effect of intravenous injection of TG(20Å)C on the cholesterol concentration in serum: PBS (500 μl, Δ) or PBS containing 56 μg (○), 180 μg (▲), 560 μg TG(20Å)C (●), or 560 μg TGlc(4Å)C (□) is injected into the vena penis of anaesthetized rats. At the indicated times, blood samples were collected by orbital punction. The blood samples were centrifuged and the sera were obtained. Total cholesterol content of the sera were determined, in duplicate, using the CHOD-PAP kit of Boehringer Mannhein, and is plotted as % of the content at t = 0 (2.37 ± 0.16, 2.04 ± 0.11, 2.16 ± 0.3, 2.19 ± 0.08 and 2.28 ± 0.2 for PBS, 56 μg TG(20Å)C, 180 μg TG(20Å)C, 560 μg TG(20Å)C, and 560 μg TGlc(4Å)C, respectively). Values are means ± s.d. of three experiments.

μg a slight initial decrease of the cholesterol level was induced. At a dose of 560 μg and at 11 hours after injection, the serum cholesterol level was reduced by 45%. Statistical analysis of the concentration/time curves for the four treatment groups by analysis of repeated measures (corrected for missing values) confirmed that the concentration/time curves of the treatment groups differed significantly ($P < 0.001$). In addition, each of the treatment groups differed significantly from the control, the significance of this difference being increased with increasing dose of TG(20Å)C (from $P = 0.076$ for rats treated with the lowest dose of TG(20Å)C to $P = 0.004$ for rats treated with 560 μg TG(20Å)C). Also, a clearcut and comparable time effect of the serum cholesterol levels was noticed for all treatment groups ($P < 0.01$). The persistence of this reduction was remarkable. At 24 hours following administration of the agent, serum levels still had not reached control values. As a control for a potential nonspecific effect of cholesterylated cluster galactosides, the effect of the cholesterol derivative of a triantennary cluster glucoside (TGlc(4Å)C) was studied. However, a bolus injection of 560 μg TGlc(4Å)C, did not affect the level of total serum cholesterol over a 24-hour period following injection (2.28 ± 0.2 mM).

The level of the various individual lipoprotein fractions was measured at 24 hours after administration of PBS or TG(20Å)C. In view of the predominant contribution of high

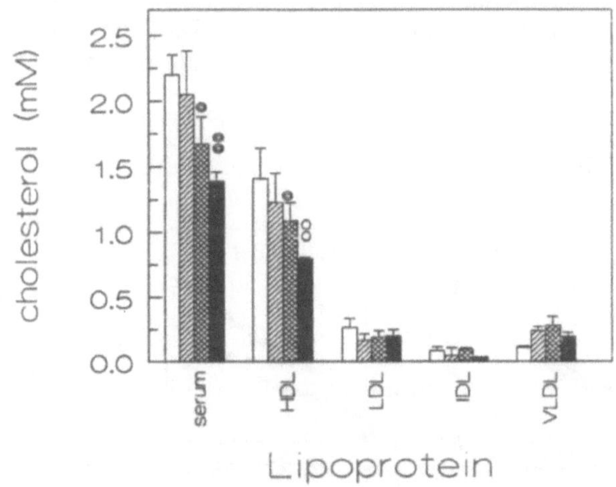

Figure 4. Effect of TG(20Å)C on the cholesterol concentration in the various lipoprotein fractions in the rat. Rats were injected with PBS (open bars) or PBS containing 56 μg (hatched bars), 180 μg (crossed bars) or 560 μg TG(20Å)C (filled bars), similarly as given in the legend for Figure 3. After 24 hours, the rats were sacrificed and blood was obtained. The sera were subjected to density-gradient ultracentrifugation and the cholesterol concentration of the lipoprotein fractions was determined, in duplicate. Values are means ± s.d. of a determination in triplicate. The statistical significance of data points relative to the control is indicated by O ($p < 0.05$) and OO ($p < 0.01$), respectively (Students T-test).

density lipoprotein (HDL) cholesterol to the total serum cholesterol level in rats, being approximately 65%, it was anticipated that the level of HDL must be affected by administration of TG(20Å)C. Indeed, the HDL level was dose-dependently reduced with maximally 35%, at a dose of 560 µg ($P = 0.0066$; one-way ANOVA) (Figure 4). The LDL level tended to decrease by 25-30% ($P = 0.036$). Surprisingly, administration of TG(20Å)C tends to enhance the VLDL level ($P = 0.07$). Serum samples of the TG(20Å)C-treated animals did not exhibit any sign of hemolysis.

EFFECT OF TG(20Å)C ON THE BILIARY SECRETION IN RATS

Subsequently, it was investigated whether administration of TG(20Å)C influenced the biliary secretion. TG(20Å)C (560 µg) was injected into unrestrained rats, equipped with catheters in bile duct, duodenum, and heart, the bile was collected for 48 hours, and both the bile flow and the biliary bile acid/cholesterol secretion were determined. The biliary secretion of cholesterol of the TG(20Å)C-treated rats was identical to that of the controls (0.41 µmol/h versus 0.37 µmol/h for the control) (Figure 5). By contrast, the secretion of bile-acids in the bile was significantly accelerated, from 72.9 ± 23 to 152 ± 22 µmol/2h, during the first two hours after injection of TG(20Å)C ($p < 0.05$, $n = 3$; students T-test) (Figure 5). After 2 hours the rate of bile acid secretion of the TG(20Å)C-treated rats stabilized at control values, i.e. 9.5 ± 2.8 and 7.7 ± 2.0 µmol/h, respectively. The biliary flow (Figure 5) was not affected by injection of TG(20Å)C (0.75 versus 0.70 ml/h, $n = 3$).

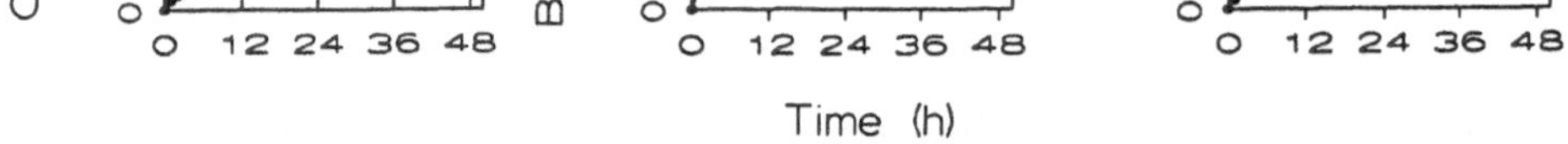

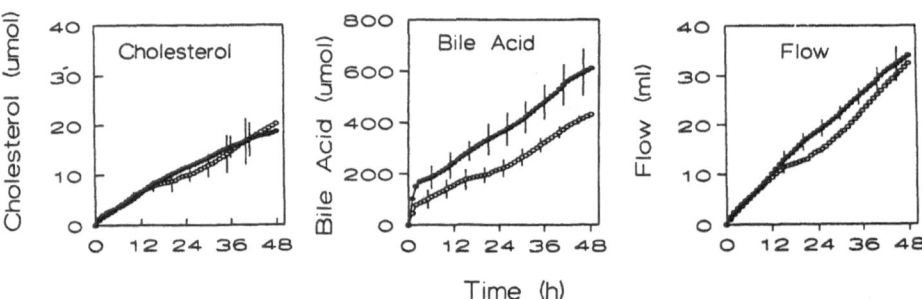

Figure 5. Effect of TG(20Å)C on the biliary secretion of cholesterol, bile acids, and the biliary flow in the rat. PBS (○), or PBS containing 560 µg of TG(20Å)C (●) was injected intracardially into unrestrained catherized rats. Bile was collected immediately after injection. The bile acid and cholesterol concentrations were determined and expressed cumulatively as µmol/h. Values represent means ± s.d. of three and four experiments, respectively. For clarity sake, error bars are only given every fifth hour.

Discussion

Previously, we have reported that lipoprotein catabolism can be enhanced by administration of lipophilized galactose-terminated galactosides, which induce uptake of lipoproteins by hepatic galactose recognizing receptors [2,3,11]. However, a prolonged infusion of relatively high doses was required in order to significantly lower the blood cholesterol content. It was rationalized that the low potency may be caused by the low affinity and specificity of the galactose-terminated cluster galactoside for the hepatic asialoglycoprotein receptor. On basis of previous studies on the prerequisites for high affinity recognition by this receptor [5,6,13], and using molecular modelling new triantennary cluster galactosides have been designed and synthesized [14]. In the present study, we demonstrate that the affinity of these new galactosides for the asialoglycoprotein receptor is markedly increased as a result of proper spacing of the terminal galactose units within a triantennary cluster galactoside. TG(20Å), in which the terminal galactose moieties were spaced at 20 Å from the branching point of the dendrite, possessed a 2000-fold higher affinity (K_i = 190 nM) than a previously utilized cluster galactoside, TG(4Å) (K_i = 390 μM) [2-4]. TG(9Å), TG(10Å), and TG(13Å) displayed intermediate affinities for the asialoglycoprotein receptor.

In contrast, elongation of the spacers within a cluster galactoside from 4Å to 20Å did not influence the affinity for the galactose/fucose receptor on the Kupffer cell, which also recognizes galactose-terminated galactosides. Hence, it can be concluded that not only the affinity but also the specificity for the asialoglycoprotein receptor as compared to the galactose/fucose receptor is dramatically enhanced upon elongation of the spacer. In view of the affinity of ASOR for the asialoglycoprotein receptor, an additional 25-fold gain in affinity and specificity may be achieved for synthetic cluster galactosides. However, the affinity of TG(20Å) for the asialoglycoprotein receptor, which is 2000-fold higher than that of TG(4Å), may indicate that the cholesterol-lowering activity of a cholesterylated galactoside correlates with an increase in the affinity of the galactoside for the asialoglycoprotein receptor; a further improvement in affinity may lead to direct clearance of the compound before any accumulation of the compound into lipoproteins can take place. Therefore we have derivatized the most selective galactoside, TG(20Å), with cholesterol. The resulting compound, TG(20Å)C, is an amphiphilic compound. Previous study has demonstrated that TG(20Å)C incorporates spontaneously into lipoproteins both upon incubation with serum [14] and upon incubation with isolated lipoproteins [15]. Subsequently we have evaluated the physiological activity of TG(20Å)C in the rat. Intravenous bolus injection of TG(20Å)C into rats resulted in a significant, dose-dependent decrease of the serum cholesterol concentration. A maximal decrease of the serum cholesterol concentration by 45% was observed after a single injection of only 560 μg of TG(20Å)C. Its hypocholesterolemic potency was at least 30-fold higher than that of a previously developed compound, TG(4Å)C [4]. In contrast to TG(4Å)C, application of TG(20Å)C did not require an infusion protocol, and did not lead to hemolysis at therapeutic doses [4]. Even intravenous injection of 6 mg TG(20Å)C/kg rat were tolerated well. The decrease in the serum cholesterol level persisted for at least 24 hours, possibly reflecting the low rate of *de novo* synthesis of HDL in the rat. Alternatively, it may arise from storage of

TG(20Å)C in and sustained release from a hydrophobic compartment in the rat (i.e. cell membranes).

At first glance, accelerating the catabolism of HDL seems to be undesired as it might result in a more atherogenic plasma lipoprotein profile. However, a compound that selectively enhances the hepatic uptake of HDL may concomitantly stimulate the HDL-mediated reverse cholesterol transport from the periphery to the liver, which of course is beneficial. In this respect it has to be verified whether chronic administration of TG(20Å)C will affect the reverse cholesterol transport of HDL, the rate of *de novo* synthesis of HDL and, thus, the lipoprotein profile.

In conclusion, the present data show that TG(20Å)C is a promising and potent serum-cholesterol lowering agent. In rats, TG(20Å)C principally induces hepatic uptake of HDL, thereby stimulating the reverse cholesterol transport. Further study of TG(20Å)C or analogues on the lipid metabolism in an animal model, that is more comparable with the human species in terms of lipoprotein profile and cholesterol metabolism, will reveal whether it is also capable of inducing significant hepatic uptake of LDL. Administration of lipoprotein uptake enhancers, like TG(20Å)C, involves a completely new approach for treating hypercholesterolemia. Its therapeutic activity does not depend on the presence of functional LDL receptors, as do conventional therapies based on HmG-CoA reductase or bile-acid sequestrants. Therefore, we surmise a therapy involving TG(20Å)C or analogues to be a promising alternative for those patients, that do not, or insufficiently, respond to the aforementioned therapies.

Acknowledgements

This work was supported by a grant from the Dutch Heart Foundation (42.005). Dr. E.A. Van de Velde is gratefully acknowledged for his help in statistical analysis.

References

1. Kempen HJM, Hoes C, van Boom JH, Spanjer HH, Langendoen A, van Berkel TJC. A water-soluble cholesteryl-containing trisgalactoside: Synthesis, properties, and use in directing lipid containing particles to the liver. J Med Chem 1984; 27:1306-1292
2. Van Berkel ThJC, Kruijt JK, Spanjer HH, Nagelkerke JF, Harkes L, Kempen HM. The effect of a water-soluble tris-galactoside-terminated cholesterol derivative on the fate of low density lipoproteins and liposomes. J Biol Chem 1985;260:2694-99.
3. Van Berkel ThJC, Kruijt JK, Kempen HJM. Specific targeting of high density lipoproteins to liver hepatocytes by incorporation of a tris-galactoside-terminated cholesterol derivative. J Biol Chem 1985;260:12203-207.
4. Kempen HJ, Kuiper F, van Berkel ThJC, Vonk RJ. Effect of infusion of "tris-galactosyl-cholesterol" on plasma cholesterol, clearance of lipoprotein cholesteryl esters, and biliary secretion in the rat. J Lipid Res 1987;28:659-66.
5. Lee YC, Townsend RR, Hardy MR, et al. Binding of synthetic oligosaccharides to the hepatic Gal/GalNAc lectin. J Biol Chem 1983;258:199-202.

6. Connolly DT, Townsend RR, Kawaguchi K, Bell WR, Lee YC. Binding and endocytosis of cluster glycosides by rabbit hepatocytes. J Biol Chem 1982;257:939-43.
7. Biessen EAL, Bakkeren HF, Beuting DM, Kuiper J, Van Berkel ThJC. Recognition of both fucose- and galactose-exposing particles by the hepatic fucose receptor depends on the particle size. Biochem J 1994;299:291-96.
8. Lehrmann MA, Haltiwanger RS, Hill RL. The binding of fucose-containing glycoproteins by hepatic lectins. J Biol Chem 1986;261:7426-32.
9. Kuiper J, Bakkeren HF, Biessen EAL, Van Berkel ThJC. Characterisation of the interaction of galactose-exposing particles with rat Kupffer cells. Biochem J 1994; 299:285-90.
10. Biessen EAL, Broxterman H, Van Boom JH, Van Berkel ThJC. The cholesterol derivative of a new triantennary cluster galactoside with high affinity for the hepatic asialoglycoprotein receptor is a potent hypocholesterolemic agent. J Med Chem 1995;38:1846-52.
11. Bijsterbosch MK, Bakkeren HF, Kempen HJM, van Berkel ThJC. A monogalactosylated cholesterol derivative that specifically induces uptake of LDL by the liver. Arteriosclerosis and Thrombosis 1992;12:1153-60.
12. Roelen HCPF, Bijsterbosch MK, Bakkeren HF, et al. Water-soluble cholesteryl-containing phosphorothioate monogalactosides: Synthesis, properties, and use in lowering blood cholesterol by directing plasma proteins to the liver. J Med Chem 1991;34:1036-42.
13. Baenziger JU, Maynard Y. The asialoglycoprotein receptor. J Biol Chem 1980;255: 4607-13.
14. Biessen EAL, Vietsch H, Van Berkel ThJC. The cholesterol derivative of a new triantennary cluster galactoside lowers serum cholesterol levels and enhances the biliary secretion of bile acids in the rat. Circulation 1995;91:1848-54.
15. Biessen EAL, Vietsch H, Van Berkel ThJC. The cholesterol derivative of a new triantennary cluster galactoside directs low- and high-density lipoproteins to the parenchymal liver cell. Biochem J 1994;302:283-89.

EFFECT OF ORAL BILE ACIDS ON SERUM LIPIDS

Goro Kajiyama, Masayumi Saeki, and Kozo Hayashi
First Department of Internal Medicine, School of Medicine, Hiroshima University, 1-2-3 Kasumi, Minami-ku, Hiroshima 734, Japan

Introduction

It is well known that hyperlipidemic patients have an abnormal bile acid pool size according to their phenotype [1] and that there is a close relationship between serum lipids and bile acids.

We investigated the effect of change in bile acid composition after oral administration of cholic acid (CA) chenodeoxycholic acid (CDCA) or ursodeoxycholic acid (UDCA) on lipid metabolism in volunteers [2] and hamsters [3].

SUBJECTS AND METHODS

Six male volunteers (22-27 years of age) who had normal serum lipid level, normal liver function tests, and no clinical symptoms of the gastrointestinal tract were asked to maintain their ordinary life style throughout the trials.

Drugs were prohibited except for the bile acids used in the experiment. Six volunteers were orally given either 400 mg/day CA, 400 mg/day UDCA, or 600 mg/day UDCA for one month. Three volunteers were orally given UDCA, CDCA, and CA and the remaining three were administered UDCA, CA, and CDCA successively. Cholesterol was collected and determined by intestinal perfusion technique using triple lumen tube [4]. Percent cholesterol absorption was calculated using the following formula:

$$\%\ \text{cholesterol absorption} = \frac{\dfrac{\text{cholesterol(B)}}{\beta\text{-sitosterol(B)}} - \dfrac{\text{cholesterol(A)}}{\beta\text{-sitosterol(A)}}}{\dfrac{\text{cholesterol(B)}}{\beta\text{-sitosterol(B)}}} \times 100$$

(A) juice from absorption syringe; (B) juice from secretion syringe; from [5].

A. M. Gotto, Jr. et al. (eds.), Drugs Affecting Lipid Metabolism, 541–546.

The composition of bile lipids and bile acid was determined by the method reported by Tazuma et al. [6] using GEL.

Sixty golden hamsters were divided into four groups. They were fed either standard chow or standard chow plus 0.1% bile acid for three weeks as shown in Table 1.

Table 1. Animal groups.

Control group:	Standard chow (0.027% cholesterol)
CA group:	Standard chow + 0.1% CA
CDCA group:	Standard chow + 0.1% CDCA
UDCA group:	Standard chow + 0.1% UDCA

Serum lipids were assayed using enzymatic methods. LDL receptor activity was assayed according to the method reported by Goldstein, Basu and Brown [7] and cholesterol 7α-hydroxylase activity was assayed by the method reported by Ogishima and Okuda [8].

Results

In the volunteers, administration of CA, CDCA, and UDCA for one month induced increase of their biliary mole percent as shown in Figure 1.

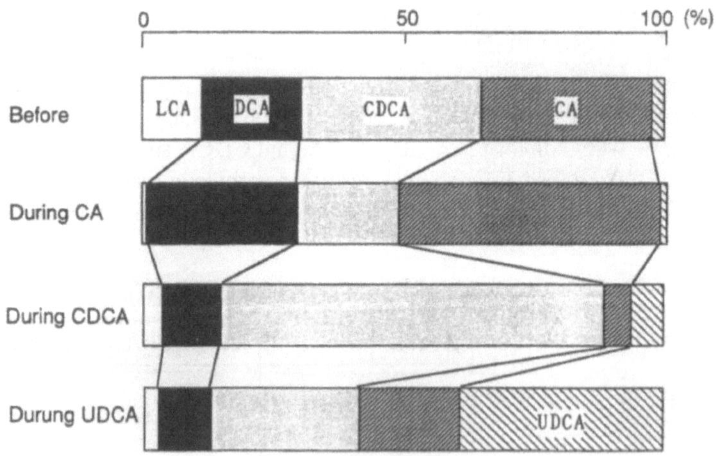

Figure 1. Change in mole percent of biliary bile acids during oral administration of CA, CDCA or UDCA in six volunteers.

CA increased percent cholesterol absorption in five of the six volunteers. CDCA had no affect, but UDCA significantly decreased percent cholesterol absorption in all cases as shown in Figure 2.

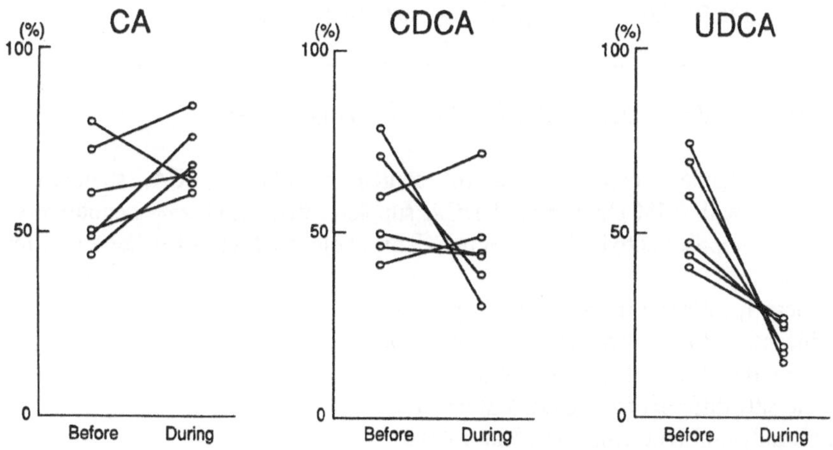

Figure 2. Change in percent cholesterol absorption during oral administration of CA, CDCA, or UDCA in six volunteers.

In hamsters, administration of CA and CDCA increased serum total and LDL cholesterol, but UDCA decreased serum total and LDL cholesterol, as shown Table 2.

Table 2. Effect of bile acids on serum lipid levels

Group[a]	Total Cholesterol	LDL Cholesterol	HDL Cholesterol	TG	Phospholipids
Control	178.3±39.8	55.6±11.8	93.4±10.6	105.2±40.7	240.5±31.6
CA	239.0±53.2[c,d]	120.0±24.5[b,d]	101.0±10.5[e,f]	137.0±97.0	276.0±76.5[c]
CDCA	193.7±40.0[e]	83.5±38.6[d]	82.0±13.4	176.4±90.1[e]	254.1±49.0
UDCA	135.8±35.0	29.7±16.0[c]	88.9±6.2	103.1±91.6	204.4±43.0

mean ± standard deviation (mg/dl) (n = 15); TG = Triglycerides.

a) Control, standard chow (cholesterol content = 0.027%); CA, standard chow supplemented with 0.1% cholic acid; CDCA, supplemented with 0.1% chenodeoxycholic acid; UDCA, supplemented with 0.1% ursodeoxycholic acid; each hamsters was fed for three weeks.
b) Significantly different from Control at $p < 0.01$.
c) Significantly different from Control at $p < 0.05$.
d) Significantly different from UDCA at $p < 0.01$.
e) Significantly different from UDCA at $p < 0.05$.
f) Significantly different from CDCA at $p < 0.01$.

Administration of CA and CDCA suppressed activities of hepatic LDL receptors and cholesterol 7α-hydroxylase but not UDCA (Figures 3, 4, and Table 3).

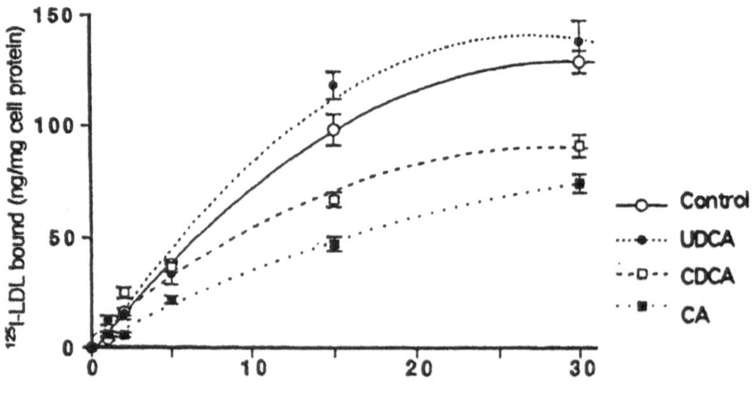

Figure 3. LDL receptor activity in cultured hepatocytes.

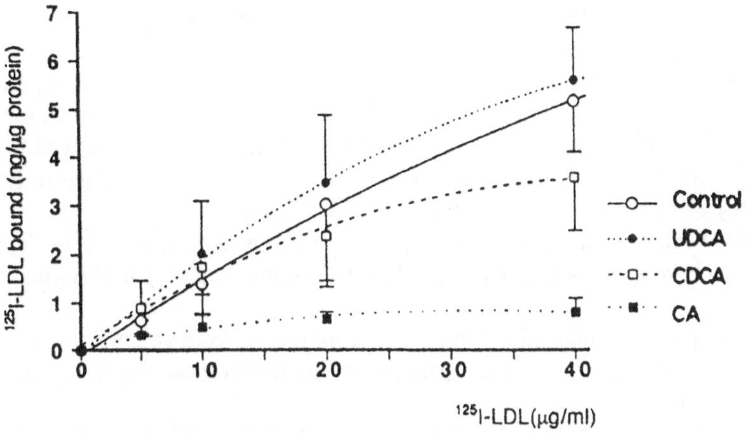

Figure 4. LDL receptor activity in liver microsomes.

Table 3. Effect of bile acids on cholesterol 7α-hydroxylase activity of the liver microsomal fraction.

Group[a]	Cholesterol 7α-Hydroxylase Activity
Control	2.24 ± 1.00
CA	0.68 ± 0.43[b,c]
CDCA	0.72 ± 0.53[b,c]
UDCA	1.98 ± 1.03

mean ± standard deviation (p mol/min/mg protein) (n = 15)

a) Control, standard chow (cholesterol content = 0.027%); CA, standard chow supplemented with 0.1% cholic acid; CDCA, supplemented with 0.1% chenodeoxycholic acid; UDCA, supplemented with 0.1% ursodeoxycholic acid; each hamster was fed for three weeks.
b) Significantly different from Control at $p < 0.01$.
c) Significantly different from UDCA at $p < 0.01$.

Discussion

It is known that oral administration of bile acids affects serum and hepatic lipid metabolism. CA increases the dietary cholesterol absorption in rats and mice. Long term administration of CDCA also increases the serum LDL level and apolipoprotein B [9] during gallstone dissolution therapy.

In our current experiment, oral administration of CA increased biliary percent CA and was considered to have induced an expanded CA pool size, resulting in an increase of intestinal cholesterol absorption in most volunteers. In hamsters, CA as well as CDCA suppressed activities of hepatic LDL receptors and cholesterol 7α-hydroxylase and consequently elevated serum total and LDL cholesterol level.

It has been previously reported that among various hyperlipoproteinemia, type IV and V patients have a very large pool size of CA when compared to that of normal subjects [1].

This report in combination with our present results from volunteers and hamsters indicates that the increased pool of CA participates in the elevation of serum cholesterol in type IV and V patients.

Unlike CA and CDCA, UDCA inhibited cholesterol absorption and did not suppress LDL receptors and cholesterol 7α-hydroxylase in our experiment. Therefore, this bile acid may be useful for the treatment of hyperlipidemia caused by abnormal bile acid metabolism.

References

1. Einarsson K and Hellström K. The formation of bile acids in patients with three types of hyperlipoproteinemia. Europe J Clin Invest 1972;2:225-30.
2. Horiuchi I. Effect of bile acids on intestinal cholesterol absorption in normal volunteers. J Japan Biliary Association 1988;2:239-47.
3. Saeki M. The effects of ursodeoxycholic acid, chenodeoxycholic acid and cholic acid on hepatic cholesterol metabolism and serum lipid levels in hamsters. Med J Hiroshima Univ 1995;43:93-102.
4. Bergmann K, Keiss O, Streicher V, et al. Effect of various bile acids on cholesterol absorption in man. In: Paumgartner, editor. Bile acids and cholesterol in health and disease. Lancaster: MTP Press, 1983:203-212.
5. Grundy SM and Mok HYI. Determination of cholesterol absorption in man by intestinal perfusion. J Lipid Res 1977;18:263-71.
6. Tazuma S, Hatsushika S, Yamashita G, et al. Simultaneous microanalysis of biliary cholesterol, bile acids and fatty acids in lecithin using capillary column gas chromatography: An advantage to assess bile lithogenesity. J Chromatograph B 1994;653:1-7.
7. Goldstein JL, Basu SK, Brown MS. Receptor mediated endocytosis of low density lipoprotein in cultured cell. Methods in Enzymology 1983;98:241-60.
8. Ogishima T and Okuda K. An improved method for assay of cholesterol 7α- hydroxylase activity. Anal Biochem 1986;158:228-32.
9. Albers JJ, Grundy SM, Cleary PA. National cooperative gallstone study-The effect of chenodeoxycholic acid on lipoproteins and apoproteins. Gastroenterology 1982;82:638-46.

EFFECTS OF A NOVEL ACAT INHIBITOR, F-1394, ON THE PROGRESSION AND REGRESSION OF ATHEROSCLEROTIC LESIONS IN THE AORTA OF CHOLESTEROL-FED RABBITS

Shizuya Yamashita, A.H.M. Waliul Islam, Masato Ishigami, Tadashi Nakamura, Jun Kusunoki*, Katsumi Aragane*, Tetsuya Kitamine*, Sakiko Higashinakagawa*, Tetsuaki Yamaura*, Haruo Ohnishi*, and Yuji Matsuzawa

*Second Department of Internal Medicine, Osaka University Medical School, 2-2 Yamada-oka, Suita, Osaka 565 and *Fujirebio Inc., Hachioji, Tokyo 192, Japan*

Introduction

The accumulation of both cholesterol and its ester in the arterial wall is one of the important features of atherosclerosis. Acyl-CoA:cholesterol acyltransferase (ACAT) is an enzyme that catalyzes the intracellular esterification of free cholesterol to cholesteryl ester (CE) and is supposed to be localized to the rough endoplasmic reticulum. ACAT has been implicated to be a key enzyme involved in the absorption of cholesterol by small intestines, the secretion of very low density lipoprotein (VLDL) from the liver, and the formation of lipid-laden foam cells in the atherosclerotic lesions [1]. Recently, Chang et al. have cloned a cDNA for ACAT and its regulation *in vitro* by cholesterol loading has been reported [2,3]. Since ACAT is involved in various aspects of cholesterol metabolism in the small intestines, liver, and arterial walls, the inhibition of ACAT may have potent hypolipidemic and antiatherosclerotic effects.

The increased absorption of cholesterol is considered to be one of the causes of hypercholesterolemia. Intestinal ACAT plays a crucial role in the absorption of cholesterol for the formation of chylomicrons. Therefore, various attempts have been made to inhibit intestinal ACAT activity for reducing cholesterol absorption. Streptozotocin (STZ)-induced rat is a model of insulin-dependent diabetes mellitus. We previously reported that plasma cholesterol was approximately 1.3-fold increased in STZ-induced diabetic rats compared with control rats, while a far more remarkable increase (5.5-fold) in plasma cholesterol was observed in STZ-rats when fed a high-cholesterol diet [4]. Intestinal ACAT activity was approximately 3 times higher in diabetic rats compared with control rats. Furthermore, insulin supplementation reduced ACAT activity to the levels of control rats. These data suggested that the enhancement of ACAT activity in the small intestines might be one of the major factors responsible for hypercholesterolemia in diabetes mellitus.

Regarding the regulatory effect of insulin *in vitro*, we reported that insulin caused

A. M. Gotto, Jr. et al. (eds.), Drugs Affecting Lipid Metabolism, 547–555.

the suppression of ACAT activity in Caco2 cells, a model of intestinal epithelium, and that ACAT activity was increased after the removal of insulin from culture medium [5]. These findings indicate that insulin acts on the enterocytes to suppress intestinal CE synthesis, thereby inhibiting the absorption of cholesterol in the small intestines.

ACAT inhibitors are a novel class of therapeutic agents currently under investigation for their hypolipidemic and antiatherosclerotic activity. Various kinds of ACAT inhibitors have been developed so far ([6] for review). Figure 1 shows the chemical structure of our novel ACAT inhibitor, (1s,2s)-2-[3-(2,2-dimethylpropyl)-3-nonylureido]aminocyclohexane-1-yl 3-[*N*-(2,2,5,5-tetramethyl-1,3-dioxane-4-carbonyl)amino]propionate (F-1394) [7,8]. It is a pantotheic derivative, and possesses a structure of acyl-CoA which is a substrate of ACAT. This drug has been obtained by screening about 400 compounds which contain the parts of acyl-CoA and inhibits ACAT activity. As reported previously [7], F-1394 inhibited ACAT activities in a dose-dependent manner in rat liver microsomes, homogenates of rabbit small intestinal mucosa and lysates of J774 macrophages with IC_{50} values of 6.4 nM, 10.7 nM, and 32nM, respectively. The kinetic studies demonstrated that F-1394 exerted a competitive-type inhibition, and the Ki values in liver and small intestinal ACAT were 4.0 nM and 9.9 nM, respectively. Therefore, the inhibitory effect of F-1394 on the ACAT activity was very potent, similar to those of other ACAT inhibitors. F-1394 had no significant effect on the activities of HMG-CoA reductase, acyl-CoA synthetase, and cholesterol esterase. F-1394 was shown to inhibit the dietary cholesterol absorption in rats fed a high-cholesterol diet [8].

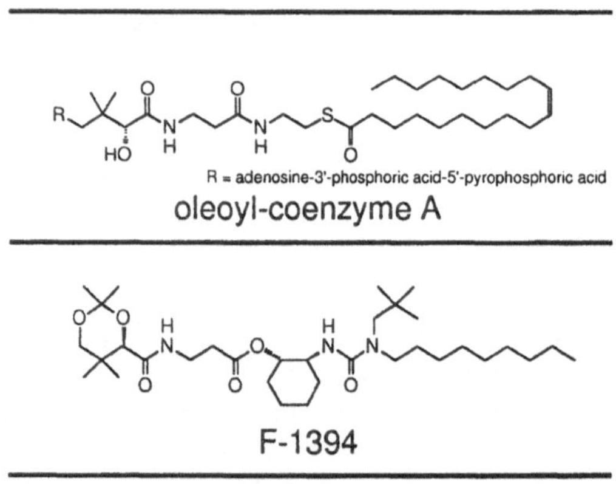

Figure 1. Chemical structure of F-1394 and oleoyl-CoA.

In the current study, we have analyzed the *in vivo* effects of F-1394 on the serum cholesterol levels in STZ-rats. Furthermore, we tested the effects of F-1394 on the accumulation of CE in macrophages as well as those on the progression and regression of atherosclerosis in cholesterol-fed rabbits.

Methods and Results

EFFECTS OF F-1394 ON LIPOPROTEIN CHOLESTEROL LEVELS IN STREPTOZOTOCIN-INDUCED DIABETIC RATS AND IN RABBITS FED A HIGH-CHOLESTEROL DIET

STZ-induced diabetic rat is an animal model of insulin-dependent diabetes mellitus. In the current study, the effect of F-1394 on the serum cholesterol levels was studied in STZ-induced diabetic rats fed a high-cholesterol diet. After injection of STZ (60 mg/kg), rats were fed a 1% cholesterol diet. At the same time, F-1394 was orally administered for 3 weeks at a dose of 3, 10, 30, and 100 mg/kg. Serum lipoproteins were ultracentrifugally separated according to the method of Havel et al. [9]. Serum total cholesterol level was increased to ~ 360 mg/dl after cholesterol feeding in STZ-rats, while F-1394 decreased serum total cholesterol levels in a dose-dependent manner; at a dose of 30 mg/kg almost no increase in serum total cholesterol was observed. The decrease in VLDL and low density lipoprotein (LDL)-cholesterol was most prominent, while high density lipoprotein (HDL)-cholesterol level was slightly increased, but the difference was not statistically significant (data not shown).

Furthermore, the hypocholesterolemic effect of F-1394 was also evaluated in rabbits fed a high-cholesterol diet. Rabbits were given a 1% cholesterol diet and F-1394 (1-100 mg/kg/day) for 5 days. F-1394 markedly reduced serum total cholesterol, VLDL-cholesterol, and LDL-cholesterol concentrations in a dose-dependent manner, while serum HDL-cholesterol was increased (data not shown). These data suggested that the inhibition of intestinal ACAT activity by F-1394 caused a decrease in serum cholesterol in cholesterol-fed animals through decreasing dietary cholesterol absorption in the intestines.

EFFECTS OF F-1394 ON THE CHOLESTEROL METABOLISM IN MACROPHAGES

Although it may be important to evaluate the effect of ACAT inhibitors on cholesterol absorption, it is also crucial to make an approach from a viewpoint of inhibiting ACAT activity in macrophages of atherosclerotic lesions. Modified LDLs such as oxidized LDLs are taken up by macrophages through the scavenger receptor or recently identified CD36 [10]. The CE is hydrolyzed and then re-esterified by ACAT, leading to the intracellular accumulation of CE and the formation of foam cells. Therefore, the inhibition of ACAT in macrophages may result in a decreased content of CE and an increased mass of free cholesterol. Free cholesterol may then be taken up by HDL, which could lead to the inhibition of foam cell formation. We tested this possibility *in vitro* by the following experiments. Mouse peritoneal macrophages were obtained by peritoneal lavage and then cultured in Dulbecco's modified Eagle's medium (DMEM) supplemented with 3% bovine serum albumin. After washing the cells with DMEM, acetyl LDL was added to the medium at a final concentration of 50 µg protein/ml and at the same time various concentrations of F-1394 was added. After incubating cells for 24 hours, macrophages were washed and the lipids were extracted as reported previously [11]. CE content was measured by an enzyme-fluorescence assay. In some experiments, HDL was added to the medium. Figure 2 shows the dose-dependent effect of F-1394 on cholesterol accumulation in macrophages. The addition of acetyl LDL caused a 10-fold increase in CE content. However, the addition of F-1394 inhibited the accumulation of CE in a dose-dependent manner. Furthermore, we examined the effect of HDL alone or in combination with F-1394 on the CE accumulation by acetyl LDL. F-1394 at a concentration of 10^{-6} M and HDL at a protein concentration of 100 μg/ml prevented the accumulation of CE to a similar extent. The combined addition of F-1394 and HDL further prevented CE accumulation in macrophages.

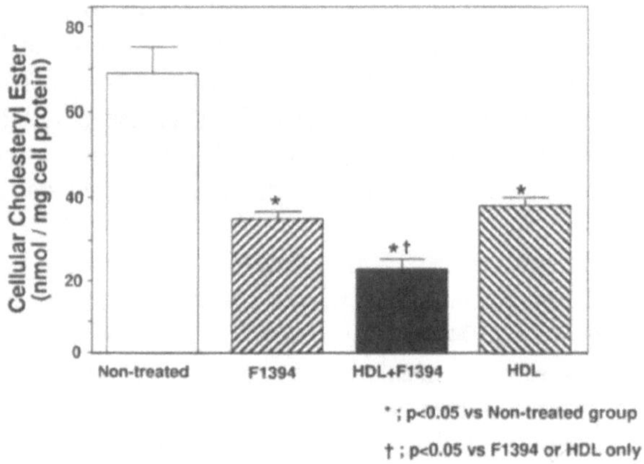

Figure 2. Preventive effect of F-1394 and HDL on cholesterol accumulation by acetylated LDL in mouse peritoneal macrophages.

Cholesterol efflux was also measured by adding F-1394 and HDL to the medium. To measure cholesterol efflux, mouse peritoneal macrophages were cultured for 24 hours in a medium containing acetyl LDL. Macrophages were then washed, and HDL alone or in combination with F-1394 was added followed by an additional incubation for 24 hours. Macrophages were then washed and their CE content was measured. Both F-1394 and HDL enhanced the cholesterol efflux from macrophages, and the combined addition of F-1394 and HDL induced more cholesterol efflux from macrophages than HDL alone. These data strongly suggested a synergistic role of ACAT inhibitor and HDL in the acceleration of reverse cholesterol transport.

Effects of F-1394 on the Progression and Regression of Atherosclerosis in Cholesterol-Fed Rabbits

These *in vitro* experiments suggested a possibility that F-1394 can be used as an antiatherosclerotic drug by inhibiting CE accumulation in macrophages and by accelerating cholesterol efflux. We tested *in vivo* the antiatherosclerotic effect of F-1394 in cholesterol-fed New Zealand White rabbits. Rabbits were fed 0.5% cholesterol diet for 3 months and then divided into 3 groups. Thereafter, rabbits were given a 0.5% cholesterol diet for additional 3 months in the control group and a normal chow in the normal-chow group, respectively. The third group was fed a high-cholesterol diet containing F-1394 at a concentration of 30 mg/kg.

First, the changes of serum cholesterol levels were evaluated after F-1394 treatment. The control group maintained serum cholesterol levels around 2,000 mg/dl. In contrast, the administration of F-1394 reduced serum cholesterol levels more markedly to the levels similar to those of the normal-chow group. Secondly, the changes in the area of atherosclerotic lesions in the aorta of rabbits were evaluated. F-1394 inhibited by ~ 20% the progression of atherosclerotic lesion area, although the difference was not statistically significant. However, thirdly, when total cholesterol content in the thoracic aorta was determined, it was significantly decreased by ~ 50% in the F-1394-treated rabbits (Figure 3). Similar inhibitory effects of F-1394 were obtained in both ascending and abdominal aorta. These results demonstrated that F-1394 may be effective for inhibiting the progression of atherosclerotic lesions in the aorta induced by cholesterol feeding. One possible mechanism for this may be the inhibition of cholesterol absorption, but an additional direct effect of ACAT inhibition in the arterial wall is also feasible.

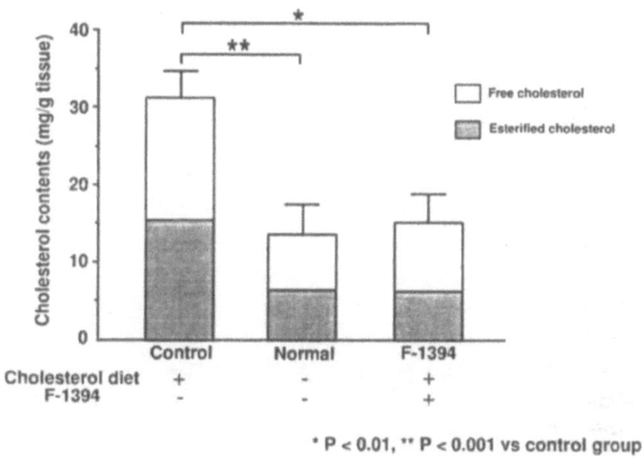

Figure 3. Cholesteryl ester content of the aorta after F-1394 treatment in cholesterol-fed rabbits.

We next examined whether F-1394 may regress the atherosclerotic lesions in the aorta that have already been developed. As shown in the experimental protocol of Figure 4A, New Zealand White rabbits were fed 0.5% cholesterol diet for 3 months to develop atherosclerosis. The diet was then changed to a normal commercial chow at this point. At the same time, F-1394 was orally administered to the rabbits at a dose of 100 mg/kg for

4A
4B
4C

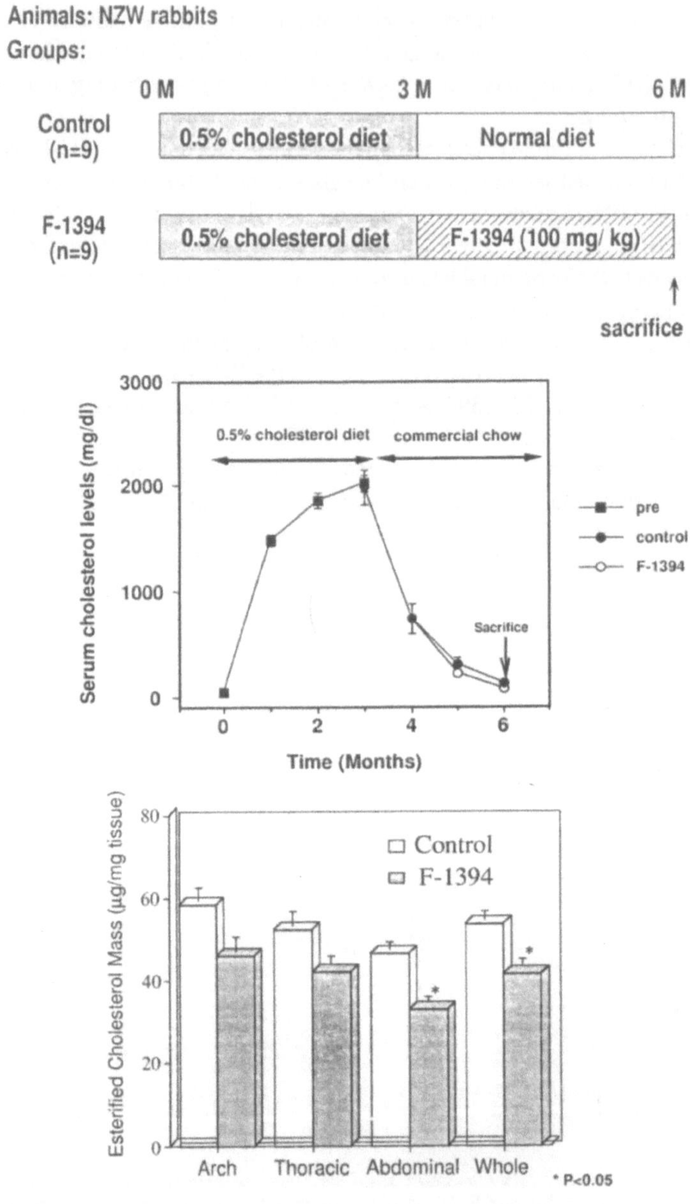

Figure 4. Study protocol for evaluation of the regression of atherosclerosis by F-1394 in cholesterol-fed rabbits (A), changes in serum total cholesterol level after F-1394 treatment (B), and those in CE content of the aorta (C).

another 3 months. Serum cholesterol levels of the control group during the regressive phase were not significantly different from those of the F-1394-treated group (Figure 4B). As shown in Figure 4C, F-1394 significantly reduced the mass of CE in the aorta, especially in the abdominal aorta. The difference was also statistically significant in the whole aorta. These results indicated that F-1394 can decrease CE mass in the aorta, independent of serum cholesterol levels.

The histological changes of aorta were evaluated in F-1394-treated rabbits in comparison with vehicle-treated control rabbits. Tissue specimens were stained with hematoxylin-eosin and oil red O. By hematoxylin-eosin staining, an intimal thickening occurred in the F-1394-treated rabbits to an extent similar to that in the control rabbits. In contrast, F-1394 markedly reduced the degree of staining by oil red O (data not shown), suggesting that F-1394 is also effective for the regression of atherosclerotic lesions that have already been established.

Discussion

Hypercholesterolemia is one of the independent risk factors for atherosclerosis in the coronary arteries and aorta. HMG-CoA reductase inhibitors, probucol, and cholestyramine have been used to reduce serum cholesterol for hypercholesterolemic patients. Although these drugs were proved to be effective for decreasing the incidence of myocardial infarction and death from cardiovascular causes in hypercholesterolemic patients, the effects have not been enough for completely preventing new cardiac events or regressing the already established atherosclerosis. Two other possible therapeutic strategies of current interest may be the prevention of the absorption of dietary cholesterol and a direct inhibition of cholesterol accumulation in the arterial wall.

In recent years, various kinds of ACAT inhibitors have been developed. Of these, only melinamide, which we previously demonstrated its efficacy in treating hypercholesterolemia in cholesterol-fed diabetic rats [12], is available for clinical use. Some of them have been eliminated from clinical use because of their side effects such as diarrhea, liver dysfunction, and atrophy of adrenal glands. In the current study, we administered F-1394 into rats and rabbits without any side effects and demonstrated that F-1394 can reduce serum total cholesterol level in cholesterol-fed STZ-rats in which ACAT activity is accelerated. Furthermore, we have shown that F-1394 strongly inhibited CE accumulation in mouse peritoneal macrophages loaded with acetylated LDL. In the presence of HDL in the medium, a more marked inhibition of CE accumulation was observed, suggesting that F-1394 could be effective *in vivo* for attenuating the progression of atherosclerosis. The *in vivo* study using cholesterol-fed rabbits clarified that F-1394 could suppress the development of atherosclerosis, although we could not rule out the possibility that a marked reduction in serum cholesterol level due to inhibition of cholesterol absorption might have played a major part. Therefore, we performed additional experiments in rabbits with established atherosclerotic plaques by cholesterol feeding. F-1394 could induce the regression of established atherosclerosis, which was histologically confirmed by oil red O staining. The free cholesterol generated by the inhibition of ACAT will be removed by HDL or other acceptors and targeted back to the liver. This mechanism provides a direct antiatherosclerotic potential for ACAT inhibitors, and thus targets the site of atherosclerosis. To obtain these direct antiatherosclerotic functions, ACAT inhibitors must be delivered into the arterial wall. We determined the concentrations of the unchanged form of F-1394 in plasma by liquid chromatography/mass spectrometry/mass spectrometry (LC/MS/MS) method and found that the drug was present in plasma with concentrations enough for inhibiting ACAT activity in macrophages. In our drug distribution study in rabbits after administering radiolabeled F-1394, the radioactivity in the aorta was 2.5 times that in the plasma 48 hours after the administration, suggesting that we could expect the inhibition of ACAT activity in the arterial wall.

In conclusion, the current study has demonstrated a potent antiatherosclerotic effect of F-1394, a novel ACAT inhibitor. The results strongly suggest that F-1394 is very effective for both prevention and regression of atherosclerotic lesions in the aorta and may have applications as a potent antiatherosclerotic drug for primary and secondary preventions of coronary heart disease. Further studies are in progress to establish the safety and usefulness of this drug for the treatment of both hypercholesterolemia and atherosclerosis.

Acknowledgments

This study was supported in part by a Grant-in-Aid from the Japanese Ministry of Education (No. 3557117 and 04404085).

References

1. Suckling KE, Stange EF. Role of acyl-CoA:cholesterol acyltransferase in cellular cholesterol metabolism. J Lipid Res 1985;26:647-71.
2. Chang CC, Huh HY, Cadigan KM, Chang TY. Molecular cloning and functional expression of human acyl-coenzyme A:cholesterol acyltransferase cDNA in mutant Chinese hamster ovary cells. J Biol Chem 1993;268:20747-55.
3. Cheng D, Chang CC, Qu X, Chang TY. Activation of acyl-coenzyme A:cholesterol acyltransferase by cholesterol or by oxysterol in a cell-free system. J Biol Chem 1995;270: 685-95.
4. Jiao S, Matsuzawa Y, Matsubara K, et al. Increased activity of intestinal acyl-CoA:cholesterol acyltransferase in rats with streptozotocin-induced diabetes and restoration by insulin supplementation. Diabetes 1988;37:342-46.
5. Jiao S, Moberly JB, Cole TG, Schonfeld G. Decreased activity of acyl-CoA: cholesterol acyltransferase by insulin in human intestinal cell line Caco-2. Diabetes 1989;38:604-609.
6. Sliskovic DR, White AD. Therapeutic potential of ACAT inhibitors and lipid lowering and anti-atherosclerotic agents. Trends Pharmacol Sci 1991;12:194-99.
7. Kusunoki J, Aragane K, Yamaura T, Ohnishi H. Studies on acyl-CoA:cholesterol acyltransferase (ACAT) inhibitory effects and enzyme selectivity of F-1394, a pantotheic acid derivative. Jpn J Pharmacol 1995;67:195-203.
8. Kusunoki J, Aragane K, Kitamine T, et al. Hypocholesterolemic action and prevention of cholesterol absorption via the gut by F-1394, a potent acyl-CoA:cholesterol acyltransferase (ACAT) inhibitor, in cholesterol diet-fed rats. Jpn J Pharmacol 1995;69:53-60.

9. Havel RJ, Eder HA, Bragdon JH. The distribution and chemical composition of ultracentrifugally separated lipoproteins in human serum. J Clin Invest 1955;34: 1345-53.
10. Endemann G, Stanton LW, Madden KS, Bryant CM, White RT, Protter AA. CD36 is a receptor for oxidized low density lipoprotein. J Biol Chem 1993;268:11811-16.
11. Ishigami M, Yamashita S, Sakai N, et al. Large and cholesteryl ester-rich high-density lipoproteins in cholesteryl ester transfer protein (CETP) deficiency can not protect macrophages from cholesterol accumulation induced by acetylated low-density lipoproteins. J Biochem 1994;116:257-62.
12. Matsubara K, Matsuzawa Y, Jiao S, et al. Cholesterol-lowering effect of N-(α-methylbenzyl)linoleamide (melinamide) in cholesterol-fed diabetic rats. Atherosclerosis 1988; 72:199-204.

GEMFIBROZIL INCREASES PLASMA LEVELS OF CHOLESTERYLESTER TRANSFER PROTEIN (CETP), BUT LOWERS CHOLESTERYLESTER TRANSFER IN HYPERTRIGLYCERIDEMIC SUBJECTS

Arie van Tol[1], Juhani Kahri[2], Bernhard Eisele[3], Timo Sane[2], and Marja-Riitta Taskinen[2]

[1]Department of Biochemistry, Cardiovascular Research Institute (COEUR), Faculty of Medicine and Health Sciences, P.O. Box 1738, Erasmus University, 3000 DR Rotterdam, The Netherlands,[2]3rd Department of Medicine, Mehlatti Hospital, Helsinki University, Helsinki, Finland, and [3]Department of Biomedical Research, Dr. Karl Thomae GmbH, Birkendorfer Strasse 65, D-88397 Biberach a/d Riss, Germany

Introduction

Hypertriglyceridemia (HTG) may be a risk factor for atherosclerosis [1], especially when caused by a prolonged plasma residence time of very low density lipoproteins (VLDL). During a prolonged stay in the circulation VLDL may become enriched in cholesterylesters (CE) via lipid transfer reactions, catalyzed by cholesterylester transfer protein (CETP). Also when increased VLDL synthesis coincides with suboptimal remnant removal (type III hyperlipoproteinemia), the triglyceride (TG)-rich lipoproteins become enriched in CE, due to increased plasma CETP activity levels as well as increased concentrations of the TG-rich acceptor lipoproteins [2]. Therefore treatment of HTG by improving the removal mechanisms of TG-rich lipoproteins will be beneficial. Lipoprotein lipase (LPL) is a key enzyme in the metabolism of TG-rich lipoproteins and it is well known that treatment of HTG patients with gemfibrozil may cause elevation of LPL activity, as measured in post-heparin plasma [3,4]. HTG often coincides with low levels of high density lipoprotein (HDL). This association may be partly explained by increased CETP-catalyzed transfer of CE out of HDL into TG-rich particles. Lowering of plasma TG concentration by gemfibrozil coincides with a raise in HDL-cholesterol and this combined effect may cause a reduction in CHD events [5]. Paradoxically, elevation of CETP activity levels (measured with excess exogenous substrate) was observed by gemfibrozil treatment on several occasions [4,6]. On the other hand CE transfer rates, measured with endogenous substrates, are increased in patients with hyperlipidemia [7-9] and can be down-regulated by gemfibrozil treatment [8]. A lowering of CE transfer was also reported in patients with hypertriglyceridemia after treatment with bezafibrate, although this fibrate had no effect on optimal CETP activity [9].

A. M. Gotto, Jr. et al. (eds.), Drugs Affecting Lipid Metabolism, 557–565.

We decided to analyze the effect of gemfibrozil treatment in HTG patients on plasma concentrations of CETP and relate the CETP concentrations with CETP activity, measured by an excess exogenous substrate method as well as with rates of CE transfer using endogenous plasma lipoproteins as substrates.

Methods

STUDY DESIGN

Twelve men with serum TG between 1.5 and 7.3 mM were included in the study. None of the patients was taking any lipid lowering drug at the start and other medication was unchanged during the study. After a six-week, single-blind placebo period, 6 patients received gemfibrozil (600 mg) twice daily and 6 patients received placebo for three months in a double-blind fashion. The groups were matched for age (range 39-57 years). Table 1 gives patient characteristics in the placebo and gemfibrozil groups at the start of the study. The patients were instructed to consume isocaloric diets (30-35% of calories as fat, 45-50% as carbohydrates, and 15-25% as protein) during the single-blind pretreatment period as well as the double-blind experimental period. The patients were informed of the purpose of the study and a written consent was obtained. The study protocol was approved by the Ethics Committee of the Mellahti Hospital in Helsinki.

SERUM LIPIDS AND LIPOPROTEIN ANALYSIS

Pre- and post-treatment samples of venous blood were collected after a 12-hour fast; serum as well as EDTA-plasma was obtained by low speed centrifugation. Serum lipoproteins (VLDL, intermediate density lipoprotein [IDL], low density lipoprotein [LDL], and HDL) were separated by sequential ultracentrifugation using a Beckman L8-70 ultracentrifuge (Beckman Incorporated, Palo Alto, California) in a Kontron TFT 45.8 rotor as previously described in detail [10].

Table 1. Patient characteristics at randomization.

	Gemfibrozil	Placebo
Age (years)	50.5 ± 4.4	49.7 ± 7.9
BMI (kgm^{-2})	28.9 ± 1.8	27.8 ± 1.5

BMI, body mass index.

DETERMINATION OF CETP MASS

Plasma CETP mass was determined by a solid phase competitive immunoassay in the presence of triton and the specific monoclonal antibody TP-2 [11]. In brief, plastic wells were coated with recombinant CETP and saturated with bovine serum albumin. Diluted samples and a limiting dilution of iodine-125-labeled TP-2 antibody were preincubated and added to the coated wells. The wells were incubated, washed and the bound radioactivity was measured. Determinations were carried out in triplicate. Cells producing recombinant CETP (CHO-E8) and the TP-2 antibody (TP-2 hybridoma cells were obtained from A.R. Tall, Columbia University, New York) and were grown in a bioreactor (Technomouse, Technomara Integra Biosciences). CETP standards were calibrated with recombinant CETP purified to electrophoretic homogeneity. Protein was determined by the BioRad method using bovine serum albumin as standard.

Assay Method of Plasma CETP Activity Level Using Exogenous Substrates

Plasma CETP activity levels, using exogenous substrates, were assayed in the supernatant fraction of plasma after removal of endogenous VLDL+LDL by phosphotungstate/Mg^{2+} precipitation [12]. The assay detects the transfer/exchange of CE between excess exogenous [^{14}C]CE-labelled LDL and excess exogenous unlabelled normal HDL, while LCAT is inhibited with 2 mmol/L of 2-nitro-benzoic acid [13]. Incubations were for 16 hours at 37° C. The reaction was stopped by cooling the tubes to 4° C and LDL was precipitated from the incubation mixture with Mg-phosphotungstate and the radioactivity measured in the HDL-containing supernatant. CETP activity was calculated as the bidirectional transfer of CE between radiolabelled LDL and HDL [13]. CE donor and acceptor lipoproteins used in the analyses were from the same lipoprotein batch and all samples were analyzed in the same run. The results were calculated and expressed as arbitrary units (% reference poolplasma). All assays were performed in duplicate and the measured activities were linear with the amount of plasma used. The within-assay coefficient of variation was 2.7%. CETP activities are stable during storage of plasma/serum at -80° C for 5-6 years [14].

Assay of CE Transfer Rates with Endogenous Plasma Lipoproteins

The rate of CE transfer with endogenous (newly synthesized) CE was determined as described [15], with minor modifications. In short, the transfer of labelled CE to VLDL+LDL was measured, during incubation of whole plasma, in the absence of LCAT inhibitors, with a trace amount of radioactive cholesterol (complexed with bovine serum albumin). After incubation, the apo B-containing lipoproteins VLDL and LDL are precipitated from plasma by phosphotungstate/Mg^{2+} and the radioactive cholesterol and CE, present in the precipitate, are separated using disposable silica columns. The CE are eluted from the column using hexane:diethylether (6:1, v/v). The activity is expressed in nmol/ml plasma/h.

Analytical Methods

Concentrations of cholesterol and triglycerides [16] were measured enzymatically using kits from Hoffman-La Roche, Basel, Switzerland (Nrs 0715166 for cholesterol and 0722138 for triglycerides) in an automated Cobas Mira analyzer (Hoffman-La Roche Basel, Switzerland).

STATISTICAL METHODS

The statistical comparisons between the gemfibrozil and placebo groups were calculated by the Mann-Whitney nonparametric test. Wilcoxon's signed rank test was used to calculate differences between pre- and post-treatment values separately in the two groups. For correlation analyses Pearson's correlation coefficient was calculated.

Results

CHANGES IN SERUM LIPIDS AND LIPOPROTEINS

The baseline values of fasting serum lipids were comparable in the gemfibrozil and the placebo groups. The mean concentration of serum total cholesterol was reduced by 14% during gemfibrozil treatment (6.33 $\pm$ 1.54 mM before and 5.46 $\pm$ 0.90 mM after treatment). This change was however not statistically significant, probably due to the relatively small number of patients in each group. Plasma cholesterol tended to increase (not significant) in the placebo group (6.32 $\pm$ 1.46 mM before and 6.89 $\pm$ 1.30 mM after treatment). The concentration of total serum TG decreased by 56% ($p < 0.03$) during gemfibrozil treatment (3.37 $\pm$ 1.25 mM before and 1.47 $\pm$ 0.15 after treatment), which was mainly due to a reduction (-63%, $p < 0.03$) in VLDL-TG (2.37 $\pm$ 0.87mM before and 0.87 $\pm$ 0.18 mM after treatment). TG concentrations (both in total plasma and in VLDL) tended to increase in the placebo group, but these changes were not statistically significant. Treatment with gemfibrozil or placebo had no significant effects on serum LDL-cholesterol and HDL-cholesterol concentrations, although the highest HDL-cholesterol levels were found after treatment with gemfibrozil, as expected (0.95 $\pm$ 0.22 mM before and 1.01 $\pm$ 0.16 mM after treatment with gemfibrozil).

RESPONSES OF PLASMA CETP CONCENTRATIONS AND CETP ACTIVITY LEVELS TO GEMFIBROZIL TREATMENT

At baseline, both plasma concentrations and activities of CETP (measured with exogenous substrates) were similar in the gemfibrozil and in the placebo groups. Plasma CETP concentrations were raised by 10.8% ($p < 0.03$) during gemfibrozil treatment and decreased significantly in the placebo group (Figure 1). Plasma CETP activity levels were raised by 8.2% ($p < 0.03$) during gemfibrozil treatment and the activity showed a tendency to decrease in the placebo group. These changes resulted in identical specific activities (expressed in % activity/µg protein) of CETP before and after treatment in both groups. Figure 2 shows that CETP mass and CETP activity levels (measured with exogenous substrates) correlate well, both before and after gemfibrozil treatment (all values, $r = 0.82$, $p < 0.01$).

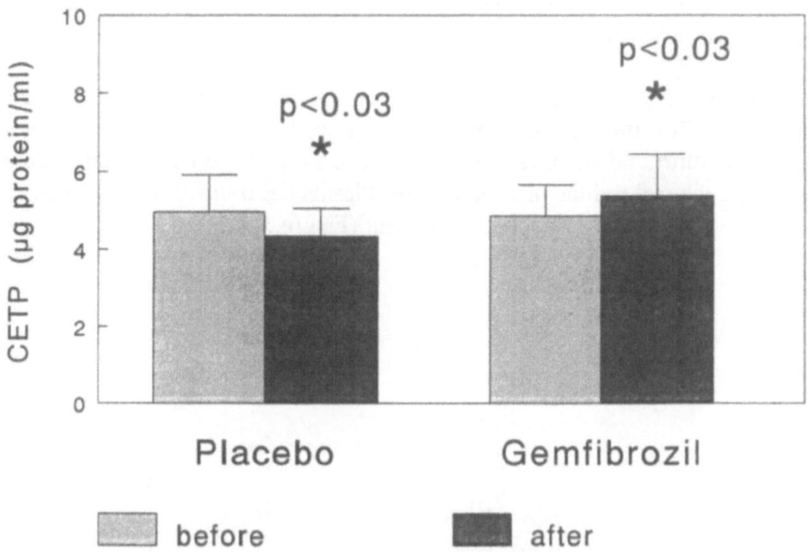

Figure 1. Plasma CETP concentration before and after treatment with gemfibrozil or placebo.

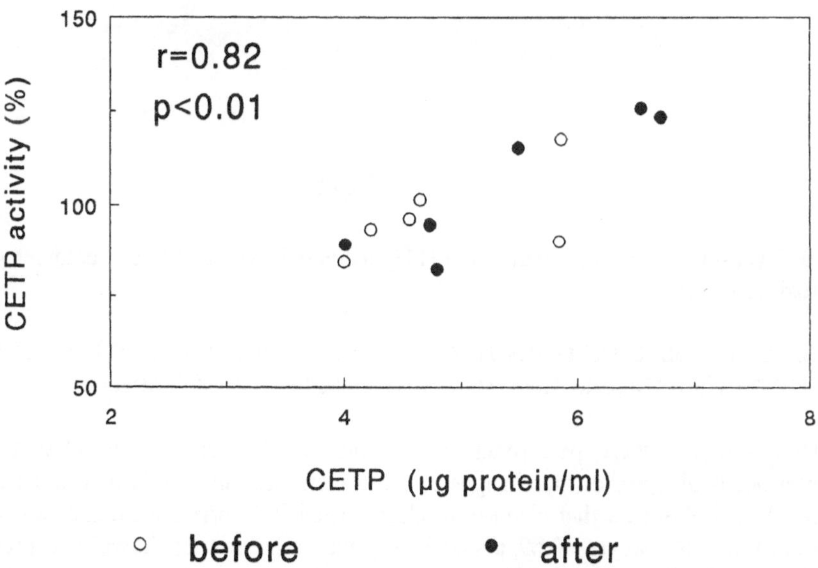

Figure 2. Correlation between plasma CETP concentrations and CETP activity levels (measured with exogenous substrates) before (○) and after (●) gemfibrozil treatment.

Effects of Gemfibrozil Treatment on Plasma CE Transfer Rates Measured Using Endogenous Lipoproteins

The CE transfer of newly synthetised CE to VLDL+LDL was measured after incubation of whole plasma with a trace amount of radioactive cholesterol, bound to bovine serum albumin, without further additions (see Methods). The baseline CE transfer rates were very similar in the gemfibrozil and the placebo groups. Plasma CE transfer rates were decreased by 29.0% ($p < 0.03$) during gemfibrozil treatment (Figure 3).

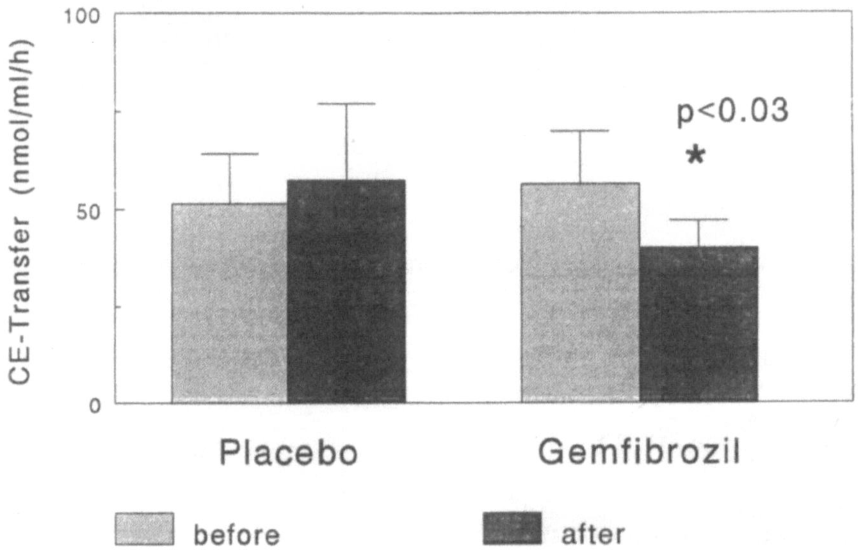

Figure 3. CE transfer rates in plasma from HTG patients before and after treatment with gemfibrozil or placebo.

Relation of Changes in CE Transfer Rates to Changes in Plasma TG and VLDL-TG Concentrations during Treatment with Gemfibrozil or Placebo

Correlation analyses were performed to examine whether changes in plasma TG concentrations could predict the changes in CE transfer during gemfibrozil or placebo treatment. Figure 4 shows that changes in plasma total TG correlate significantly with changes in CE transfer rates ($r = 0.69$, $p < 0.02$). A similar relation (not shown) was present between changes in plasma VLDL-TG concentrations and changes in CE transfern ($r = 0.79$, $p < 0.01$).

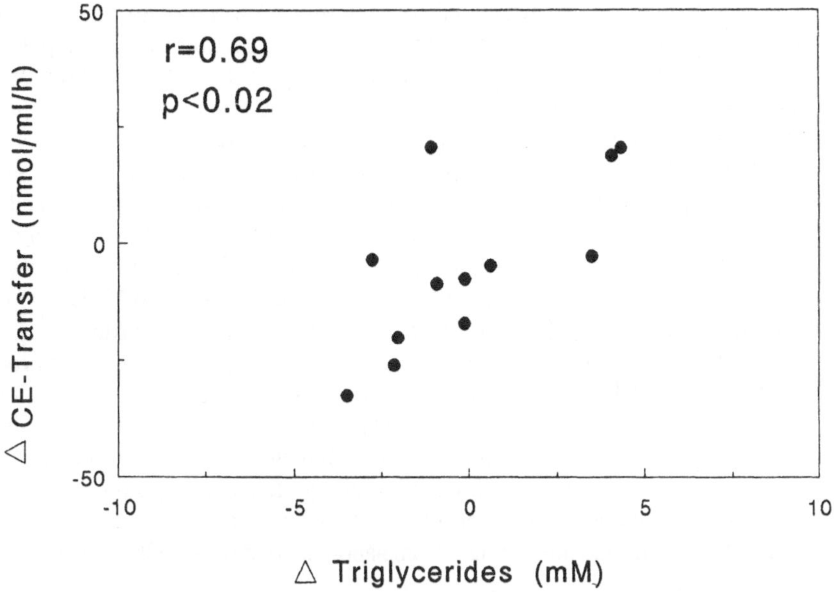

Figure 4. Correlation between the changes in plasma triglyceride concentration and in CE transfer during gemfibrozil or placebo treatment.

Discussion

The present study was performed to evaluate the apparent contradiction in published observations on effects of gemfibrozil treatment on CETP activities measured with exogenous substrates (increase, [4,6]) and CETP-catalysed CE transfer with endogenous substrates (decrease, [8]). In addition we measured plasma CETP mass using an immunoassay. The latter method revealed increased plasma concentrations of CETP by gemfibrozil treatment (by 11%) and allowed us to conclude that the specific activity of CETP is not affected by gemfibrozil treatment. On the other hand, a 29% decrease was found in the transfer rate of endogenously LCAT-generated CE. The latter decrease correlated with the changes occurring in total plasma TG and VLDL-TG concentrations. This shows once more that CE transfer rates are not only dependent on CETP mass, but also on VLDL-TG concentration and VLDL composition [c.f. 17]. Our observation, that the CE transfer rate can be decreased by drug treatment in the light of an increased CETP concentration, shows that the availability of active acceptor lipoproteins (VLDL) is more important than the plasma level of the catalyst CETP, at least in the present group of patients with HTG. Mann et al. [9] added partially purified CETP to plasma enriched with VLDL and found net mass CE transfer to increase 2-3 fold. Therefore it seems that increasing plasma levels of CETP by a factor of 2 or more will stimulate CE transfer rates, while CE transfer catalysed by CETP levels in the normal range is regulated by acceptor lipoprotein concentrations rather than CETP concentrations. The absolute values of CETP concentrations measured in the present study are relatively high, if compared with published values [18]. This is likely to be due to the standardization procedure. We used the BioRad protein assay to measure pure CETP standards. CETP was found to give lower protein values using this method, if compared with the Lowry procedure.

Gemfibrozil treatment has multiple effects on plasma lipoproteins and affects lipolytic activities (both hepatic lipase and extrahepatic LPL, [3,4,6]) and apo A-I and A-II synthesis rates [19], in addition to the effects on CETP described in the present and earlier reports [4,6]. HDL concentrations are increased by gemfibrozil and it is clear now that gemfibrozil causes a preferential rise of the HDL_3 subfraction (relative to HDL_2) [4,6,20]. Also, apoA-II containing lipoproteins increase more than LpA-I particles [6]. The consequences of these changes for cholesterol fluxes between plasma and tissues remain unclear at present. Results of the Helsinki Heart Study have shown that gemfibrozil treatment may reduce coronary heart disease [21]. The combined effects of gemfibrozil (increased synthesis of HDL apolipoproteins, lowering of TG-rich lipoproteins due to enhanced LPL activity and decreased CE transfer into apo B-containing lipoproteins) may enhance the net flux of cholesterol out of the periphery into the liver (reverse cholesterol transport) and at the same time prevent the accumulation of atherogenic, CE-rich VLDL and LDL.

Acknowledgements

The authors acknowledge the technical assistance of T. van Gent and P. van den Berg in performing the lipid transfer activity assays. This work was supported by grants from the Netherlands Heart Foundation (nr 89.094), Aarne Koskelo Foundation, the Meilahti Foundation, the Orion Corporation Research Foundation, Finnish State Medical Research Council (The Academy of Finland), and the Sigrid Juselius Foundation, Finland and from Warner-Lambert Company, Ann Arbor, Michigan, USA.

References

1. Brunzell JD, Schrott HG, Motulsky AG, Bierman EL. Myocardial infarction in the familial forms of hypertriglyceridemia. Metabolism 1976;25:313-20.
2. Zhao S-P, Smelt AHM, Van den Maagdenberg AMJM, et al. Plasma lipoprotein profiles of normocholesterolemic and hypercholesterolemic homozygotes for apolipoprotein E2($Arg_{158} \rightarrow$ Cys) compared. Clin Chem 1994;40:1559-66.
3. Nikkilä EA, Ylikahri R, Huttunen JK. Gemfibrozil: Effect on serum lipids, lipoproteins, postheparin plasma lipase activities and glucose tolerance in primary hypertriglyceridemia. Proc Royal Soc Medicine 1976;69(2):58-63.
4. Kahri J, Vuorinen-Markkola H, Tilly-Kiesi M, Lahdenperä S, Taskinen M-R. Effect of gemfibrozil on high-density lipoprotein subspecies in non-insulin dependent diabetes mellitus. Relations to lipolytic enzymes and to the cholesteryl ester transfer protein activity. Atherosclerosis 1993;102:79-89.
5. Tenkanen L, Pietilä K, Manninen V, Mänttäri M. The triglyceride issue revisited: Findings

from the Helsinki Heart Study. Arch Intern Med 1994;154:2714-20.

6. Kahri J, Sane T, Van Tol A, Taskinen M-R. Effect of gemfibrozil on the regulation of HDL subfractions in hypertriglyceridemic patients. J Intern Med 1995;238:429-36.

7. Van Tol A, Scheek LM, Groener JEM. Cholesterol esterification and net mass transfer of cholesterylesters and triglycerides in plasma from healthy subjects and hyperlipidemic coronary heart disease patients In: Malmendier CL, Alaupovic P, editors. Eicosanoids, apolipoproteins, lipoprotein particles and atherosclerosis. Adv Expl Med Biol 243. New York: Plenum Press, 1988:231-37.

8. Bhatnagar D, Durrington PN, Mackness M, Arrol S, Winocour PH, Prais H. Effect of treatment of hypertriglyceridemia with gemfibrozil on serum lipoproteins and the transfer of cholesteryl esters from high-density lipoprotein to low density lipoproteins. Atherosclerosis 1992;92:49-57.

9. Mann CJ, Yen FT, Grant AM, Bihain BE. Mechanism of plasma cholesteryl ester transfer in hypertriglyceridemia. J Clin Invest 1991;88:2059-66.

10. Taskinen M-R, Kuusi T, Helve E, Nikkilä EA, Yki-Järvinen H. Insulin therapy induces antiatherogenic changes of serum lipoproteins in noninsulin-dependent diabetes. Arteriosclerosis 1988;8:168-77.

11. Marcel YL, McPherson R, Hogue M, et al. Distribution and concentration of cholesteryl ester transfer protein in plasma of normolipemic subjects. J Clin Invest 1990;85:10-17.

12. Speijer H, Groener JEM, Van Ramshorst E, Van Tol A. Different locations of cholesterylester transfer protein and phospholipid transfer protein activities in plasma. Atherosclerosis 1991; 90:159-68.

13. Groener JEM, Pelton RW, Kostner GM. Improved estimation of cholesteryl ester transfer/exchange activity in serum or plasma. Clin Chem 1986;32:283-86.

14. Van Tol A, Zock PL, Van Gent T, Scheek LM, Katan MB. Dietary trans fatty acids incease serum cholesteryl ester transfer protein activity in man. Atherosclerosis 1995;115:129-34.

15. Channon KM, Clegg RJ, Bhatnagar D, Ishola M, Arrol S, Durrington PN. Investigation of lipid transfer in human serum leading to the development of an isotopic method for the determination of endogenous cholesterol esterification and transfer. Atherosclerosis 1990; 80:217-26.

16. Wahlefeld AW. Triglyceride determination after enzymatic hydrolysis. In: Bergmeyer HV, editor. Methods of enzymatic analysis, 2nd edition. New York: Academic Press,1974:1831-41.

17. Dullaart RPF, Groener JEM, Erkelens DW. Effect of the composition of very low and low density lipoproteins on the rate of cholesterylester transfer from high density lipoproteins in man, studied in vitro. Eur J Clin Invest 1987;17:241-48.

18. McPherson R, Mann CJ, Tall AR, et al. Plasma concentrations of cholesterylester transfer protein in hyperlipoproteinemia. Arterioscl Thromb 1991;11:797-804.

19. Saku K, Gartside PS, Hynd BA, Kashyap ML. Mechanism of action of gemfibrozil on lipoprotein metabolism. J Clin Invest 1985;75:1702-12.

20. Mänttäri M, Koskinen P, Manninen V, Huttunen, JK, Frick MH. Effect of gemfibrozil on the concentration and composition of serum lipoproteins. Atherosclerosis 1990;81:11-17.

21. Manninen V, Elo MO, Frick MH. Lipid alterations in the incidence of coronary heart disease in the Helsinki Heart Study. JAMA 1988;260:641-51.

CONTROL OF LIPOPROTEIN LEVELS IN CORONARY HEART DISEASE TODAY: A FOCUS ON HIGH-DOSE FLUVASTATIN AND COMBINATION THERAPIES

Eran Leitersdorf
The Center for Research, Prevention and Treatment of Atherosclerosis, Hadassah University Hospital, 91120 Jerusalem, Israel

Introduction

Patients with ischemic heart disease (IHD) have a multitude of underlying risk factors, some of which have been demonstrated to be causally linked to the development of the disease. Among them, the most important risk parameters, a variety of dyslipidemias, may be present. In many cases, it is impossible to achieve the target lipid and lipoprotein levels as recently defined by international authorities [1,2]. In these cases, a "joint effort" which includes life style modification and pharmacological treatment is used.

During the last six years, we performed a series of clinical trials using multi-modality therapy for the treatment of patients with the monogenic disorder familial hypercholesterolemia (FH). All patients were instructed to adhere to the American Heart Association Step II diet [3], and reassessment of the dietary status was regularly performed. An initial single-blind dose finding study which examined the therapeutic potential of fluvastatin (up to 40 mg/d dose) as a cholesterol reducing agent [4,5] was followed by a double-blind study which defined the possible advantage of increasing the dose of up to 60 mg/d [6]. The therapeutic potential related to the possible combination of fluvastatin with either cholestyramine or with bezafibrate was analyzed in a short-term double-blind double-dummy experiment which defined the possible advantage of each combination [7,8]. The possibility of using triple therapy for this dyslipidemia was subsequently studied [9]. An open-label study has recently being initiated in order to examine the potential use of fluvastatin at the 80 mg/d dose either alone or in combination with bezafibrate 200-400 mg/d. The initial results were recently reported [10] and the present paper describes the final results of this 88-week study.

Discussion

Twenty-two patients with severe familial hypercholesterolemia whose plasma low density lipoprotein cholesterol (LDL-C) concentrations did not achieve the target levels [1,2] while

A. M. Gotto, Jr. et al. (eds.), Drugs Affecting Lipid Metabolism, 567–570.

on treatment with a combination of fluvastatin 60 mg/d, bezafibrate 200 mg/d, and cholestyramine 8 g/d were included in the present study. This open-label study included 6 weeks of monotherapy with 40 mg fluvastatin twice daily, at breakfast and at bedtime. In the second period (weeks 7-12), the patients received in addition to the fluvastatin, bezafibrate 200 mg/d at lunch time. During the third period (weeks 13-88), the patients received 80 mg/d of fluvastatin (40 mg at breakfast and 40 mg at bedtime) and 400 mg/d of bezafibrate in a slow release form which was administered at lunchtime. All patients signed an informed consent and the study was approved by the Hadassah University Hospital Ethics Committee and by the Israel Ministry of Health.

Dietary compliance was monitored throughout the study using an analysis of three days food records. All patients had to observe a strict low cholesterol diet instructed according to the American Heart Association Step II [3]. Compliance with the study medications was recorded at each visit. All patients underwent routine physical examinations, vital signs, and electrocardiography at regular intervals. Standard laboratory evaluations included blood chemistry and lipid profiles which were analyzed at the same laboratory. All possible adverse events were carefully recorded using specific questionnaires.

The efficacy results obtained up to week 88 of the study are presented (Figure 1). It is noteworthy that at week 6 (following monotherapy with 80 mg/d fluvastatin) the mean plasma LDL-C level was 30.8% lower than at baseline, at week 12 (following combination therapy of 80 mg/d fluvastatin and 200 mg/d of bezafibrate) it was 34.8% lower than at baseline, and at weeks 18-88 (while the patients were on the maximal dose) the level was kept at the 33.1%-37.4% lower than at baseline. Plasma high density lipoprotein cholesterol (HDL-C) levels increased by 4.0% when the patients were treated with fluvastatin alone, 14.3% when they received the addition of 200 mg/d of bezafibrate, and by 9.8%-21.1% when they were maintained on the highest dose of this combination treatment. The impact on the LDL-C/HDL-C ratio, a well-recognized risk parameter for IHD, was substantial. The three treatment periods resulted in 32.6%, 42.2%, and 39.6%-45.9% decrease from baseline. The treatment resulted in a decrease of plasma LDL-C levels to below 200 mg/dl in 72.7% (16/22) of the patients who participated in the study.

Fluvastatin alone and the combination with bezafibrate was extremely well tolerated. The compliance to the study medications was 91.9%-95.9% and 83.1%-100.0% for fluvastatin and bezafibrate, respectively. All patients participated in the study to its end and underwent all clinical and laboratory examinations. Safety analysis revealed no new abnormalities in renal and liver function tests.

In conclusion, this relatively long-term study suggests that in patients with heterozygous FH, the use of combination therapy, which includes the HMG-CoA reductase inhibitor fluvastatin with the fibric acid-derivative bezafibrate, provides a highly effective as well as well-tolerated and safe treatment aimed at the prevention of IHD.

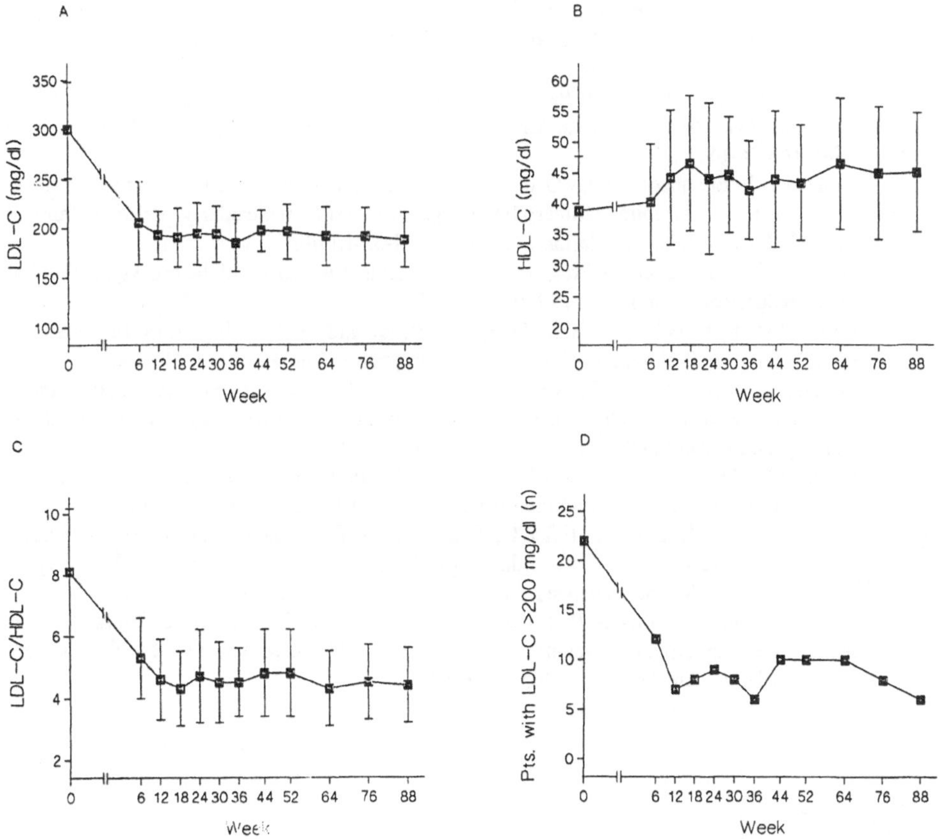

Figure 1. The response of plasma lipoprotein concentrations (A, LDL-C; B, HDL-C; C, LDL-C/HDL-C; D, percent of patients with LDL-C > 200 mg/dl) to the study medications. Week 0, baseline was obtained after 4 weeks of placebo treatment [4]. The results shown for weeks 6, 12, and 18-88 correspond to treatment with fluvastatin 80 mg/d, fluvastatin 80 mg/d plus bezafibrate 200 mg/d, and fluvastatin 80 mg/d plus 400 mg/d of bezafibrate, respectively.

References

1. Prevention of coronary heart disease: Scientific background and new clinical guidelines. Recommendations of the European Atherosclerosis Society prepared by the international task force for prevention of coronary heart disease. Nut Metab Cardiovasc Dis 1992;2:113-56.

2. Summary of the second report of the National Cholesterol Education Program (NCEP) expert panel on detection, evaluation, and treatment of high blood cholesterol in adults (adult treatment panel II). J Am Med Ass 1993;269:3015-23.
3. The Expert Panel. Report of the national cholesterol education program expert panel on detection, evaluation, and treatment of high blood cholesterol in adults. Arch Int Med 1988;148:36-69.
4. Leitersdorf E, Eisenberg S, Eliav O, et al. Genetic determinants of responsiveness to the HMG CoA reductase inhibitor fluvastatin in patients with molecularly defined familial hypercholesterolemia. Circulation 1993;87(III):III-35-III-44.
5. Leitersdorf E. Gender-related response to fluvastatin in patients with heterozygous familial hypercholesterolaemia. Drugs 1994;47(2):54-58.
6. Leitersdorf E, Eisenberg S, Eliav O, et al. Efficacy and safety of high dose fluvastatin in patients with familial hypercholesterolemia. European J Clin Pharmacol 1993;45:513-18.
7. Leitersdorf E, Muratti EN, Eliav O, et al. Efficacy and safety of a combination fluvastatin-bezafibrate treatment for familial hypercholesterolemia: Comparative analysis to a fluvastatin-cholestyramine combination. Am J Med 1994;96:401-407.
8. Muratti EN, Peters TK, Leitersdorf E. Fluvastatin in familial hypercholesterolemia: A cohort analysis of the response to combination treatment. Am J Cardiol 1994;73:30D-38D.
9. Leitersdorf E, Muratti EN, Eliav O, Peters TK. Efficacy and safety of triple therapy (fluvastatin-bezafibrate-cholestyramine) for patients with severe familial hyper-cholesterolemia: A cohort analysis. Am J Cardiol 1995;76:84A-88A.
10. Eliav O, Schurr D, Pfister P, Friedlander Y, Leitersdorf E. High dose fluvastatin and bezafibrate combination treatment of patients with heterozygous familial hyper-cholesterolemia. Am J Cardiol 1995;76:76A-79A.

THE FUTURE: ELEVATING HIGH DENSITY LIPOPROTEIN

James R. Paterniti, Jr.*, Robert E. Damon, J. Bruce Eskesen, and David B. Weinstein
*Preclinical Research Department, Sandoz Research Institute, E. Hanover, New Jersey 07936 and *Department of Cardiovascular Research, Ligand Pharmaceuticals, 9393 Towne Center Drive, San Diego, California 92121, USA*

Introduction

No less than fifteen epidemiological and clinical studies have demonstrated an inverse correlation between low levels of plasma high density lipoprotein (HDL) cholesterol and the major HDL protein component apolipoprotein A-I (apo A-I), with the risk of coronary disease and atherosclerosis [1]. Current management for treatment of dyslipidemias focuses largely on the ability to decrease low-density lipoprotein (LDL) cholesterol levels with potent, safe, and very effective HMG-CoA reductase inhibitors [2]. Aggressive approaches to raising HDL-cholesterol level or HDL particle number could be useful primary or suitable adjunctive therapy in many dyslipidemias. Current approaches to clinical management of hypoalphalipoproteinemias include changes in dietary intake and the saturated/polyunsaturated fatty acid composition of the diet; exercise in sedentary individuals; cessation of smoking; postmenopausal estrogen replacement; moderate intake of alcohol; and with drugs that may elevate HDL levels by either primary or secondary mechanisms [3].

Primary drug-based regimens to raise HDL, include nicotinic acid and its derivatives which can produce a 15-35% elevation of HDL cholesterol associated with potential hepatotoxicity and many other adverse effects. The mechanism of action is complex involving inhibition of fatty acid mobilization, decrease in VLDL production, elevation of lipoprotein lipase activity, and a decrease in apo A-I catabolism. Other primary drug-based regimens include gemfibrozil and other fibric acid derivatives for which a 10-30% elevation of HDL-cholesterol is well-documented. The mechanism of action is complex and poorly understood involving increased catabolism of triglyceride-rich lipoproteins and increased lipoprotein lipase activity.

Other lipid-altering therapies that produce elevations in HDL levels include HMG-CoA reductase inhibitors that raise HDL-cholesterol by 8-11%. These safe and effective first-line therapeutics for hypercholesterolemia also lower plasma triglycerides but the mechanism(s) for effects on HDL are not understood. Additionally bile acid sequestrants in use for lowering of LDL-cholesterol may raise HDL-cholesterol by 5-8% in some patients.

A. M. Gotto, Jr. et al. (eds.), Drugs Affecting Lipid Metabolism, 571–579.

Other drugs that may secondarily raise HDL levels include phenytoin, terbutaline, cimetidine, and some alpha-adrenergic agents [3]. Novel first-line therapeutics for elevation of plasma HDL-cholesterol levels have not surfaced in the past 15 years, despite the growing interest in HDL metabolism and the relationship between HDL and coronary disease over that time period. In the last 18 months, approximately 2,000 references have appeared in the biological literature on all aspects of HDL metabolism, structure, function, clinical trials, and assorted topics. Of these recently published studies on HDL, information on new clinical studies related to pharmacotherapeutic approaches to elevating HDL levels are reported for 14 classes of compounds or complex mixtures of agents (Table 1).

Table 1. Agents reported to increase HDL levels in clinical studies (from the 1995 biological literature).

"War Horses"	Other Drugs	Natural Product Derivatives
Estrogens	Dexfenfluramine	Red Wine
Fish Oil	Fludiazepam	No. 90 Dasheng Jiangya Oral Liquid
Antiepileptic Drugs	Lifibrol (Fibrate-Like Phenoxy Acid)	Vitamin C
Niceritrol		Green Tea
HMG-CoA Reductase Inhibitors		Oral Pryridoxine (Vitamin B6)
		Jiangzhi Zhongyno Pian (Chinese Herbal)

If we eliminate the "war-horses" such as estrogen, fish oil, antiepileptic drugs, nicotinic-acid derivatives, and HMG-CoA reductase inhibitors, then the list can be reduced by half. Lifibrol is a fibrate-like agent that has been in clinical studies for over 5 years and raises HDL-cholesterol by a maximum of 10% in patients with primary hypercholesterolemia [4] but shows a biphasic dose-response curve. Phenytoin, a microsomal enzyme inducer, was shown to raise plasma HDL cholesterol subfractions by as much as 40-50% in a dose-dependent manner in normal subjects and the effects were coincident with large decreases in cholesteryl ester transfer activity levels in plasma [5]. However, in patients with hypoalphalipoproteinemia, these changes were not observed. More than half of the remaining reports are of the use of ethnopharmacologic herbal medications that have been known in Eastern societies for centuries. Why are there so few novel contributions describing efforts to raise HDL levels from the pharmaceutical industry in this period? One must always consider the requirement for protection of proprietary information in any pharmaceutical drug development project. A more formidable obstacle is the current limited information base on the mechanisms that are responsible for determining either HDL-cholesterol or apo A-I levels in plasma. Both the production and removal of HDL particles from plasma are dependent upon multiple pathways, several major tissue sites, and diverse mechanisms regulating these processes. Some studies have suggested that the catabolic rate of apo A-I is elevated in hypoalphalipoproteinemics, while others suggest that the apo A-I synthetic or transport rate is the major determinant of HDL levels [6]. Human HDL levels may be partially determined by insulin sensitivity, adiposity, lipase activities, lipid transfer proteins, plasma triglyceride levels, and as yet poorly understood genetic factors [7-9]. All of these potential determinants of steady state HDL levels increase the complexity and difficulty of selecting a metabolic pathway or specific target for novel therapeutic agents. In addition, the biosynthesis of HDL particles by the liver cannot be readily modeled in hepatic cells that are maintained in culture. Drugs or hormones that are known to alter HDL levels *in vivo* may occasionally generate alterations in apo A-I synthesis, transport, or gene expression in cell models. However, the effects are not robust and cannot be maintained for long-term analysis of dose-response activities. The absence of a high capacity *in vitro* screening model is a major hurdle to rapid and economical development of new therapeutic agents designed to increase HDL production rate. At the other end of the scale is the complex dissociation of HDL cholesterol ester uptake from apo A-I removal and degradation [10]. It would be difficult, at best, to model HDL removal pathways and screen these processes *in vitro* or *in vivo* for the large number of new chemical entities that are required for the discovery and development of new therapeutics. Finally, it is not clear that small animal models can be effectively used to predict either the metabolic effects, or the human dose range, for new therapeutic agents that alter HDL levels. The rodent models that best define alterations of lipoprotein levels in response to experimental therapies (rats and mice) differ from humans in the regulation of HDL metabolism. For example, rats have more than 70% of their plasma cholesterol in HDL particles; very low levels of LDL-cholesterol; very large HDL particles rich in apolipoprotein E; and an absence of cholesteryl ester transfer protein activity. A best example of the difficulties in modeling HDL parameters in rodents is nicotinic acid. This efficacious HDL-elevating drug in humans, can be shown to rapidly alter plasma fatty acid transport and lipolysis after administration to rodents. However, HDL cholesterol elevation is not observed under any practical dose regimens [11]. These and other factors have been major impediments to the development of novel therapies for the elevation of HDL.

Beecham Pharmaceuticals in the mid-1980s embarked on a program to develop HDL-elevating agents using rats fed on sucrose-rich, semisynthetic diets designed to lower intrinsic plasma HDL levels and thus provide a larger window of response for use in a structure-activity screening program [12]. A variety of chemical derivatives of phenylalanine and tyrosine were prepared with HDL elevating activities of 50-125% compared to untreated control rats. While the mechanism of action of the lead development compound of this series (BRL 26314) has not been published, it also increased HDL phospholipid and apolipoprotein levels, and was shown to inhibit atherosclerosis in a diet+aortic de-endotheliazation rabbit model at high dose (100 mg/kg body weight for 28 days). While the Beecham program did not continue development of this series of highly active HDL-elevating compounds, it was shown that a structure-activity screen *in vivo* in rats could generate active compounds.

In 1988, the Sandoz Lipoprotein Metabolism group began a program to identify agents to raise HDL levels from a large library of lipid altering compounds that had been tested during 20 years of earlier Sandoz screening programs. No suitable lead candidates were found until the search parameters were changed to include compounds that raised total plasma cholesterol levels in normal, chow-fed rats. Since plasma HDL is the major carrier of cholesterol in normal rats, agents that significantly raise total plasma cholesterol may do so by raising HDL-cholesterol levels. In this manner, a series of active thiourea derivatives, such as SDZ 265-855 were developed. In the cholesterol and cholic acid-fed rat model, SDZ 265-855 produced a dose-related increase in HDL-cholesterol (Figure 1A) of approximately twice that produced by gemfibrozil (Figure 1B) at its maximum effect dose in this rat model. A dose-dependent increase in rat serum apo A-I levels with a half maximum increase of 41% was obtained at a dose of SDZ 265-855 of 47 umoles or 11 mg/kg/day (Figure 1C). Figure 1D shows the comparison with gemfibrozil for elevation of serum apo A-I in this model. There was no effect on thyroid hormone levels (T_3 orT_4) at doses of SDZ 265-855 that significantly elevated HDL cholesterol levels. SDZ 265-855 lowered serum triglycerides in non-fasted rats to a greater extent than gemfibrozil. During the testing of this chemical series, it was determined that SDZ 265-855 increased the size of HDL particles isolated from rat serum. This can be seen in Figure 2 as a large shift to the left of the HDL peak after Superose-6 gel permeation chromatography. SDZ 265-855 also effectively elevated HDL cholesterol levels in chow-fed rats and hamsters (data not shown). Studies on the mechanism of action of SDZ 265-855 indicated that both steady state levels of hepatic apo A-I mRNA and the plasma half-life of apo A-I were increased by treatment with this agent. The specific mechanisms that regulate both changes in apo A-I production and increased plasma residence time of apo A-I are unknown. This profile differs from that of known fibric acid derivatives and is unique for an agent that alters plasma HDL levels. More detailed studies on the lead compound from this thiourea series, SDZ HDL 376, will be presented elsewhere (in preparation).

Human HDL contains at least two classes of apo A-I-containing particles that differ in the presence or absence of apo A-II and may have different metabolic, functional, and clinical significance [13]. In insulin-resistant normolipidemic populations large LDL particle size and reduced HDL_2 cholesterol levels are associated with increased disease risk, independent of other plasma lipoprotein levels [14]. These complexities in the heterogeneity of human HDL subclasses cannot be monitored or screened in small animal models of lipoprotein metabolism. The use of nonhuman primate models for such studies must generally await late-stage preclinical development of any pharmacotherapeutic agents. Despite these difficulties and complexities, at least two other HDL drug discovery programs are in progress. A series of thiazolopyrimidines, that are chemically related to the thiourea SDZ 265-855 series, has been described by Hoechst AG [15]. The most potent compound (30 mg/kg/d for 7 days) increased HDL cholesterol in normal rats by 101% and in the hypothyroid-lipid-fed rat by 152%. No further information is available about the development of this chemical series. Otsuka Pharmaceuticals has discovered a novel

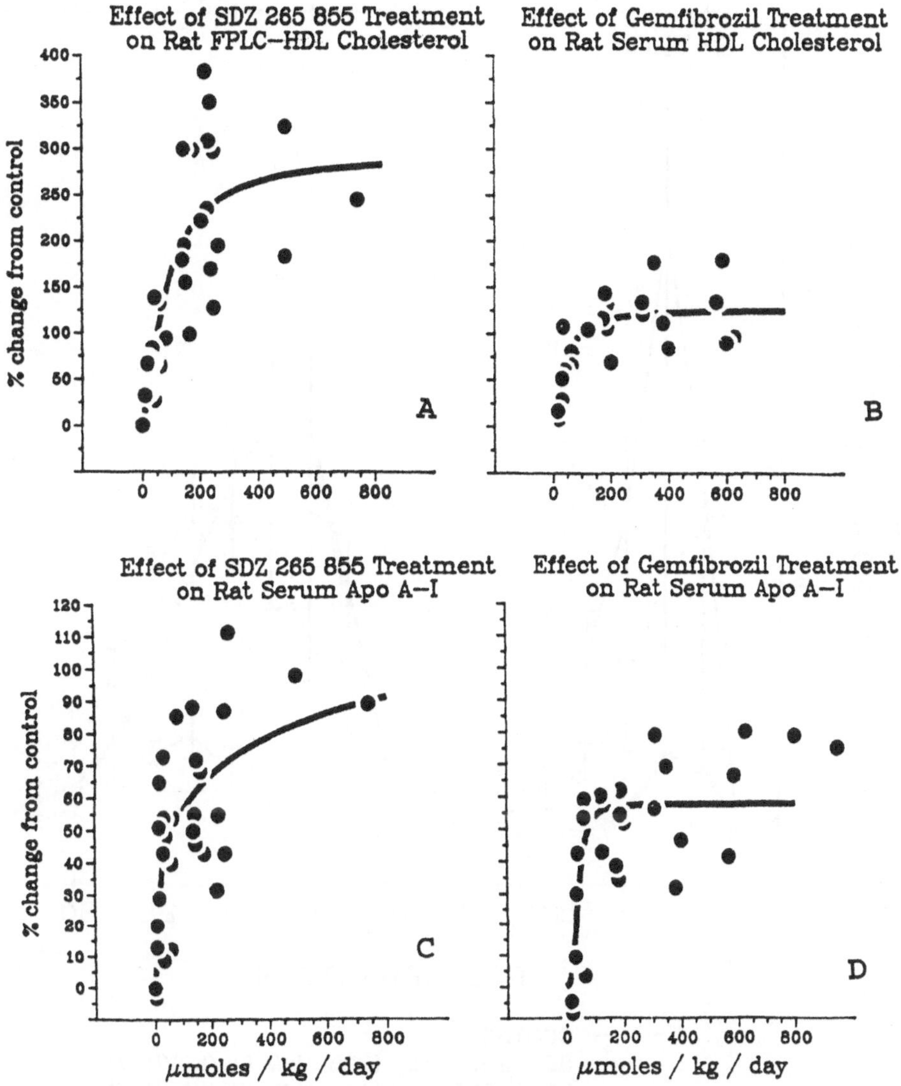

Figure 1. Effects of SDZ 265-855 (Panels A and C) and gemfibrozil (Panels B and D) on HDL-cholesterol and serum apoA-I levels in cholesterol+cholic acid-fed rats. Analysis by FPLC of HDL after treatment with SDZ 265-855 is shown in Panel A since treatment increases the size and decreases the bouyant density of rat HDL.

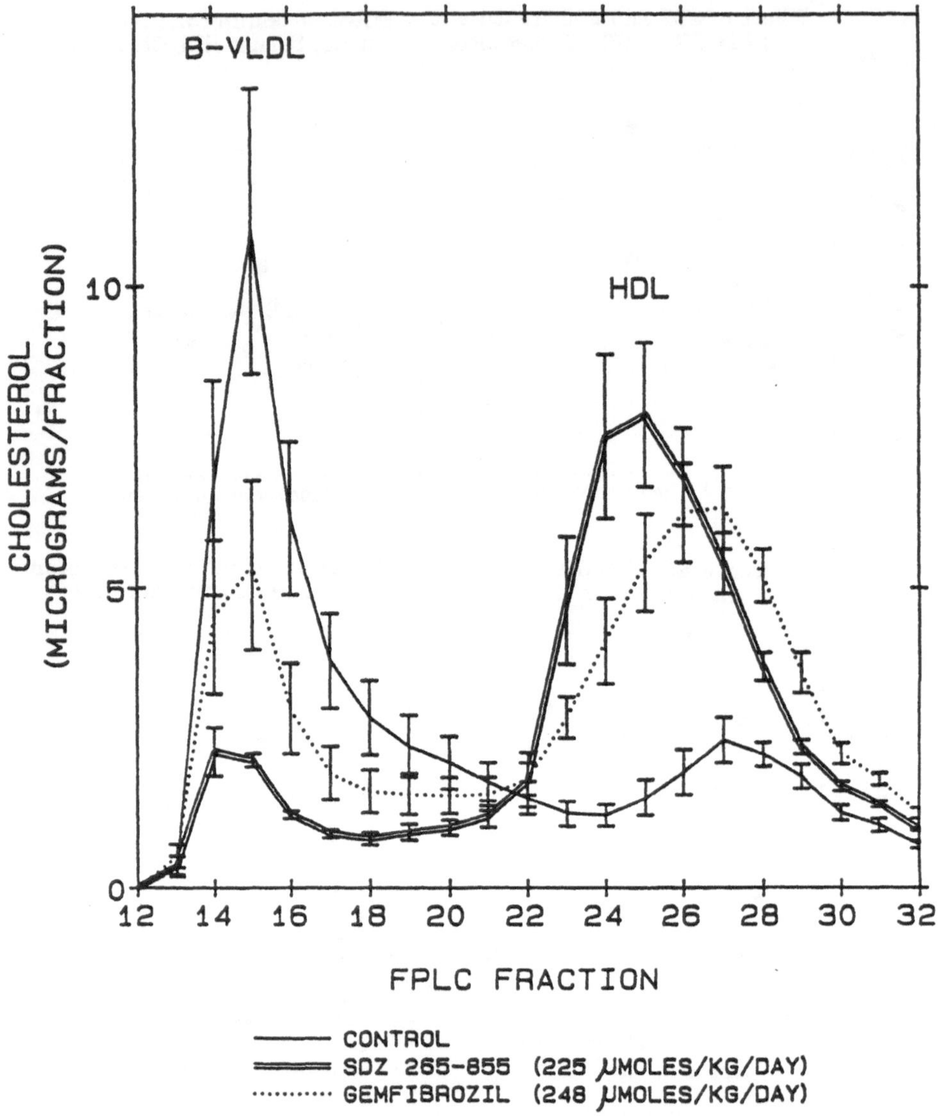

Figure 2. FPLC profile of rat serum lipoproteins after 8 day treatment with SDZ 265-855 and gemfibrozil.

compound, NO-1886, that increases lipoprotein lipase activity in postheparin plasma, adipose tissue and myocardium of rats, and produces reductions in triglyceride levels along with elevation of HDL cholesterol levels [16]. At a dose of 25 mg/kg/d for 8 days, there was a 37% increase in HDL-cholesterol in normal rats. NO-1886 also decreased the atherosclerotic changes induced in rats by Vitamin D_2 toxicity and corrected the hypertriglyceridemia in streptozotocin-induced diabetes in rats while doubling HDL-cholesterol levels [17]. It is not known whether such changes in HDL levels can be induced by NO-1886 in other species. Finally, it is apparent that several pharmaceutical companies have been struggling with attempts to develop inhibitors of cholesteryl ester transfer protein. The very high degree of hydrophobicity of this protein and its ability to nonspecifically interact with many hydrophobic chemical species and proteins has been a major deterrent to drug discovery.

Where will the HDL active drugs of the future come from? There may be many useful mechanisms involving production, transport, and catabolism of HDL particles that are capable of raising HDL plasma levels with beneficial effects on the risk of development of coronary disease. However, our current drug discovery modeling systems cannot predict which methods of raising HDL pool size are the preferred ones, if any. The development of HDL active drugs is at present a high risk effort with little assurance of success until early clinical studies indicate that elevation of HDL particles or beneficial changes in particle composition can be achieved in human populations. Even then, we must await long-term clinical trials to determine whether any clinical benefit can be derived from changes in the plasma HDL pool.

Nevertheless, it is comforting to note that the new approaches of molecular biology may provide the tools and designs to expand the current screening approaches to drug discovery in the HDL field. For example, Shimada et al. [18] have shown that overexpression of lipoprotein lipase in transgenic mice inhibited diabetes-associated hypertriglyceridemia and hypercholesterolemia. Fan et al. [19] have shown that overexpression of hepatic lipase in transgenic rabbits leads to a marked reduction of plasma high density lipoprotein and intermediate density lipoprotein. Mutations in the genes for apo A-I, apo A-II, Apo A-IV, apo C-III, lecithin-cholesterol acyltransferase, and cholesterol ester transfer protein are associated with low levels of HDL cholesterol, although the changes may not necessarily correlate with risk of coronary disease [20]. Future opportunities in the treatment of hypoalphalipoproteinemia may derive from current experimental efforts on the regulation of expression of the apo A-I gene. It is apparent that polymorphisms in the apo A-I gene promoter may be responsible for determination of the decreased production rate of apo A-I [21]. Recent studies have shown that overexpression of orphan nuclear receptors ARP-1 or Ear-1 repress hepatic expression of the human apo A-I gene while other members of the nuclear receptor superfamily such as HNF-4 can increase apo A-I gene expression [22]. Vu-Dac et al. [23] have shown that the negative regulation of the human apolipoprotein A-I promoter by fibrates can be attenuated by the interaction of the peroxisomal proliferator-activated receptor with its response elements. A new set of targets for therapeutic intervention are emerging from the growing knowledge and interest in regulation of the genes that control HDL metabolism.

References

1. Patsch W, Gotto Jr AM. High-density lipoprotein cholesterol, plasma triglyceride, and coronary heart disease: pathophysiology and management. Adv Pharmacol 1995;32:375-426.
2. Levy RI, Troendle AJ, Fattu JM. A quarter century of drug treatment of dyslipoproteinemia, with a focus on the new HMG-CoA reductase inhibitor fluvastatin. Circulation 1993;87(III):III-45-III-53.
3. Rosenson RS. Low levels of high-density lipoprotein cholesterol (hypoalphalipoproteinemia). An approach to management. Arch Intern Med 1993;153:1528-38.
4. Locker PK, Jungbluth GL, Francom SF, Hughes GS Jr., for the Lifibrol Study Group. Lifibrol: A novel lipid-lowering drug for the therapy of hypocholesterolemia. Clin Pharmacol Ther 1995;57:73-88.
5. Franceschini G, Werba JP, D'Acquarica AL, Gianfranceschi G, Michelagnoli S, Sirtori CR. Microsomal enzyme inducers raise plasma high-density lipoprotein cholesterol levels in healthy control subjects but not in patients with primary hypoalphalipoproteinemia. Clin Pharmacol Ther 1995;57:434-40.
6. Gylling H, Vega GL, Grundy SM. Physiologic mechanisms for reduced apolipoprotein A-I concentrations associated with low levels of high density lipoprotein cholesterol in patients with normal plasma lipids. J Lipid Res 1992;33:1527-39.
7. Brinton EA, Eisenberg S, Breslow JL. Human HDL cholesterol levels are determined by apoA-I fractional catabolic rate, which correlates inversely with estimates of HDL particle size. Effects of gender, hepatic and lipoprotein lipases, triglyceride and insulin levels, and body fat distribution. Arterioslcer Thromb 1994;14:707-20.
8. Tall AR. Plasma cholesteryl ester transfer protein and high-density lipoproteins: new insights from molecular genetic studies. J Intern Med 1995;237:5-12.
9. Mahaney MC, Blangero J, Rainwater DL, et al. A major locus influencing plasma high-density lipoprotein cholesterol levels in the San Antonio Family Heart Study. Arterioscler Thromb Vasc Biol 1995;15:1730-39.
10. Glass C, Pittman RC, Weinstein DB, Steinberg D. Dissociation of tissue uptake of cholesterol ester from that of apolipoprotein A-I of rat plasma high density lipoprotein: Selective delivery of cholesterol ester to liver, adrenal and gonad. Proc Natl Acad Sci USA 1983;80:5435-39.
11. Olivier P, Plancke MO, Marzin D, Clavey V, Sauzieres J, Fruchart JC. Effects of fenofibrate, gemfibrozil and nicotinic acid on plasma lipoprotein levels in normal and hyperlipidemic mice. Atherosclerosis 198; 70:107-14.
12. Fears R, Esmail A, Walker P, Rush WR, Ferres H. Hyperalpha-lipoproteinemic activity of BRL 26314. II. Inhibition of atherosclerosis in rabbits. Biochem Pharmacol 1984;33:219-28.
13. Fruchart JC, Ailhaud G, Bard JM. Heterogeneity of high density lipoprotein particles. Circulation 1993;87(III):III-22-III-27.
14. Campos H, Roederer GO, Lussier-Cacan S, Davignon J, Krauss RM. Predominance of large LDL and reduced HDL2 cholesterol in normolipidemic men with coronary artery disease. Arterioscler Thromb Vasc Biol 1995;15:1043-48.
15. Furrer H, Granzer E, Wagner R. A new class of potent hypolipemic agents raising high-density lipoproteins. Synthesis, reactions and pharmacological properties. Eur J Med Chem 1994;29:819-29.
16. Tsutsumi K, Inoue Y, Shima A, Iwasaki K, Kawamura M, Murase T. The novel compound

NO-1886 increase lipoprotein lipase activity with resulting elevation of high density lipoprotein cholesterol, and long-term administration inhibits atherogenesis in the coronary arteries of rats with experimental atherosclerosis. J Clin Invest 1993;92:411-17.

17. Tsutsumi K, Inoue Y, Shima A, Iwasaki K, Murase T. Correction of hypertriglyceridemia with low high-density lipoprotein cholesterol by the novel compound NO-1886, a lipoprotein lipase-promoting agent, in STZ-diabetic rats. Diabetes 1995;44:414-17.

18. Shimada M, Ishibashi S, Gotoda T, et al. Overexpression of human lipoprotein lipase protects diabetic transgenic mice from diabetic hypertriglyceridemia and hypercholesterolemia. Arterioscler Thromb Vasc Biol 1995;15:1688-94.

19. Fan J, Wang J, Bensadoun A, et al. Overexpression of hepatic lipase in transgenic rabbits leads to a marked reduction of plasma high density lipoproteins and intermediate density lipoproteins. Proc Natl Acad Sci USA 1994;91:8724-28.

20. Assmann G, von Echardstein A, Funke H. High density lipoproteins, reverse cholesterol transport of cholesterol, and coronary artery disease. Insights from mutations. Circulation 1993;87(III):III-28-III-34.

21. Smith TD, Brinton EA, Breslow JL. Polymorphism in the human apolipoprotein A-I gene promoter region: association of the minor allele with decreased production rate in vivo and promoter activity *in vitro*. J Clin Invest 1992;89:1796-1800.

22. Malik S, Karathanasis S. Transcriptional activation by the orphan nuclear receptor ARP-1. Nucleic Acids Res 1995;23:1536-43.

23. Vu-Dac N, Schoojans K, Laine B, Fruchart JC, Auwerx J, Staels B. Negative regulation of the human apolipoprotein A-I promoter by fibrates can be attenuated by the interaction of the peroxisomal proliferator-activated receptor with its response elements. J Biol Chem 1994;269:31012-18.

OXIDATIVE MODIFICATION OF LDL: EPIDEMIOLOGIC AND CLINICAL CONSIDERATIONS

Daniel Steinberg
University of California, San Diego, Department of Medicine 0682, 9500 Gilman Drive, La Jolla, California 92093-0682, USA

Introduction

As discussed elsewhere in this Symposium [1], the hypothesis that oxidative modification of LDL plays an important role in the pathogenesis of atherosclerosis is strongly supported by a variety of experimental findings and by direct demonstration that antioxidants can inhibit atherogenesis in animal models of several kinds. Does it necessarily follow that appropriate antioxidant treatment of humans will slow the progression of their atherosclerosis? Maybe and maybe not. Let us begin by summarizing the evidence we have with respect to the role of oxidized LDL in the human disease.

EVIDENCE THAT OXIDATION OF LDL DOES INDEED TAKE PLACE IN HUMANS

Demonstration of oxidized LDL in extracts of human atheromata. LDL gently extracted from human arterial lesions, obtained either from organ donors or within a few hours of death, has many of the properties of oxidized LDL generated in *vitro* [2,3]. These include an increased electropheretic mobility, an increased hydrated density, and, most important, more rapid uptake by macrophages *in vitro* [4-6].

Demonstration of immunoreactive materials in human lesions using antibodies generated against oxidized LDL. At all stages from the fatty streak to the late, complicated lesion, antibodies against oxidized LDL react with materials in atherosclerotic lesions both experimental and human [2,3,7]. In some cases the modified LDL against which the antibody was raised has a reasonably well-defined structure. For example, malondialdehyde-treated LDL yields antibodies that are reactive with "epiptopes" in human lesions. However, the precise antigenic structure (and therefore the precise targets in the lesions) are not known with certainty because even treatment with malondialdehyde can generate a variety of derivatives, primary and secondary. It should also be pointed out that the presence of the "oxidized LDL" in a lesion does not necessarily mean that it was generated there. It could in theory have been generated elsewhere in the body and then been transported to the vessel.

A. M. Gotto, Jr. et al. (eds.), Drugs Affecting Lipid Metabolism, 581–589.

This seems unlikely for highly oxidized LDL in view of the extremely rapid uptake of extensively oxidized LDL (or acetyl LDL) into the liver. Minimally oxidized LDL (MM-LDL), on the other hand, because it is not recognized by scavenger receptors [8], would be expected to have a normal or even a longer than normal lifetime in the plasma and could easily be generated at any site of inflammation and transported through the plasma into developing lesions. Additional oxidation within the wall of the artery could then generate the materials recognized by antibodies against oxidized LDL.

Demonstration of autoantibodies against oxidized LDL in human plasma. Significant titers of autoantibodies against oxidized LDL have been found in the plasma of both normal subjects and patients with clinically evident atherosclerosis [3,9].

THE BASIC PATHOBIOLOGY OF HUMAN ATHEROGENESIS, AT LEAST UP TO FATTY STREAK FORMATION, APPEARS TO BE VERY CLOSELY SIMILAR TO THAT OF THE RABBIT AND THE NONHUMAN PRIMATE

The morphology and the early evolution of human lesions are closely mirrored by those of the most commonly used animal models of atherosclerosis [10-14]. The resemblance is less convincing in the later stages of lesion evolution. The levels of hyperlipoproteinemia needed to induce fatty streaks in animal models are in the same range as those that predispose to the human disease; the cellular composition of the lesions and the progressive changes that occur in them are very similar in the human and in the animal diseases. Thus it seems reasonable to extrapolate from the large body of evidence that oxidation is involved in fatty streak formation in the animal models and assume that the same will be true in the human disease.

A major caveat is that the time scale of the animal and of the human disease processes are quite different. Studies in animals are generally designed to produce lesions within weeks or months whereas the human disease evolves over decades. Conceivably, such an enormous quantitative difference could play itself out as a qualitative difference. Specifically, the effects of oxidized LDL (in generation of foam cells, in stimulation of cytokine release, cytotoxicity) may be much more important in the animal model systems where all of the events are compressed in time. In contrast, when the disease evolves very slowly over many decades, there may be time for "repair" or antiatherogenic processes of one kind or another which may make the impact of oxidized LDL much less important. Even if we discount this kind of difference we cannot rule out the possibility that other elements in the pathogenesis are sufficiently different so that antioxidants will work in animal models and yet not work in humans.

EPIDEMIOLOGIC DATA CORRELATING INTAKE OF ANTIOXIDANT VITAMINS AND A DECREASE IN CHD RISK

Negative correlations have been reported between CHD risk and estimated intake of vitamin E, beta carotene, vitamin C, and some other antioxidants. In other studies, tissue content or plasma levels of antioxidants have been taken as indicators of dietary habits and again negative correlations have been noted. However, not all epidemiologic studies have yielded such correlations (see ref [15] for review). In any case, epidemiologic correlation does not, of course, in itself constitute proof of a cause-and-effect relationship. Studies of this kind can be confounded. For example, persons with certain dietary habits (e.g. high intake of fruits and vegetables) may also be individuals who exercise regularly and who do not smoke cigarettes. Epidemiologic studies can at the most suggest hypotheses but it remains for appropriate clinical trials to determine whether the relationship is or is not causal.

INCREASING DIETARY INTAKE OF ANTIOXIDANTS DOES PROTECT CIRCULATING HUMAN LDL AGAINST *EX VIVO* OXIDATIVE MODIFICATION

The same antioxidants that have been shown to inhibit progression of atherosclerosis in animal models can protect human LDL against ex vivo oxidation. For example, probucol at the same doses used to lower lipid levels strongly protects circulating LDL against oxidative modification [16,17]. Administration of vitamin E supplements in doses above 100 to 200 units per day also confers protection although less striking than that seen in the case of probucol administration [18]. Beta carotene is frequently lumped together with vitamin E as an antioxidant. Actually it is rather different, being a very good trapper of singlet oxygen but far less effective than vitamin E as a chain-interrupting free radical trap at least at ambient oxygen tensions [19,20]. Reaven et al. [18,21] showed that administration of beta carotene to humans even at very high doses did not increase the resistance of circulating LDL to oxidative modification even though the LDL content of beta carotene was increased almost ten-fold and even when oxidation was determined at low oxygen tensions. Reaven's results are in conflict with those of Jialal et al. [22] but in accordance with those of van Hinsbergh et al. [23], Morel et al. [24], and Princen et al. [25]. While the extent of such studies is still limited, it is clear that one can achieve in humans the degree of protection afforded LDL in the animal studies using probucol or vitamin E. Thus clinical trials can be designed and carried out with the antioxidants available. An important question is whether or not the level of protection needed in humans will be greater than that needed in the animal studies because of the chronic, indolent progression of the human disease.

Another area of concern with respect to the clinical trials is the length of the studies, as discussed elsewhere [26]. The results of the animal studies tell us only that antioxidants can inhibit the initiation and progression of fatty streak lesions; they do not tell us whether antioxidants will have any effect on the progression of lesions during the later stages nor whether they will affect the probability of expression clinically. If antioxidants only affect initiation and progression of fatty streaks, then a trial based on clinical events would have to last much longer than the canonical five years in order to demonstrate a significant effect. This should be kept in mind in designing clinical endpoint trials. On the other hand, antioxidants may be more likely to have an effect on the appearance of new lesions or on the development of intima/media thickness in the common carotid artery, a measurement that correlates well with more advanced lesions in the coronary bed.

Clinical Trials of Antioxidants

Over the past five years there have been several reports of clinical trials in which antioxidants have been administered and in which cardiovascular events have been recorded. None of these, however, was designed with coronary heart disease as a primary end point. Most of them were designed to test the question of whether antioxidants might reduce risks of cancer. The only exception is the Swedish PQRST study [27] designed to test whether probucol (through its cholesterol-lowering effect or its antioxidant effect or both) could influence the progression of femoral atherosclerosis assessed angiographically. The clinical trial results reported thus far are briefly summarized below with some comments on their interpretation.

The Physicians' Health Study

This study was begun in 1983 with more than 22,000 participating physicians to test the efficacy of aspirin in the primary prevention of cardiovascular disease and the efficacy of beta carotene in the primary prevention of cancer. Aspirin proved to be highly effective and was discontinued early because of a clearly positive result. The beta carotene arm (50 mg every other day) was continued. In 1990 Gaziano et al. [28] analyzed the results in a subset of 333 men who had had evidence of coronary heart disease (CHD) at the time they entered the study. Pre-existing CHD was an exclusion criterion but somehow these men were entered into the study and followed (although presumably not constituting a part of the formal data base for the central study). The analysis of this subset showed a 54% reduction in risk of major coronary events (nonfatal myocardial infarction, fatal CHD, or coronary revascularization; P = 0.014). The full cohort was continued on beta-carotene until near the end of 1995. The results have not yet been formally published but a press conference was held early in 1996 to announce that the results of the full study showed no effect of beta carotene either on cancer or on CHD. At the same press conference it was reported that the results of the CARET study (Carotene And Retinol Efficacy Trial), a test of the efficacy of beta carotene and vitamin A in prevention of cancer in chronic smokers or men with asbestos exposure, were also negative. The latter study involved over 17,000 men followed for up to nine years [29]. In the CARET study there was enough of a suggestion of a harmful effect from beta carotene supplementation that the NIH has recommended deletion of beta carotene from ongoing clinical trials until the data can be more definitely evaluated.

The CARET Trial (see above)

The Alpha-Tocopherol, Beta Carotene (ATBC) Cancer Prevention Study

The Alpha-Tocopherol, Beta Carotene (ATBC) Cancer Prevention Study [30] was designed to test whether alpha-tocopherol, beta carotene, or a combination of the two would reduce incidence of lung cancer and other cancers. Over 29,000 heavy smokers (20 cigarettes per day for 36 years on average) were followed for a period of five to eight years. Neither beta carotene nor vitamin E reduced incidence of either lung cancer or any other cancers (with the possible exception of a slightly reduced number of cases of prostrate cancer in those taking alpha-tocopherol). Actually there was a suggestive increase in incidence of lung cancer in the men receiving beta carotene. While not a primary end point, deaths from ischemic heart disease and other cardiovascular diseases were recorded. Neither beta carotene nor alpha-tocopherol had any significant effect.

Several points should be noted about this study. First, the dose of vitamin E (50 mg daily) is far below that needed to confer significant protection on LDL against *ex vivo* oxidative modification. Studies by Reaven et al. [18,31], by Esterbauer et al. [32], and by Jialal et al. [33] show that supplements must be at least 200 mg daily to effect significant protection against oxidation and that the effectiveness increases progressively with doses up to 800 mg daily. Thus this study did not represent an adequate test of the efficacy of vitamin E as an antioxidant in prevention of CHD. The dose of beta carotene (20 mg daily), on the other hand, was very similar to the dose used in the Physicians' Health Study (50 mg every other day). This dose is enough to increase plasma beta carotene levels many-fold, yet direct studies show that, despite the marked increase in beta carotene content of LDL, the LDL is not protected against *ex vivo* oxidation at these levels of beta carotene [18,21].

With respect to the absence of an effect on lung cancer it should be noted that these men had been heavy smokers for more than 30 years in most cases. Our current understanding of carcinogenesis is that it entails multiple hits. The "trigger reaction" that laid the groundwork for lung cancer in these men may have occurred years ago, long before the antioxidant intervention was initiated. In other words intervention with vitamin E was both "too little" and "too late."

Despite these limitations and qualifications of the interpretation, the negative results with respect to CHD in the beta carotene arm, together with the negative results of the Physicians' Health Study and the failure of beta carotene supplementation to protect LDL against oxidation call for a complete reevaluation of beta carotene as an antioxidant.

THE PROBUCOL QUANTITATIVE REGRESSION SWEDISH TRIAL (PQRST)

This study in 303 patients with angiographically confirmed femoral atherosclerosis was designed to determine whether probucol would slow disease progression as assessed by repeated femoral angiography [27]. All of the subjects were treated with cholestyramine and half were randomized either to placebo or to probucol, 0.5 gm twice daily. Probucol treatment lowered total serum cholesterol by 12%, LDL cholesterol by 12%, and HDL cholesterol by 24% compared to the values in subjects receiving cholestyramine only. Over the three-year period of observation probucol did not have any significant favorable effect on progression of the disease, assessed in terms of changes in total angiographically determined volume of a defined segment of the femoral artery.

The design of this study called for all candidate subjects to participate in a pre-randomization trial on cholestyramine (8-16 gm daily) for two months after which probucol (0.5 gm twice daily) was added. Only subjects who showed more than an 8% decrease in total cholesterol on cholestyramine and then at least an additional 8% change upon addition of probucol were eligible for randomization. Because of this design, both the "placebo" group (actually, the "cholestyramine only" group) and the "active" group (the "cholestyramine plus probucol group") showed a marked decrease in total and LDL cholesterol compared to the pre-randomization levels on no treatment. The total cholesterol in the "placebo" group was about 22% below the pre-randomization level and it was 35% lower in the "active drug" group. LDL cholesterol levels were also 25 to 30% lower than pre-randomization values in both groups. In other words, in both groups the vessel wall was exposed during the study to cholesterol levels well below the pre-trial values. Over the three years the mean lumen volume in the "placebo" group actually increased by 4.2% ($p < 0.001$). It also increased in the "probucol" group but only by 0.6% ($p = 0.61$). Perhaps the most striking difference between the two groups was the expected large fall in HDL cholesterol due to probucol (20 to 30% below pre-randomization values) while the "placebo" group had only marginal changes in HDL cholesterol.

Several difficult questions arise in connection with this study. By its design the study could not detect changes in early lesions. Early lesions would contribute only minimally to the restriction of lumen volume and changes in early lesions would contribute little or nothing to any observed overall changes in lumen volume. In other words, even a significant reduction in the size of a set of small lesions would only minimally influence the overall volume of the measured segment. Second, femoral lesions in humans are the most advanced (just the opposite of the situation in rabbits) and therefore less likely to show regression. As mentioned above, the only thing the animal model studies tell us so far is that probucol and other antioxidants can slow the initiation and progression of fatty streak lesions. All of the patients in this study were followed for three years with total cholesterol levels and LDL cholesterol levels well below those that had characterized them for the preceding decades. While it is true that the levels in the cholestyramine-only group were not as low as those in the probucol plus cholestyramine group, those differences were less striking than the differences between the pre-randomization values and the study values. Nevertheless, if probucol were effective through its antioxidant activity, one should have expected a difference. It was shown explicitly that the LDL from the probucol-treated subjects was significantly protected against *ex vivo* oxidative modification [34]. In summary, the study fails to show an effect of probucol on the basis of its antioxidant activity when tested with respect to progression/regression of advanced femoral arterial lesions. The marked drop in HDL cholesterol may be relevant but we do not have enough evidence to conclude that. Other studies have shown xanthoma regression in probucol-treated patients even in the face of markedly lower HDL levels [35]. In fact, the regression of xanthomas appeared in this study to be positively correlated with the decrease in HDL cholesterol levels in that study.

Are We Doing the Right Thing?

As I have discussed in detail elsewhere [26], the intervention trials to test the efficacy of antioxidant treatment may or may not be properly designed. The advice of the group assembled by the National Heart Lung and Blood Institute to discuss the question of clinical intervention trials was to limit them initially to the use of natural antioxidants because they are less likely to cause deleterious side effects [36]. Whether or not they give sufficient protection against oxidative modification of LDL in humans is not really known. Certainly they do confer a reasonably high level of protection but not as high as that conferred, for example, by probucol. As discussed above, we know really very little about the level of protection against atherogenesis, on the one hand, and the level of protection of LDL against *ex vivo* oxidation, on the other hand, even in animal models let alone in humans.

At the moment there is no direct evidence that antioxidants influence the later stages of atherogenesis, specifically the events that lead to the fatal thrombosis, although in theory there are ways that they might. Consequently, the clinical event trials may not be properly designed. If the effects of antioxidants are indeed limited to initiation and early progression of lesions, with no effects on the late, clinically important events, it may take longer than the canonical five years to see an impact on clinical event rates. It is true that intervention through drastically lowered LDL levels has an impact on event rates well within five years but the evidence becomes increasingly strong that these early effects relate not to regression of stenosis but to stabilization of unstable plaques. Whether or not antioxidants also have such an effect is not known. Finally, the epidemiologic evidence is strongest for a correlation with antioxidant vitamin intake in the form of fruits and vegetables. Individual antioxidant supplements may or may not be effective in isolation.

Summary

Because antioxidants have been effective in slowing the progression of experimental atherosclerosis does not necessarily mean that antioxidants will be effective in the human disease, for reasons discussed above. At the same time, there is a very good possibility that they may be effective and so the clinical trials must go on. The design of these clinical trials should draw on those things we have learned from the animal studies. Specifically, they should include and stress the measurement of early lesions either by direct assessment (e.g. carotid intima/media thickness progression) or by following the cohort long enough to allow the effects of the antioxidants to begin to show an impact on event rate. The negative results of clinical event trials reported thus far do not disprove the oxidative modification hypotheses. Most were not designed with coronary heart disease or atherosclerosis as a primary end point and the patient populations may not have been appropriate. Nevertheless, these negative results suggest that antioxidants may not have an enormous impact on atherogenesis or events and that the trial designs may have to be very carefully crafted to see smaller effects.

References

1. Steinberg D. Oxidized LDL, its receptors, and its role in atherosclerosis. In: Gotto AM, Jr., Paoletti R, Smith LC, Catapano AL, editors. Drugs Affecting Lipid Metabolism. Dordrecht, The Netherlands: Kluwer Academic Publishers, 1996: in press.
2. Yla-Herttuala S, Palinski W, Rosenfeld ME, et al. Evidence for the presence of oxidatively modified low density lipoprotein in atherosclerotic lesions of rabbit and man. J Clin Invest

1989;84:1086-95.

3. Yla-Herttuala S, Palinski W, Rosenfeld ME, Steinberg D, Witztum JL. Lipoproteins in normal and atherosclerotic aorta. Eur Heart J 1990;11(E):88-99.
4. Henriksen T, Mahoney EM, Steinberg D. Enhanced macrophage degradation of low density lipoprotein previously incubated with cultured endothelial cells: Recognition by receptors for acetylated low density lipoproteins. Proc Natl Acad Sci USA 1981;78:6499-503.
5. Henriksen T, Mahoney EM, Steinberg D. Interactions of plasma lipoproteins with endothelial cells. Ann N Y Acad Sci 1982;401:102-16.
6. Henriksen T, Mahoney EM, Steinberg D. Enhanced macrophage degradation of biologically modified low density lipoprotein. Arteriosclerosis 1983;3:149-59.
7. Haberland ME, Fong D, Cheng L. Malondialdehyde-altered protein occurs in atheroma of Watanabe heritable hyperlipidemic rabbits. Science 1988;241:215-18.
8. Berliner JA, Schwartz DS, Territo MC, et al. Induction of chemotactic cytokines by minimally oxidized LDL. Adv Exp Med Biol 1993;351:13-18.
9. Palinski W, Rosenfeld ME, Yla-Herttuala S, et al. Low density lipoprotein undergoes oxidative modification in vivo. Proc Natl Acad Sci USA 1989;86:1372-76.
10. Witmer-Pack MD, Veselinovitch D. Experimental models of human atherosclerosis. Ann NY Acad Sci 1968;149:907-22.
11. Faggiotto A, Ross R, Harker L. Studies of hypercholesterolemia in the nonhuman primate. I. Changes that lead to fatty streak formation. Arteriosclerosis 1984;4:323-40.
12. Faggiotto A, Ross R. Studies of hypercholesterolemia in the nonhuman primate. II. Fatty streak conversion to fibrous plaque. Arteriosclerosis 1984;4:341-56.
13. Rosenfeld ME, Tsukada T, Chait A, Bierman EL, Gown AM, Ross R. Fatty streak expansion and maturation in Watanabe heritable hyperlipemic and comparably hypercholesterolemic fat-fed rabbits. Arteriosclerosis 1987;7:24-34.
14. Tsukuda T, Rosenfeld M, Ross R, Gown AM. Immunocytochemical analysis of cellular components in atherosclerotic lesions. Use of monoclonal antibodies with the Watanabe and fat-fed rabbit. Arteriosclerosis 1986;6:601-13.
15. Jha P, Flather M, Lonn E, Farkouh M, Yusuf S. The antioxidant vitamins and cardiovascular disease. A critical review of epidemiologic and clinical trial data [see comments]. Ann Intern Med 1995;123:860-72.
16. Parthasarathy S, Young SG, Witztum JL, Pittman RC, Steinberg D. Probucol inhibits oxidative modification of low density lipoprotein. J Clin Invest 1986;77:641-44.
17. Reaven PD, Parthasarathy S, Beltz WF, Witztum JL. Effect of probucol dosage on plasma lipid and lipoprotein levels and on protection of low density lipoprotein against in vitro oxidation in humans. Arterioscler Thromb 1992;12:318-24.
18. Reaven PD, Khouw A, Beltz WF, Parthasarathy S, Witztum JL. Effect of dietary antioxidant combinations in humans. Protection of LDL by vitamin E but not by beta-carotene. Arterioscler Thromb 1993;13:590-600.
19. Krinsky NI. Antioxidant functions of carotenoids. Free Radical Biology and Medicine 1989;7: 617-35.
20. Stocker R, Yamamoto Y, McDonagh AF, Glazer AN, Ames BN. Bilirubin is an antioxidant of possible physiological importance. Science 1987;235:1043-46.
21. Reaven PD, Ferguson E, Navab M, Powell FL. Susceptibility of human LDL to oxidative modification. Effects of variations in beta-carotene concentration and oxygen tension. Arterioscler Thromb 1994;14:1162-69.
22. Jialal I, Norkus EP, Cristol L, Grundy SM. Beta-carotene inhibits the oxidative modification

of low-density lipoprotein. Biochim Biophys Acta 1991;1086:134-38.
23. van Hinsbergh VW, Scheffer M, Havekes L, Kempen HJ. Role of endothelial cells and their products in the modification of low-density lipoproteins. Biochim Biophys Acta 1986;878:49-64.
24. Morel DW, Hessler JR, Chisolm GM. Low density lipoprotein cytotoxicity induced by free radical peroxidation of lipid. J Lipid Res 1983;24:1070-76.
25. Princen HMG, VanPoppel G, Vogelezang C. Supplementation with vitamin E but not beta-carotene protects low density lipoprotein from lipid peroxidation in vitro: Effects of cigarette smoking. Arterioscler Thromb 1992;12:554-62.
26. Steinberg D. Clinical trials of antioxidants in atherosclerosis: Are we doing the right thing? Lancet 1995;346:36-38.
27. Walldius G, Erikson U, Olsson AG, et al. The effect of probucol on femoral atherosclerosis: the probucol quantitative regression Swedish trial (PQRST). Am J Card 1994;74:875-83.
28. Gaziano JM, Manson JE, Ridker PM, Buring JE, Hennekens CH. Beta Carotene Therapy for Chronic Stable Angina. Circulation 1990;82:III-201
29. Thornquist MD, Omenn GS, Goodman GE, et al. Statistical design and monitoring of the Carotene and Retinol Efficacy Trial (CARET). Controlled Clinical Trials 1993;14:308-24.
30. Alpha-Tocopherol, Beta-Carotene Cancer Prevention Study Group. The effect of vitamin E and beta-carotene on the incidence of lung cancer and other cancers in male smokers. N Engl J Med 1994;330:1029-35.
31. Reaven PD, Witztum JL. Comparison of supplementation of RRR-alpha-tocopherol and racemic alpha-tocopherol in humans. Effects on lipid levels and lipoprotein susceptibility to oxidation. Arterioscler Thromb 1993;13:601-608.
32. Dieber-Rotheneder M, Puhl H, Waeg G, Striegl G, Esterbauer H. Effect of oral supplementation with D-alpha-tocopherol on the vitamin E content of human low density lipoproteins and resistance to oxidation. J Lipid Res 1991;32:1325-32.
33. Jialal I, Grundy SM. Effect of combined supplementation with alpha-tocopherol, ascorbate, and beta carotene on low-density lipoprotein oxidation [see comments]. Circulation 1993;88:2780-86.
34. Regnstrom J, Walldius G, Carlson LA, Nilsson J. Effect of probucol treatment on the susceptibility of low density lipoprotein isolated from hypercholesterolemic patients to become oxidatively modified in vitro. Atherosclerosis 1990;82:43-51.
35. Yamamoto A, Matsuzawa Y, Yokoyama S, Funahashi T, Yamamura T, Kishino B. Effects of probucol on xanthomata regression in familial hypercholesterolemia. Am J Cardiol 1986;57:29H-35H.
36. Steinberg D. Antioxidants in the prevention of human atherosclerosis. Summary of the proceedings of a National Heart, Lung, and Blood Institute Workshop: September 5-6, 1991, Bethesda, Maryland. Circulation 1992;85:2337-44.

REBOUND CURVE FOLLOWING LDL-APHERESIS REFLECTS CATABOLIC RATE OF PLASMA CHOLESTEROL AND THE SYNTHETIC RATE OF LP(a)

Mariko Harada-Shiba, Taku Yamamura, Yasushi Toyota, Motoo Tsushima, Shunichi Kojima*, and Akira Yamamoto
*National Cardiovascular Center Research Institute, 5-7-1 Fujishiro-Dai, Suita, Osaka 565, Japan, and *National Tosei Hospital, 762-1 Nagasawa, Shimizu-cho, Shunto-gun, Shizuoka 411, Japan*

Introduction

Hypercholesterolemia is one of the major risk factors for atherosclerosis. In order to prevent the development of atherosclerosis, there have been many attempts to reduce plasma cholesterol levels including antilipidemic drugs, LDL-apheresis, and liver transplantation. The development of LDL-apheresis has enabled us to reduce plasma cholesterol levels to an extremely low level even in homozygotes and in severe cases of heterozygotes with familial hypercholesterolemia (FH). We have already reported that the repeated treatment of LDL-apheresis was useful not only in the prevention of progression of atherosclerosis, but also in some cases, could achieve regression of atheromatous lesions [1].

Plasma cholesterol levels decreased within one operation of LDL-apheresis, but increased again by the next one. The rebound after LDL-apheresis is different from one individual to another among the homozygous and heterozygous cases probably due to the difference in expression of the residual activity of the LDL-receptor. Unless there is a proper way to suppress the rebound, it is necessary to repeat the operation more frequently for the purpose of increasing the efficiency of the treatment. To determine the appropriate interval of the operation and also to evaluate the effect of the apheresis in comparison to the drug treatment in heterozygous cases, we have established a noninvasive method for estimating cholesterol kinetics using the rebound curves of plasma cholesterol levels following LDL-apheresis treatment [2]. The kinetics of cholesterol were analyzed by the application of a two-compartment model. The adequacy of the kinetic parameters for cholesterol obtained by this method was examined by comparing these values with the urinary excretion rate of mevalonate, an intermediate on the biosynthesis of cholesterol. Since the synthetic rate of cholesterol was significantly correlated with the urinary mevalonate excretion rate, it was suggested that the calculated values were appropriate.

Lp(a) has also been reported to be a strong atherogenic factor independent of LDL. It was reported that Lp(a) has an affinity to LDL receptors *in vitro* [3], and is catabolized

A. M. Gotto, Jr. et al. (eds.), Drugs Affecting Lipid Metabolism, 591–597.

via LDL receptors *in vivo* [4]. However, homozygous patients for FH do not always have high levels of serum Lp(a) whereas normolipidemic individuals sometimes have high levels of Lp(a). It is still not clear which factors determine serum levels of Lp(a). While Lp(a) is removed by LDL-apheresis, we also analyzed the kinetics of Lp(a) using the rebound curves.

Materials and Methods

PATIENTS

Four homozygous patients with FH, 8 heterozygous patients, and one healthy volunteer were enrolled in this study. The homozygous FH patients were diagnosed by their LDL receptor activity in cultured fibroblasts, and all of them belonged to the LDL-receptor negative type. The heterozygous FH patients were diagnosed by their plasma cholesterol levels, family history, and the thickness of their Achilles tendons.

LDL-APHERESIS

To remove LDL from the plasma by LDL-apheresis, one of the two techniques was used, double-membrane filtration method or the LDL-absorption method [5]. Plasma cholesterol and Lp(a) levels were determined by the enzymatic method and the latex method, respectively, for more than at least 10 times during the 14 days following the LDL-apheresis operation.

KINETIC ANALYSIS

To estimate the kinetics for cholesterol and Lp(a), the time courses of the plasma cholesterol and Lp(a) were analyzed applying the two-compartment model (Figure1). The model demonstrates that cholesterol and Lp(a), flow into the plasma at a rate R (production rate), are cleared from the plasma at a rate k (fractional catabolic rate, FCR), and exchange between the plasma and tissue pools at rates k_{12} and k_{21}. The quantitative relations are expressed as follows:

$$dC_1/dt=R/V_1-(k+k_{12})C_1+k_{21}C_2$$
$$dC_2/dt=k_{21}(C_1-C_2)$$

C_1 is the concentration of plasma substrate and C_2 is the concentration of substrate in the tissue. V_1 is the plasma volume. Each parameter was calculated by the nonlinear regression program of the Multi-Runge-Kutta-Gill as described [6].

MEASUREMENT OF URINARY MEVALONATE EXCRETION RATE

Urine samples were taken by every 24 hours and collected under acidic conditions, and stored at -20° C. The urine samples were neutralized with 6 N NaOH and absorbed by an ion-exchange resin. The mevalonate was eluted with 0.1 N formic acid and quantified by gas chromatography-mass spectrometry.

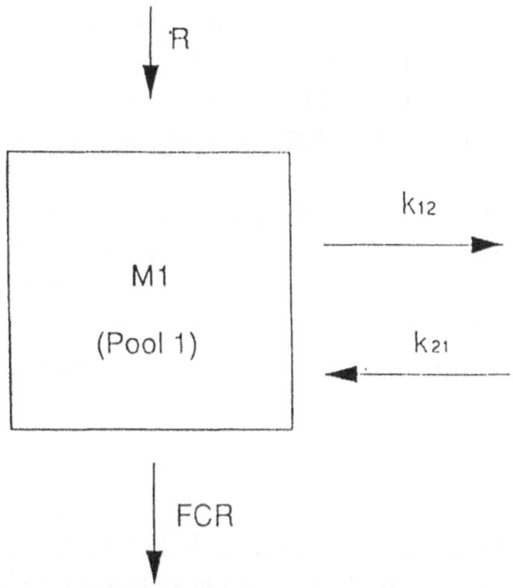

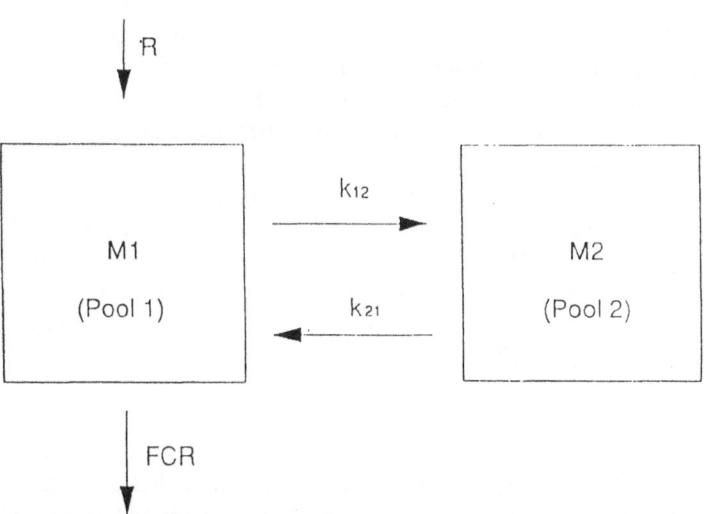

Figure 1. Schema of two-compartment model. Pool 1 is the intravascular (plasma) substrate, and pool 2 is the extravascular substrate pool. M1 and M2 demonstrate the size of pools 1 and 2, respectively. R is the production rate of substrate. k shows the fractional catabolic rate (FCR). k_{12} and k_{21} are substrate transfer rates between pool 1 and 2.

Results

The FCR of cholesterol FH was 0.206 $\pm$ 0.060 pools/day (mean $\pm$ SD) in heterozygous patients with FH, (0.160 $\pm$ 0.074 pools/day) in homozygous patients, and (0.262 pools/day) in the control subject. The FCR of cholesterol in the homozygous patients in FH was significantly lower than that of the heterozygous patients, indicating that the degradation pathway is more severely disturbed in homozygous patients than in heterozygous patients. The production rates of cholesterol in heterozygous patients were 21.9 $\pm$ 5.1 mg/kg/day, which were significantly lower than that of the homozygous patients (30.8 $\pm$ 7.5). These values were in good agreement with the data in a previous report obtained by use of isotope labeled-lipoproteins [7]. The production rates of cholesterol were significantly correlated to urinary mevalonate excretion rates (r = 0.69), which were reported to be a good marker for the intrinsic cholesterol synthesis. These results suggest that our method is useful for the estimation of cholesterol kinetics.

The expressed plasma cholesterol levels were calculated by simulation using parameters obtained from the observed rebound curves in 2 heterozygous FH patients (HT and TF). The simulation values fit well with the actual levels (Figures 2 [a] and [b]). In HT, the integral average of the plasma cholesterol level was 180 mg/dl on the 3rd day after the procedure, and 250 mg/dl on the 9th day. Assuming that the extraction of plasma cholesterol is achieved more intensively with the postapheresis level 80 mg/dl, the calculated cholesterol level was 200 mg/dl on the 6th day, and 250 on the 12th day.

Lp(a) is also removed by LDL-apheresis. The plasma Lp(a) levels increased more rapidly and reached the steady state earlier than cholesterol, indicating that the kinetics of Lp(a) are quite difference from that of cholesterol. The FCR of Lp(a) in each patients had not correlation with that of cholesterol (r = 0.28). The production rates of Lp(a) in each patients had no correlation with that of cholesterol. These results suggest that Lp(a) has its own metabolic pathway independent of LDL.

In order to study which factors determine the plasma Lp(a) levels, the kinetic parameters were compared with plasma Lp(a) levels which were measured in a period without treatment. The Lp(a) levels were not correlated with their FCR (f = 0.29), but were significantly correlated with their production rate (r = 0.76). This suggests that the production rate of Lp(a), rather than the degradation rate, is the major factor that determines plasma Lp(a) levels.

Discussion

Several methods have been reported for the measurement of cholesterol kinetics. Among these, tracer studies by use of isotope-labeled lipoproteins have been thought to be the most effective. However, it is very difficult to perform this kind of study in Japan. We established a method for estimating cholesterol kinetics from the rebound curve of cholesterol following LDL-apheresis treatment. We chose a two-compartment model as a model for cholesterol kinetics. Because Bilheimer et al. reported that after injection of isotope labeled LDL [7], the decay curve was biphasic. This shows that two or more compartments are required for the cholesterol kinetic model. In order to simulate the changes in concentration of substrate, the more the number of parameters are used, the better the curve fits. However, as the number of parameters increases, the reliability of each parameter decreases. Therefore, it is best to find the least number of parameters that fit the curve well. We calculated the index based on "an information criterion" [8], for each person and the index values were lowest in the two-compartment model (data not shown). The two-compartment model seems to be the most appropriate model for cholesterol kinetics.

We determined the production rate and FCR of cholesterol as a constant value, R and k, respectively (Figure 1). The production rate and FCR were assumed to be constant by this model, despite the change in the pool size of cholesterol by LDL-apheresis.

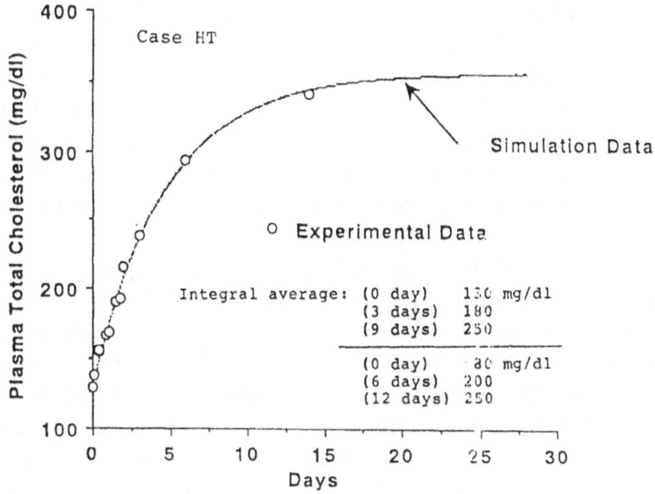

2a

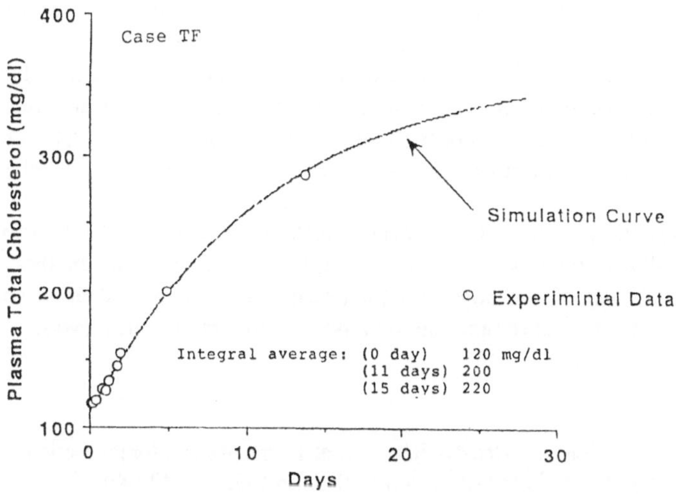

2b

Figure 2. The simulation curves and actual levels of plasma cholesterol following LDL-apheresis. Total plasma cholesterol levels were determined following LDL-apheresis treatment shown as dots. Simulated curves were shown as lines. (a) Heterozygous patient for FH (HT). (b) Heterozygous patient for FH (TF).

Thompson et al. reported that the degradation rate of cholesterol had no correlation to its pool size in homozygous and heterozygous patients of FH [9]. Souter et al. reported that the synthetic rate of Apo B is not affected by an operation of LDL-apheresis [10]. These reports suggest that the model of Figure 1 is appropriate for the kinetics of cholesterol. The parameters obtained here were close to the value studied by Bilheimer using isotope-labeled lipoproteins. The calculated values of the production rate of cholesterol were significantly correlated with the urinary mevalonate excretion rates. These results suggest that the calculated values reflected well the *in vivo* state.

Lp(a), known as one of the atherogenic lipoproteins, has been a matter of interest. Lp(a) contains apo B combined with apo (a) by disulfide bond. It is not clear whether Lp(a) is metabolized via LDL receptors or not. It has been reported that Lp(a) is bound to and internalized and degraded by fibroblasts and HepG2 cells via LDL receptors [11,12]. Utermann reported that the patients with FH had higher serum Lp(a) levels in all the phenotypes of Lp(a) [13]. This suggested that LDL receptors are somewhat involved in the metabolism of Lp(a). Hypocholesterolemic drugs, such as cholestyramine or HMG-CoA reductase inhibitors, decrease serum cholesterol levels by increasing LDL receptor activity. These drugs have no effect on serum levels of Lp(a) [14,15]. Rhesus monkey which had a defect in its LDL receptors had the same levels of Lp(a) [16]. These reports suggest that the LDL pathway is not a major pathway in the metabolism of Lp(a).

The pattern of the rebound curve of Lp(a) following LDL-apheresis is completely different from that of cholesterol, and the calculated degradation rates of Lp(a) and cholesterol had no correlation between each other. These results suggest that the major metabolic pathways of Lp(a) and cholesterol are different. Serum Lp(a) levels did not correlate with degradation rates. They did however correlate with their production rates. Therefore, serum Lp(a) levels appear to be determined by their production rates. These results were in good agreement with the report by Rader in which isotope labeled Lp(a) was used.

In this paper, we reported a noninvasive method for estimating cholesterol and Lp(a) kinetics by analyzing rebound curves following LDL-apheresis. This method is useful in deciding the interval of the apheresis treatment and also in evaluating the effect of antilipidemic drugs on suppressing the rebound of serum cholesterol levels.

References

1. Yamamoto A, Kojima S, Harada-Shiba M, et al. Plasmapheresis for prevention and regression of coronary atherosclerosis. Ann New York Acad 1995;748:429-40.
2. Harada-Shiba M, Tajima S, Miyake Y, et al. Siblings with normal LDL receptor activity and severe hypercholesterolemia. Arterioscl Throm 12;1071-78.
3. Armstrong VW, Walli AK, Seidel D, et al. Isolation, characterization and uptake in human fibroblasts of an apo(a)-free lipoprotein obtained on reduction of lipoprotein (a). J Lipid Res 1985;26:1314-23.
4. Krempler F, Kostner GM, Roscher A, et al. Studies on the rate of specific cell surface receptors in the removal of the lipoprotein (a) in man. J Clin Invest 1983;71:1431-41.
5. Yokoyama S, Hayashi R, Satani M, Yamamoto A. Selective removal of low density

lipoprotein by plasmapheresis in familial hypercholesterolemia. Arteriosclerosis 1985;5:613-22.
6. Yamaoka K, et al. A nonlinear least squares program based on differential equations, MULTI (RUNGE), for microcomputers. J Pharmacodyn 1983;6:595-606.
7. Bilheimer DW, Stone NJ, Grundy SM. Metabolic studies in familial hypercholesterolemia, evidence for a gene-dosage effect in vivo. J Clin Invest 1979;64:524-533.
8. Akaike H. A new look at the statistical model identification. IEEE Trans Automat Contr 1974;19:716-23.
9. Thompson GR, Myant NB. Low density lipoprotein turnover in familial hypercholesterolemia after plasma exchange. Atheroscl 1976;23:371-77.
10. Souter AK, Myant NB, Thompson GR. Metabolism of apoplipoprotein B containing lipoprotein in familial hypercholesterolaemia. Atheroscl 1979;32: 315-27.
11. Steyrer E, Kostner GM. Interaction of lipoprotein Lp(a) with the B/E-receptor: A study using isolated adrenal cortex and human fibroblast receptors. J Lipid Res 1990;31:1247-53.
12. Williams KJ, Fless GM, Petrie ML, et al. Mechanisms by which lipoprotein lipase alters cellular metabolism of lipoprotein(a), low density lipoprotein, and nascent lipoproteins. Roles for low density lipoprotein receptors and heparan sulfate proteoglycans. J Biol Chem 1992; 267:13284-92.
13. Vessby B, Kostner GM, Lithell H, et al. Diverging effects of cholestyramine on apolipoprotein B and lipoprotein Lp(a). A dose-response study of the effects of cholestyramine in hypercholesterolemia. Atheroscl 1982;44:61-71.
14. Kostner GM, Gavish D, Leopold B, et al. HMG CoA reductase inhibitors lower LDL cholesterol without reducing Lp(a) levels. Circulation 1989;80:1313-19.
15. Neven L, Khalil A, Pfaffinger D, et al. Rhesus monkey model of familial hyper-cholesterolemia: Relation between plasma Lp(a) levels, apo(a) isoforms, and LDL-receptor function. J Lipid Res 1990;31:633-43.
16. Rader DJ, Cain W, Tally G, et al. The inverse association of plasma lipoprotein (a) concentrations with apolipoprotein(a) isoform size is not due to differences in Lp(a) catabolism but to differences in production rate. J Clin Invest 1994;93:2758-63.

ENZYMES AND PROTEINS THAT ARE ASSOCIATED WITH HIGH DENSITY LIPOPROTEIN AND THEIR ROLE IN THE ANTI-INFLAMMATORY CAPACITY OF HDL

Susan Y. Hama, Trung Nguyen, Thao Nguyen, Gregg C. Fonarow, Davis C. Drinkwater, Hillel Laks*, Mohamad Navab, and Alan M. Fogelman
Divisions of Cardiology and Cardio-thoracic Surgery, School of Medicine, University of California, Los Angeles, California 90095-1679, USA*

In population studies the risk for an atherosclerotic event is very strongly and inversely related to high density lipoprotein (HDL) levels [1]. However, individual patients often deviate from the prediction. Some patients with normal levels of HDL have severe coronary artery disease and conversely, some patients with low levels of HDL never develop clinically significant coronary artery disease. The role of HDL in preventing atherosclerosis has long been thought to be due to its role in reverse cholesterol transport. Recent evidence from Rothblat's laboratory is consistent with this hypothesis when the results from a whole population are considered [2]. However, Rothblat and colleagues noted that there was often individual variation of a substantial degree that deviated from the prediction. Moreover, over the range of nearly a four-fold difference in HDL levels there was only about a half-fold difference in cholesterol efflux (50% versus 400%) [2]. Thus, there remains the possibility that certain properties of HDL other than its ability to promote cholesterol efflux may play a role in its protective effect. A role for oxidation of low density lipoprotein (LDL) lipids in the development of atherosclerotic lesions has been firmly established over the past 15 years [3-7] and a role for lipid oxidation in the causation of plaque rupture and thrombosis has recently been suggested [8]. HDL has been found to protect against the oxidation of LDL by metal ions *in vitro* [9,10] and was found to prevent the production of mildly oxidized LDL by artery wall cells in co-culture [11]. However, HDL obtained either from patients undergoing surgery or after myocardial infarction in which apolipoprotein AI was displaced from the HDL by the acute phase reactant, serum amyloid A, were not only not protective against LDL modification but actually enhanced LDL modification by the co-cultures [12]. Two enzyme systems associated with normal HDL have been reported to inhibit the oxidation of LDL *in vitro*. Stafforini and colleagues [13] reported that the platelet activating factor acetylhydrolase (PAF hydrolase) was effective in preventing metal ion-dependent oxidation of LDL. Mackness and colleagues [14] reported that a second enzyme associated with HDL, paraoxonase, also inhibited LDL oxidation *in vitro*. Both of these enzymes have been found to protect against LDL modification in the co-culture system

A. M. Gotto, Jr. et al. (eds.), Drugs Affecting Lipid Metabolism, 599–601.

[15,16]. Thus, the inverse relationship between risk for atherosclerotic events and HDL levels may be due to enzymes associated with HDL that protect against LDL oxidation as well as the putative role of HDL in reverse cholesterol transport. Moreover, since these enzymes are associated with only a small fraction of HDL particles, this may, in part, explain why some patients with low levels of total HDL cholesterol may not have clinically significant atherosclerosis and others with relatively normal levels of HDL cholesterol may have premature atherosclerosis.

We suggest that the inverse correlation of high density lipoproteins with risk for atherosclerotic disease is at least partly due to enzymes and proteins that are associated with HDL subpopulations that are antioxidant or pro-oxidant in nature.

References

1. Gordon DJ, Probstfield JL, Garrison RJ, et al. High density lipoprotein cholesterol and cardiovascular disease. Circulation 1989;79:8-15.
2. de la Llera Moya M, Atger V, Paul JL, et al. A cell culture system for screening human serum for ability to promote cellular cholesterol efflux. Relations between serum components and efflux, esterification, and transfer. Arterioscler Thromb 1994;14:1056-65.
3. Steinberg D, Parthasarathy S, Carew TE, Khoo JC, Witztum JL. Beyond cholesterol. Modifications of low density lipoproteins that increase its atherogenicity. N Engl J Med 1989;320:915-24.
4. Witztum JL, Steinberg D. Role of oxidized low density lipoprotein in atherogenesis. J Clin Invest 1991;88:1785-92.
5. Parthasarathy S. Modified lipoproteins in the pathogenesis of atherosclerosis. R.G. Landes Co.: Austin, TX, 1994:91-119.
6. Witztum JL. The oxidation hypothesis of atherosclerosis. Lancet 1994;344:793-95.
7. Young SG, Parathasarthy S. Why are low density lipoproteins atherogenic? West J Med 1994;160:153-64.
8. Berliner JA, Navab M, Fogelman AM, et al. Atherosclerosis: Basic Mechanisms. Oxidation, inflammation, and genetics. Circulation 1995;in press.
9. Hessler JR, Robertson AL, Jr, Chisolm GM. LDL-induced cytotoxicity and its inhibition by HDL in human vascular smooth muscle and endothelial cells in culture. Atherosclerosis 1979;32:213-29
10. Parthasarathy S, Barnett J, Fong LG. High density lipoprotein inhibits the oxidative modification of low-density lipoprotein. Biochim Biophys Acta 1990;1044:275-83
11. Navab M, Imes SS, Hama SY, et al. Monocyte transmigration induced by modification of low density lipoprotein in co-cultures of human aortic wall cells is due to induction of monocyte chemotactic protein 1 synthesis and is abolished by high density lipoprotein. J Clin Invest 1991;88:2039-46
12. Hama SY, Navab M, de Beer FC, Fogelman AM. Acute-phase high density lipoprotein does not prevent but amplifies the modification of low density lipoprotein. Circulation 1992;86:I-423, abstract.
13. Stafforini DM, Zimmerman GA, McIntyre TM, Prescott SM. The platelet activating factor acetylhdrolase from human plasma prevents oxidative modification of low density lipoprotein. Trans Amer Assoc Phys 1993;106:44-63
14. Mackness MI, Arrol S, Durrington PN. Paraoxonase prevents accumulation of lipoperoxides

in low-density lipoprotein. Febs Lett 1991;286:152-54

15. Watson AD, Navab M, Hama SY, et al. Effect of platelet activating factor-acetylhydrolase on the formation and action of minimally oxidized-low density lipoprotein. J Clin Invest 1995;95:774-82.
16. Watson AD, Navab M, Hough GP, et al. Biologically active phospholipids in MM-LDL are transferred to HDL and are hydrolyzed by HDL-associated esterases. Circulation 1994;90:I-353, abstract.

OXIDIZED LDL TRIGGER THE EXPRESSION OF HSP70 IN CULTURED ENDOTHELIAL CELLS

Paola Roma[1], Angela Pirillo[1], Weimin Zhu[1], and Alberico Luigi Catapano[1,2]
[1]Institute of Pharmacological Sciences, University of Milan, Via Balzaretti 9, Milan 20133, Italy and [2]Centro per lo Studio delle Vasculopatie Periferiche, Ospedale Bassini, Milan, Italy

Introduction

A growing body of evidence indicates that oxidative modification of low density lipoprotein (LDL) can affect several cellular functions in a proatherogenic way [1,2]. Because oxidized LDL (OxLDL) are cytotoxic [3], particularly to proliferating cells [4], their presence in the subendothelial space, where they are believed to form, may contribute to lesion formation.

It may be conceived that, especially during the initial steps of lesion formation, cells of the vasculature, like endothelial cells, smooth muscle cells, and eventually monocyte/macrophages, activate some mechanisms of defense. These would increase their potential of surviving in a toxic environment. It is known that the presence of environmental stressors induces the expression of heat shock genes [5], which encode for a family of polypeptides called "heat shock proteins" [hsps] or, more generally, stress proteins. The "stress response" is a common feature of living organisms, from bacteria to complex multicellulars, and the structure of hsps is highly conserved [5]. The function of stress proteins is essential to cell survival, not only in the presence of environmental stressors, when the synthesis of the inducible forms is activated, but also under physiologic conditions. In fact, the constitutive cognates of hsps ensure the acquirement and the keeping of a functional folding of proteins, during both synthesis and intracellular translocation. Because of this role, stress proteins have been defined as molecular chaperons [6,7].

Recently, hsp70 has been detected in human atherosclerotic plaques [8-10], particularly in endothelial cells and macrophages. These observations suggest that hsp70 may play a role in atherosclerosis. With our recent research we investigated whether, because of their toxicity, oxidized LDL are able to induce the expression of heat shock proteins in cultured human endothelial cells.

Methods

CELLS

Human umbilical vein endothelial cells (HUVEC) were isolated according to established

A. M. Gotto, Jr. et al. (eds.), Drugs Affecting Lipid Metabolism, 603–612.

procedures [11] and cultured under standard conditions in M-199, with the addition of heparin (15 U/mL) and endothelial cell growth factor (ECGF) (20 μg/mL). The EAhy-926 [12] line was cultured under standard conditions in minimal essential medium (MEM) + 10% fetal calf serum (FCS) and 1% hypoxanthine aminopterin thymidine (HAT). Parallel experiments were performed with both sparse cultures and postconfluent cultures, in which cells acquire a typical "cobblestone" morphology.

LIPOPROTEINS

LDL (1.019-1.063 g/mL) were isolated from freshly obtained human plasma, by preparative ultracentrifugation [13], and dialyzed in 0.15 M NaCl, 0.01% ethylene diaminetetraacetic acid (EDTA). Before oxidation EDTA was removed by gel filtration in PBS on a Sephadex G-25 column. Protein was measured by the Lowry method [14]. LDL (200 μg lipoprotein protein /mL) were oxidized in sterile conditions for 24 hours, at 37° C, in PBS containing $CuSO_4$ 20 μM, concentrated by ultrafiltration under N_2 pressure, desalted in PBS on Sephadex G-25 columns and sterile filtered. LDL modification was assessed by nondenaturing gel electrophoresis in 0.8% agarose [15]. In order to test the influence of the interaction between receptors and protein ligands on hsp70 expression aliquots of medium containing LDL or OxLDL were boiled for 15' in sterile conditions. Lipids were extracted from LDL and OxLDL with chloroform:methanol 2:1 (vol:vol) [16]. Extracts were evaporated to dryness under a N_2 stream and lipids were redissolved in absolute ethanol. The solution was filtered through a 0.45 μm pore filter to decrease turbidity and aliquots were added to the incubation medium. The volume of ethanol never exceeded 1% of total medium volume. Control medium containing 1% ethanol did not affect cell viability or hsp70 expression.

CELL VIABILITY

Cell viability was assessed by the release of ^{3}H-adenine into the culture medium [17], as described [18]. Percent ^{3}H-adenine release was expressed as the ratio of medium radioactivity to medium plus cell radioactivity.

UPTAKE AND DEGRADATION OF IODINATED LIPOPROTEINS

Lipoproteins were labeled with ^{125}I-NaI according to Bilheimer et al. [19]. EAhy-926 cells were incubated for 6 hours at 37° C in MEM containing essential fatty acid-free bovine serum albumin (EFAF-BSA) (2 mg/mL) and ^{125}I-OxLDL (10-100 μg/mL), or in the same medium containing ^{125}I-OxLDL and 30-fold unlabeled lipoprotein. Specific uptake and degradation were calculated as described [20]. Uptake was also measured in cells incubated with ^{125}I-OxLDL in the presence of fucoidin (20 μg/mL), which binds to scavenger receptors with high affinity.

IMMUNOCYTOCHEMISTRY

Sparse or confluent cultures were incubated with OxLDL (400 μg/mL) for different times (up to 24 hours) or with different concentrations (200-800 μg/mL) of the modified lipoprotein. Cells were fixed and processed for immunostaining, as described [18]. Antibodies used were: a) mouse monoclonal antibody specific for hsp72, the inducible form of hsp70, followed by biotinylated anti-mouse IgG and fluorescein-conjugated streptavidin; b) mouse monoclonal antibody against BrdU, followed by rhodamine-conjugated anti-mouse IgG. For double labeling, staining for BrdU was performed after staining for hsp70 [21]. Samples were examined with a fluorescence microscope and photographed using a 400 ASA film. To evaluate, within the same culture plate, the response of sparse and confluent cells to a challenge with OxLDL, a wounding experiment was performed. HUVEC were cultured to a postconfluent state, as judged on the basis of their "cobblestone" morphology; the monolayer was then wounded with a Teflon cell lifter and the cells were allowed to recover for 24 hours in M-199 containing FCS (20%). After recovery, BrdU (10 μM final concentration) was added to the culture medium for a further incubation of 6 hours. The medium was then replaced by M-199 containing OxLDL (400-600 μg/mL) for a period of 12 hours. At the end of the incubation cells were processed for immunostaining of hsp70 and BrdU [22].

IMMUNOBLOTTING

Sparse or confluent cultures were incubated with OxLDL for different times (up to 24 hours) or with different concentrations (200-800 μg/ml) of the modified lipoprotein.

Cells were lysed in tris(hydroxymethyl)aminomethane (TRIS)-glycine buffer (0.25 M TRIS, 0.173 M glycine, pH 8.5) containing sodium dodecyl sulfate (SDS) (3%) and protein was measured by the Lowry method [14]. Equal amounts of protein from the different samples were subjected to sodium dodecyl sulfate-polyacrylamide gel electrophoresis (SDS-PAGE) on a 10% polyacrylamide gel, in reducing conditions [23], and transferred onto nitrocellulose [24]. The membrane was incubated with anti-hsp70 antibody, then with peroxidase-conjugated goat anti-mouse IgG. Immunocomplexes were detected by an enhanced chemiluminescence method followed by autoradiography and were quantified by the Image program (ISF 1.47). Data were expressed as area units (AU).

Results

Results on the cytotoxicity of OxLDL to endothelial cells (EAhy-926 line) are presented in Table 1. This shows that, as opposed to native LDL and BSA, OxLDL affect cell viability. Acetylated LDL, which like OxLDL bind to scavenger receptors, did not significantly affect cell viability. When confluent cells were incubated with OxLDL [^{3}H]-adenine release was similar to that observed in the presence of the other lipoproteins or BSA. Table 1 also shows that sparsely grown cells are more sensitive than confluent cells to OxLDL toxicity. The cytotoxic effect of OxLDL was accompanied by the induction of hsp 70 expression, as

Table 1. [^{3}H]-Adenine labeled EAhy-926 cells were incubated for 24 h at 37° C with either OxLDL, AcLDL, LDL or BSA (200 ug/mL) and [^{3}H]-adenine release was evaluated as described in Methods. Values are the mean ± SE of triplicates and are representative of 4 separate experiments.

Effect of cell density on OxLDL cytotoxicity. [^{3}H]-Adenine Release[%]				
	OxLDL	AcLDL	LDL	BSA
Sparse Cells	52.4 ± 7.10	20.2 ± 0.85	21.3 ± 0.42	21.3 ± 0.10
Confluent Cells	20.0 ± 1.74	19.5 ± 0.57	22.6 ± 1.07	21.1 ± 0.49

was observed by both immunofluorescence (Figure 1) and imunoblotting experiments (data not shown). Furthermore, the response of sparse cells to a challenge with OxLDL was time-dependent and concentration-dependent (Figure 2). One possible explanation for the different sensitivity of cells at different densities to OxLDL toxicity might be a different degree of expression of scavenger receptors involved in OxLDL binding and internalization [25-27].

The role of scavenger receptors in the stress response activated by OxLDL was assessed by uptake/degradation studies. The extent of uptake and degradation of ^{125}I-OxLDL was similar for sparse and confluent endothelial cells (Table 2).

Table 2. Sparse and confluent cultures of EAhy-926 cells were incubated for 6 hours at 37° C in MEM containing EFAF-BSA (2 mg/mL) and the indicated concentrations of ^{125}I-OxLDL, with or without a 30-fold excess of unlabeled OxLDL. Specific degradation was evaluated as described in Methods.

Effect of cell density on the specific degradation of ^{125}I-OxLDL (ng/mg cell protein)		
^{125}I-OxLDL (μg/mL)	Sparse Cells	Confluent Cells
10	200 ± 2*	224 ± 16
30	345 ± 18	319 ± 22
50	370 ± 51	336 ± 16
100	421 ± 8	448 ± 40

* mean ± SD of triplicates

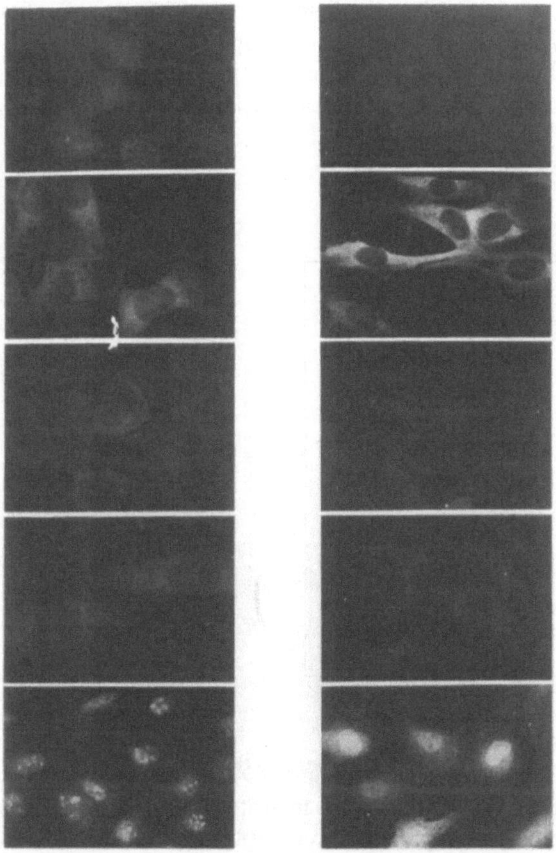

Figure 1. Sparse and confluent monolayers of EAhy-926 cells (a-e) and HUVEC (f-j) were incubated at 37° C for the indicated times in fresh medium without FCS, containing OxLDL or LDL (200 µg/mL), or heat shocked at 45° C for 15'. Cells were then processed for immunofluorescence with anti hsp70, as described in Methods, examined with a fluorescence microscope and photographed. Panels refer to: 0 h incubation (a, f); 7 h incubation with OxLDL (b, g: sparse monolayers and c, h: confluent monolayers); 7 h incubation with LDL (d, i); heat shock (e, j).

Furthermore, fucoidin did not hamper the expression of hsp70 triggered by these lipoproteins, although competing with OxLDL for uptake via scavenger receptors. In fact, in the presence of fucoidin (20 µmg/mL) uptake of ^{125}I-OxLDL decreased markedly in both sparse and confluent EAhy-926 cells. Fucoidin alone did not trigger hsp70 expression (data not shown). Because the role of scavenger receptors is probably not relevant to the effect of OxLDL on the expression of hsps we tested the possibility that the lipid moiety of the lipoprotein, which includes several oxidized lipids, may be the actual inducer of the stress response. In fact, as opposed to the lipid moiety of native LDL, lipids extracted from OxLDL markedly induced the expression of hsp70 in endothelial cells (not shown). The possibility that oxysterols, which are present in OxLDL lipids and are known to be cytotoxic, are the actual inducers is presently being explored.

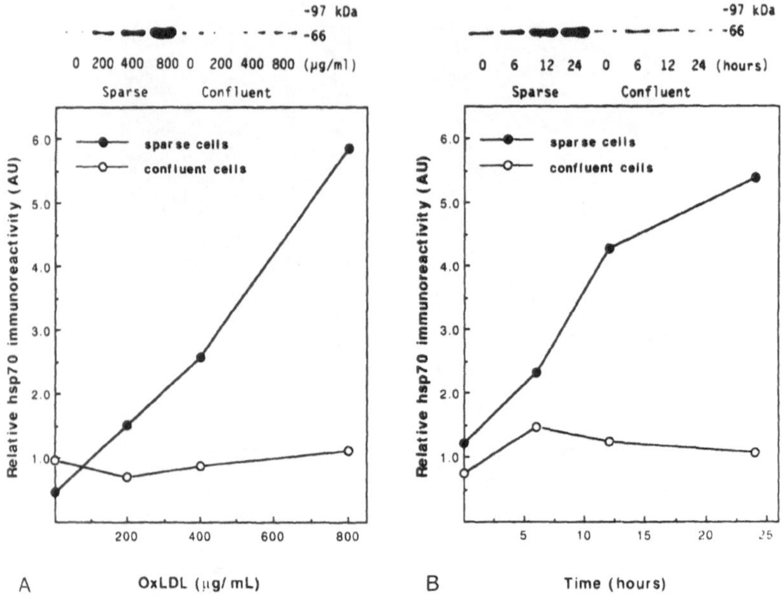

Figure 2. Panel A. Sparse (●) and confluent (○) cultures of HUVEC were incubated for 12 hours at 37° C in M-199 containing the indicated concentrations of OxLDL. At the end of the incubation cellular proteins were subjected to SDS-PAGE in 10% gels. Immunoblotting with anti-hsp70 antibody was then performed. Bands relative to hsp70 were analyzed by densitometry and the intensity of hsp70 staining was plotted as area units (AU). Panel B. Sparse (●) and confluent (○) cultures of HUVEC were incubated at 37° C in M-199 containing OxLDL (400 μg/mL) for the indicated times. Cells were then processed as above.

After wounding a confluent monolayer, we allowed enough time for the cells closest to the lesion to start healing it by proliferating and/or migrating. Cells were then incubated with a cytotoxic concentration of OxLDL, known to markedly inhibit proliferation and to induce hsp70 expression. Figure 3 shows the results of immunostaining. Only cells located on the edge of the wound and healing the lesion displayed hsp70 staining, while staining of confluent cells was very faint (Figure 3, panel a). The majority of these cells were positive for both hsp70 (Figure 3, panel b) and BrdU (Figure 3, panel c); this indicated that cells on the edge of the injured area expressed hsp70 (Figure 3, panels b and d) upon challenge with OxLDL and were actively cycling (Figure 3, panels c and d). In fact, since recovery took place in serum-containing medium, healing of the wounded monolayer was most likely due to cell proliferation. Immunostaining of a wounded monolayer that was allowed to recover and then incubated in complete medium without OxLDL was negative, indicating that injury and recovery *per se* were not able to induce the expression of hsp70 in cells on the edge of the lesion (not shown). This result indicated that actively dividing or/and migrating cells involved in wound repair, as sparse cells are likely to be, were more sensitive to OxLDL than relatively quiescent and stationary cells. Furthermore, immunoblotting results also indicated that hsp70 expression was highly inducible in sparse cells (not shown) and the extent of expression was dependent on the concentration of OxLDL during the challenge.

Discussion

Synthesis of stress proteins is generally regarded as a defense response triggered by toxic environmental conditions [5], and cytoprotection provided by hsps appears to be relevant in several pathologies [28]. It is conceivable that hsps have a role also in atherosclerosis, since increased expression of hsp70 has been observed in human atherosclerotic lesions [8-10]. The finding that OxLDL induce the expression of hsp70 in cultured endothelial cells reinforces the hypothesis that these lipoproteins may trigger a defense response in cells of the arterial wall. This may confer a relative resistance to repeated challenges driven by OxLDL or, possibly, other toxic challenges. Our data indicate that the activity of the scavenger receptors does not influence the expression of hsp70, suggesting that internalization and degradation of the lipoprotein are not necessary for it.

Hsp70 expression mostly depended on whether cells exposed to OxLDL were in a postconfluent or in a nonconfluent state, that is, whether they were quiescent or proceeding through the cell cycle. After a "cobblestone" monolayer of endothelial cells was wounded and allowed to recover only the cells at the edge of the wound, which were proliferating and most probably responsible for healing the lesion, expressed hsp70 upon incubation with OxLDL. The vast majority of the cells expressing hsp70 were also labeled by BrdU. This observation suggests a close relation between cell cycle and hsp70 expression as driven by OxLDL. Cell cycle dependence of hsp70 expression has been observed in heat-shocked CHO cells [29]. It appears that the induction of hsp72 is essential for the accomplishment of the early S phase and is also necessary in G1 [29]. Furthermore, OxLDL toxicity to fibroblasts appears to be selective for the S phase of the cell cycle [4]. Under normal conditions, endothelial cells are quiescent and form an antithrombogenic monolayer. Different types of injury can cause endothelial activation/denudation and adhesion of platelets to the subendothelium. Areas of blood vessels which are prone to lesion formation are characterized by enhanced endothelial regeneration and by an increased permeability [30], which allows the diffusion of plasma lipoproteins into the subendothelial space and their subsequent oxidation. Therefore, *in vivo*, the risk of being challenged by OxLDL is higher for cells healing an injured vessel wall than for cells of unaffected areas. On the basis of the above *in vitro* results, and of similar results obtained with cultured smooth muscle cells [31], we speculate that the increased expression of the inducible form of hsp70 may

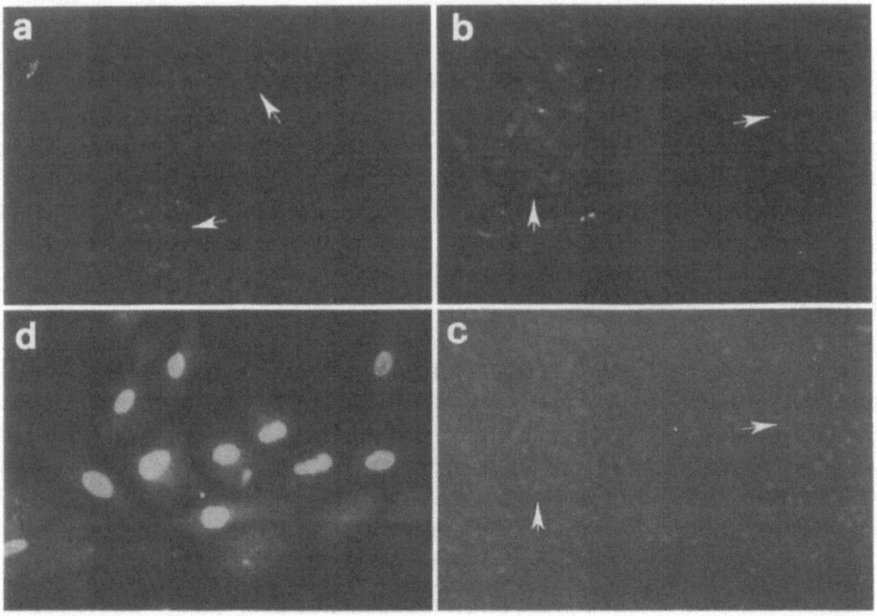

Figure 3. HUVEC were cultured to a post-confluent state (judged by their "cobblestone" morphology). The monolayer was then wounded by mean of a Teflon spatula and cells were allowed to recover for 24 hours in M-199 + 20% FCS. After recovery, BrdU (10 µM final concentration) was added to the culture medium for a further incubation of 6 hours. The medium was then replaced with M-199 containing OxLDL (600 µg/mL) for an incubation of 12 hours. Cells were then processed for immunostaining of hsp70 (a,b,d) or of BrdU (c,d). Original magnification: (a,b,c) 100 x; (d) 400 x.

represent a defense mechanism against cytotoxic proatherogenic stress sustained by OxLDL. Cytoprotection afforded by stress proteins may allow these healing cells a higher chance of surviving further toxic stimuli. Overexpression of hsp70 has been shown to increase the threshold for the release of stress mediators (IL-1, IL-6) induced by UV light and oxidants [32]. If this is a more general mechanism it can be speculated that at early stages of atherosclerosis hsp expression allows cells to cope with oxidative damage while repeated oxidative insults will result in a lower ability to cope with them and eventually lead to cell death. In summary, we have demonstrated that OxLDL can trigger the expression of hsp70 (inducible form) only in nonconfluent endothelial cells, and that cell proliferation is responsible for this finding. Whether this effect has *in vivo* relevance remains to be addressed; we speculate that cells rapidly growing are more sensitive to cytotoxicity of OxLDL and that expression of hsp70 could allow a better chance of survival. This observation might also have therapeutic applications in atherosclerosis

Acknowledgments

The authors are grateful to Miss M. Marazzini for typing the manuscript. This work was supported, in part, by a grant from CNR, Progetto Finalizzato Invecchiamento (Publication No. 963667) and by a Research Grant of the European Community (PL931790).

References

1. Steinberg D, Parthasarathy S, Carew TE, Khoo JC, Witztum JL. Beyond cholesterol. Modifications of low-density lipoprotein that increase its atherogenicity. New Engl J Med 1989;320:915-24.
2. Parthasarathy S, Rankin SM. Role of oxidized low density lipoprotein in atherogenesis. Prog Lipid Res 1992;31:127-43.
3. Hessler JR, Morel DW, Lewis LJ, Chisholm GM. Lipoprotein oxidation and lipoprotein-induced cytotoxicity. Arteriosclerosis 1983;3:215-22.
4. Kosugi K, Diane WM, Morel DW, Di Corleto PE, Chisolm GM. Toxicity of oxidized low-density lipoprotein to cultured fibroblasts is selective for S phase of the cell cycle. J Cell Physiol 1987;130:311-20.
5. Lindquist S. The heat-shock response. Ann Rev Biochem 1986;55:1151-91.
6. Georgopulos C, Welch WJ. Role of the major heat shock proteins as molecular chaperons. Annu Rev Cell Biol 1993;9:601-34.
7. Hendrick JP, Hartl FU. Molecular chaperon functions of heat-shock proteins. Annu Rev Biochem 1993;62:349-84.
8. Berberian PA, Myers W, Tytell M, Challa V, Bond G. Immunoistochemical localization of heat shock protein-70 in normal-appearing and atherosclerotic specimens of human arteries. Am J Pathol 1990;136:71-80.
9. Johnson AD, Berberian PA, Tytell M, Bond G. Atherosclerosis alters the localization of HSP70 in human and macaque aortas. Exp Mol Pathol 1993;58:155-68.
10. Johnson AD, Berberian PA, Tytell M Bond MG. Arterioscler Thromb Vasc Biol 1995;15:27-36.
11. Jaffe EA, Nachman RL, Becker CJ, Minick CR. Culture of human endothelial cells derived from umbilical veins: Identification by morphological and immunological criteria. J Clin Invest 1973;52:2745-49.
12. Edgell CJS, Mc Donald CC, Graham JB. Permanent cell line expressing human factor VIII-related antigen established by hybridization. Proc Natl Acad Sci USA 1983;80:3734-37.
13. Havel RJ, Eder HA, Bragdon JH. The distribution and chemical composition of ultracentrifugally separated lipoproteins in human serum. J Clin Invest 1955;34:1345-53.
14. Lowry OH, Rosebrough NJ, Farr AL, Randall RJ. Protein measurement with the folin phenol reagent. J Biol Chem 1951;193:265-75.
15. Noble RP. Electrophoretic separation of plasma lipoproteins in agarose gels. J Lipid Res 1968;9:693-700.
16. Bligh EG, Dyer WJ. A rapid method of total lipid extraction and purification. Can J Biochem Physiol 1959;37:911-17.
17. Kishi Y, Numano F. In vitro study of vascular endothelial injury by activated platelets and its prevention. Atherosclerosis 1989;76:95-101.
18. Zhu WM, Roma P, Pellegatta F, Catapano AL. Oxidized low density lipoprotein induce the

expression of heat shock protein 70 in human endothelial cells. Biochem Biophys Res Commun 1994;200:389-94.
19. Bilheimer DW, Eisenberg S, Levy RI. The metabolism of very low density lipoprotein proteins. I. Preliminary in vitro and in vivo observations. Biochim Biophys Acta 1973; 250:212-21.
20. Goldstein JL. Ho YK, Basu SK, Brown MS. Binding site on macrophages that mediate the uptake and degradation of acetylated low density lipoprotein, producing massive cholesterol deposition. Proc Natl Acad Sci USA 1979;76:333-37.
21. Zhu WM, Roma P, Pirillo A, Pellegatta F, Catapano AL. Human endothelial cells exposed to oxidized LDL express hsp70 only when proliferating. Arterioscler Thromb Vasc Biol; in press.
22. Houck DW, Loken MR. Simultaneous analysis of cell surface antigens, bromodeoxyuridine incorporation and DNA content. Cytometry 1993;6:531-38.
23. Laemmli UK. Cleavage of structural proteins during the assembly of the head of bacteriophage T4. Nature 1970; 227:680-85.
24. Towbin H, Staehelin T, Gordon J. Electrophoretic transfer of proteins from polyacrylamide gels to nitrocellulose sheets: Procedure and some applications. Proc Natl Acad Sci USA 1979; 76:4350-54.
25. Sparrow CP, Parthasarathy S, Steinberg DA. A macrophage receptor that recognizes oxidized low density lipoprotein but not acetylated low density lipoprotein. J Biol Chem 1989;264: 2599-604.
26. Endemann G, Stanton LW, Madden KS, Bryant CM, White RT, Protter AA. CD36 is a receptor for oxidized low density lipoprotein. J Biol Chem 1993;268:11811-16.
27. Ottnad E, Parthasarathy S, Sambrano GR, et al. A macrophage receptor for oxidized low density lipoprotein distinct from the receptor for acetyl low density lipoprotein: Partial purification and role in recognition of oxidatively damaged cells. Proc Natl Acad Sci USA 1995;92:1391-95.
28. Minowada G, Welch WJ. Clinical implications of the stress response. J Clin Invest 1995;95:3-12.
29. Hang H, Fox MH. Expression of HSP70 induced in CHO cells by 45.0° C hyperthermia is cell cycle associated and DNA synthesis dependent. Cytometry 1995;19:119-25.
30. Caplan BA, Schwartz CJ. Increased endothelial cell turnover in areas of in vivo Evans Blue uptake in the pig aorta. Atherosclerosis 1973;17:401-17.
31. Zhu WM, Roma P, Pirillo A, Pellegatta F, Catapano AL. Oxidized LDL induce hsp70 expression of heat shock protein 70 in human smooth muscle cells. FEBS Letters 1995;372:1-5.
32. Simon MM, Reikerstorfer A, Schwarz A, et al. Heat shock protein 70 overexpression affects the response to ultraviolet light in murine fibroblasts. Evidence for increased cell viability and suppression of cytokine release. J Clin Invest 1995;95:926-33.

LYSOPHOSPHATIDYLCHOLINE-INDUCED GENE EXPRESSION OF ENDOTHELIAL PLATELET-DERIVED GROWTH FACTOR-B-CHAIN AND INTERCELLULAR ADHESION MOLECULE-1

T. Kita, N. Kume, H. Ochi, E. Nishi, K. Ichii, Y. Nagano, and M. Yokode
Department of Molecular Medicine for Adult and Geriatric Diseases, Graduate School of Medicine, Kyoto University, 54 Kawahara-cho, Shogoin, Sakyo-ku, Kyoto 606-01, Japan

Introduction

The atherosclerosis is indicated by many complex characteristics, including infiltration of inflammatory leukocytes, accumulation of cholesterol-laden macrophages, proliferation of smooth muscle cells, deposition of extracellular matrix, and thrombosis [1,2]. Vascular endothelium in particular plays a pivotal role in the early stage of atherosclerosis, expressing endothelial-leukocyte adhesion molecules, growth factors, and cytokines in response to various pathophysiological stimuli [3]. Lysophosphatidylcholine (lyso-PC) is a prominent phospholipid component of atherogenic lipoproteins and is generated also in inflammatory lesions by extracellular phospholipase A_2 activities [3]. Lyso-PC has been shown to differentially upregulate vascular cell adhesion molecule (VCAM)-1 and intercellular adhesion molecule (ICAM)-1 expression in various cultured endothelial cells, showing its potential role in mononuclear leukocyte recruitment into these lesions [4]. Lyso-PC also has been demonstrated to induce gene expression of potent smooth muscle growth factors such as platelet-derived growth factor (PDGF-B chains and heparin-binding epidermal growth factor-like growth factor (HB-EGF) in cultured human endothelial cells [5]. The effects of lyso-PC on endothelial genes appear to be specific and distinct from those elicited by cytokines, such as interleukin (IL)-1 and tumor necrosis factor (TNF)-α since neither E-selection nor IL-8 was upregulated in the same cells stimulated with lyso-PC. Lyso-PC stimulates transcription of these genes; however, signal transduction mechanisms responsible for the gene induction of adhesion molecules and growth factors by this lyso-PC stimulus have not been fully understood.

A. M. Gotto, Jr. et al. (eds.), Drugs Affecting Lipid Metabolism, 613–618.

Materials and Methods

CELL

Cultured human umbilical vein endothelial cells (HUVECs) were isolated by collagenase digestion and grown in medium 199 with 20% (vol/vol) heat-inactivated FBS. All experiments were carried out within 3 days after HUVECs reached confluence. Cells (passage numbers between 2 and 4) were incubated with or without test stimuli in medium 199.

NORTHERN BLOT ANALYSIS [6]

Total cellular RNA, isolated from HUVECs by the acid guanidinium-phenol-chloroform method, was electrophoresed through 1% agarose gels containing formaldehyde, transferred onto 0.45-μm nylon membranes (Zeta-Probe, Bio-Rad), and fixed by ultraviolet cross-linking. Northern membranes were hybridized with human ICAM-1 and PDGF-B cDNA probes, which were labeled with [α-^{32}P] deoxycytidine triphosphate (dCTP) (DuPont NEN) by using random hexanucleotide primers (Pharmacia) at 65°C for 18 hours in a mixture containing 1 mmol/l ethylenediamine tetracetic acid (EDTA), 0.25 mol/l Na_2HPO_4 (pH 7.2), and 7% sodium dodecyl solution (SDS). The filters were subsequently washed at 65°C twice with 1 mmol/l EDTA, 40 mmol/l Na_2HPO_4 (pH 7.2), and 1% SDS and exposed to x-ray films. A 1.3-kb *Xho*I fragment of human ICAM-1, kindly provided by Dr. Brian Seed (Massachusetts General Hospital, Boston, Massachusetts), was used to detect ICAM-1 mRNA. A 2.1-kb *Bam*HI fragment of human PDGF-B cDNA, obtained from American Type Culture Collection, and a *Pst* I-*Eco*RI fragment of human PDGF-B, kindly provided by Dr. Tucker Collins (Brigham and Women's Hospital, Boston, Massachusetts) were used as hybridization probes. Northern analyses using these PDGF-B cDNAs gave similar results. Some blots were rehybridized with radiolabeled human β-actin cDNA to control the amounts of RNA loaded. Densitometric scanning was performed to quantify the amounts of mRNA; and Image Master laser densitometer (Pharmacia) was used. Relative amounts of mRNA for PDGF-B and ICAM-1 were normalized to β-actin mRNA levels.

WESTERN BLOT ANALYSIS

Laemmli sample buffer (2% SDS, 10% glycerol, 60 mmol/l Tris [pH 6.8], and 0.001% bromophenol blue) was directly poured into HUVEC culture plates, and the cell lysates were passed through 25-gauge needles 10 times. After heating at 98°C for 10 minutes, samples were subjected to SDS-polyacryl-amide (1% to ~20% gradient) gel electrophoresis in nonreducing conditions and transferred onto nitro-cellulose filters (Hybond ECL filter, Amersham Corp.) by electroblotting. After preincubation with Tris-buffered saline (TBS) (50 mmol/l Tris-Ll [pH 8.0], 2 mmol/l $CaCl_2$, 100 mmol/l Nacl, and 5% [wt/vol] nonfat dry milk) for 3 hours at room temperature, filters were incubated with a rabbit polyclonal antibody directed to PDGF-BB homodimer (Genzyme Corp.) diluted in TBS at room temperature for 2 hours, followed by washing twice with TBS without nonfat dry milk. Filters were then incubated with the horseradish peroxidase-conjugated anti-rabbit immunoglobulin G (IgG) antibody (Amersham Corp.) diluted in TBS for 2 hours at room temperature, washed twice in TBS without nonfat dry milk, and visualized by use of a chemiluminescence reagent (ECL Kit, Amersham Corp.).

Results and Discussion

PDGF-B mRNA is upregulated by lyso-PC, depending on *de novo* protein synthesis. However, in case of ICAM-1, upregulation of ICAM-1 mRNA by lyso-PC does not require *de novo* protein synthesis using cycloheximide, which blocks protein synthesis. Cycloheximide completely blocked lyso-PC induced increases in PDGF mRNA levels, but not ICAM-1 mRNA. Inhibition of nascent protein synthesis by cycloheximide provided contrasting results between PDGF-B chain and ICAM-1 gene regulation. PDGF-B mRNA induction by lyso-PC, as well as that elicited by phorbol 12-myristate 12-acetate (PMA), requires *de novo* protein synthesis, but ICAM-1 does not. In fact, cycloheximide enhanced the accumulation of ICAM-1 mRNA in both lyso-PC treated and untreated HUVECs. This finding appears to be similar to the previous finding with PMA-treated and TNF-α-treated HUVECs [7]. These results clearly indicate that signal transduction mechanisms responsible for lyso-PC-induced gene expression might be different between PDGF-B and ICAM-1. To investigate the potential role of protein kinase C (PKC) in PDGF-B chain and ICAM-1 mRNA induction by lyso-PC, we used two different ways. Pretreatment with PMA for 24 hours, which depleted PKC activities by prolonged exposure to PMA and inhibited PKC actions by a pharmacological dose, significantly blocked PDGF-B mRNA induction elicited by the subsequent stimulation with PMA (63 $\pm$ 18% reduction).

However, this PMA pretreatment did not inhibit lyso-PC-induced increases in PDGF mRNA nor ICAM-1 mRNA. We also used staurosporine (10nmol/l), which is inhibitor of PKC activities, significantly reduced PMA-induced increases in PDGF-B mRNA level (44 $\pm$ 12% reduction), but this agent did not inhibit those elicited by lyso-PC. These results indicate that signal transduction mechanisms responsible for PDGF-B and ICAM-1 mRNA upregulation elicited by lyso-PC in HUVECs appear to be dissociated from PMA-regulatable PKC activation. Previous reports by others, using PMA and staurosporine, have indicated that ICAM-1 upregulation by TNF-α also is dissociated from PKC activation [8], thus supporting the existence of PKC-independent mechanisms of ICAM-1 gene induction. Transient increases in cytosolic calcium levels and turnover of phosphoinositides have been detected in lyso-PC-treated cultured endothelial cells and are reported to be involved in the inhibitory actions of lyso-PC on endothelium-dependent vasorelaxation. However, our preliminary experiments, have revealed that the calcium ionophore ionomycin did not induce PDGF-B or ICAM-1 mRNA, suggesting that calcium mobilization alone is not sufficient to induce endothelial genes such as PDGF-B and ICAM-1.

To explore the potential role of cAMP in lyso-PC-induced PDGF-B and ICAM-1 gene expression, we studied the effects of forskolin, which elevates the intracellular cyclic adenosine monophosphate (cAMP) level, and Bt_2 cAMP. We treated HUVECs with or without lyso-PC or PMA in the presence or absence of forskolin and measured mRNA levels for PDGF-B and ICAM-1 by northern blot analysis. Forskolin significantly reduced lyso-PC induced, as well as PMA-induced, increases in PDGF-B mRNA (59 $\pm$ 19% and 68 $\pm$ 19% reduction, respectively). In contrast, this agent inhibited only lyso-PC induced increases in ICAM-1 mRNA (67 $\pm$ 22% reduction), but not block those induced by PMA. Bt_2 cAMP exhibited effects similar to those observed with forskolin. Upregulated expression of PDGF-B chain mRNA elicited by lyso-PC, as well as PMA, was significantly prohibited by Bt_2 cAMP (54% and 30% reduction, respectively). However, Bt_2 cAMP (2mmol/l) blocked only lyso-PC-induced ICAM-1 mRNA upregulation (46% reduction), but did not show any significant inhibition on PMA-induced ICAM-1 mRNA expression. Since forskolin or Bt_2 cAMP inhibited lyso-PC-induced ICAM-1 mRNA upregulation but did not affect that induced by PMA, these effects of cAMP-elevating agents do not appear to result from general inhibitory action. Although previous reports have demonstrated that elevated levels of intracellular cAMP can also antagonize the effects of thrombin or TGF-β on PDGF-B mRNA levels but do not suppress ICAM-1 expression induced by TNF-α, our results appear to be the first to demonstrate that elevated levels of cAMP can counteract the effect of lyso-PC on both PDGF-B and ICAM-1 expression. Lyso-PC has been shown to increase the amounts of mRNA for PDGF-B chain [5]. To examine the effects of lyso-PC on PDGF-B protein levels, we performed western blot analyses using cell lysate from lyso-PC treated HUVECs. Multiple bands with approximate molecular weight between 38 and 43 kD, which appear to be compatible with previous reports [9,10] were detected by treatments with lyso-PC for 8 hours and continuously increased for at least 20 hours. Similar bands were detectable in HUVECs treated with PMA for 8 hours. All these bands disappeared when excess amounts of recombinant human PDGF-BB homodimer were included in the incubation buffer containing antihuman PDGF-B antibody.

Previous studies [5] with nuclear runoff assays and northern blot analyses using actinomycin D have demonstrated that lyso-PC does not appear to act on ICAM-1 and PDGF-B genese by stabilizing mRNA but rather by stimulating gene transcription. Consensus sequences for binding of known transcription factors, including activating protein-1, have been identified in 5' promoter regions of ICAM-1 [11,12] and PDGF-B chain gene [13,14,15].

In the present study, we have shown for the first time that cell- and matrix-associated forms of PDGF-B protein and its mRNA are increased by lyso-PC treatment in HUVECs. We have partially characterized potential signal transduction mechanisms responsible for endothelial gene induction elicited by lyso-PC; PDGF-B chain and ICAM-1 gene induction by lyso-PC appears to depend on signal transduction mechanisms other than PMA-regulatable PKC, which can be suppressed by elevated levels of cAMP. Dependence of *de novo* protein synthesis on PDGF-B chain is different from that for ICAM-1, suggesting that lyso-PC might stimulate multiple and diverse signaling pathways. Further studies related to signal transduction pathways and transcriptional regulatory mechanisms involved in this lipid stimulus relevant to atherogenesis and inflammation may provide new insights into endothelial activation in these pathophysiological settings and might provide potential therapeutic targets in preventing vascular disease.

Summary

Lysophosphatidylcholine (lyso-PC) is a major phospholipid component of atherogenic lipoproteins, such as oxidized LDL and β-VLDL. Lyso-PC has been shown to differentially upregulate VCAM-1, and ICAM-1, and also PDGF-A, B chains and HD-EGF gene expression in various cultured endothelial cells. In this paper, we demonstrate increased expression of cell- and matrix-associated forms of PDGF-B protein elicited by lyso-PC and further characterized potential signal transduction mechanisms responsible for lyso-PC-induced human umbilical vein endothelial cell. Cycloheximide inhibited PDGF-B but not ICAM-1 mRNA induction by lyso-PC, suggesting the dependence on *de novo* protein synthesis for PDGF-B, but not ICAM-1. A protein kinase C(PKC) inhibitor did not block lyso-PC-induced increases in PDGF-B or ICAM-1 mRNA. The elevated level of cAMP blocked both PDGF-B and ICAM-1 upregulation by lyso-PC. However, cAMP-elevating agents did not suppress ICAM-1 upregulation by PMA. Taken together, PDGF-B and ICAM-1 gene induction by lyso-PC may involve different signaling mechanisms; however, both appear to be independent of PMA-regulatable PKC activation but are suppressed by increased levels of intracellular cAMP.

Acknowledgments

This study was supported by a research grant from the Ministry of Education, Science, and Culture of Japan (No. 07557073, 05404039, 07044255), a Research Grant for Health Sciences from Japanese Ministry of Health and Welfare, and Grants for Cardiovascular Disease (5A-2, 6B-1) from Japanese Ministry of Health and Welfare.

References

1. Ross S. The pathogenesis of atherosclerosis: A perspective for the 1990s. Nature 1993;362:801-809.
2. Kume N, Arai H, Kawai C, Kita T. Receptors for modified low-density lipoproteins on human endothelial cells: Different recognition for acetylated low-density lipoprotein and oxidized low-density lipoprotein. Biochem Biophys Acta 1991;1091:63-67.
3. Gimbrone MA Jr, Kume N, Cybulsky MI. Vascular endothelial dysfunction and the pathogenesis of atherosclerosis. In: Wever PC, Leaf A, editors. Atherosclerosis Reviews. New York: Raven Press Publishers, 1993;25:1-9.
4. Kume N, Cybulsky MI, Gimbrone MA Jr. Lysophosphatidylcholine, a component of atherogenic lipoproteins, induces mononuclear adhesion molecules in cultured human and rabbit arterial endothelial cells. J Clin Invest 1992;90:1138-44.
5. Kume N, Gimbrone MA Jr. Lysophosphatidylcholine transcriptionally induces growth factor gene expression in cultured human endothelial cells. J Clin Invest 1994;93:907-911.
6. Ochi H, Kume N, Nishi E, Kita T. Elevated levels of cyclic AMP inhibits protein kinase-C independent mechanisms of endothelial PDGF-B chain and ICAM-1 gene induction by lysophosphatidylcholine. Circulation Research 1995;77:530-35.
7. Wertheimer SJ, Myers CL, Wallace RW, Parks TP. Intercellular adhesion molecule-1 gene

expression in human endothelial cells: Differential regulation by tumor necrosis factor-α and phorbol myristate acetate. J Biol Chem 1992;267:12030-35.
8. Ritchie AJ, Johnson DR, Ewenstein BM, Pober JS. Tumor necrosis factor induction of surface antigen is independent of protein kinase C activation or inactivation: Studies with phorbol myristate acetate and staurosporine. J Immunol 1991;146: 3056-62.
9. Kelly JL, Sanchez A, Brown GS, Chesterman CN, Sleigh MJ. Accumulation of PDGF B and cell-binding forms of PDGF A in the extracellular matrix. J Cell Biol 1993;121:1153-63.
10. Raines EW, Ross R. Compartmentalization of PDGF on extracellular binding sites dependent on exon-6-encoded sequences. J Cell Biol 1992;116:533-43.
11. Degitz K, Kian-Jie L, Caughman SW. Cloning and characterization of the 5'-transcriptional regulatory region of the human intercellular adhesion molecule 1 gene. J Biol Chem 1991;266:14024-14030.
12. Voraberger G, Schafer R, Stratowa C. Cloning of the human gene for intercellular adhesion molecule 1 and analysis of its 5'-regulatory region: induction by cytokines and phorbol ester. J Immunol 1991;147:2777-86.
13. Ratnerl L, Thielan B, Bollins T. Sequences of 5' portion of the human c-sis gene: Characterization of the transcriptional promoter and regulation of expression of the protein product by 5' untranslated mRNA sequence. Nuclein Acids Res 1987;15: 6017-36.
14. Pech M, Rao CD, Robbins KC, Aaronson SA. Functional identification of regulatory elements within the promoter region of platelet-derived growth factor 2. Mol Cel Biol 1989;9:396-405.
15. Khachigian LM, Fries JWU, Benz MW, Bonthron DT, Collins T. Novel cis-acting elements in the human platelet-derived growth factor B-chain core promoter that mediate gene expression in cultured vascular endothelial cells. J Biol Chem 1994;269:22647-56.

MULTIPLE FUNCTIONAL DOMAINS OF MACROPHAGE SCAVENGER RECEPTORS

Takefumi Doi[1], Yoichiro Wada[2], Liao Hai-Sun[2,3], Akiyo Matsumoto[2,3], and Tatsuhiko Kodama[2]
[1]Department of Pharmaceutical Sciences, University of Osaka, [2]The Third Department of Internal Medicine, University of Tokyo, and [3]Department of Clinical Nutrition, National Institute of Health and Nutrition, Tokyo, Japan

Introduction

Macrophage scavenger receptors (MSR) are trimeric membrane glycoproteins implicated in the pathologic deposition of cholesterol during the atherogenesis through receptor mediated uptake of modified lipoproteins [1]. The molecular cloning of type I and type II MSR indicates that the receptor consist form 6 characteristic domains [2,3]. The structure is well conserved among four animal species, bovine human, murine and rabbit [4-7]. The detailed structure function analysis using protein engineering indicates that MSR is a mosaic of functional domains encoded by each exons [8-10]. MSR mediate (a) endocytosis of a wide range of negatively charged macromolecules; (b) phagocytosis of apoptotic cells; (c) EDTA resistant macrophage adhesion; and (d) cell-cell interaction. Each of these functions are mediated by the interaction of a specific domain to their ligands, antibodies, and intracellular apparatus. The multiple functions are well dissected by the analysis of each domains, but several remaining problems are related to the conformational changes mediated by the allosterical effect between different domains. In this paper we would like to summarize the recent advances in the understanding of functional domains of MSR.

Domain Structure of Macrophage Scavenger Receptors

Comparison of the amino acid sequences of bovine, human, murine, and rabbit scavenger receptors, as determined by cDNA cloning indicated that the 6 functional domain structure proposed [2] was conserved in all animal species studied. The receptor contains a single hydrophobic stretch of 26 amino acids, but does not have a typical N-terminal signal sequence. The polarity of amino acids immediately next to this hydrophobic domain and the location of all seven potential N-terminal sugar attachment sites strongly indicate that the receptor is an integral membrane protein with a single membrane spanning domain and an N-terminal cytoplasmic domain. N-linked sugars account for as much as 15-20 K of the

A. M. Gotto, Jr. et al. (eds.), Drugs Affecting Lipid Metabolism, 619–630.

mature monomer subunit. Signals were not observed at the two relevant asparagine locations during sequencing of peptides, indicating that these sites are glycosylated. The hypothesis that C-terminal domains locate in extracellular space, was finally confirmed with experiments using truncated mutant receptors expressed on COS cells. The truncation of the C-terminal domain resulted in a loss of ligand-binding activity, although the trimeric receptor appeared on the cell surface (see below). In this paper we wish to report the detailed structure of each domain.

DOMAIN 1: N-TERMINAL CYTOPLASMIC DOMAIN

The N-terminal cytoplasmic domain consists of about 50 amino acid residues. MSR mediate the binding and uptake of modified LDL and a wide range of other negatively charged macromolecules. Immunoelectron microscopic studies revealed that at 4° C, MSR gathered in the coated pit, but when the temperature is raised to 37° C, MSR are internalized and accumulated in the endosome of macrophages. We generated a series of deletion mutant cDNAs that are expressed in COS cells. The results of degradation experiments shown in Figure 1 suggested that residues 11-23 are important for the endocytosis of MSR. In the case of LDL receptor and several other endocytotic receptors, the NPXY sequence is essential for internalization [11] and the YXRF sequence is essential for the endoccytosis of transferrin receptor [12]. In both cases, these sequences can form the tight turn structure. On the other hand, MSR cytoplasmic domain dose not have these sequences. Therefore, MSR may have a new signal motif sequence for endocytosis. Because the computer analysis of the secondary structure of MSR, cytoplasmic domain indicated that there existed two possible turn structure sequences (residue 13-21 and residue 34-41), these sequence might be related with this event. The addition of YXRF motif in either right or opposite orientation to MSR cytoplasmic domain showed the reduction of degradation activity indicating that tissue specific factors might be related with endocytosis and/or that more than two factors might be responsible for this event.

We also carried out point mutation experiments. The results shown in Figure 1 indicated that the residues 21, 22, and 23 are essential for the ligand degradation. In order to elucidate the structure determining the internalization activity, we made the mutant receptor constructs whose amino acids were substituted into alanine. These cDNAs were transfected into COS cells, and the internalization index of acetyl-LDL in these cells was measured (T. Doi et al., unpublished observation). Substitution of amino acid residue 16 to 23 did not alter the internalization index, although substitution of valine 21 into alanine, lysine 22 into alanine, and phenylalanine 23 into alanine markedly reduced both cell surface expression and degradation activities. These results indicated that the residues 21,22, and 23 is essential for the cell surface appearance of MSR. There is a potential protein kinase substrate site, RXXS/T, in the middle of this domain, which is well conserved. The point mutation introduced around this region reduced the internalization index (T. Doi et al., unpublished observation). Further characterization about the structure of cytoplasmic domain will be needed. When bovine MSR protein was expressed into COS cells or CHO cells, expressed MSR was mainly detected ER and/or Golgi apparatus and only small portion of receptor molecules were expressed in the cell surface [13,14]. These results suggested that intracellular transport of MSR is mediated by macrophage specific mechanism. When CHO cells expressing MSR were cultivated MAC medium (40 μM compactin, 200 μM mevalonate, 3 μg/ml acetyl-LDL in 3% lipoprotein deficient serum), which is the selection medium for cells expressing MSR, the number of receptors expressed on the cell surface increased (S. Gordon , T. Kodama et al., unpublished). The cells selected by MAC selection indicated high degradation activity for acetyl-LDL. This may be related not only to the increase in the number of receptor molecule, but also to the increased effective transport to the cell surface.

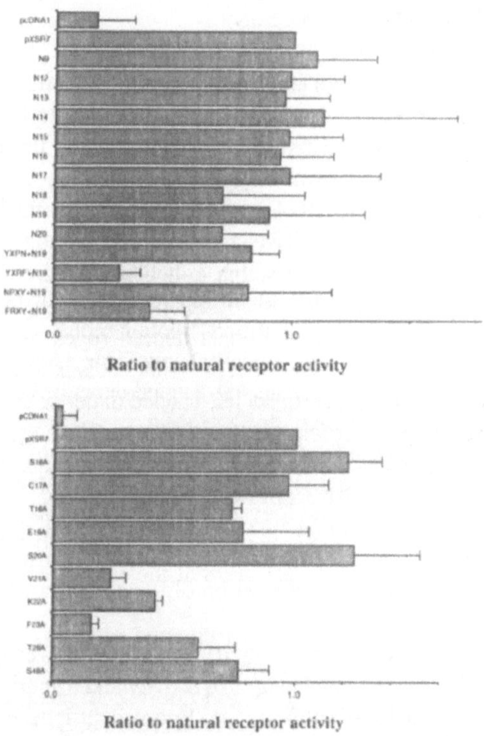

Figure 1. Acetyl-LDL degradation activity of COS cells expressing cytoplasmic mutant MSR. Upper panel: Wild type and mutant bovine MSR were expressed in COS cells and the acetyl-LDL degradation activity was measured. N-terminal portion of cytoplasmic domain of each mutant receptors were deleted. The numbers indicate the length of deleted amino acid residues from N-terminus. Effects of the additions of NPXY or YXRF in either right or opposite direction are also indicated. Lower panel: Effect of amino acid substitution of cytoplasmic domain of MSR. Each amino acid residues as indicated by the residue number was substituted to alanine, and the degradation activity of COS cells expressing both wild type and mutant receptors were measured.

DOMAIN 2: MEMBRANE SPANNING DOMAIN

The transmembrane domain consists of a stretch of 26 hydrophobic amino acids.

DOMAIN 3: SPACER DOMAIN

A 32 amino acid domain connects the membrane spanning domain to the long fibrous coiled coil domain. There are two possible N-linked sugar attachment sites, one of which is not conserved in the murine receptor.

DOMAIN 4: A-HELICAL COILED COIL DOMAIN

Domain 4 contains as many as 23 seven amino-acid 'heptad' repeats. From the sequences of these repeats we strongly predict an α-helical coiled coil structure held together by an interhelical hydrophobic core of aliphatic residues at the first and third or fourth position of the heptad. The α-helical coiled coil was originally proposed by Crick [15]. Recently, the leucine zipper motif was proposed as DNA binding proteins that facilitate dimer formation [16]. Studies of the short peptides which have leucine repeats in the transcriptional regulator GCN4 showed that these peptides form stable α-helical coiled coil dimers with parallel orientations [17], and NMR and x-ray analysis of this peptide confirmed this structure [18]. Many leucine zipper sequences have additional heptad repeat amino acids at the next position of the Leu/Ile repeat on the helical wheel schema. This additional interaction makes a right-handed α-helical monomer unit parallel left-handed dimer or trimer bundles as shown by myosin, intermediate filament protein, gp17 protein, or fibrinogen [19].

The heptad repeats of MSR are divided into two groups due to the disruption of repeats by a skip at 204-211. An analysis of the exon/intron organization of the human gene revealed that the junction of exons 4 and 5 exactly matches this skip position, indicating that the α-helical coiled coil domain of MSR consists of two coil structures encoding different exons and that the junction generates a distortion of the coiled-coil which may be important for its function.

We generated a series of C-terminally truncated mutant receptors (Figure 2). These are expressed in COS cells, and their ligand uptake activity and trimeric structure were studied using a trimer specific monoclonal antibody and fluorescent labelled acetyl-LDL. IgG-D2, which recognizes only the trimeric form of this receptor, recognized a deletion mutant protein constructed from 221 amino acids from the N-terminus (N221) and longer proteins. This result indicates that the collagen-like domain is not required for the trimer formation, and suggests that an α-helical coiled coil structure perhaps mediates the assembly of the functional trimeric receptor.

Among these leucine or isoleucine repeats on scavenger receptors, two histidine residues, which are conserved in human, bovine, rabbit, and mouse, exist side by side in each repeat and disrupt both leucine/isoleucine motifs. Because one of the pKa of histidine is 6.0, we hypothesized that these His residues must play a role in receptor function by changing the structure of the α-helical coiled coil domain in the acidified endosomes [2]. Immunoelectron

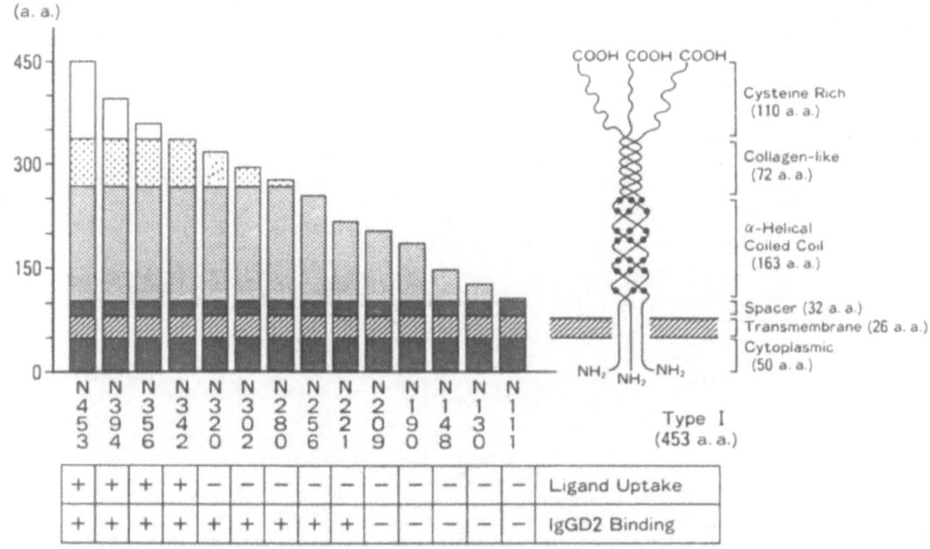

Figure 2. Schematic representation of the C-terminal deletion of mutant MSR. Each of the six domain is distinguished by a type of shadowing. The ligand uptake activities determined by fluorescent labeled DiI-acetyl-LDL and the trimer formation determined by cell surface IgG-D2 binding of the mutants are shown as positive (+) or negative (-), respectively.

microscopic studies had already shown that the scavenger receptors dissociate their ligands in the endosomes and enter the recycling pathway [20].The presence of histidines at positions 168 and 260 is another conserved characteristics of this domain. This result raises the possibility that the stability of the structure which exhibits pH dependance could be involved at physiologically relevant pH. Immunoelectron microscopic studies revealed that after internalization, MSR dissociate their ligands in the endosome and recycle them through transgolgi to the cell surface (Figure 3). We substituted His168 and His260 into leucine, a hydrophobic amino acids, and measured their abilities to dissociate their ligands at an acidic pH. The 260His → Leu substitution results in the loss of acid-dependent ligand dissociation activity, whereas the 268His → Leu substitution does not affect it. Immunoelectron microscopic studies indicated that the 260His → Leu mutant receptors appeared in the lysosome compartments with their ligands, 30 minutes after warm up, whereas normal receptors had already dissociated their ligands and appeared in transgolgi and other recycling pathways. These results signified that His260 is essential for the pH-dependent conformational change of MSR, which leads to the dissociation of their ligands at an acidic pH [10].

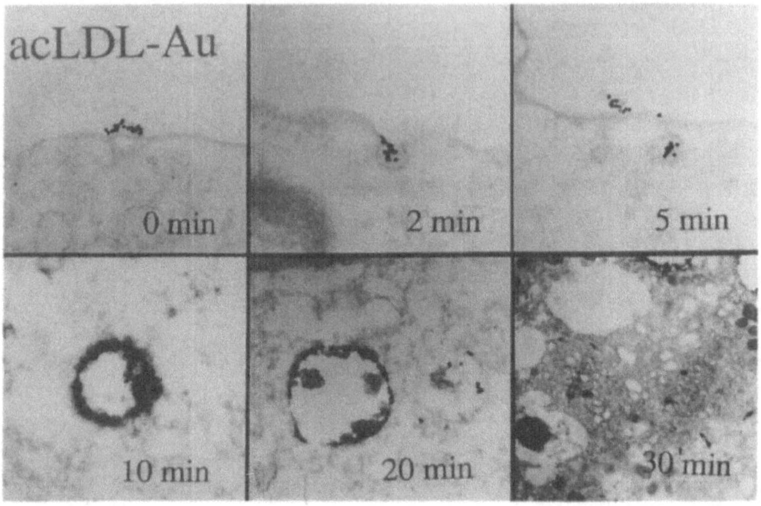

Figure 3. Recycling pathway or MSR in bovine alveolar macrophages. After a 2-hour incubation at 4° C, acetyl LDL-Au particles and positive reactions of anti-MSR monoclonal antibody, IgG D2 are found on the cell surface membrane. After warming up to 37° C, both of these are concentrated in coated pits and coated vesicles. At 20 minutes, MSR still remained in endosome, and the acetyl ldl-Au was detected in lysosome. MSR is the detected in trans cisterna of the Golgi complex (30 minutes) and is observed in the secretory vesicle.

One of the most important recent progress is the finding by Gordon and colleagues [21]. They established an monoclonal antibody 2F8 which effectively blocks the cation independent macrophage adhesion to bacterial plastic dish. Later they indicated that 2F8 is also effectively inhibits adhesion in liver or spleen tissue slice. The antigen of 2F8 was appeared to be MSR. The binding site of 2F8 to MSR was determined using truncated murine receptor expressed in CHO cells. Mutated murine receptor lacking complete collagenous domain still can bind 2F8 (S. Gordon and T. Kodama, unpublished). Current results suggest that MSR mediate the cation independent adhesion function through the interaction of α-helical coiled-coil domain and plasma component (S. Gordon et al., personal communication).

DOMAIN 5: COLLAGEN-LIKE DOMAIN

Domain 5 consists of 23 to 24 uninterrupted Gly-X-Y tripeptide repeats that form a collagenous triple helix. In collagens, residue Y is often either proline or lysine, which is frequently hydroxylated post-translationally to stabilize the trimeric structure. In the bovine receptor, 14 out of 24 Y residues were proline or lysine.

One of the most distinctive features of MSR is their broad ligand-binding specificity. High affinity ligands include some LDL modified to increase their negative charge, maleylated bovine serum albumin, certain polyribonucleotides, some polysaccharides, and other various negatively charged macromolecules [1]. MSR ligand-binding is unusual not only because of its broad specificity but also because it exhibits nonreciprocal cross-competition. Non-reciprocal cross-competition of acetyl LDL and oxidized LDL was first observed in macrophages [22,23]. Oxidized LDL which is a physiological ligand for MSR [24], is detected in atherosclerotic lesions, and plays a critical role in the cholesterol accumulation in these lesions. The experiments using C-terminally deleted receptors indicated that the 22 C-terminal amino acids of domain 5 are essential for ligand binding and uptake. Comparison of the amino acid sequences among human, mouse, rabbit, and bovine receptors revealed that this domain is highly conserved, and in particular, the C-terminal 10 amino acids are identical. The other conspicuous feature is that four basic amino acids (Lys 327, 334, 337, and 340) in this region are conserved. Considering that this receptor recognizes a wide range of negatively charged macromolecules, these positively charged residues should be extremely significant. We prepared point mutant receptors with lysines at the above positions and investigated their ligand binding and uptake activities. Substitution of lysine 337 into alanine abolished the acetyl-LDL degradation and binding at 37° C, but did not abolish the 4° C binding. In contrast, substitution of more than 2 lysines in this region were needed to abolish the oxidized LDL degradation and 37° C binding. This observation is consistent with reported nonreciprocal cross competition [25]. The results of direct binding experiments show that the binding activities of certain mutants at 4° C were different at 37° C. In general, collagen molecules dissolve in solution at 4° C and aggregate at 37° C because the hydrophobic interaction at 37° C is stronger than at 4° C. With our results reported here, we wish to propose the importance of 37° C binding experiments in comparison to 4° C binding experiments.

Based on the computational model of this domain using the coordinates of backbone atoms given by X-ray fiber diffraction for poly (L-prolyl-glycyl-L-proline), we built a structure of this domain, and named it the "charge collagen" model (Figure 4). This model is characterized by three coiled grooves containing nine lysines. We selected the polynucleic acids, because poly (I) and poly (G) can inhibit actyl-LDL binding to MSR but poly (A) and poly (C) cannot. When a phosphate backbone of poly (G) is placed into the modelled ligand binding groove, alternative phosphate groups are fitted to interact with the lysine residues, and the poly (G) chain winds around the collagen structure along the three turn coiled groove. Since the bases of the nucleotide chain seem to be recognized by the receptor, syn orientation about the glycosyl bond is necessary for the proposed phosphate backbone structure so that the bases interact with the peptides. It is well known that anti conformers dominate over syn for polypyrimidines and that syn and anti are about equally abundant for polypurines [26]. This may explain why polypyrimidines are not binding competitors to acetyl LDL in our model. Considering the structural difference between poly (G) or (I) and poly (A), 6-carbonyl groups of guanine and inosine bases could be recognized by the lysine and the preceding glutamine residues. In order to inhibit acetyl-LDL binding, the molecular weight of polynucleotide must be more than 8300 [27]. In the charged collagen model, 7 bases wind around the coiled groove for each turn. Thus, more than 21 nucleotides are necessary to make three turns and form a tight complex, which is consistent with the results of the inhibition studies.

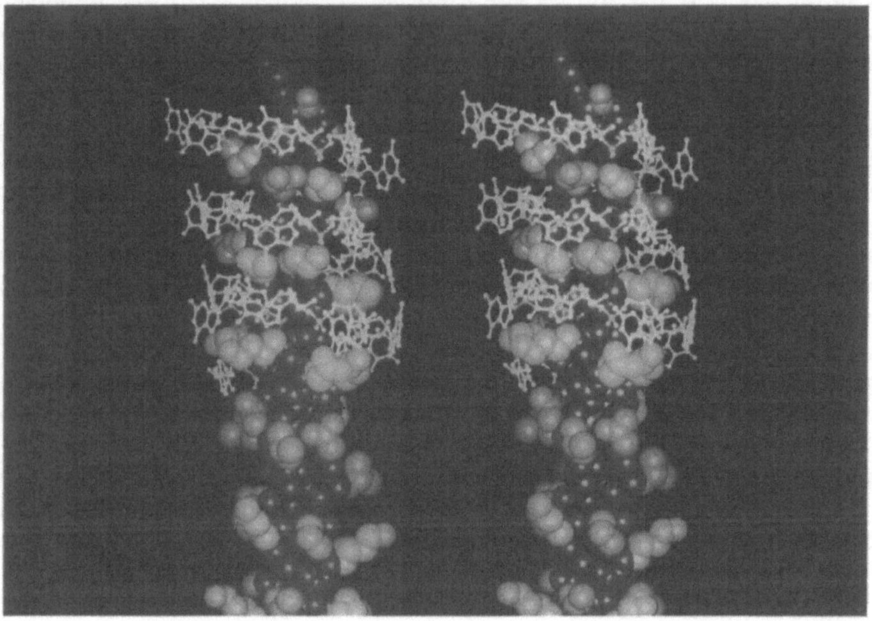

Figure 4. Computer graphics model of the interaction between collagen structure of MSR and polynucleic acids. Stereo drawing van der Waarls model of the ligand-binding domain of MSR and its possible interaction with poly (G) is indicated (for details, see [10]).

The oxidation of LDL results in an increase of their binding to collagen [28,29]. Deposited lipoproteins are initially trapped in the extracellular matrix of arteries. The charged collagen structure of MSR can compete for modified lipoproteins with the arterial collagens, which may lead to foam cell formation in atheromatous lesion. In addition to the extracellular matrix collagens, other proteins including complement C1q, pulmonary surfactant apoprotein, acetylcholine esterase, and serum mannose-binding protein, have collagenous domains.

A transmembrane molecule named MARCO (macrophage receptor with a collagenous structure) [30] closely resembling MSR was reported. This trimeric receptor has 270 amino-acids G-X-Y repeats. MARCO also contains a SRCR domain at the N-terminus. MARCO can bind acetyl-LDL and bacteria, but not yeast or Ficoll. MSR is expressed in most macrophage lineage cell types including Kupffer cell of the liver and lung alveolar macrophages. The expression of MARCO is limited to marginal zone macrophages of lymph node and spleen, which is implicated in the host defense, especially bacterial recognition and phagocytosis.

Sequence identities between domain 5 and other molecules that contain Gly-X-Y repeats except MARCO in the national Biomedical Research Foundation database were not particularly high (for example 51.4% identity over 74 residues of human type IV collagen a1), considering that one-third of these residues are glycine, and many are proline or lysine. The amino acid sequence mimicking the "charged collagen structure" of MSR (GPKGQKGEKG) appeared at the N-terminus of collagenous domain of MARCO (GQKGEKGQKGE).

DOMAIN 6: C-TERMINAL TYPE-SPECIFIC DOMAIN

By alternative splicing of 3'exons, two C-terminally different receptor subunits were generated. Type I C-terminal domain contains six conserved cysteins, consisting of scavenger receptor cystein-rich (SRCR) domains. A group of genes encodes a domain highly identical to the SRCR domain has been reported by Krieger and colleagues. The proteins with SRCR domains, the number of SRCR domain per molecule, and their distribution (indicated in parentheses) are as follows: MSR type I, 1 (macrophages); MARCO, 1, (a subset of macrophages); Cyclophilin/MAC 2 binding protein , 1 (bone marrow stromal cells, macrophages, breast cancer); sea urchin speract receptor, 4 (sea urchin sperm); complement factor 1,1; WC1 (gd T cell antigen), 11; M130 (human macrophage antigen), 9; CD6 (T cell antigen), 3; and CD5 (T cell antigen), 3. The distribution suggests that protein having SRCR domain are mainly expressed in lymphocyte and macrophages, and may be related to particular ligand recognition or host defense mechanism [31], which is yet still unknown.

The domain structure Type II C-terminal domain lacks cystein and differs among the animal species studied. When transfected separately, both type I and type II receptors mediated the scavenger function. Double immunostaining studies indicated that both type I and type II receptors are coexpressed in the same human macrophages [20]. The expression of type I mRNA and protein increased during differentiation from monocytes to macrophages, which was associated with an increase in receptor activity, whereas type II expression did not change as dramatically [32].

Conclusion

Figure 5 summarizes the domain structure of MSR. The receptor is a trimeric membrane glycoprotein with a single transmembrane domain. MSR mediates 1) a wide range of ligand binding; 2) ligand internalization; 3) acid dependent ligand dissociation; 4) cell adhesion; and 5) cell-to-cell interaction. The mechanism by which the scavenger receptor is regulated and the internalization, recycling, and adhesion functions remain an open question. Several possible explanations may exist. When a ligand binds to domain 5, the internalization may occur, and on the other hand binding a ligand or antibody to domain 4 may result in the adhesion function or inhibition of adhesion.

The other possibility is as follows. If the ligand is free in liquid, it will be internalized. If the ligand is too big for endocytosis, the binding of many MSR molecules may enhance the phagocytosis, and if the ligand is fixed on the extracellular matrix, adhesion may occur. If the ligand is on the cell surface, MSR may mediate cell-to-cell interaction. A further understanding of MSR will provide new insight into various macrophage-mediated physiological processes, and also macrophage-related pathological processes, including atherosclerosis.

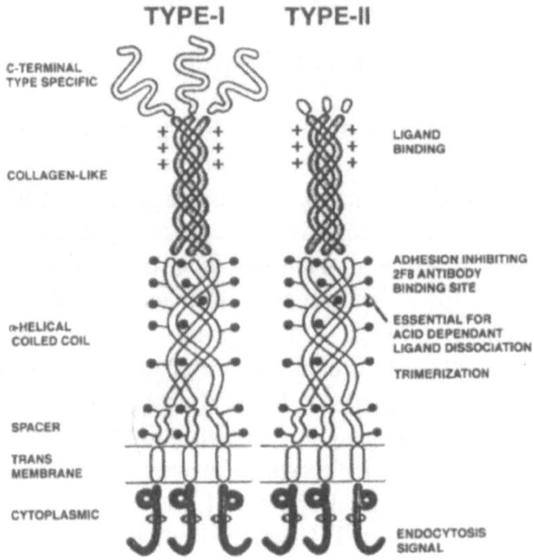

Figure 5. Functional domains of MSR

References

1. Brown MS, Goldstein JL. Lipoprotein metabolism in macrophage. Annu Rev Biochem 1983;52:223-61.
2. Kodama T, Freeman M, Rohrer L, Zabrecky J, Matsudaira P, Krieger M. Type I macrophage scavenger receptor contains Éø-helical and collagen-like coiled coils. Nature 1990;343:531-35.
3. Rohrer L, Freeman M, Kodama T, Penman M, Krieger M. Coiled-coil fibrous domains mediate ligand binding by macrophage scavenger receptor type II. Nature 1990;343:570-72.
4. Freeman M, Ashkenas J, Rees DJ, et al. An ancient, highly conseved family of cystein-rich protein domains revealed by cloning type I and type II murine macrophage scavenger receptors. Proc Natl Acad Sci USA 1990;87:8810-14.
5. Matsumoto A, Naito M, Itakura H, et al. Human macrophage scavenger receptors: Primary structure, expression, and localization in atherosclerotic lesions. Proc Natl Acad Sci USA 1990;87:9133-37.
6. Kurihara Y, Matsumoto A, Itakura H, Kodama T. Macrophage scavenger receptors. Curr Opinion Lipidol 1990;2:295-300.

7. Bickel PE, Freeman M. Rabbit aortic smooth muscle cells express inducible macrophage scavenger receptor messenger RNA that is absent from endothelial cells. J Clin Invest 1992; 90:1450-57.
8. Doi T, Higashino K, Kurihara Y, et al. Charged collagen structure mediates the recognition of negatively charged macromolecules by macrophage scavenger receptors. J Biol Chem 1993; 268:2126-33.
9. Emi M, Asaoka H, Matsumoto A, et al. Structure, organization and chromosomal mapping of the human macrophage scavenger receptor gene. J Biol Chem 1993;268:2120-2125.
10. Doi T, Kurasawa M, Higashino K, et al. The histidine interruption of an a-helical coiled coil allosterically mediates a pH dependent ligand dissociation from macrophage scavenger receptors. J Biol Chem 1994;268:25598-604.
11. Chen W, Goldstein JL, Brown MS. NPXY, a sequence often found in cytoplasmic tails, is required for coated pit-mediated internalization of the low density lipoprotein receptor. J Biol Chem 1990;265:3116-32.
12. Collawn JF, Stangel M, Kuhn LA, et al. Transferrin receptor internalization sequence YXRE implicates a tight turn as the structural recognition motif for endocytosis. Cell 1990;63:1061-72.
13. Naito M, Kodama T, Matsumoto A, Doi T, Takahashi K. Tissue distribution, intracellular localization, and in vitro expression of bovine macrophage scavenger receptors. Am J Pathol 1991;139:1411-23.
14. Naito M, Suzuki H, Mori T, Matsumot A, Kodama T, Takahashi K. Coexpression of type I and type II human macrophage scavenger receptors in macrophages of various organs and foam cells in atherosclerotic lesions. Am J Pathol 1992;141:591-99.
15. Crick FHC. Structure of collagen. Acta Crystallogr 1953;6:689-97.
16. Landschulz WH, Johnson PF, McKnight SL. The leucine zipper: A hypothetical structure common to a new class of DNA binding proteins. Science 1988;240:1759-64.
17. O'Shea EK, Klemm JD, Kim PS, Alber T. X-ray structure of the GCN4 leucine zipper, a two stranded, parallel coiled coil. Science 1991;254:539-44.
18. Oas TG, McIntosh LP, O'Shea EK, Dahlquist FW, Kim PS. Secondary structure of leucine zipper determined by nuclear magnetic resonance spectroscopy. Biochemistry 1990;29:2891-94.
19. Cohen C, Parry DAD. Structure of collagen. Proteins 1990;7:1-15.
20. Mori T, Takahashi K, Naito M, et al. Endocytic pathway of scavenger receptor vi trans-Golgi system in bovine alveolar macrophages. Lab Invest 1994; in press.
21. Fraser I, Hughes D, Gordon S. Divalent cation independent macrophage adhesion inhibited by monoclonal antibody to murine scavenger receptor. Nature 1993;364:343-46.
22. Arai H, Kita T, Yokode M, Narumiya S, Kawai C. Multiple receptors for modified low density lipoproteins in mouse peritoneal macrophages. Biochem Biophys Res Commun 1989;159: 1375-82.
23. Sparrow CP, Parthasarathy S, Steinberg, D. A macrophage receptor that recognizes oxidized low density lipoprotein but not acetylated low density lipoprotein. J Biol Chem 1989;264: 2599-2604.
24. Steinberg D, Parthasarathy S, Carew TE, Khoo JC, Witztum JL. Beyond cholesterol. modification of low-density lipoprotein that increase its atherogenecity. N Engl J Med 1989; 320:915-24.
25. Freeman M, Ekkel Y, Rohrer L, et al. Expression of type I and type II bovine scavenger receptors in CHO cells. Proc Natl Acad Sci USA 1991;88:4931-35.

26. Seanger W. In: Principle of nucleic acid structure. New York: Springer Verlag, 1984:69-78.
27. Brown MS, Basu SK, Falck JR, Ho YK, Goldstein JL. The scavenger cell pathway for lipoprotein degradation. J Supramol Struc 1980;13:67-81.
28. Hoover GA, McCorkick S, Kalant N. Interaction of native and modified low density lipoprotein with collagen gel. Arteriosclerosis 1988;8:525-34.
29. Jimi S, Sakata N, Matunaga A, Takebayashi S. Low density lipoproteins bind more to type I and III collagens by negative charge dependent mechanism. Atherosclerosis 1994;107:109-16.
30. Elooma O, Kangas M, Sahlberg C, et al. Cloning of a novel bacteria-binding receptor structurally related to scavenger receptors and expressed in a subset of macrophages. Cell 1995;80:603-609.
31. Resnick D, Pearson A, Krieger M. The SRCR superfamily. Trend Biochem Sci 1994;19:5-8.
32. Geng Y, Kodama T, Hansson G. Differential expression of scavenger receptor isoforms during monocyte-macrophage differentiation and foam cell formation. Arterioscler Thromb 1994;14: 798-806.

APOLIPOPROTEIN C-III, AN IMPORTANT PLAYER IN LIPOPROTEIN METABOLISM

J.C. Fruchart, V. Clavey, G. Luc, J. Dallongeville, B. Staels, and J. Auwerx
Serlia et Inserm U325, Institut Pasteur, 1 rue du Pr Calmette, 59019 Lille Cédex, France

Introduction

Apolipoprotein (apo) C-III is a component of several classes of plasma lipoproteins such as triglyceride-rich particles (chylomicrons, very low density lipoproteins [VLDL], intermediate density lipoproteins [IDL]) and high density lipoproteins (HDL) [1]. Apo C-III is a 79 aminoacid glycoprotein produced predominantly in the liver and to a lesser extent in the intestine.

When triglyceride-rich lipoproteins enter the circulation, they acquire apo C-III from HDL [2,3] and apo C-III is usually present in multiple copies on each triglyceride-rich particle [4]. Several studies suggest that apo C-III modulates the metabolism of these triglyceride-rich particles, but its exact function *in vivo* is not yet fully understood.

In vitro, apo C-III has been shown to inhibit hydrolysis of triglycerides by lipoprotein lipase [5,6]. It also inhibits apo E-mediated clearance of lipoproteins *in vitro* and *in vivo* [7,8]. The importance of apo C-III becomes evident from the correlation between apo C-III levels with triglyceride concentrations in plasma from normal or dyslipoproteinemic subjects. Patients deficient in apo C-III exhibit an increased catabolism of VLDL and an unusually efficient conversion of VLDL to IDL and low density lipoproteins (LDL) [9]. In contrast, elevated apo C-III synthetic rates have been observed in hypertriglyceridemic patients [10]. Furthermore, genetic studies have identified several apo C-III gene polymorphisms, which may be associated with increased plasma apo C-III levels and hypertriglyceridemia [11,12].

The strongest evidence for a role of apo C-III in lipid homeostasis comes from studies in transgenic animals. In animals overexpressing apo C-III, marked hypertriglyceridemia was found [13,14], whereas in animals mutant for both apo C-III alleles, hypotriglyceridemia was observed [15]. The animals with a targeted disruption of the apo C-III gene were furthermore protected from postprandial hypertriglyceridemia, a predisposing factor for the development of atherosclerotic vascular disease [15].

This review will focus on the interaction of apo C-III- and apo B-containing particles with the LDL receptor, the role of apo C-III-containing particles in the susceptibility to the atherogenic process and the effect of drugs affecting the metabolism of apo C-III-containing

A. M. Gotto, Jr. et al. (eds.), Drugs Affecting Lipid Metabolism, 631–638.

lipoprotein.

Modulation of Lipoprotein B Binding to the LDL Receptor by Apolipoprotein C-III

We have recently shown that apo B-containing lipoproteins isolated by immunoaffinity chromatography bind to the LDL receptor of HeLa cells with an affinity dependent on their apo C-III and apo E content [16]. We showed that apo C-III when present diminished the binding of apo B-containing particles. Removal of apo C-III affects the accessibility and conformation of apo B100 near the residue 3249 which is the primary thrombin cleavage site. These results suggest that the receptor domain of apo B100 may be masked either by lipids or by apo C-III [17].

Naturally occurring lipoproteins are very heterogeneous and cannot be used to study the role of each parameter separately. Therefore we purified LpB by immunoaffinity and enriched these lipoproteins either in lipids or in apolipoproteins [18]. The increased content of triglycerides reduced LpB binding to the LDL receptor. Addition of apo C-III to triglyceride-enriched LpB almost completely abolished the interaction with the receptor, indicating a synergistic effect of lipids and apo C-III (Figure 1).

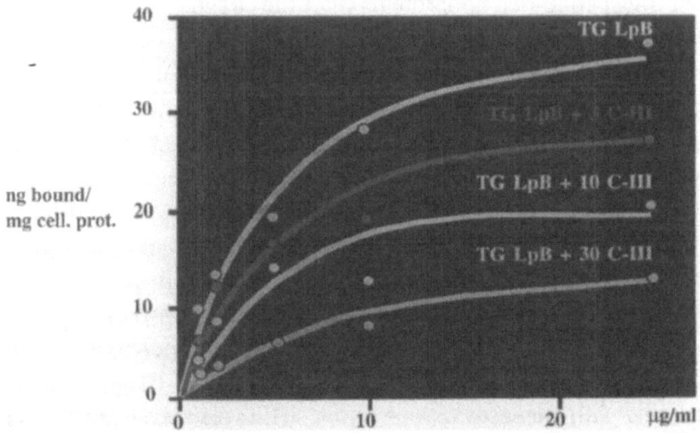

Figure 1. Interaction at 4° C with the LDL receptor of TG LpB incubated with different amounts of apo C-III.

The apo C-III effect was specific and cannot be obtained with apo C-I. With apo C-II, an inhibitory effect was also observed, but to a lesser extent than with apo C-III. At 37° C, apo C-III decreased the catabolism of triglyceride-enriched LpB by the LDL receptor of fibroblasts. Simultaneous addition of apo C-III and apo E impaired the stimulating effect of apo E (Figure 2).

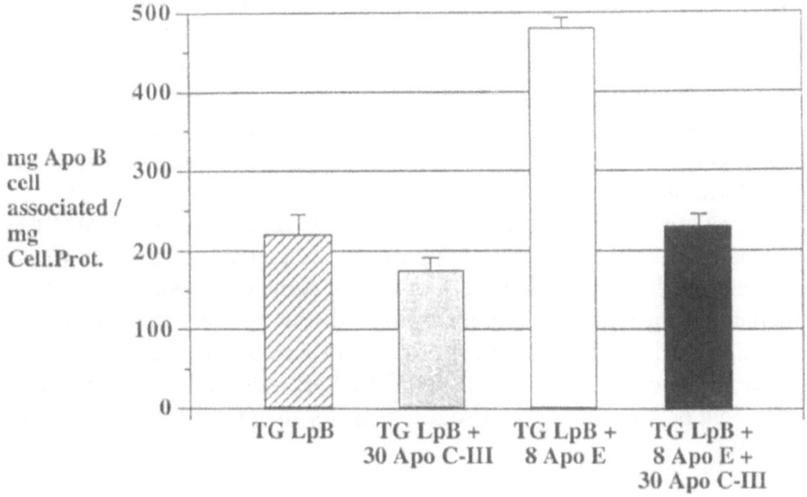

Figure 2. Specific cell association at 37°C (binding and internalization) of TG LpB complexed with apolipoproteins to the LDL receptor on fibroblasts.

Our approach, which presents the advantage of allowing us to dissociate the effect of lipids and apolipoproteins without interference of endogenous apolipoproteins other than apo B, confirms previous experiments showing that the degree of cell metabolism is determined by the ratio of apo E to apo C-III [19].

Role of Apolipoprotein C-III in the Susceptibility to the Atherogenic Process

Using a procedure combining immunoprecipitation and rocket immunoelectrophoresis, we compared the distribution of apo C-III between apo B-containing lipoproteins (apo C-III-LpB) and lipoproteins which do not contain apo B (apo C-III-Lp non-B) [20].

A case control study of apo C-III-containing particles has been performed in two populations at contrasting risk for coronary artery disease (ECTIM Study). The ECTIM Study offered the opportunity to compare the distribution of apo C-III in 360 survivors of myocardial infarction (MI) and 489 controls in France and in Northern Ireland (where the mortality and the incidence of coronary heart disease is more than three times as great as in France) [21].

The mean values of lipoparticle levels of MI and controls in each country and between controls of both countries were compared by an analysis of variance after adjustment for covariates (age, body mass index, alcohol consumption, drug intake, cigarette smoking). None of the subjects were treated with hypolipidemic drugs. Apo C-III-

LpB appeared significantly higher in survivors of MI than in controls in both countries, while apo C-III-Lp non-B were not statistically different in both groups in each country (Table 1). Therefore, the apo C-III ratio (apo C-III-LpB non-B/apo C-III-LpB) was significantly lower in MI than in controls, both in France and in Northern Ireland. The comparison between French and Irish controls showed that the two populations differed for apo C-III-Lp non-B and apo C-III ratio which were higher in France and for apo C-III-LpB which were lower in France (Table 1).

Multivariate analysis showed that the apo C-III ratio was a better means of discriminating between the two control populations than conventional risk factors. These differences between the two control populations are of particular interest with regard to the large difference of the incidence in coronary heart disease between the two countries and suggest that apo C-III ratio is a risk marker for MI. In accordance with our results, several clinical studies showed that the increase of apo C-III-LpB and/or the decrease of apo C-III-Lp non-B could be a marker for atherogenesis or for the progression of atherosclerotic lesions [22-25].

Drugs Affecting Apo C-III Containing Lipoprotein Metabolism

We have recently demonstrated that different hypolipidemic drugs such as fibrates or n-3 fatty acids and, to a lesser extent, statins, can reduce significantly apo C-III and apo B containing particles [26-29]. In contrast, no effect was observed with cholestyramine [26,27].

Recent studies performed in our laboratory have shown that fibrates down-regulate apo C-III gene expression at the transcriptional level [30]. In primary cultures of rat and human hepatocytes, fenofibric acid lowered apo C-III mRNA in a time and dose-dependent manner. This reduction in apo C-III mRNA levels was accompanied by a decreased secretion of apo C-III in the culture medium of human hepatocytes (Figure 3).

This decrease in apo C-III gene expression by fenofibrate provides a potential mechanism by which this drug induces a less atherogenic plasma lipoprotein profile.

Conclusion

Accumulating evidence indicates that apo C-III decreases plasma triglyceride-rich lipoprotein catabolism. This implies decreased *in vivo* lipolysis and tissue uptake.

Epidemiological and angiographic trials have demonstrated the clinical importance of the quantitation of apo C-III containing particles, but further studies, particularly prospective studies, are needed to confirm and establish the atherogenic potential of these parameters.

Lipid lowering medications appear to have specific effects on apo C-III containing lipoproteins. Further investigations are necessary to determine how these parameters may be used to adapt therapy to the individual.

Table 1. Mean (SD) levels of lipids, apolipoproteins and apo C-III-containing particles in survivors of Myocardial Infarction (MI) and Control subjects © in France and in Northern Ireland.

	France			Northern Ireland			Between Controls
	MI mg/dl	C mg/dl	p	MI mg/dl	C mg/dl	p	p
Cholesterol	226.5(38.0)	321.3(41.1)	ns	240.1(39.4)	235.1(42.2)	ns	ns
Triglycerides	174.9(82.4)	159.8(83.7)	0.01	199.4(87.8)	160.0(89.9)	0.0001	ns
VLDL-cholesterol	29.8(19.6)	26.2(16.9)	0.01	34.6(14.8)	27.8(16.1)	0.0001	0.03
LDL-cholesterol	154.8(33.4)	151.6(38.0)	ns	163.2(35.9)	155.9(39.0)	ns	ns
HDL-cholesterol	42.5(10.4)	53.7(16.1)	0.0001	41.8(13.0)	51.4(14.8)	0.0001	0.05
Apo A-I	126.6(19.7)	151.1(27.4)	0.0001	123.4(20.3)	145.6(26.2)	0.0001	0.02
Apo B	134.0(29.3)	127.9(30.9)	0.05	145.8(30.0)	131.7(32.3)	0.0001	0.04
Apo C-III Lp non-B	18.9(7.2)	19.9(7.1)	ns	18.2(6.6)	18.2(7.8)	ns	0.02
Apo C-III Lp B	10.3(5.4)	9.3(5.9)	0.01	14.9(8.1)	11.3(6.9)	0.02	0.0001
Apo C-III ratio*	2.27(1.54)	2.99(3.53)	0.004	1.43(0.68)	2.17(3.56)	0.02	0.0001

*Apo C-III ratio = apo C-III Lp non-B / apo C-III Lp B. p, values represent significant levels after adjustment for age, body mass index, alcohol intake and cigarette smoking. ns, not significant ($p > 0.05$).

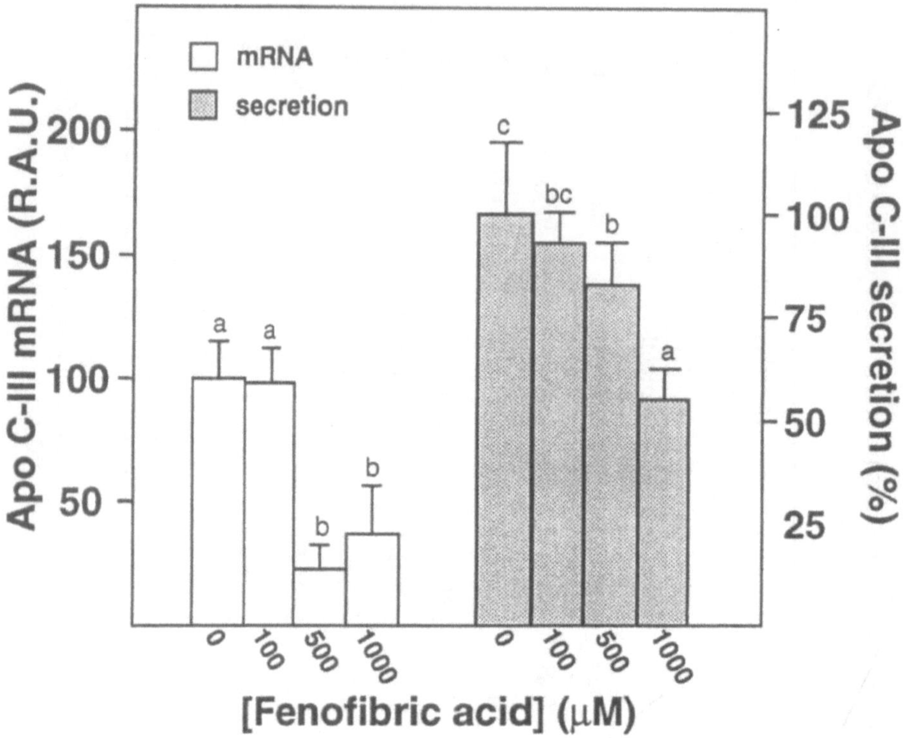

Figure 3. Dose-dependent effects of fenofibrate on apo C-III mRNA and secretion in primary cultures of adult human hepatocytes.

References

1. Mahley RW. Plasma lipoprotein : Apolipoprotein structure and function. J Lipid Res 1984;25:1277-94.
2. Havel RJ, Kane JP, Kashyap ML. Interchange of apolipoprotein between chylomicrons and high density lipoproteins during alimentary lipemia in man. J Clin Invest 1973; 52:328.
3. Berman M, Hall M, Levy RI, et al. Metabolism of apo B and apo C lipoproteins in man: Kinetic studies in normal and hyperlipoproteinemic subjects. J Lipid Res 1978; 19:38-56.
4. Kane JP, Sata T, Hamilton RL, Havel RJ. Apoprotein composition of very low density lipoproteins of human serum. J Clin Invest 1975;56:1622-34.
5. Wang CS, McConathy WJ, Kloer HU, Alaupovic P. Modulation of lipoprotein lipase activity by apolipoproteins. Effect of apolipoprotein C-III. J Clin Invest 1985;75:384-90.
6. McConathy WJ, Gesquière JC, Bass H, Tartar A, Fruchart JC, Wang CS. Inhibition of lipoprotein lipase activity by synthetic peptides of apolipoprotein C-III. J Lipid Res 1992;33/7:995-1003.
7. Windler E, Chao Y, Havel RJ. Regulation of the hepatic uptake of triglyceride-rich

lipoproteins in the rat. J Biol Chem 1980;255:8303-7.

8. Quarfordt SH, Michalopoulos G, Shirmer B. The effect of human C apolipoproteins on the *in vitro* hepatic metabolism of triglyceride emulsions in the rat. J Biol Chem 1982;257:14642-47.

9. Ginsberg HN, Le NA, Goldberg IJ, et al. Apolipoprotein B metabolism in subjects with deficiency of apolipoproteins C-III and A-I : Evidence that apolipoprotein C-III inhibits catabolism of triglyceride-rich lipoproteins by lipoprotein lipase *in vivo*. J Clin Invest 1986;78:1287-95.

10. Malmendier CL, Lontie JF, Delcroix C, Dubois DY, Magot T, De Roy L. Apolipoproteins C-II and C-III metabolism in hypertriglyceridemic patients. Effect of a drastic triglyceride reduction by combined diet restriction and fenofibrate administration. Atherosclerosis 1989;77:139-49.

11. Rees A, Shoulders CC, Stocks J, Galton DJ, Baralle FE. DNA polymorphism adjacent to human apoprotein A-I gene: Relation to hypertriglyceridemia. Lancet 1983;1:444-46.

12. Dammerman M, Sandkuijl LA, Halaas JL, Chung W, Breslow JL. An apolipoprotein C-III haplotype protective against hypertriglyceridemia is specified by promoter and 3' untranslated region polymorphisms. Proceedings of the National Academy of Sciences USA 1993;90:4562-66.

13. Ito Y, Azrolan N, O'Connell A, Walsh A, Breslow JL. Hypertriglyceridemia as a result of human apo C-III gene expression in transgenic mice. Science 1990;249: 790-93.

14. De Silva HV, Lauer SJ, Wang J, et al. Overexpression of human apolipoprotein C-III in transgenic mice results in an accumulation of apolipoprotein B48 remnants that is corrected by excess apolipoprotein E. J Biol Chem 1994;269:2324-35.

15. Maeda N, Li H, Lee D, Oliver P, Quarfordt SH, Osada J. Targeted disruption of the apolipoprotein C-III gene in mice results in hypertriglyceridemia and protection from postprandial hypertriglyceridemia. J Biol Chem 1994;269:23610-16.

16. Agnani G, Bard JM, Candelier L, Delattre S, Fruchart JC, Clavey V. Interaction of LpB, LpB:E, LpB:C-III and LpB:C-III:E lipoproteins with the low density lipoprotein receptor on HeLa cells. Arterioscler 1991;11/4:1021-29.

17. Yang CY, Gu ZW, Valentinova N, et al. Human very low density lipoprotein structure : Interaction of the C apolipoproteins with apolipoprotein B100. J Lipid Res 1993;34:1311-21.

18. Clavey V, Lestavel-Delattre S, Copin C, Bard JM, Fruchart JC. Modulation of lipoprotein B binding to the LDL receptor by exogenous lipids and apolipoproteins C-I, C-II, C-III and E. Arterioscler 1995;15:963-71.

19. Sehayek E, Eisenberg S. Abnormal composition of hypertriglyceridemic very low density lipoprotein determines abnormal cell metabolism. Arterioscler Thromb 1990;10:1088-96.

20. Parra HJ, Arveiler D, Evans AE, et al. A case-control study of lipoprotein particles in two populations at contrasting risk for coronary heart disease : The ECTIM Study. Arterioscler Thromb 1992;12:701-7.

21. Who Monicia Projet Principal Investigators. The World Health Organization MONICA Project (Monitoring trends and determinants in Cardiovascular disease) : A major international collaboration. J Clin Epidemiol 1988;41:105-14.

22. Blankenhorn DH, Alaupovic P, Wickham E, Chin HP, Azen SP. Prediction of angiographic change in native human coronary arteries and aortocoronary bypass grafts: Lipid and nonlipid factors. Circulation 1990;81:470-76.

23. Hodis HN, Mack WJ, Azen SP, et al. Triglyceride- and cholesterol-rich lipoproteins have a differential effect on mild/moderate and severe lesion progression as assessed by quantitative

coronary angiography in a controlled trial of lovastatin. Circulation 1994;90:42-9.
24. Hodis HN, Mack WJ, Knight-Gibson C, Alaupovic P. The role of triglyceride-rich lipoprotein families in the progression of coronary artery atherosclerotic lesions. J Am Coll Cardiol 1995;195A: submitted for publication.
25. Chivot L, Mainard F, Bigot E, et al. Logistic discriminant analysis of lipids and apolipoproteins in a population of coronary bypass patients and the significance of apolipoproteins C-III and E. Atherosclerosis 1990;82:205-11.
26. Bard JM, Parra HJ, Douste-Blazy P, Fruchart JC. Changes in lipoprotein particles defined by their apolipoprotein composition on pravastatin or cholestyramine therapy. J Drug Dev 1990;3/1:111-15.
27. Bard JM, Ose L, Hagen E, et al. for the European Fluvastatin Study Group. Changes in plasma apolipoprotein B-containing lipoparticle levels following therapy with fluvastatin and cholestyramine. Am J Cardiology 1995;76:65A-70A.
28. Bard JM, Luc G, Douste-Blazy P, et al. Effect of simvastatin on plasma lipids, apolipoproteins and lipoprotein particles in patients with primary hyper-cholesterolaemia. Eur J Clin Pharmacol 1989;37:545-50.
29. Fruchart JC. Particules riches en triglycérides et athérosclérose. Rôle des acides gras Oméga 3. Symposium " Omega 3, lipoprotéines et Athérosclérose " Grenade du 13-14 octobre 1995.
30. Staels B, Vu Dac N, Kosykh VA, et al. Fibrates downregulate apolipoprotein C-III expression independent of induction of peroxisomal acylcoenzyme A oxidase. A potential mechanism for the hypolipidemic action of fibrates. J Clin Invest 1995;95:705-12.

FIBRINOGEN BINDING OF LIPOPROTEIN(a) DOES NOT REQUIRE AN ACTIVE LYSINE BINDING SITE IN APOLIPOPROTEIN(a) KRINGLE IV-10

Angelo M. Scanu[†*], Olga Klezovitch[†], and Celina Edelstein[†]
Departments of Medicine[†], Biochemistry and Molecular Biology, University of Chicago, Chicago, Illinois 60637, USA*

Introduction

We have previously shown that rhesus monkey Lp(a) has an impaired lysine binding capacity which we attributed to the replacement of Trp72 by Arg in the lysine binding site (LBS) of apo(a) kringle IV-10 [1]. Subsequently, we identified lysine-binding defective human mutants with the Trp72→ Arg substitution in the LBS of kringle IV-10 [2]. The relationship between lysine and fibrin(ogen) binding in apo(a) is still unclear [3-5]. In order to shed light on this subject, we studied the fibrinogen binding capacity of wild-type and mutant Lp(a) particles, isolated from either human or rhesus monkey plasma, as well as the free apo(a)s each separated from the parent lipoprotein by a mild reductive procedure able to promote the cleavage of the interchain disulfide between apo(a) and apoB100 [6]. We also studied the fibrinogen binding capacity of human wild-type (Trp72) and mutant (Arg72) apo(a) kringle IV-10 expressed both in *E. coli* and Chinese hamster ovary (CHO) cells [7]. The overall results show that the fibrinogen binding capacity of both Lp(a) and apo(a) does not require the activity of the LBS of kringle IV-10 and that this binding resides in a domain which is to a large extent masked in apo(a) when it is a constituent of the Lp(a) particle.

MATERIALS AND METHODS

The wild-type and the mutant subjects with the Trp72→ Arg substitution were described before as well as the methods for the phenotyping and genotyping of apo(a) [2]. In wild-type subjects, the Lp(a) was isolated from the plasma by combining ultracentrifugal techniques and lysine-Sepharose column chromatography [8]. In mutant subjects the isolation of Lp(a) was modified as previously described [1,6]. Free apo(a) was prepared by subjecting each parent Lp(a) to mild reductive conditions using 2 mM dithioerythritol in the presence of 100 mM ϵ-aminocaproic acid (EACA) as previously described [6]. The conditions for the expression of wild-type and mutant human kringle IV-10 in *E. coli* and CHO cells were those reported by Klezovitch and Scanu [7]. The lysine binding properties of Lp(a), apo(a), and recombinant kringles were examined by affinity chromatography on

A. M. Gotto, Jr. et al. (eds.), Drugs Affecting Lipid Metabolism, 639–647.

lysine-Sepharose [2]. In the fibrinogen binding assay, fibrinogen was immobilized on microtiter plates and either used as such or after treatment with plasmin (PM-fibrinogen) following the method described by Harpel et al., [9]. The quantification of apo(a) was carried out by ELISA as previously reported [10].

Results

STUDIES WITH RECOMBINANT HUMAN WILD-TYPE AND MUTANT KRINGLE IV-10

The nonglycosylated wild-type kringle IV-10 expressed in *E. coli* and the glycosylated form expressed in CHO cells bound to lysine-Sepharose and were eluted from the column by 200 mM EACA, indicating that the binding was lysine dependent and was not influenced by the state of glycosylation of the kringle. In turn, the mutant kringle IV-10 expressed in either *E. coli* or CHO cells, had no affinity for lysine-Sepharose supporting the critical role played by the Trp72 of kringle IV-10 in the binding.

Wild-type kringle IV-10 exhibited a bimodal binding to PM-fibrinogen: one component was saturable with an apparent Kd of 23 μM and inhibitable by 200 mM EACA. The other component, which represented about 60% of the total binding, was nonsaturable and was unaffected by EACA. The total binding to PM-fibrinogen by mutant kringle IV-10 was markedly less than that of its wild-type counterpart and was only represented by the nonlysine mediated component (data not shown). Moreover, L-proline, which had an inhibitory action on the binding of Lp(a) and apo(a) to PM-fibrinogen (see below), had no effect on the fibrinogen binding of kringle IV-10.

STUDIES ON HUMAN LP(A) AND DERIVED FREE APO(A)

Lysine binding studies. We have previously reported that mutant apo(a), which is lysine binding defective when a member of the Lp(a) particle, binds to lysine-Sepharose when studied as free apo(a) due to the unmasking of the 'Lys-Pro sensitive domain' (LPSD) [6]. In the current studies we compared the binding capacity to lysine-Sepharose of mutant free apo(a) having a non-functional LBS and an open LPSD with that of native Lp(a) having an open functional LBS but a masked LPSD. For this purpose, we used a 0-200 mM EACA elution gradient. The elution of free mutant apo(a) occurred at 50 mM EACA whereas that of wild-type Lp(a) required a much higher EACA concentration, (100 mM), indicating that in the open state, the affinity for lysine of the LBS is two-fold higher than that of LPSD.

Fibrinogen binding studies. In the case of the wild-type subjects, both Lp(a) and derived free apo(a) bound to PM-fibrinogen. However, the total binding of free apo(a) was about three-fold higher than that of Lp(a). In both cases, the binding was concentration-dependent and approached saturation at 120 nM protein (Figure 1). The binding to PM-fibrinogen was hampered by the presence of either EACA or L-proline, each at 200 mM although the inhibitory action was about 2-fold higher with EACA (Figure 2). Moreover, the specific lysine- and proline-mediated binding of free apo(a) for fibrinogen was about four-fold higher than that of Lp(a). This was due to differences in Bmax (Figure 1), since the Kd values (Table 1) were in comparable ranges, 35-87 nM.

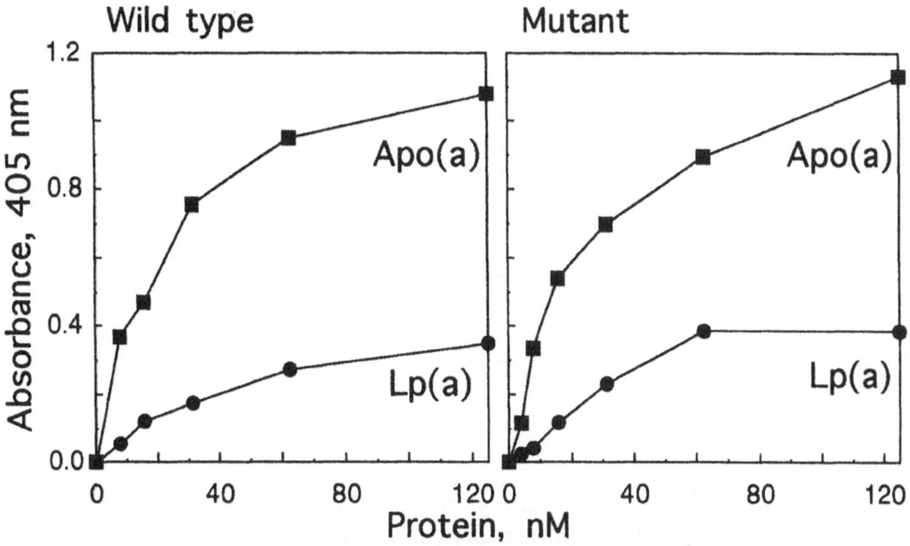

Figure 1. Binding to PM-fibrinogen of human wild-type and mutant Lp(a) species and derived free apo(a)s. The proteins were incubated with immobilized PM-fibrinogen overnight at 22° C. The bound protein was detected with an antibody specific for apo(a). Apo(a), ■; Lp(a), ●.

In the case of the lysine binding defective mutant subjects, Lp(a) and derived free apo(a) bound to PM-fibrinogen in a manner similar to that exhibited by wild-type Lp(a) and apo(a) in terms of both total and lysine- and proline-mediated binding (Figures 1 and 2). There was also a significant difference in the Bmax values (Figure 1) between apo(a) and Lp(a) whereas the apparent Kds were in the same range (Table 1).

STUDIES ON RHESUS LP(A) AND DERIVED FREE APO(A)

Rhesus Lp(a) and derived free apo(a) bound to PM-fibrinogen in a manner similar to that of the corresponding human products. Similar to the results with the human Lp(a) mutant, the binding of free apo(a) was about four-fold higher than that of Lp(a). The binding parameters, Kd and Bmax, were also similar to those observed with the human counterparts (data not shown).

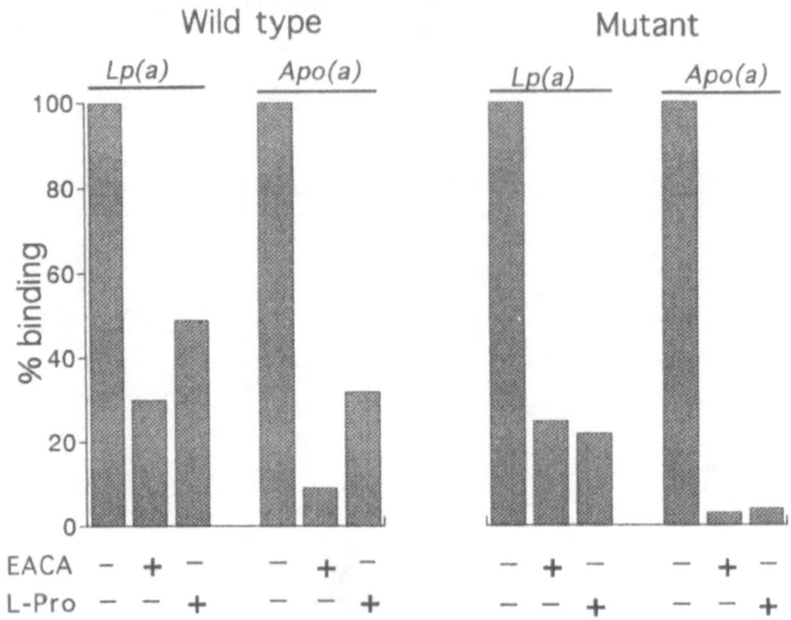

Figure 2. Effect of EACA and L-proline, each 200 mM, on the binding to PM-fibrinogen of human wild-type and mutant Lp(a) species and derived free apo(a)s.

Table 1. PM-fibrinogen binding affinities of human Lp(a) and free apo(a).

Sample	Total	Lys-mediated*	Pro-mediated**
	Kd, nM‡		
Wild type			
Lp(a)	35.1 ± 17.1 (8)	43.5 ± 30.0 (8)	71.7 ± 32.8 (2)
apo(a)	87.2 ± 27.3 (8)	85.5 ± 29.1 (8)	35.3 ± 12.1 (4)
Mutant			
Lp(a)	99.9 ± 18.3 (4)	93.8 ± 49.2 (4)	85.3 ± 19.2 (2)
apo(a)	33.3 ± 8.3 (2)	34.3 ± 15.2 (2)	35.4 ± 12.3 (2)

*Lys-mediated binding was obtained by subtracting the binding in the presence of 0.2 M EACA from the total binding. **Pro-mediated binding was obtained by subtracting the binding in the presence of 0.2 M proline from the total binding. ‡Dissociation constants (Kd) are expressed as a mean ± SD. The values in parenthesis represent the number of experiments.

Discussion

In these studies we have shown that a functional LBS in kringle IV-10 is not required for the binding of Lp(a) and apo(a) to fibrinogen. We have also demonstrated that free apo(a) binds to fibrinogen more avidly than its parent Lp(a) and attributed this difference to the activity of the LPSD which we previously identified in the course of *in vitro* reassembly studies [6]. This binding domain (Figure 3) which is sensitive to lysine and proline, is still poorly characterized and is presumed to extend between kringles IV-4 and IV-9 [6].

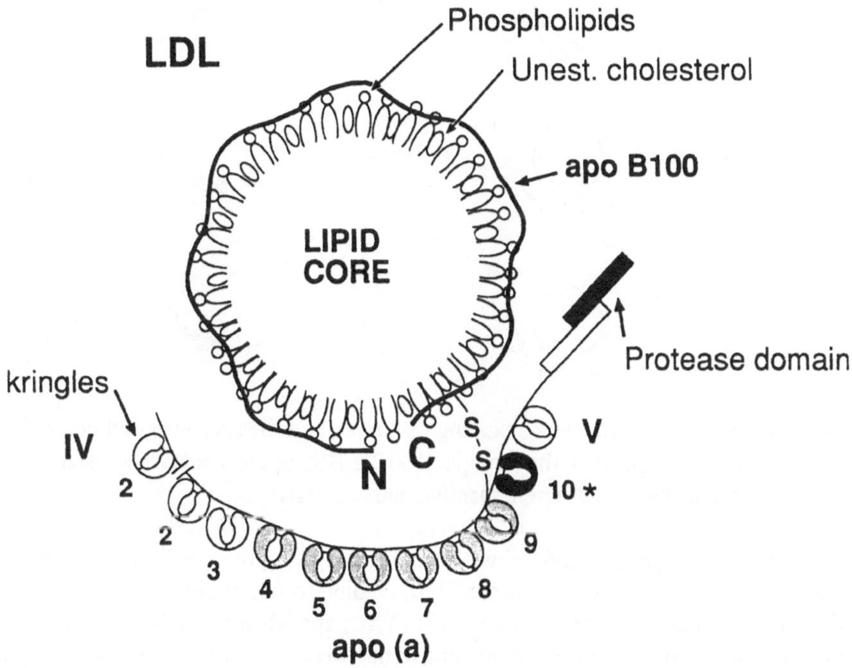

Figure 3. Model of Lp(a) showing kringle IV-10 (black) which contains the LBS involved in binding to lysine-Sepharose and the LPSD (shaded) involved in fibrinogen binding.

In terms of lysine binding, our data showed the following (Figure 4): 1) human wild-type Lp(a) binds to lysine via the LBS of apo(a) kringle IV-10 without a significant involvement of the masked LPSD indicating that an active LBS is open for ligand interaction; 2) both human mutant and rhesus Lp(a) are lysine binding negative because the open LBS is nonfunctional due to the presence of Arg72 instead of Trp in the LBS of kringle IV-10 [1,2]; 3) free apo(a), derived from wild-type human Lp(a), binds to lysine-Sepharose via the activity of both the LBS of kringle IV-10 and the unmasked LPSD; 4) free apo(a) derived from mutant Lp(a) or rhesus Lp(a) binds to lysine via the unmasked LSBD. In addition, we now show that the binding affinity for lysine-Sepharose of the LPSD of apo(a) is markedly less than that of the LBS of kringle IV-10, likely an indication that none of the kringles comprising the LPSD has an LBS as competent as that of kringle IV-10.

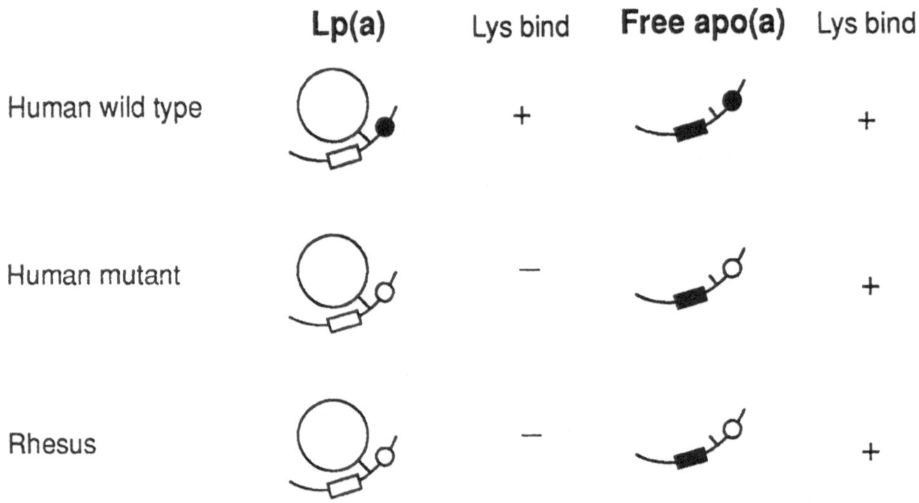

Figure 4. Schematic view of the lysine binding of human and rhesus Lp(a) and derived free apo(a). Small circles represent the kringle IV-10 LBS: open, inactive; closed, active. Rectangles represent the LPSD: open, inactive; closed, active.

In terms of fibrinogen binding, we made the following observations (Figure 5): 1) human wild-type, mutant Lp(a) and rhesus Lp(a) all bind to fibrinogen to the same extent, indicating that the binding occurs via the LPDS; 2) free apo(a)s derived from either human wild-type, or mutant Lp(a) or rhesus Lp(a), bind to fibrinogen with a comparable affinity but with a more marked avidity (higher Bmax) than their respective parents. This indicates that the extent of fibrinogen binding in apo(a) is related to the portion of LPSD which becomes functional when apo(a) is freed from Lp(a).

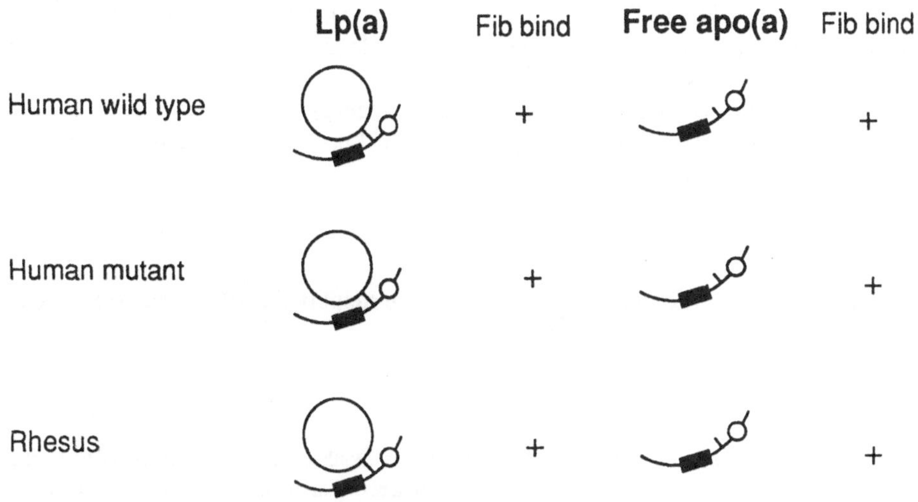

Figure 5. Schematic view of the fibrinogen binding of human and rhesus Lp(a). The symbols are the same as in the legend to Figure 4.

Taken together our current findings provide strong evidence that in the whole Lp(a) particle, the site which plays a role in the binding to lysine-Sepharose is distinct from that involved in fibrinogen binding. This conclusion may appear to be at variance with our previous results indicating that recombinant wild-type kringle IV-10 has the capacity to bind to fibrinogen [7]. However, the fibrinogen binding capacity of the individual recombinant kringle was quantitatively modest and of a low affinity (micromolar) in contrast to the nanomolar range exhibited by apo(a) either free or as a constituent of Lp(a). Thus, we may conclude that the binding of apo(a) to fibrinogen can be essentially accounted for by the activity of the LPSD.

On an *in vivo* level, the above results suggest that in the plasma, apo(a) which mostly circulates as a constituent of Lp(a), binds to fibrinogen via the partially masked LPSD. On the other hand, at the tissue level the situation may be different due to the presence of lipid-free apo(a). For instance, the presence of free apo(a) has been reported in the arterial wall [11-13]. This apo(a), by having a fully functional LPSD, would bind more avidly than Lp(a) to fibrin and, in consequence, enhance the accumulation of the latter in the atherosclerotic plaque. Moreover, such an accumulation may be contributed by the potential interfering action of apo(a) on the activity of plasmin at the fibrin surface. In support of these hypotheses are the studies showing that fibrin/apo(a) complexes are present in atherosclerotic lesions [14] and that Lp(a) and recombinant apo(a) may compete for the binding of plasminogen to the fibrin surface [5]. From previous studies *in vitro* it had been proposed that Lp(a) may enhance fibrin accumulation by retarding the process of plasmin generation through a kringle IV- mediated mechanism [3-5]. Thus, Lp(a) may contribute to the formation and growth of the atherosclerotic plaque by several mechanisms not necessarily exclusive of each other and possibly acting synergistically. On the basis of these considerations, the knowledge of the fibrin(ogen) binding capacity of free apo(a) should prove to be very useful in establishing the role that Lp(a) plays in the pathogenesis of atherothrombotic disorders.

Acknowledgments

The original studies carried out in this laboratory were supported by Program Project NIH-HL 18577.

References

1. Scanu AM, Miles LA, Fless GM, et al. Rhesus monkey lipoprotein(a) binds to lysine-Sepharose and U937 monocytoid cells less efficiently than human lipoprotein(a) - evidence for the dominant role of kringle 4-37. J Clin Invest 1993; 91:283-91.
2. Scanu AM, Pfaffinger D, Lee JC, Hinman J. A single point mutation (Trp72→ Arg) in human apo(a) kingle 4-37 associated with a lysine binding defect in Lp(a). Biochim Biophys Acta 1994;1227:41-45.
3. Miles LA, Fless GM, Scanu AM, et al. Interaction of Lp(a) with plasminogen binding sites on cells. Thromb Haemost 1995;3:458-65.
4. Edelberg JM, Pizzo SV. Lipoprotein(a): The link between impaired fibrinolysis and atherosclerosis. Fibrinol 1991;5:135-43.
5. Harpel PC, Hermann A, Zhang X, Ostfeld I, Borth W. Lipoprotein(a), plasmin modulation and atherogenesis. Thromb Haemost 1995;74:382-86.
6. Edelstein C, Mandala M, Pfaffinger D, Scanu A.M. Determinants of lipoprotein(a) assembly: A study of wild-type and mutant apolipoprotein(a) phenotypes isolated from human and rhesus monkey lipoprotein(a) under mild reductive conditions. Biochemistry 1995;34:16483-92.
7. Klezovitch O, Scanu AM. Lysine and fibrinogen binding of wild-type (Trp72) and mutant (Arg72) human apolipoprotein(a) kringle IV-10 expressed in E. coli and CHO cells. Arter Thromb Vasc Biol; in press.
8. Fless GM, Rolih CA, Scanu AM. Heterogeneity of human plasma lipoprotein(a) isolation and characterization of lipoprotein subspecies and their apoproteins. J Biol Chem 1984;259:11470-78.
9. Harpel CH, Gordon BR, Parker TS. Plasmin catalyzes binding of lipoprotein(a) to immobilized fibrinogen and fibrin. Proc Natl Acad Sci USA 1989;86:3847-51.
10. Fless GM, Snyder ML, Scanu AM. Enzyme-linked immunoassay for Lp(a). J Lipid Res 1989;30:651-62.
11. Cushing GL, Gaubatz JW, Nava ML, et al. Quantitation and localization of apolipoproteins(a) and B in coronary artery bypass vein grafts resected at re-operation. Arteriosclerosis 1989;9:593-603.
12. Pepin JM, O'Neil JA, Hoff HF. Quantification of apo(a) and apoB in human atherosclerotic lesions. J Lipid Res 1991;32:317-27.

13. Rath M, Neindorf A, Reblin T, Dietel M, Krebber H, Beisiegel U. Detection and quantification of lipoprotein(a) in the arterial wall of 107 coronary bypass patients. Arteriosclerosis 1989;9:579-92.
14. Smith EB, Cochran S. Factors influencing the accumulation in fibrous plaques of lipid derived from low density lipoproteins. II. Preferential immobilization of lipoprotein(a) (Lp(a)). Atherosclerosis 1990;84:173-81.

IN VITRO STUDIES ON HUMAN CHYLOMICRON CATABOLISM

Ulrike Beisiegel, Annette Krapp, Jörg Heeren, and Wilfried Weber
University Hospital Eppendorf, Medical Clinic, Martinistraße 52, 20246 Hamburg, Germany

Introduction

The catabolism of human chylomicrons (CM) has not been extensively studied in the past. Most of the knowledge on CM catabolism is derived from experiments with rat chylomcirons [1-3]. We were interested in the composition of human CM and the mechanism by which the particles are taken up into liver cells. The best known mediator of chylomicron remnant (CR) catabolism is apolipoprotein E (apo E), but recently other proteins have been shown to be involved in this process.

Our studies were based on the concept that chylomicorns are hydrolyzed by lipoprotein lipase (LpL) after they entered the blood stream and that the enzyme then stays associated with the CR, as first indicated by Felts et al. [4] and later confirmed by Goldberg et al. [5]. The LpL was shown to mediate the uptake of lipoproteins into several cell types [6-9] and it could be demonstrated that it directly binds to the LDL receptor-related protein (LRP) [7]. Next to the LpL, hepatic lipase (HL) was proposed to be involved in CR catabolism and we [10] and others [11-13] recently showed that HL also binds to LRP and is able to mediate the uptake of lipoproteins into cells. It has therefore been proposed that HL might also play a role in CR catabolism. Both enzymes bind to the cell surface proteoglycans first [13,14] and then mediate the uptake of the lipoprotein particle via lipoprotein receptors. This receptor has been shown in vitro to be LRP, but *in vivo* studies in mice demonstrated a role in CR catabolism for both the LDL receptor (LDLR) and the LRP.

In our studies we characterized human CM derived from the plasma of patients with LpL or apo C-II deficiency. We hydrolyzed these CM *in vitro* with LpL and performed uptake experiments on human hepatoma cells. Cellular consequences of the uptake were studied in the same cells.

Characterization of Human Chylomicrons and Chylomicron Remnants

We obtained human CM from patients with LpL or apo C-II deficieny, who cannot hydrolize the CM *in vivo*. The composition of the particles as they are isolated from the

A. M. Gotto, Jr. et al. (eds.), Drugs Affecting Lipid Metabolism, 649–655.

patients plasma is given in Table 1 and the apoprotein pattern is shown in Figure 1. Next to apo B-48 some apo B-100 can be detected, indicating that the fraction does also contain some VLDL. The main apolipoprotein was apo E, and we observed in addition to the known apoproteins A-I, A-VI, and the C-apoproteins, a 110 kDa protein which has not been described before. This protein has been characterized and found to be a member of the family of complement factor H related proteins (Zipfel and Beisiegel, manuscript in preparation).

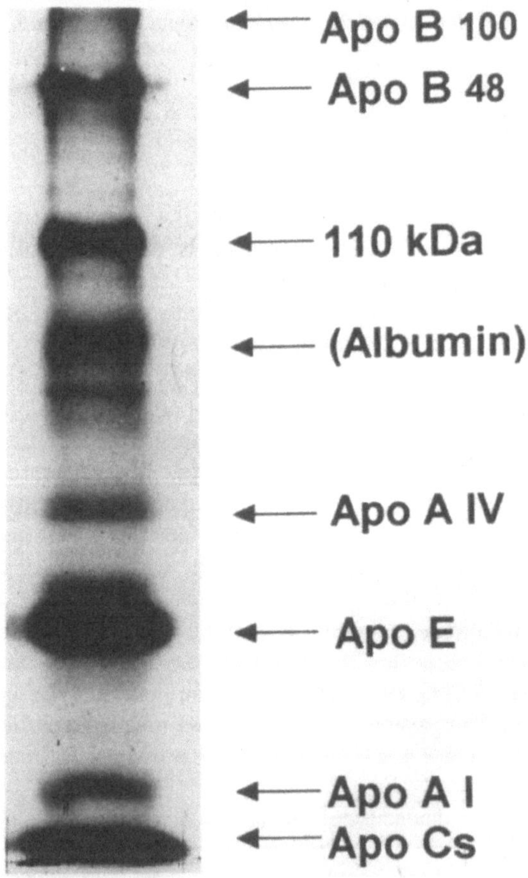

Figure 1. Autoradiography of the apoproteins of ^{125}I-CM. CM were isolated from a LpL-deficient patient and iodinated by the ICL-method. After precipitation with chloroform/methanol, the protein fraction was separated in a 12% SDS page, blotted on nitrocellulose and exposed to an x-ray film for 24 hours. In addition to the apoproteins some albumin can be detected on the particles.

Table 1. Composition of chylomicrons. The composition of CM is given as the mean value of ten preparations. Phospholipides were not determined. The sum of triglycerides, cholesterol, cholesterolesters, and proteins was set to 100%.

Triglycerides (%)	Cholesterol/Cholesterolester (%)	Proteins (%)
93 ± 2	6 ± 2	1 ± 0.8

The CM were incubated with purified bovine LpL to obtain a 30-40% hydrolysis, and the CR were then re-isolated in a sucrose spin. The isolated CR were analyzed on SDS-gelelectrophoresis and found to contain LpL detectable on immunoblots (data not shown). The CM and CR were radiolabeled with ^{125}iodine and used for uptake experiments.

Uptake Studies

Our main interest was to study the function of lipoprotein receptors, rather then only binding to the cell surface. For this reason we performed uptake experiments at 37° C. In earlier studies we have seen that the uptake is already at a maximum level after 90 minutes of incubation. All uptake experiments were performed in presence of Orlistat® (LaRoche, Basel) [15], a potent inhibitor of LpL activity, to avoid hydrolysis of the particles while the incubation.

Since CR catabolism mainly occurs in the liver we peformed the first series of experiments on human hepatoma cells (Hep3b). These cells have a low level of LDLR expression and have been shown to express LRP. A clear increase of CM uptake could be observed when LpL was added to the incubation medium, and CR, containing LpL, were also taken up more efficiently then CM alone. The addition of LpL to the LpL containing CR resulted in a further increase in the uptake (Table 2).These experiments with CR confirm earlier data obtained with rabbit β-VLDL as a model ligand [6].

Hepatic Lipase Can Mediate Chylomicron Remnant Uptake

HL-deficient patients have been described to accumulate CR. This might not only be due to the missing enzyme activity, but the lack of HL protein can affect the mediation of lipoprotein uptake. We performed uptake experiments with HL in the same way as described for LpL.

HL is secreted by human hepatoma cells, particularly by HUH_7 cells, and we used this cell line to obtain human HL free from LpL. We isolated the enzyme from the cell culture supernatant by a heparin column.

The isolated HL was used in the uptake experiments with human CM on hepatoma cells (Hep3b and HuH_7) and fresh human hepatocytes. As shown in Table 3 there is an increase in the CM uptake in all experiments. Even though the basic uptake of CM might already be increased by the HL secreted of the cells, the HL-mediated increase is in the same range as observed for the LpL. Therefore we propose an important role for this hepatic enzyme in CR clearance.

Table 2. Uptake of human chlylomicrons and chylomicron remnants. CR were produced by in vitro hydrolysis using 0.2 μg/ml bovine LpL for 30 minutes at 37° C. The amount of hydrolysis was determined by measuring the released fatty acids (free fatty acids half-micro test, Boehringer, Mannheim). The hydrolysis was around 30-40%. Specific uptake of the CR was determined in presence and absence of LpL on Hep3b. The experiments were performed at 37° C for 90 minutes. The bound ligands were released by heparin and the amount of uptake was measured in the cell lysate (NaOH). The values for the uptake without LpL were set to 100%. The number of experiments included in this table is given in brackets.

Ligands	% Uptake (n) [CM uptake = 100%]
CR w/o LpL	271 ± 30 (4)
CM + LpL	670 ± 80 (4)
CR + LpL	704 ± 50 (4)

Table 3. Effect of HL on the uptake of chylomicrons into human hepatoma cells and hepatocytes. Specific uptake of CM was determined in presence and absence of HL on the different cell lines and the values for the uptake without HL were set to 100%. The experiments were performed as decribed for Table 2. The number of experiments included in this table is given in brackets, two experiments were performed on hepatoctyes and both values are presented.

Cells	% Uptake (n) [CM uptake = 100%]
Hep3b	200 ± 51 (5)
HuH_7	176 ± 48 (4)
Hepatocytes	156 / 206

Role of Proteoglycans in Lipoprotein Uptake

All ligands described to be involved in the uptake of CR into liver cells, apo E, LpL, and HL, are known to be heparin binding proteins. And it is also known that these proteins bind to the proteoglycans on the cell surface. Therefore several authors proposed an important role of these proteoglycans in lipoprotein uptake [16]. We used normal Chinese hamster ovary cells (CHO) and CHO cells which are deficient in proteoglycans to study the lipase-mediated uptake of CM. The experiments showed (Table 4) that proteoglycans are necessary for cellular interaction, since the uptake is nearly abolished in the proteoglycan deficient cells. Studies with heparinase on other cells, also demonstrated that the proteoglycans are necessary for the binding to the cell surface however, the proteoglycans do not mediate the uptake [17].

Table 4. Influence of proteoglycans on the lipase-mediated uptake of chylomicrons. The specific uptake was determined in presence and absence of LpL or HL on the different cell lines as described for Table 2. The uptake without the addition of LpL or HLwas set to 100%. One representative experiment is shown for LpL. Two experiments were performed with HL and both values are presented.

	CHO Control Cells [CM uptake = 100%]	CHO PG Deficient Cells [CM uptake = 100%]
CM + LpL	350	102
CM + HL	349 / 320	110 / 102

Cellular Consequences

The uptake of CM and CR into heptoma cells does not lead to a total degradation as described for the LDL. Moreover we could show that around 50% of the radioactivity taken up by the cells was resecreted in the media in a chase incubation. In the presence of fetal calf serum or human serum this radioactivity was mainly found associated with the HDL-density fraction. We analyzed this fraction on SDS-PAGE and found that the apo E as well as the apoproteins A and C were resecreted from the cells. Similar observations have been made by Deckelbaum et al. [18]. We therefore propose that the liver cells do not degrade the apoprotein constituents of the CR but rather reuse them for secretion. We did not yet characterize whether the apo E is secreted alone or in a lipid particle.

Conclusion

In vitro hydrolysis of human CM produces CR containing LpL which are effectively taken up into hepatoma cells by an apo E and LpL mediated process. HL can also mediate the uptake of CM and therefore it might play an important role in the CR removal *in vivo*. Both enzymes fulfill this ligand function independently from their enzymatic activity.

Proteoglycans are important for the fast and effective initial binding of CR to the liver cells and seem to facilitate the subsequent receptor-mediated uptake. The receptors, responsible for the CR uptake are the LDLR and the LRP. The LRP mediates the particle uptake via an endocytotic pathway, different from this of the LDLR. This uptake mechanism for CR seems to allow a dissociation of the CR particle leading to a retroendocytosis of some apoproteins, while others are degraded in the cells.

Acknowledgements

We thank Nicolette Meyer for excellent technical assistance. This study was supported by grant Gr 258/10-1 of the Deutsche Forschungsgesellschaft.

References

1. Imaizumi K, Fainaru M, Havel RJ. Composition of proteins of mesenteric lymph chylomicrons in the rat and alterations produced upon exposure of chylomicrons to blood serum and serum proteins. J Lipid Res 1978;19:712-17.
2. Schaefer EJ, Jenkins LL, Brewer HB, Jr. Human chylomicron apolipoprotein metabolism. Biochem Biophys Res Commun 1978;80(2):405-12.
3. Pattnaik NM, Zilversmit DB. Effect of size and competition by lipoproteins and apolipoproteins on the uptake of chylomicrons and chylomicron remnants by hepatoma cells in culture. Biochim Biophys Acta 1980;617:335-46.
4. Felts JM, Itakura H, Crave JC. The mechanisms of assimilation of constituents of chylomicrons, very low density lipoproteins and remnants - a new theory. Biochem Biophys Res Commun 1975;66(4):1467-75.
5. Goldberg IJ, Kandel JJ, Blum CB, Ginsberg HN. Association of plasma lipoproteins with postheparin lipase activities. J Clin Invest 1986;78(6):1523-28.
6. Beisiegel U, Weber W, Bengtsson Olivecrona G. Lipoprotein lipase enhances the binding of chylomicrons to low density lipoprotein receptor-related protein. Proc Natl Acad Sci USA 1991;88:8342-46.
7. Nykjaer A, Bengtsson Olivecrona G, Lookene A, et al. The alpha 2-macroglobulin receptor/low density lipoprotein receptor-related protein binds lipoprotein lipase and beta-migrating very low density lipoprotein associated with the lipase. J Biol Chem 1993;268(20):15048-55.
8. Chappel DA, Fry GL, Waknitz MA, Iverius PH, Williams SE, Strickland DK. The low density lipoprotein receptor-related protein/a2-macroglobulin receptor binds and mediates catabolism of bovine milk lipoprotein lipase. J Biol Chem 1992;267: 25764-67.
9. Williams SE, Inoue I, Tran H, et al. The carboxyl-terminal domain of lipoprotein lipase binds to the low density lipoprotein receptor-related protein/alpha 2-macroglobulin receptor (LRP) and mediates binding of normal very low density lipoproteins to LRP. J Biol Chem 1994;269(12):8653-58.
10. Beisiegel U, Krapp A, Weber W, Olivecrona G. The role of alpha 2M receptor/LRP in chylomicron remnant metabolism. Ann NY Acad Sci 1994;737:53-69.
11. Bu X, Warden CH, Xia YR, et al. Linkage analysis of the genetic determinants of high density lipoprotein concentrations and composition: Evidence for involvement of the apolipoprotein A-II and cholesteryl ester transfer protein loci. Hum Genet 1994;93(6):639-48.
12. Diard P, Malewiak MI, Lagrange D, Griglio S. Hepatic lipase may act as a ligand in the uptake of artificial chylomicron remnant-like particles by isolated rat hepatocytes. Biochem J 1994;299(Pt 3):889-94.
13. Krapp A, Ahle S, Kersting S, et al. Hepatic lipase mediates the uptake of chylomicrons and b -VLDL into cells via the LDL receptor-related protein (LRP). J Lipid Res 1996; in press.
14. Eisenberg S, Sehayek E, Olivecrona T, Vlodavsky I. Lipoprotein lipase enhances binding of lipoproteins to heparan sulfate on cell surfaces and extracellular matrix. J Clin Invest 1992;90(5):2013-21.
15. Hadvary P, Siedler W, Meister W, Vetter W, Wolfer H. The lipase inhibitor tetrahydrolipstatin binds covalently to the putative active serine of pancreatic lipase. J Biol Chem 1996;266:2021-27.
16. Ji ZS, Brecht WJ, Miranda RD, Hussain MM, Innerarity TL, Mahley RW. Role of heparan sulfate proteoglycans in the binding and uptake of apolipoprotein E-enriched remnant

lipoproteins by cultured cells. J Biol Chem 1993;268(14): 10160-67.
17. Hilpert J, Willnow TE, Jonat S, Herz J. The role of the low density lipoprotein lipase receptor-related protein versus low density lipoprotein receptor in chylomicron catabolism. Circulation 1995;92:Suppl I-691.
18. Chen CM, Al-Haideri M, Presley JF, et al. Apoprotein E on model triglyceride-rich particles, incomparison to apoprotein B on LDL, remains relatively intact after cell uptake. Circulation 1995;92:Suppl I-691.

DIFFERENTIAL ACTIVITY OF APO AI AND APO AII IN REVERSE CHOLESTEROL TRANSPORT

Claire Benetollo[1], Corinne Talussot[1], Didier Rouy[2], Berlinda Vanloo[1], Patrice Denèfle[2], Robert Brasseur[3], and Maryvonne Rosseneu[1]
[1]Laboratory Lipoprotein Chemistry, Department of Biochemistry, University of Gent, Hospitaalstr. 13, 9000 Gent, Belgium, [2]Rhone-Poulenc Rorer, Centre Recherches Vitry, 13 Quai Jules Guesdes, 94403 Vitry/Seine, France, and [3]Centre Biophysique Moléculaire Numérique, Facultés Sciences Agronomiques, 5060 Gembloux, Belgium

Introduction

Reverse cholesterol transport is one of the major mechanisms involved in a decrease of the progression or in the regression of atherosclerotic lesions [1]. This process includes several steps: cholesterol is first desorbed from the cellular plasma membrane and incorporated into acceptor particles; this is followed by the esterification of the absorbed cholesterol and finally by the transport of the cholesteryl esters either to other lipoproteins and/or to the liver where they are catabolized. The first step of this process probably occurs through a passive diffusion of cholesterol into the acceptor phospholipid-apoprotein complexes [2]. The subsequent steps involve the action of the lecithin cholesterol acyl transferase enzyme (LCAT) for cholesterol esterification, of the cholesteryl esters transfer protein for cholesterol exchange between lipoproteins and of putative hepatic receptors for cholesterol catabolism [1].The relative contribution of the two major apoproteins apo AI and apo AII of the high density lipoproteins (HDL), to the reverse cholesterol transport is still controversial [2]. Apo AI-phospholipid and apo AII-phospholipid complexes are both acceptors of cellular cholesterol, although literature reports disagree about their relative efficiency [2]. In this report we compare the efficiency of apo AI- and apo AII-lipid complexes to promote cellular cholesterol efflux and subsequent cholesterol esterification. We further identify a domain of apo AII responsible for the displacement of lipid-associated apo AI and for the modulation of the LCAT activation of apo AI in the acceptor particles.

Materials and Methods

All experiments were carried out in a 10 mM Tris-HCl standard buffer pH 8.0, containing 150 mM NaCl, 0.01% EDTA. Human apo AI, apo AII, and apo E were purified to

A. M. Gotto, Jr. et al. (eds.), Drugs Affecting Lipid Metabolism, 657–665.

homogeneity as previously described [3]. The apo AII peptides corresponding to the amphipathic helices of apo AII, identified using the method proposed by Brasseur et al. [4], i.e. residues 13-29, 34-50, and 54-70 were synthesized by solid-phase synthesis using the F-moc protection method [5]. The peptides were purified by reverse-phase HPLC and their purity and mass controlled by sequencing and mass spectrometry.

PREPARATION OF R-HDL PARTICLES

The complexes were prepared by the sodium cholate dialysis method as described by Matz and Jonas [6]. For the cellular efflux experiments, complexes of dipalmitoyl-phosphatidylcholine (DPPC), and apoprotein were prepared at a DPPC-apoprotein ratio of 3/1 (w/w). For the LCAT activity measurements, complexes were prepared with palmitoyl-linoleyl-phosphatidylcholine (PLPC), cholesterol and apo AI at a PLPC/C/apo AI initial ratio of 2.5/0.125/1 (w/w), in order to increase the sensitivity of the detection for polyunsaturated cholesteryl esters [7]. The protein/lipid mixtures were incubated for 24 hours at 43° C and 4° C for the DPPC and PLPC complexes respectively, and the cholate was removed by extensive dialysis. The homogeneity of the complexes was assessed by gel chromatography on a Superose 6 PG column in 0.01 M Tris-HCl buffer, pH 7.6, in a FPLC system (Waters). The complexes were detected by continuous monitoring of the absorbance at 280 nm and the Trp fluorescence emission at 330 nm. The composition of the complexes was determined by quantitation of phospholipids and cholesterol using enzymatic colorimetric kits (Boehringer, Mannheim). Protein content was assayed by the method of Lowry [8], in the presence of sodium deoxycholate, using bovine albumin as a standard.

REACTION OF THE R-HDL WITH LCAT

The activity of the LCAT enzyme towards the different lipid/apoprotein complexes used as substrates, was determined by measuring the amount of cholesteryl esters by HPLC, as previously described [7]. The assay mixture consisted of a constant amount of complex at a cholesterol concentration of 20 µM. After a preincubation of 20 minutes at 37° C, the enzymatic reaction was initiated by adding 5 µl of the semi-purified LCAT enzyme. The reaction was stopped by extraction of the incubation mixture with hexane/isopropanol (3:2, v/v) containing cholesteryl heptadecanoate, as internal standard. Cholesteryl esters (CE) were quantified by isocratic HPLC on a reversed-phase Zorbax ODS column, eluted with acetonitrile/isopropanol (1:1, v/v). Detection was performed at 210 nm.

CELLULAR CHOLESTEROL EFFLUX

J774 macrophages cells were incubated with acetylated low density lipoprotein (LDL) (100 µg/ml apoB) for 16 hours and the cellular cholesterol levels were quantified by HPLC after lipid extraction. The cholesterol level in the cells (expressed as µg cholesterol/2.10^6 cells) increased from 8.7 up to 44 µg. The esterified cholesterol represented 35% of the total cholesterol in the loaded cells. Cholesterol efflux was measured after 16 hours of incubation of the J774 macrophages with increasing amounts of apoprotein/phospholipid complexes. The cholesterol content in the medium was subsequently measured by HPLC and represented the net cholesterol efflux, as spontaneous efflux was negligible in the absence of acceptors.

DISPLACEMENT OF APO AI FROM PHOSPHOLIPID/CHOLESTEROL/APO AI COMPLEXES

PLPC/C/apo AI complexes were incubated with increasing amounts of either apo AII or the synthetic peptides for two hours at 23° C. The apo AII/apo AI molar ratios varied between 0 and 4 for native apo AII, and between 0 and 16 for the synthetic apo AII peptides. Complexes were detected by measuring the absorbance at 280nm and Trp emission at 330 nm. Phospholipids were quantified as described above. Apo AI and apo AII were assayed by immunonephelometry and peptides by Phe quantitation by HPLC [9].

Results

CHOLESTEROL EFFLUX BY APOPROTEIN/PHOSPHOLIPID COMPLEXES

Cholesterol efflux from the laden J774 macrophages to the acceptor complexes was observed after 16 hours of incubation (Figure 1). The maximal cholesterol efflux was observed with the apo AI/phospholipid complexes. The cholesterol efflux induced by the apoE- and the apoAII-lipid complexes was comparable and about 40% lower than with the apoAI complexes. A plateau was reached around 100 µg for the three apoproteins after 16 hours of incubation with the cells.

DISPLACEMENT OF APO AI BY APO AII AND BY THE HELICES OF APO AII

We previously demonstrated before that plasma and recombinant apo AII are able to displace apo AI both from native HDL and from reconstituted phospholipid/apo AI complexes [9,10]. In order to locate the domain of the protein responsible for this effect, we synthesized the helical segments of apo AII: residues 13-29, 34-50, and 54-70. The characteristics of these segments are described in Table I. The helical repeats of apo AI are mainly hydrophilic with a mean hydrophobicity of -0.35, an hydrophobic moment of the same magnitude and a mean hydrophobic angle of around 125°. The N-terminal helices of apo AII have comparable characteristics to the repeats of apo AI, whereas the C-terminal helix is predominantly hydrophobic with a mean hydrophobicity of 0.22 and an hydrophobic angle of 200°.

Incubation of either plasma HDL or of apo AI/phospholipid complexes with any of the two N-terminal helices of apo AII did not affect either the size or the composition of the native particles. After separation of the mixture components by gel filtration, the elution volume, the A280 and the Trp fluorescence intensity of HDL and r-HDL remained unchanged. After incubation of the C-terminal apo AII helix with either plasma HDL (Figure 2B) or with r-HDL (Figure 2A) consisting of PLPC, cholesterol and apo AI, apo AI was displaced from HDL and r-HDL. This was demonstrated by the decrease of the Trp fluorescence, due only to apo AI as apo AII has no Trp residues, in the major HDL peak and the appearance of an extra apo AI peak at larger elution volume. This effect was accompanied by an increased size of the original plasma HDL and r-HDL, at ratios where apo AI and the C-terminal apo AII peptide coexist in the same particle. When apo AI had been completely displaced and substituted by the apo AII peptide, the plasma HDL recovered their original size (Figure 2B). The displacement of apo AI by the apo AII peptide occured at lower peptide/apo AI ratios in plasma HDL than in the discoidal r-HDL particles, as apo AI was completely displaced by the peptide at a molar ratio of 16/1 in HDL, whereas only 15% displacement occured in the discoidal particles at this particular ratio. Addition of a larger excess of peptide, up to a 32/1 peptide/apo AI molar ratio, enhanced the displacement of apo AI from the complexes, but the total amount of free apo AI did not increase above 40%, a value significantly lower than with plasma HDL [10]. Compared to the displacement induced by native apo AII, the molar amount of C-terminal peptide required was about eight times that of native dimeric apo AII [9,10].

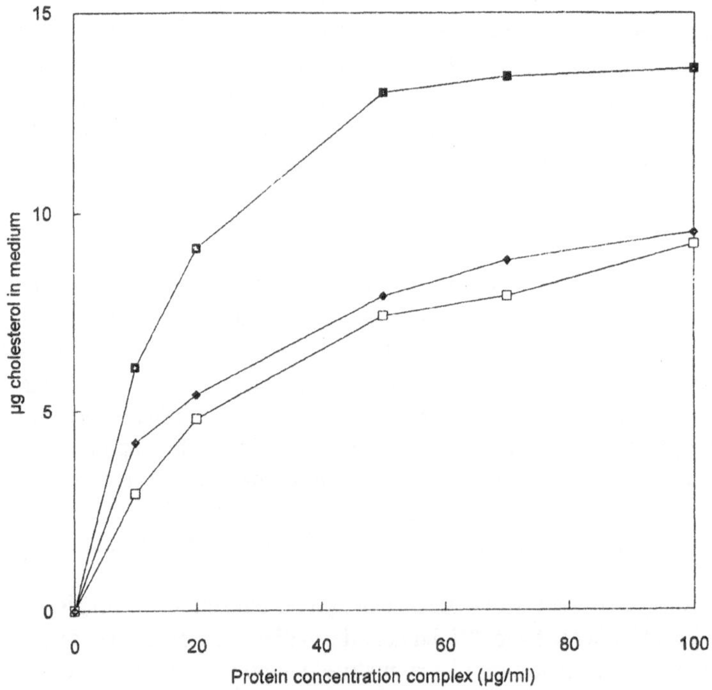

Figure 1. Cholesterol efflux from cholesterol-laden J774 macrpohages induced by DPPC/apoprotein complexes. (■): DPPC/apo AI; (♦): DPPC/apo AII; (□): DPPC/apo E.

Table 1. Properties of the helices of apo AI and AII.

Helical Repeat	$\langle H_o \rangle$	$\langle \mu_H \rangle$	Pho (°)
apo A-I 69-85	-0.38	0.36	116
apo A-I 102-118	-0.56	0.53	114
apo A-I 124-140	-0.38	0.37	121
apo A-I 146-162	-0.55	0.53	121
apo A-I 168-184	-0.44	0.41	125
apo A-I 190-206	-0.13	0.12	123
apo A-I 223-239	-0.043	0.087	134
apo A-II 13-29	-0.08	0.07	170
apo A-II 34-50	-0.23	0.24	140
apo A-II 54-70	0.22	0.26	200

$\langle H_o \rangle$ mean hydrophobicity according to Eisenberg's consensus scale
$\langle \mu_H \rangle$ mean hydrophobic moment

MODULATION OF THE LCAT ACTIVATION OF APO AI BY THE C-TERMINAL PEPTIDE OF APO AII

As we previously reported [3], the LCAT activation properties of apo AII are negligible compared to those of apo AI, as the Vmax and Km of activation by discoidal phospholipid/cholesterol/apoprotein complexes differ by a factor 10 when apo AII is compared to apo AI. In the course of the displacement of apo AI from apoAI/PLPC/cholesterol complexes by the apo AII C-terminal peptide, a mixed apo AI/peptide/lipid complex is generated. The activation of LCAT by this complex was followed as a function of percentage of displacement of apo AI by the peptide and compared to that of the original PLPC/cholesterol/apo AI complex (Figure 3). The kinetics of activation of the enzyme became slower as the amount of apo AI decreased and that of apo AII peptide increased in the mixed complex. When 40 % apo AI had been released from the discoidal particle, the percentage esterified cholesterol by the mixed apo AI/apo AII complex had decreased by 80 % compared to the esterification by the apo AI/lipid substrate (Figure 4, lower part). The decrease in total esterification was accompanied by a comparable decrease of the initial reaction rate Vo (Figure 4, upper part).

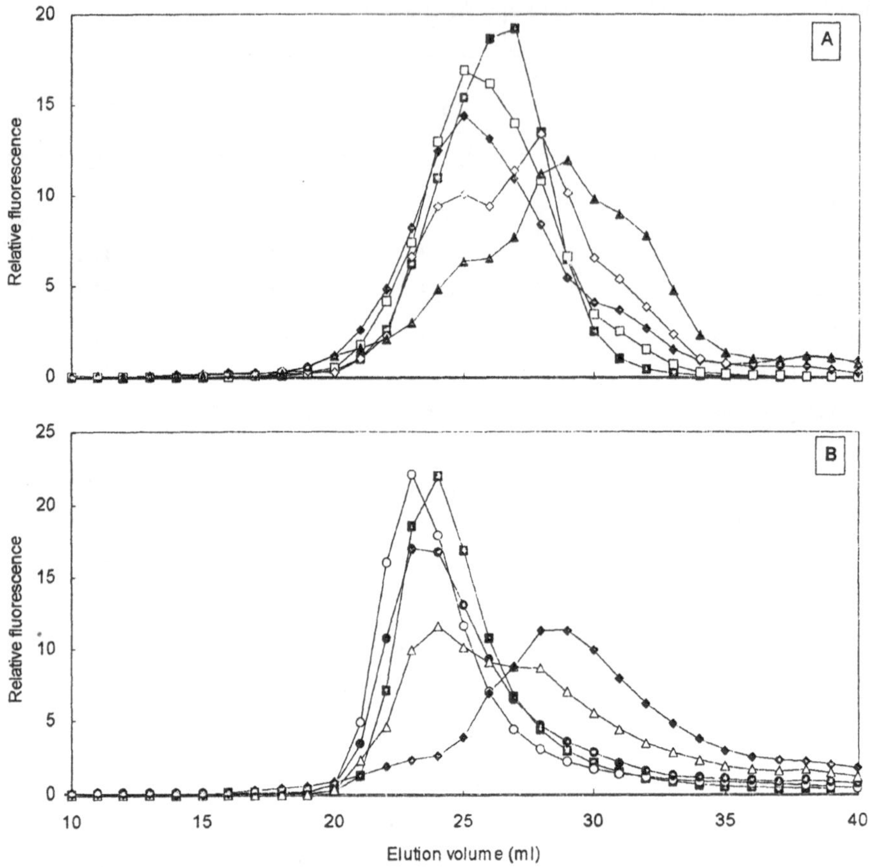

Figure 2. Displacement of apo AI from PLPC/cholesterol/apo AI complexes (A) by the apo AII C-terminal 53-70 peptide at apo AI/peptide molar ratios of : (■): 0/1; (□): 8/1; (◆): 16/1; (◇): 24/1; (▲) 32/1 and from HDL (B) and at apo AI/peptide molar ratios of : (■): 0/1; (○): 4/1; (●): 8/1; (Δ): 12/1; (◆): 16/1.

Conclusions

The reverse cholesterol transport process involves several steps; the first step consists in the efflux of cholesterol from the plama membrane of the cells, a process occuring probably through passive diffusion of the lipid to the smaller discoidal particles which are the most efficient acceptors [1,2]. During this step, cholesterol becomes incorporated into the complexes and the morphology of the acceptor particle seems more critical than its protein composition; at comparable dimensions of the complexes, the apo AI, AII, and E act as

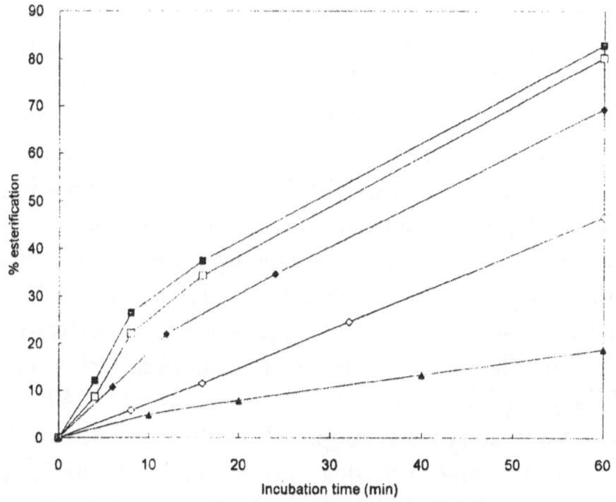

Figure 3. Cholesterol esterification by the lecithin cholesterol acyl transferase enzyme (LCAT) of mixed complexes consisting of PLPC/cholesterol/apo AI/apo AII C-terminal 53-70 peptide at peptide/apo AI ratios of: (■):0/1; (□): 8/1; (◆): 16/1; (◇): 24/1; (▲) 32/1.

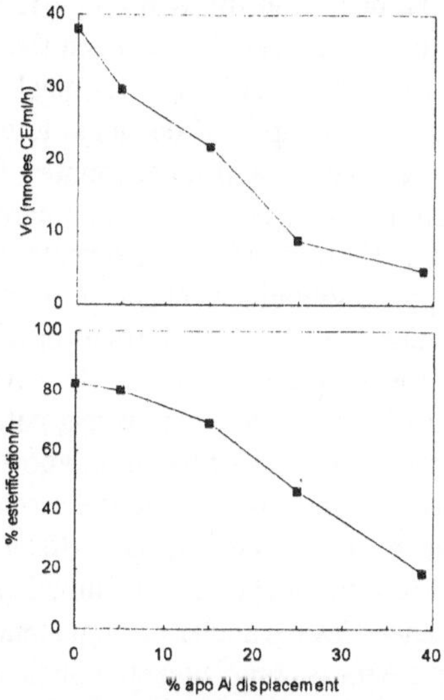

Figure 4. LCAT activation parameters, initial velocity Vo (upper curve) and percentage of cholesterol esterification after 60 minutes (lower curve) as a function of the percentage of apo AI displacement from PLPC/cholesterol/apo AI complexes by the C-terminal 54-70 peptide of apo AII.

efficient cholesterol acceptors, even though apo AI seems more efficient. Synthetic amphipathic peptides mimicking those of the apoproteins have comparable efficiency [11], stressing the lack of specificity of the helical residues surrounding the lipid bilayer for cholesterol incorporation into the discoidal complexes [2]. The second step of the reverse cholesterol transport process consists in the esterification of the cholesterol incorporated into the discoidal acceptor particle by the LCAT enzyme. This is accompanied by a transformation of the acceptor particles from discs into spheres. In contrast to the lack of specificity at the level of cholesterol capture and incorporation into the acceptor complexes, the LCAT activation properties of the complexes are modulated by the nature of their apoprotein component. While apo AI is the most potent LCAT activator, together with apo AIV, apo AII is unable to efficiently activate the enzyme. In mixed apo AI/AII particles, the apo AI content of the complexes and as a consequence their LCAT activating properties, is modulated by apo AII which displaces apo AI from these particles. Within apo AII, the C-terminal helix is responsible for this displacement, probably due to its higher hydrophobicity. This particular helix has the highest hydrophobicity of all helical repeats identified in the apoproteins, although an hydrophobicity of 0.29 is low compared to protein transmembrane segments, generally around 1.0 on the Eisenberg's scale [6]. The displacement of apo AI from plasma HDL by this peptide requires 16 moles peptide/apo AI compared to only two moles native apo AII [10]. However when expressed as number of helices, this corresponds to 12 helices in the two apo AII dimers and the difference in stoechiometry is probably due to cooperativity between the three helices of the apo AII monomer compared to the isolated helices of the C-terminal peptide. The displacement of apo AI by either the peptide or by native apo AII occurs at lower apo AII/AI ratios in HDL than in the discoidal complexes. This could be accounted for by the different mode of association between apo AI and phospholipid in a disc compared to a spherical particle. We had previously shown [12] by ATR infrared measurements that the helical repeats of apo AI are oriented parallel to the phospholipid acyl chains around a disc whereas they become perpendicular to the acyl chains after the transformation of a discoidal into a spherical particle under the action of the LCAT enzyme. As the surface of contact between the hydrophobic face of the apo AI helices and the lipids is greater in the discoidal than in the spherical particles, the displacement of apo AI by either apo AII or the C-terminal peptide requires larger amount of this protein. Moreover in the arrangement of the helices of apo AI around the discoidal complexes, there might be space for intercalation of single apo AII helices in-between the helical repeats of apo AI. The mobility of the central hinge domain of apo AI might further enhance this particular arrangement. This could account for the increased size of the mixed apo AI/AII complexes. In conclusion, no precise physiological function had been assigned to apo AII yet, except for an effect on the hepatic lipase activity [13]. The above data suggest that it plays a key role as modulator of the LCAT activation by apo AI in discoidal apo AI/AII particles through the ability of its C-terminal domain to displace apo AI from both discoidal and spherical HDL. Apo AII would thereby directly control the fate of the cellular cholesterol incorporated into the nascent HDL particles, a rate-limiting step in the reverse cholesterol transport.

References

1. Fielding CJ, Fielding PE. Molecular physiology of reverse cholesterol transport. J Lipid Res 1995;36:211-28.
2. Johnson WJ, Mahlberg FH, Rothblat GH, Phillips M. Cholesterol transport between cells and high density lipoproteins. Biochim Biophys Acta 1991;1085:273-98.
3. Vanloo B, Taveirne J, Baert G, et al. Activation of lecithin cholesterol acyltransferase (LCAT) by the CNBr fragments of human apo AI and conversion of the discoidal complexes into spherical particles. Biochim Biophys Acta 1992;1128:258-66.
4. Brasseur R, Lins L, Vanloo B, Ruysschaert JM, Rosseneu M. Molecular modelling of the amphipathic helices of the plasma apolipoproteins. Proteins:Structure, Function, and Genetics. 1992;13:246-57.
5. Corijn J, Deleys B, Labeur C, et al. Characterisation of the discoidal complexes generated between phospholipids and synthetic model peptides for apolipoproteins. Biochim Biophys Acta 1993;1170:8-16.
6. Matz CE, Jonas A. Micellar complexes of human apolipoprotein A-I with phosphatidylcholine and cholesterol prepared from cholate-lipid dispersions. J Biol Chem 1982;257:4535-40.
7. Vercaemst R, Union A, Rosseneu M. Separation and quantitation of free cholesterol and cholesteryl esters in a macrophage cell line by high performance liquid chromatography. J Chromatography 1989;494:43-52.
8. Lowry OH, Rosebrough NJ, Farr AC, Randall RJ. Protein measurement with the Folin phenol reagent. J Biol Chem 1951;193:265-75.
9. Lopez J, Latta M, Collet X, et al. Purification and characterization of recombinant human apolipoprotein A-II expressed in E Coli. Eur J Biochem 1994;225:1141-50.
10. Van Tornout P, Caster H, Lievens MJ, Rosseneu M, Assmann G. "In vitro" interaction of human HDL with apolipoprotein AII. Synthesis of AII-rich HDL. Biochim Biophys Acta 1981;663:630-36.
11. Brouillette CG, Anantharamaiah GM. Structural models of human apolipoprotein A-I. Biochim Biophys Acta 1995;1256:103-29.
12. Brasseur R, De Meutter J, Vanloo B, Goormaghtigh E, Ruysschaert JM, Rosseneu M. Mode of assembly of amphipathic helical segments in model high density lipoproteins. Biochim Biophys Acta 1990;1043:245-52.
13. Lacko AG. The metabolism of high density lipoproteins. Trends Cardiovasc Med 1994;4:84-88.

N-3 FATTY ACID ETHYL ESTERS LOWER TRIGLYCERIDEMIA WITHOUT INCREASING THE DIABETIC RISK: ITALIAN FISH OIL MULTICENTER STUDY

Giuseppe Abate, Renato Alessi, Canterin A. Antonin, Carlo A. Azzini, Stefano Bertolini, Gabriele Bittolo Bon, Enrico Bologna, Giandomenico Bompiani, Paolo Brunetti, Antonio Capurso, Luigi Cattin, Luigi Colombo, Domenico M. Cucinotta, Domenico Cucinotta, Luigi Cucurachi, Felice D'Onofrio, Giuseppe Erle, Fabrizio Fabris, Domenico Fedele, Renato Fellin, Sandro Forconi, Antonio Gaddi, Riccardo Giorgino, Mario Lingetti, Mario Mancini, Gianfranco Manzini, Pierluigi Mattioli, Guido Menzinger, Luciano Motta, Michele Muggeo, Sergio Muntoni, Renzo Navalesi, Alberto Notarbartolo, Giorgio Pagani, Gianfranco Pagano, Annibale Papa, Mario Passeri, Livio Perotti, Luigi Pisano, Guido Pozza, Giuseppe Realdi, Franco Rengo, Giorgio Ricci, Luigi Saccá, Gianfranco Salvioli, Sergio Sensi, Mario Serio, Saverio Sgambato, Cesare R. Sirtori*, Antonio Tiengo, Antonio Trinchera, Mario Velussi, Alessandro Ventura, Carlo Vergani, Paolo Viglierchio, Flavio Vigneri, Flavio Virgili, Silvana Zoppi, for the Italian Fish Oil Multicenter Study

**Institute of Pharmacological Sciences, Via Balzaretti 9, Milan 20133, Italy*

Introduction

Intake of n-3 polyunsaturated fatty acids from fish exerts a favorable effect on atherosclerosis development and progression [1-3]. This protective effect is believed to be mediated by changes in plasma lipids, particularly triglycerides (TG) [4], prostaglandin metabolism [5], reduced formation of growth factors [6], and stimulated endothelial relaxation [7].

While in the presence of these favorable lipid, prostaglandin, and tissue changes, caution has been warned against the use of n-3 fatty acids in patients with glucose intolerance or clear cut diabetic conditions [8-11]. In these, significant rises were reported in plasma glucose [9], with reduced insulinemia and increased requirements for both insulin and/or hypoglycemic agents [10,11]. According to a number of clinical reports, however, n-3 fatty acids do not seem to impair glycemic control, either in type I [12] or in noninsulin-dependent diabetes (NIDDM) [13-15].

N-3 fatty acids are frequently used in patients with lipid disorders characterized by hypertriglyceridemia, where hyperinsulinemia/insulin resistance as well as arterial hypertension (syndrome X) may often be detected [16]. A large controlled multicenter study

A. M. Gotto, Jr. et al. (eds.), Drugs Affecting Lipid Metabolism, 667–673.

was therefore designed for patients with hypertriglyceridemia (Fredrickson's types IIB and IV), in a large percentage with the constellation of symptoms characteristic of syndrome X. These were randomized to receive, in double-blind conditions, either n-3 fatty acids, under the form of ethyl esters (EE) or a corresponding placebo.

Patients and Methods

Patients of both sexes were selected, aged between 45-75 years old for males and 55-80 years old for females, presenting with hyperlipoproteinemias type IIb or IV, associated to at least one further risk factor:

- glucose intolerance (IGT);
- NIDDM; and /or
- arterial hypertension.

The multicenter study involved 63 clinical groups, distributed throughout Italy. The selected centers were invited to treat the first 16-20 cases, presenting with the requirements for admission to the study. The study design did not foresee standard treatment criteria for each single risk factor, since it was not the study's objective to interfere with the normal behavior of each single participating clinician, except for the use of n-3 EE or corresponding placebo.

The start of the active treatment/placebo was preceded by a run-in and wash-out period of at least 4 weeks, during which concomitant therapy (e.g. hypotensive/antidiabetic) was stabilized and no hypolipidemic drugs were prescribed. Following this, a double-blind phase was started. In the first two months all patients received their conventional therapy with, in addition, 1 g of ESAPENT® (Pharmacia-Upjohn, Milan, Italy) corresponding to 465 mg of eicosapentaenoic acid (EPA) and 290 mg of docosahexaenoic acid (DHA), or a corresponding placebo (olive oil), both given three times a day. After the first two months the doses of both ESAPENT® and placebo were reduced to 1 capsule twice daily, up to the end of the sixth month.

All subjects underwent a complete laboratory evaluation, including urinalysis and hematology before the run-in period, at the time 0 visit and at the end of the sixth month of controlled investigation. At all visits (basal, 2, 4, and 6 months), patients underwent a complete lipid/lipoprotein evaluation as well as the determination of fasting glucose levels and, only in patients with IGT or NIDDM, glycosylated hemoglobin and serum insulin. An oral glucose tolerance test with 75 g of glucose was carried out in the patients with IGT and NIDDM, with the determination of glucose and insulin at all time points. Levels of EPA and DHA in plasma and in red blood cells (RBC) were monitored in all the patients of three of the participating centers.

Results

The 63 participating centers provided a total of 935 patients, 470 assigned to n-3 EE, and 465 to placebo. The majority (62.4%) of the patients were males, similarly distributed between the two treatment groups. Hyperlipidemias were also evenly distributed between

Table 1. Characteristics of the participating patients.

		EPA + DHA (n = 470)	Placebo (n = 465)
Sex			
	Female	176	176
	Male	294	289
Age (yr)			
	Female	62.2 ± 7.12	61.8 ± 7.06
	Male	55.8 ± 9.35	57.0 ± 9.54
	Mean	58.2 ± 9.09	58.8 ± 8.99
Body Weight (kg)			
	Baseline	74.0 ± 10.44	73.7 ± 10.08
	6 Months	73.5 ± 10.38	73.2 ± 10.10
Height (cm)		167.3 ± 8.68	166.8 ± 8.53
Type of Hypercholesterolemia			
	Type II B	65%	65%
	Type IV	35%	35%
Additional Risk Factors			
	NIDDM	44%	45%
	IGT	11%	11%
	Arterial Hypertension	68%*	68%*

NIDDM: Noninsulin dependent diabetes mellitus
IGT: Impaired glucose tolerance

Values are Means ± SD
*Alone or combined with one of the other risk factors

the n-3 EE and placebo groups. The majority of patients (65%) had a type IIb hyperlipoproteinemia, versus 35% with type IV. Fifty-five percent of the selected patients, evenly distributed between the two treatment groups, had a pathological glycemic control (11% IGT and 44% NIDDM) (Table 1). These last were considered all together in the final analyses (IGT/NIDDM). Sixty-eight percent had arterial hypertension, almost all on drug treatment. Plasma lipid, lipoprotein levels, fasting glucose, and blood pressure values are reported for the two groups in Table 2.

Table 2. Baseline lipid, fasting glucose, and blood pressure levels in all patients.

	EPA + DHA (n = 470)	Placebo (n = 465)
Total Cholesterol (mg/dl)	234.0 ± 32.5	233.7 ± 33.1
HDL-C (mg/dl)	39.9 ± 9.7	39.8 ± 9.7
Triglycerides (mg/dl)	294.3 ± 79.2	297.3 ± 84.7
Fasting Glucose (mg/dl)	119.8 ± 38.0	120.0 ± 36.6
Blood Pressure (mmHg)		
Systolic	145.7 ± 14.5	144.8 ± 14.9
Diastolic	86.5 ± 8.2	85.5 ± 8.1

Values are Mean ± SD

The treatments exerted no significant effect on total cholesterolemia; the calculated low density lipoprotein-cholesterol (LDL-C) levels, likewise, before and after 6 months of controlled investigation also behaved similarly. Conversely, triglyceridemia was significantly lowered (-21.53 versus -6.54% in the placebo group after 6 months; $p < 0.0001$), with an apparent tendency to a progressive reduction of levels with time. Patients with impaired glucose metabolism (IGT/NIDDM), did not show a different hypotriglyceridemic response versus normoglycemics.

No effect of n-3 EE treatment was observed on any of the major glycemic parameters: fasting glucose, HbA_{1C}, insulinemia, and oral glucose tolerance. These were essentially identical before and after treatment in the whole group of IGT/NIDDM patients. In addition, mean values of systolic blood pressure and diastolic blood pressure were not modified either during or at the end of the 6 months, both in the whole group and in the IGT/NIDDM patients.

Discussion

Concern about use of n-3 fatty acids has recently been raised, following the reported increase in cardiovascular morbidity in subjects with the highest n-3 fatty acid consumption in the Health Professionals' Follow up Study [17]. While the intake of fish and particularly of n-3 fatty acids may be associated with a reduction of both basal and postprandial levels of TG and very low density lipoprotein (VLDL)-cholesterol, reduced platelet aggregability and improved vasodilatation, the analysis of the direct effects of n-3 intake on parameters underlying glycemic control, has been followed by divergent responses. Studies in diabetic patients, either on dietary treatment or receiving sulfonylureas, showed a rise of glucose levels, at times associated with reduced insulinemia. These findings led, in some cases, to the suggestion that n-3 intake should be restricted in diabetics [10,11]. More recent studies, carried out mainly with relatively lower daily doses of n-3 fatty acids, in similar proportions as in the present study, failed to see significant changes in the glycemic control [13-15], with the possible exception of a small reduction of fasting insulin in n-3 fatty acid treated, moderately hypertriglyceridemic patients [18]. In addition, some favorable changes were noted, among which reduced blood pressure, in patients with insulin resistance [19].

The present study allows, for first time, evaluation of a very large sample of patients, more than half of which complied with the definition of syndrome X [20]: hypertriglyceridemia, IGT/NIDDM, low HDL-C and, in almost all cases, arterial hypertension. The study thus had the proper size and patient selection to clarify some of the questions that have emerged from the smaller, frequently noncontrolled studies, on patients with combined alterations of lipid and glucose metabolism. In addition, a relatively low daily dose of n-3 EE was selected.

Administration of the n-3 EE resulted in a significant lowering of plasma TG levels, in a similar range as reported by most investigators in the field [4] using higher doses of either n-3 EE or of fish oil triglycerides, without changes of LDL-C levels. The present study also offered an insight into the effect of the n-3 EE intake on lipid/lipoprotein parameters in patients with normal glycemic control vs IGT/NIDDM. There was essentially no effect on any of the parameters indicative of glycemic control, and patients with IGT/NIDDM appeared to have a similar sensitivity to the hypotriglyceridemic effect of n-3 EE as normoglycemics.

The lack of effect on glucose metabolism of n-3 EE administration in patients with impaired glycemic control is noteworthy and rules out any concern about the prescription of these products to diabetics. Prior investigations suggested that insulin secretion might be reduced after n-3 intake, because of changes in membrane fluidity and responsiveness of islet cells to normal stimuli, possibly due to impaired calcium flux across cell types, exposed to marine lipids [21]. The present study failed to provide any evidence of impaired insulin secretion, in addition to ruling out any activity on peripheral insulin action. While diabetics experienced a significant improvement in lipoprotein metabolism, there was no evidence for a correction of other typical traits of syndrome X, particularly in the case of blood pressure. Studies on blood pressure changes after n-3 fatty acids have shown clear effects only after high doses of n-3 fatty acids in nondrug treated hypertensives with arterial disease [22]. In the present study most of the hypertensive patients were already on some form of drug therapy and n-3 intake failed to cause a significant blood pressure reduction.

Acknowledgements

The support of the Medical Direction of Pharmacia-Upjohn (Dr. Maurizio Lavezzari, Dr. Eduardo Stragliotto, and Dr. Franco Pamparana) is gratefully acknowledged.

References

1. Leaf A, Weber PC. Cardiovascular effects of n-3 fatty acids. N Engl J Med 1988; 318:549-57.
2. Kromhout D. Bosschieter EB, de Lezenne Coulander C. The inverse relation between fish consumption and 20-year mortality from coronary heart disease. N Engl J Med 1985;312:1205-209.
3. Schmidt EB, Dyerberg J. Omega-3 fatty acids: Current status in cardiovascular medicine. Drugs 1994;47:405-24.
4. Harris WS. Fish oils and plasma lipid and lipoprotein metabolism in humans: A critical review. J Lipid Res 1989;30:785-807.
5. Von Shacky C, Fisher S, Weber PC. Long term effects of dietary marine ω-3 fatty acids upon plasma and cellular lipids, platelet function and eicosanoid formation in humans. J Clin Invest 1985;76:1626-31.
6. Tremoli E, Eligini S, Colli S, et al. n-3 fatty acid ethyl ester administration to healthy subjects and to hypertriglyceridemic patients reduces tissue factor by adherent monocytes. Arterioscl Thromb 1994;14:1600-608.
7. McVeigh GE, Brennan GM, Cohn JN, Finkelstein SM, Hayes RJ, Johnston GD. Fish oil improves arterial compliance in non-insulin-dependent diabetes mellitus. Arterioscl Thromb 1994;14:1425-29.
8. Glauber H, Wallace P, Griver K et al. Adverse effects of ω-3 fatty acids in non-insulin-dependent diabetes mellitus. Ann Inter Med 1988;108:663-68.
9. Kassim S, Stern B, Khilnani S, McLin P, Baciorowski S, Jen C. Effect of omega-3 fish oils on lipid metabolism, glycemic control and blood pressure in type II diabetic patients. J Clin Endocrinol Metab 1988;67:1-5.
10. Zambon S, Friday KE, Childs MT, Fujimoto WY, Bierman EL, Ensinck JW. Effect of glyburide and ω-3 fatty acid dietary supplements on glucose and lipid metabolism in patients with non-insulin-dependent diabetes mellitus. Am J Clin Nutr 1992;56: 447-54.
11. Friday KE, Childs MT, Tsunehara CH, Fujimoto WY, Bierman EL, Ensinck JW. Omega-3 fatty acid supplementation raises plasma glucose while lowering triglyceride levels in type II diabetes. Diabetes Care 1989;12:276-81.
12. Rillaerts EG, Engelmann GJ, Van Camp KM, De Leeuw I. Effect of omega-3 fatty acids in diet of type I diabetic subjects on lipid values and hemorheological parameters. Diabetes 1989;38:1412-16.
13. Bagdade JD, Buchanan WE, Levy RA, Subbaiah PV, Ritter MC. Effects of ω-3 fish oils on plasma lipids, lipoprotein composition, and postheparin lipoprotein lipase in women with NIDDM. Diabetes 1990;30:426-31.
14. Annuzzi G, Rivellese A, Capaldo B, et al. A controlled study on the effects of n-3 fatty acids on lipid and glucose metabolism in non-insulin-dependent diabetic patients. Atherosclerosis

1991;87:65-73.
15. Westerveld HT, de Graaf JC, van Breugel HHFI, et al. Effects of low-dose EPA-E on glycemic control, lipid profile, lipoprotein(a), platelet aggregation, viscosity, and platelet and vessel wall interaction in NIDDM. Diabetes Care 16;683-88.
16. DeFronzo RA, Ferrannini E. Insulin resistance: A multifaceted syndrome responsible for NIDDM, obesity hypertension, dyslipidemia, and atherosclerotic cardiovascular disease. Diabetes Care 1991;14:173-94.
17. Ascherio A, Rimm EB, Stampfer MJ, Giovannucci EL, Willett WC. Dietary intake of marine n-3 fatty acids, fish intake, and the risk of coronary disease among men. N Engl J Med 1995;332:977-82.
18. Eritsland J, Deljeflot I, Abdelnoor M, Arnesen H, Torjesen PA. Long-term effects of n-3 fatty acids on serum lipids and glycaemic control. Scand J Clin Lab Invest 1994;54:273-80.
19. Grundt H, Nilsen DWT, Hetland Ø, et al. Improvement of serum lipids and blood pressure during intervention with n-3 fatty acids was not associated with changes in insulin levels in subjects with combined hyperlipidaemia. J Int Med 1995;237: 249-59.
20. Moller DE, Flier JS. Insulin resistance - mechanisms, syndromes, and implications. N Engl J Med 1991;325:938-48.
21. Hallaq H, Smith TW, Leaf A. Modulation of dihydropyridine sensitive calcium channels in heart cells by fish oil fatty acids. Proc Natl Acad Sci USA 1992;89: 1760-64.
22. Bonaa K, Bjerve K, Straume B, Gram I, Thelle D. Effect of eicosapentaenoic and docosahexaenoic acids on blood pressure in hypertension. N Engl J Med 1990;322:795-801.

A METABOLIC MODEL FOR THE HYPOLIPIDEMIC AND ANTI-ATHEROGENIC EFFECTS OF N-3 FATTY ACIDS: EFFECT OF OMACOR ON PLASMA LIPIDS

Henry J. Pownall, Danièle Brauchi, Cumhur Kılınç, Christie M. Ballantyne, Barry J. McKeone, Karin Osmundsen, Quein Pao, and Antonio M. Gotto, Jr.
Department of Medicine, Baylor College of Medicine and The Methodist Hospital, 6565 Fannin, Houston, Texas 77030, USA

Introduction

Although the mechanism by which lipid disorders contribute to premature atherosclerosis and vascular disease is not clear, several possibilities have been proposed. There is continued interest in establishing a mechanistic link between coronary artery disease and elevated plasma triglycerides (TG) [1]. If an unequivocal correlation could be found, it would give added direction to attempts to identify underlying causes of atherosclerosis and possible interventions. Even if a significant correlation were proven, it is possible that the elevation in plasma TG is not directly linked to the disease process but is a function of some underlying disorder that independently contributes to atherogenesis and hypertriglyceridemia (HTG). Thus, an elevation in TG might be diagnostic for atherosclerosis without being causally linked. To confound the picture even more, elevated plasma TG are part of a syndrome (Syndrome X) found in noninsulin dependent diabetes mellitus (NIDDM). Syndrome X includes a cluster of risk factors for atherosclerosis [2]. These include small, dense, apoB-rich low density lipoproteins (LDL) (B phenotype according to [3,4]), low high density lipoprotein cholesterol (HDL-C) (near absence of HDL_2-C), and enhanced postprandial lipemia, particularly in the late postprandial phase [5,6]. The small, dense LDL have a higher than normal TG-to-cholesteryl ester (CE) ratio and exhibit defective binding to the LDL receptor on human skin fibroblasts [7]. In contrast, conversion of normal LDL to small, dense LDL leads to enhanced uptake by HepG2 cells [8].

Evidence reviewed by Krauss [9] suggests that plasma lipoprotein lipase (LPL) activity is associated with increased levels of larger LDL (A phenotype) and HDL_2 caused by transfer of surface lipids and apolipoproteins during chylomicron and very low-density-lipoprotein (VLDL)-TG hydrolysis. It is notable that B phenotype occurs more frequently in NIDDM and is associated with hypertriglyceridemia and low HDL-C [10]. B phenotype is also found more frequently in normolipemic NIDDM subjects than in matched nondiabetics. Other studies support the association of impaired lipolysis with hypertri-

A. M. Gotto, Jr. et al. (eds.), Drugs Affecting Lipid Metabolism, 675–680.

glyceridemia and increased risk for cardiovascular disease. One study found that the plasma triglycerides observed 4-8 hours postprandially were the best predictors of coronary artery disease [6]. Another report [11] found that the postprandial plasma levels of chylomicron remnants correlated best with the rate of progression of coronary lesions. In addition, remnant clearance is also reduced in subjects with insulin-dependent diabetes mellitus (IDDM) [12]. Havel [13] concluded that chylomicron and VLDL remnants are atherogenic lipoproteins. However, these studies only produced associations, and as with many other lipid markers, it is not clear whether impaired triglyceride clearance is causal or merely diagnostic for cardiovascular disease or for one of its underlying causes.

A Metabolic Model for the Clustering of Lipid Risk Factors in HTG

One underlying cause that could contribute to the atherogenic profile is impaired control of plasma nonesterified fatty acid (NEFA) levels. According to this model, increased lipolysis in adipose tissue or impaired uptake of fatty acids by adipose tissue could raise the NEFA levels in the plasma compartment (Figure 1). When plasma NEFA levels are normal, a small fraction is extracted by the liver for VLDL-TG synthesis and secretion. If the NEFA levels are sufficiently low, it is possible that some of the apoB that is synthesized is degraded prior to assembly into VLDL [14]. As a consequence, a small number of VLDL particles, which are TG-poor, are secreted into plasma. With such a small pool of plasma TG-containing particles, there is efficient conversion of the VLDL to LDL by the successive activities of LPL and hepatic lipase (HL) and very little transfer of TG molecules to other lipoproteins.

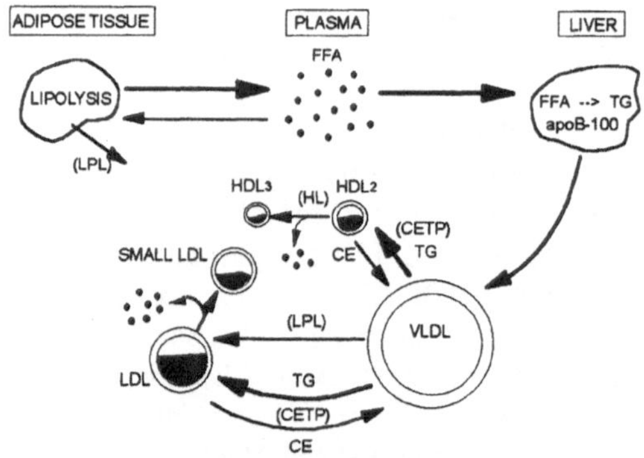

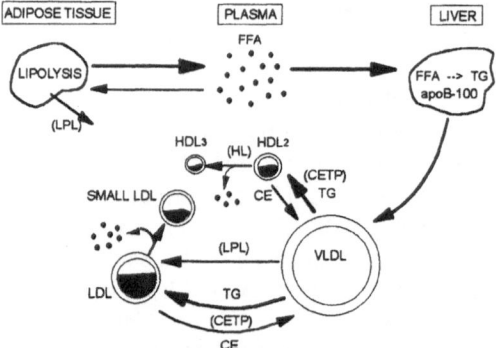

Figure 1. Schematic representation of a mechanism by which elevations of plasma NEFA derived from hypersecretion or impaired uptake by adipose tissue could lead to derangements in the plasma profiles of all lipoprotein subclasses.

However, when plasma NEFA levels are elevated, large amounts of NEFA are extracted by the liver and used to propel the hyper synthesis of VLDL-TG. Most if not all of the apoB-100 that is synthesized is incorporated into large, TG-rich VLDL that are secreted into the plasma compartment [14]. In plasma the VLDL accumulate because of 1) hypersecretion, 2) the low LPL activity that is found with hypertriglyceridemia, and 3) inhibition of lipolysis by excessive plasma NEFA levels.

In plasma, the combined actions of HL, LPL, and CETP, form small, dense LDL in the following way (Figure 2). Although some TG is removed from VLDL through the lipolytic cascade, a steady state is reached in which plasma VLDL-TG levels remain very high. The TG in this cascade is exchanged for the CE of the HDL cascade, resulting in TG-rich HDL. Similarly, there is an exchange of VLDL-TG for LDL-CE (not shown). Because the plasma pool of VLDL-TG is so large, there is a nearly inexhaustible supply of TG to exchange for the CE of LDL and HDL. After the TG enter the HDL and LDL, some are removed by further lipolysis by hepatic lipase resulting in a reduction in the size of the particle. This process forms the so-called small, dense LDL and converts HDL_2 to HDL_3. The HDL and LDL continue to acquire additional TG some of which is removed by hydrolysis. Some TG, however, stays with the particles so that they remain TG-rich. As a consequence of the loss of CE and gain of TG by LDL and HDL, the weight ratio of TG as a fraction of total neutral lipid in HDL and LDL is increased (WR = TG/[CE + TG]) (see preliminary results). This gives rise to abnormal HDL and LDL particles. Within the LDL particles the structure of apoB-100 is altered to the extent that it is not properly recognized by the LDL-receptor [8]. The TG-rich HDL have a lower cholesterol-carrying capacity because they have less neutral lipid and the fraction of neutral lipid that is CE is low. The reduced fraction of HDL and LDL neutral lipid would be expected to produce a commensurate reduction of cholesterol transport through this pathway. This is thought to impair its role in reverse cholesterol transport.

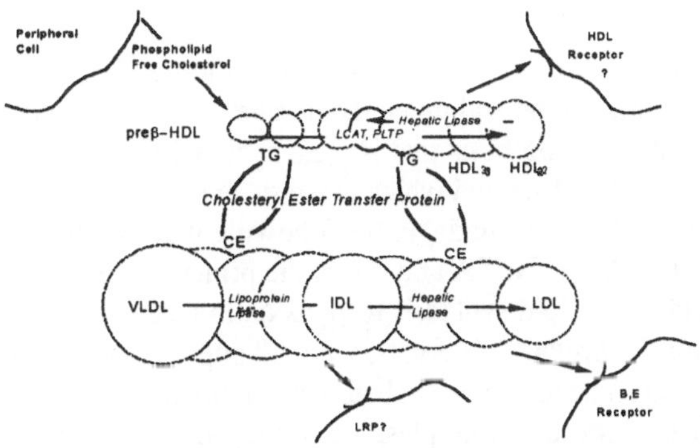

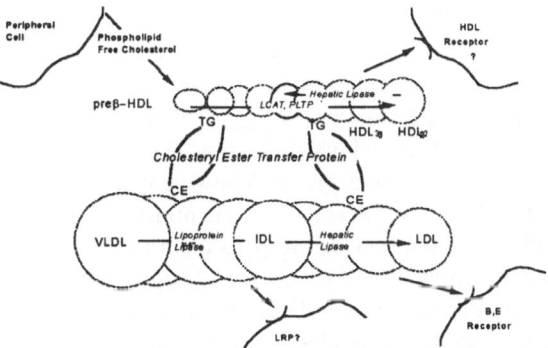

Figure 2. Schematic representation of the processes occurring within and between the HDL and VLDL cascades.

Although it is not possible to directly prove the hypothetical role of NEFA outlined above, there is some supporting evidence based on the effects of n-3 fatty acids on plasma lipid levels; n-3 fatty acids are thought to divert fatty acids from lipid synthesis by increased hepatic β-oxidation. Studies in animal models show that plasma NEFA levels are lowered by dietary n-3 fatty acids [15,16], and we hypothesized that any reduction in serum TG would be accompanied by reduced serum NEFA levels. In a recent study, the effects of Omacor, which is an 85% concentrate of n-3 fatty acid ethyl esters, on fasting serum NEFA, TG, total cholesterol, HDL-C, LDL-C, VLDL-C, HDL-WR and LDL-WR were reported [17]. These data are summarized in Table 1.

Table 1. Changes in plasma lipid levels during treatment.

	Before Treatment		After Omacor (6 wk)	
Plasma Analyte/Parameter	Mean	SEM	Mean	SEM
TG (mg/dL)	831.	74	516.	44.
Total Cholesterol (mg/dL)	343.	24.	289.	12.
HDL-C (mg/dL)	18.8	1.4	22.3	2.6
LDL-C (mg/dL)	44.2	4.1	58.8	7.2
VLDL-C (mg/dL)	221.	21.6	147.	13.3
NEFA (mg/dL)	0.93	0.10	0.74	0.07
HDL-WR	0.51	0.03	0.41	0.03
LDL-WR	0.43	0.03	0.35	0.03

These data do not prove the models shown in Figures 1 and 2. However, they are highly consistent with the model and given the number of variables involved, it is difficult to put forth an alternative hypothesis that is reasonable within the context of our current understanding of lipid metabolism and which is consistent with all the data. We view these data within the framework of our model in the following way. With the Omacor treatment there was a reduction in plasma NEFA and this is the primary effect that may be due to the diversion of fatty acids from lipid synthesis to β-oxidation. As a consequence, there is less fatty acid available for TG synthesis; in addition, not all copies of apolipoprotein B-100 may be fully lipidated so that some are degraded before assembly into VLDL. As a consequence, fewer VLDL particles are secreted into plasma and they are relatively TG-poor. In plasma, the amount of VLDL-TG available for exchange with LDL and HDL is lower so that the TG content of both HDL and LDL are decreased. There are two consequences of this. One is that both LDL and HDL are cholesteryl ester rich (i.e. WR is lower), LDL-C and HDL-C increase. Since there is less TG in the HDL and LDL, they are poorer substrates for hepatic lipase so thatneither are converted to their smaller denser forms.

Our data are consistent with hypertriglyceridemia and CETP being the two major determinants of altered HDL and LDL structure in hypertriglyceridemia. Omacor, appears to change the lipoprotein profile of hypertriglyceridemic subjects to one that may be less atherogenic. Decreasing the TG content of LDL alters its structure [7,8], enhances its binding to the LDL receptors on fibroblasts [8,18], and reduces its intracellular degradation [19,20]. Omacor increases the cholesterol content of HDL and makes it resistant to the hepatic lipase-mediated conversion to smaller more dense HDL particles. Still, in some subjects, it may be desirable to lower serum TG while controlling LDL-C. This might be achieved through an intervention that lowers both plasma TG and cholesterol.

References

1. Austin MA. Plasma triglyceride and coronary heart disease. Arteriosclerosis 1991;11:2-14.
2. Reaven GM. The fourth musketeer--from Alexander Dumas to Claude Bernard. Diabetologia. 1995;8:3-13.
3. Austin MA, King MC, Vranizan KM, Krauss RM. Atherogenic lipoprotein phenotype. A proposed genetic marker for cornary heart disease risk. Circulation 1990;82:495-506.
4. Austin MA, Brunzell JD, Fitch WL, Krauss RM. Inheritance of low desity lipoprotein subclass patterns in familial combined hyperlipidemia. Arteriosclerosis 1990;10:520-30.
5. Patsch JR, Karlin JV, Scott LW, Gotto AM Jr. Inverse relationship between blood levels of high density lipoprotein subfraction 2 and magnitude of postprandial lipemia. Proc Natl Acad Sci (USA) 1983;80:1449-53.
6. Patsch JR, Miesenbock G, Hopferwieser T, Muhlberger V, Knapp E, Dunn JK, Gotto AM Jr, and Patsch W. Relationship of triglyceride metabolism and coronary artery disease: Studies in the postprandial state. Arteriosclerosis Thromb 1992;12:1336-45.
7. Aviram M, Lund-Katz S, Phillips MC, Chait A. The influence of the triglyceride component of low density lipoprotein on the interaction of apolipoprotein B-100 with cells. J Biol Chem 1988;263:16842-48.
8. McKeone BJ, Patsch JR, Pownall HJ. Plasma triglycerides determine low density lipoprotein composition, physical properties, and cell-specific binding in cultured cells. J Clin Invest 1993;91:1926-33.
9. Krauss RM. Heterogeneity of plasma low-density lipoproteins and atherosclerosis risk. Current Opinion Lipidology 1994;5:339-49.
10. Feingold KR, Grunfeld C, Pang M, Doerrler W, Krauss RM. LDL subclass phenotypes and triglyceride metabolism in non-insulin-dependent diabetes. Arteriosclerosis Thrombosis 1992;12:1496-1502.
11. Karpe F, Steiner G, Uffelman K, Olivercrona T, Hamsten A. Postprandial lipoproteins and progression of coronary atherosclerosis. Atherosclerosis 1994;106: 83-97.
12. Georgopoulos A, Phair RD. Abnormal clearance of postprandial Sf 100-400 plasma lipoproteins in insulin-dependent diabetes mellitus. J Lipid Res 1991;32:1133-41.
13. Havel RJ. Postprandial hyperlipidemia and remnant lipoproteins. Current Opinion Lipidology 1994;5:102-109.
14. Dixon JL, Furukawa S, Ginsberg HN. Oleic acid stimulates secretion of apolipoprotein B-containing lipoproteins from HepG2 cells by reducing intracellular degradation of apolipoprotein B. Arteriosclerosis 1990;10:763a.
15. Otto DA, Tsai CE, Baltzell JK, Wooten JT. Apparent inhibition of hepatic triacylglycerol

secretion, independent of synthesis, in high-fat fish oil-fed rats: Role for insulin. Biochim Biophys Acta 1991;1082:37-48.

16. Otto DA, Baltzell JK, Wooten JT. Reduction in triacylglycerol levels by fish oil correlates with free fatty acid levels in *ad libitum* fed rats. Lipids 1992;27:1013-17.
17. Pownall HJ, Brauchi D, Kılınç C, Ballantyne CM, Osmundson K, Pao Q, Gotto, AM, Jr. A double blind placebo-controlled study of the effects of Omacor™ in patients with severe hypertriglyceridemia. Arterioscler Thromb 1996; submitted.
18. Kleinman Y, Eisenberg S, Oschry, Gavish D, Stein O, Stein Y. Defective metabolism of hypertriglyceridemic low density lipoprotein in cultured human skin fibroblasts. J Clin Invest 1985;75:1796-1803.
19. Glick JM, Adelman SJ, Phillips MC, Rothblat GH. Cellular cholesterol clearance: relationship to the physical state of cholesterol ester inclusions. J Biol Chem 1983; 258:13425-30.
20. Adelman SJ, Glick JM, Phillips MC, Rothblat GH. Lipid composition and physical state effects on cellular cholesterol ester clearance. J Biol Chem 1984;259:13844-50.

LIPID PEROXIDATION AND OMEGA-3 FATTY ACIDS

Christian A. Drevon, Ingeborg R. Brude, and Marit S. Nenseter
Institute for Nutrition Research, University of Oslo, PO Box 1046 Blindern, 0316 Oslo, Norway

Introduction

One of the concerns with the intake of omega-3 fatty acids has been the high degree of unsaturation of the fatty acids and thereby the possibility of promoting increased peroxidation of low density lipoproteins (LDL). The potentially higher level of modified LDL might then be endocytosed by macrophages and initiate development of atherosclerosis. Ylä-Herttuala et al. [1] found oxidatively modified LDL in atherosclerotic lesions of rabbit and man, whereas Parthasarathy et al. [2] showed that LDL rich in oleic acid was more resistant to oxidative modification, as compared to LDL enriched with omega-6 fatty acids. Thus, it is important to investigate whether dietary supplementation with marine omega-3 fatty acids renders human LDL particles more susceptible to oxidative modification and thereby make the development of atherosclerosis more likely.

We have reviewed the published papers concerning peroxidation of lipoproteins during feeding with fish oil or highly purified esters of very long-chain omega-3 fatty acids to man or primates. Some experiments performed on human cells *in vitro* are also discussed. See Table 1.

OMEGA-3 FATTY ACID SUPPLEMENTATION IN MAN

Nenseter et al. [3] studied normolipidemics with the skin diseases, psoriasis, and atopic dermatitis. These patients received supplements of 6 capsules daily for 4 months, each capsule containing 1 g of either highly concentrated ethyl esters of omega-3 fatty acids (with 85% EPA and DHA; Omacor, Pronova Biocare, Oslo, Norway) (n = 12) or corn oil (56 % linoleic and 26 % oleic acid) (n = 11). Each gelatine capsule contained 4 IU of α-tocopherol and the content of lipid peroxides was low. The amount of omega-3 fatty acids was higher in fish oil-enriched LDL as compared to corn oil-enriched LDL (104.0 versus 29.4 µg/mg LDL protein). Similarly, the unsaturation index in LDL was higher (6.64 versus 5.49). Peripheral blood mononuclear cells from the two supplementation groups were able to take up a similar amount of LDL, regardless of the source of LDL. LDL isolated from four individuals in the fish oil and corn oil groups showed similar susceptibility to copper-

A. M. Gotto, Jr. et al. (eds.), Drugs Affecting Lipid Metabolism, 681–687.

Table 1. Studies on omega-3 fatty acids and lipid peroxidation in man.

Authors	Supplement	Placebo	Time	Subjects	Oxidizability
Nenseter MS et al.	5g EPA/DHA (24 IU E/d)	Corn oil	4 mo	12 normolipid	LPO: ↔ MØ: ↔
Nenseter MS et al.	5g EPA/DHA (18 mg E/d)	Normal FAP	6 w	16 normolipid	CD: ↔ MØ: ↔
Harats D et al.	FO 10g ± 400 mg E/d	-	4 w	22 ± smokers	TBARS: ↑ MØ: ↑
Lussier-Cacan S et al.	5g EPA/DHA/d ± Probucol	-	6 w	10 hyperTG	TBARS: ↑
Harris WS et al.	64 mg/kg/d cross over	Olive oil	4 w	10 hyperTG	TBARS: ↑
Bittolo-Bon G et al.	2.6g EPA/DHA (1.2 mg E/d)	Olive oil	4/12 w	15 type IIb	Vit E/TBARS/FU ↔
Frankel EN et al.	2.3 g n-3 fatty acids/d (25 IU vit E)		6 w	9 hyperTG	Propanal: ↑ FO vs unsuppl diet Hexanal: ↓ FO vs unsuppl diet Total volatiles: ↔
Oostenbrug GS et al.	FO 2.4 g n-3 fatty acids/d ± vit E 300 IU/d	Usual diet	3 w	11 healthy	Lag time: ↔ FO vs Ctr Rate: ↔ FO vs Ctr Max Conj Dienes: ↑ FO vs Ctr
Suzukawa M et al.	3.4 g n-3 fatty acids/d (2.0 mg/ml α-tocopherol)	CO 4 g/d (2.2 mg/E)	Cross-over 2 x 6 w	20 hypertensive	Lag time: ↓ FO vs CO or bs Rate: ↓ FO vs CO or bs TBARS: ↑ FO vs CO or bs MØ: ↑ FO vs CO or bs

FO, fish oil; EPA, eicosapentaenoic acid; DHA, docosahexaenoic acid; LPO, lipid peroxides; CD, conjugated dienes; TBARS, thiobarbituric-acid reactive substances; IU, international units; E, vitamin E; hyperTG, hypertriglyceridemic; FAP, fatty acid pattern; CO, cornoil; MØ, uptake by macrophages; FU, fluorescence units (excitation 360 nm, emission 430 nm of LDL); ↔, no significant difference; ↑, increased; ↓, decreased.

catalyzed lipid peroxidation, as indicated by the amount of lipid peroxides formed during the oxidation period, and the degradation rate of oxidatively modified LDL in J774 macrophages.

To obtain more extensive data, another study was performed on 16 healthy women receiving either 5 g of EPA and DHA (EPAX 6000 ethyl esters, with 18 mg of α-tocopherol, JC Martens A/S, Oslo, Norway) per day for 6 weeks, or an equal amount of oil with a fatty acid pattern similar to that of an average Norwegian diet (41% saturated, 38% monounsaturated, and 21% polyunsaturated fatty acids) [4]. The extent of copper-catalyzed oxidation of LDL was determined by measuring the formation of conjugated dienes, the relative electrophoretic mobility of LDL in agarose gels, and the degradation of LDL by J774 cells. There was increased lipid peroxidation among subjects with intake of omega-3 fatty acids after 3 weeks as compared to the baseline, but no significant difference between baseline and omega-3 fatty acid-exposed LDL fractions after 6 weeks of supplementation. These data support the previous findings [3].

Harats et al. [5] studied the effect of fish oil ingestion (10 g MaxEPA/day for 4 weeks) on the susceptibility of plasma lipoproteins to peroxidation in smokers and nonsmokers. In nonsmokers, the baseline values of thiobarbituric acid reactive substances (TBARS) were lower than in smokers. Peroxidation of LDL isolated from smokers and nonsmokers fed fish oil resulted in significantly higher TBARS and its metabolism by macrophages was higher as compared to the baseline values. When dietary supplementation with 400 mg vitamin E/day was given with the fish oil, vitamin E counteracted the effect of fish oil more effectively in the nonsmokers than in the smokers.

Lussier-Cacan et al. [6] studied LDL from hypertriglyceridemic men (5 type III and 5 type IV) at baseline on a low-saturated fat, low-cholesterol diet, after 6 weeks of dietary supplementation with fish oil (Promega, 12 g/d), and after 6 weeks of fish oil combined with probucol (500 mg twice a day). With fish oil alone, TBARS production after exposure of LDL to copper for 5 hours was increased 17% compared with corresponding baseline values, whereas a marked reduction from the previous period was observed with fish oil and probucol.

Harris et al. [7] performed a study with 10 mildly hypertriglyceridemic patients in a randomized, placebo-controlled, double-blind, crossover trial. Patients were given capsules (1 per 10 kg body weight) containing 640 mg/g of omega-3 fatty acids or olive oil placebo for two 4-week periods, separated by a one-week washout phase. Apo-B containing lipoproteins were isolated by precipitation with dextran sulphate and $MgCl_2$. The susceptibility of apoB-containing lipoproteins to oxidation was increased during the omega-3 fatty acid supplementation as compared to the olive oil period, as measured by changes in TBARS levels.

Bittolo-Bon et al. [8] gave 2.6 g of highly concentrated ethyl esters (85%) supplied with 1.2 mg of vitamin E daily to 15 type IIb hyperlipidemic subjects for 4 and 12 weeks, using olive oil as a double-blind placebo control. Vitamin E, TBARS, and fluorescence were measured in LDL isolated from the patients; there was no difference in either of the parameters between the two supplementation groups.

In a study conducted by Frankel et al. [9], fish oil supplementation with 5.1 g/d for 6 weeks (providing 2.4 g omega-3 fatty acids/d) to hypertriglyceridemic subjects increased the propanal formation during copper-catalyzed LDL oxidation, and decreased the hexanal formation as compared to LDL from the same subjects on unsupplemented diet. Propanal formation was highly correlated with the omega-3 fatty acid content of LDL. However, since total volatile oxidation products remained unchanged, Frankel and colleagues concluded that omega-3 fatty acid supplementation did not alter the total oxidative susceptibility of LDL.

Oostenbrug et al. [10] studied the effects of fish oil and vitamin E supplementation on copper-catalyzed oxidation of LDL. Healthy male volunteers received 2.4 g omega-3 fatty acids per day $\pm$ 300 IU vitamin E, or no supplement for 3 weeks. Fish oil increased the maximum amount of conjugated dienes formed during oxidation. No significant difference in the lag time and the formation rate of conjugated dienes was observed. The authors concluded that fish oil supplementation increased the susceptibility of LDL to lipid peroxidation.

Suzukawa et al. [11] reported that supplementation with highly purified ethyl esters of EPA and DHA (Omacor, Pronova Biocare providing 3.4 g omega-3 fatty acids per day) for 6 weeks to hypertensive subjects increased the LDL oxidative susceptibility over that of subjects supplemented with corn oil. Fish oil reduced the lag time before onset of copper-induced oxidation, and also the propagation rate, but increased the production of TBARS and the uptake of modified LDL by macrophages. Furthermore, macrophages supplemented with omega-3 fatty acids *in vitro* showed higher capacity to oxidize LDL than either control cells or corn oil fatty acid-enriched cells.

From these clinical trials we may conclude that there are variable results regarding altered susceptibility of LDL to lipid peroxidation during supplementation with omega-3 fatty acids, when similar methods are applied. In addition, it is possible that the simple copper-catalyzed *in vitro* oxidation of LDL after supplementation with omega-3 fatty acids is not representative of what is happening *in vivo*. In the following we will review some studies where other potential mechanisms involved in lipid peroxidation are evaluated.

OMEGA-3 FATTY ACIDS AND LIPID PEROXIDATION IN HUMAN CELLS

Sirtori et al. [12] reported that 12 type II hypercholesterolemic patients were randomly allocated to three different diets providing omega-6 fatty acids (corn oil), monounsaturated fatty acids (olive oil), or omega-3 fatty acids, to a prudent diet. The omega-3 fatty acid supplementation significantly reduced superoxide anion generation by adherent monocytes.

Fisher et al. [13] supplemented subjects with 3.6 g of EPA from 30 ml of cod liver oil for 6 weeks. Phagocytosing polymorphonuclear leukocytes showed a 27% decrease in chemiluminescence and a 64% decrease in superoxide anion production after supplementation. Similar findings were observed in human monocyte preparations [14]. The cellular fatty acid pattern exhibited a marked increase in EPA and a significant reduction in arachidonic acid.

Vossen et al. [15] cultured human umbilical endothelial cells long term (weeks) with different fatty acids, before membrane phospholipids were isolated and incorporated into liposomes. When peroxidation was induced with a mixture of $CuSO_4$ and H_2O_2, the amount of conjugated dienes formed was highest with 18:2, n-6 and lowest in the presence of 18:1, n-9. The amount of conjugated dienes was linearly correlated to the unsaturation index (total number of double bonds x mole % of PUFA in the phospholipids), with 18:2, n-6 forming exceptionally high amounts of dienes far above the general linear relation, whereas incubation of cells with EPA and DHA promoted particularly low formation of conjugated dienes.

OMEGA-3 FATTY ACIDS AND LIPID PEROXIDATION IN WHOLE ANIMAL EXPERIMENTS

Demoz et al. [16] compared the effect of oral administration of purified (95%) EPA with that of mice fed palmitic acid to parameters related to lipid peroxidation. After 10 days of feeding a dose of 1 g EPA per day/kg body weight, the hepatic content of glutathione (GSH) increased as did the activities of glutathione transferase, glutathione peroxidase, and glutathione reductase. The levels of hepatic lipid peroxides were lower after EPA feeding, whereas no change was observed in mice fed palmitic acid.

Thomas et al. [17] carried out a study with LDL obtained from nonhuman primates fed diets enriched in cholesterol and one of four types of fatty acids: saturates, monoenes, omega-6 fatty acids, or omega-3 fatty acids. Linoleic acid was the predominant PUFA in all the different LDL fractions. The rates of oxidation were linearly dependent on the concentration of PUFA. When the water-soluble initiator azobis(2-amidinopropane) dihydrochloride (ABAP) was used to initiate oxidation, the lag time was linearly related to the amount of α-tocopherol. However, with copper catalysis no linear correlation was evident. If the different enrichments were analyzed independently, it was observed that copper-catalyzed oxidation of LDL enriched with omega-6 fatty acids or omega-3 fatty acids showed a linear correlation between the lag time and the amount of α-tocopherol, but LDL enriched with saturates or monoenes did not show correlation. Thus, the rate of oxidation was dependent on the concentration of PUFA in LDL. The ability of α-tocopherol to inhibit oxidation depended on the lipid environment and the mode of initiation.

Using miniature pigs, Whitman et al. [18] observed that fish oil supplementation to an atherogenic diet decreased the lag time for formation of conjugated dienes during copper-induced oxidation of LDL for 0.5 to 12 hours, and increased the relative electrophoretic mobility, as compared to control oil supplementation. However, when LDL was oxidized for 18 to 24 hours, similar extent of oxidation was observed for LDL enriched with fish oil and control oil. Furthermore, morphological examination of all major blood vessels showed no difference between the fish oil and the control oil groups with respect to atherosclerotic lesion development. Although omega-3 fatty acid enriched-LDL might be more susceptible to oxidation *in vitro*, it was not more atherogenic *in vivo* than control-LDL.

Concluding Remarks

From the reported data in this review it may be relevant to point out that the number of double bonds, the type of polyunsaturated fatty acids, the type and amount of antioxidants, the background diet, tissue response to different fatty acids, smoking, tissue lipoprotein concentration, and the amount of lipid peroxides in the diet, are of importance for the potential oxidation of LDL. Although there are some reports suggesting that intake of omega-3 fatty acids promote increased peroxidation of LDL *in vivo* and *in vitro*, there are also reports on unaltered or reduced peroxidation in the presence of omega-3 fatty acids in the diet. We are currently performing a clinical trial in which smoking men with combined hyperlipidemia are supplemented with omega-3 fatty acids ± antioxidants. LDL are oxidized by the subjects' own peripheral blood mononuclear cells. Since omega-3 fatty acids are incorporated into cell membranes as well as into LDL, this oxidation model will most likely better reflect the *in vivo* situation for oxidation of LDL than just the susceptibility of isolated LDL to lipid peroxidation.

References

1. Ylä-Herttuala S, Palinski W, Rosenfeld ME, et al. Evidence of the presence of oxidatively modified low density lipoprotein in atherosclerotic lesions of rabbit and man. J Clin Invest 1989;84:1086-95.
2. Parthasarathy S, Khoo JC, Miller E, Barnett J, Witztum JL, Steinberg D. Low density lipoprotein rich in oleic acid is protected against oxidative modification: Implications for dietary prevention of atherosclerosis. Proc Natl Acad Sci USA 1990;87:3894-98.
3. Nenseter MS, Rustan AC, Lund-Katz S, et al. Effect of dietary supplementation with n-3 polyunsaturated fatty acids on physical properties and metabolism of low density lipoprotein in humans. Arterioscler Thromb 1992; 12:369-79.
4. Nenseter MS, Rustan AC, Lund-Katz S, Søyland E, Drevon CA. Dietary supplementation with n-3 and n-6 polyunsaturated fatty acids in humans. Effects on chemical composition, cellular metabolism and susceptibility of low density lipoprotein to lipid peroxidation. In: Drevon CA, Baksaas I, Krokan HE, editors. Omega-3 fatty acids: Metabolism and biological effects. Basel: Birkhäuser, 1993:41-50.
5. Harats D, Dabach Y, Hollander G, et al.. Fish oil ingestion in smokers and nonsmokers enhances peroxidation of plasma lipoproteins. Atherosclerosis 1991;90:127-39.
6. Lussier-Cacan S, Dubreuil-Quidoz S, Roederer G, et al. Influence of probucol on enhanced LDL oxidation after fish oil treatment of hypertriglyceridemic patients. Arterioscler Thromb 1993;13:1790-97.
7. Harris WS, Windsor SL, Caspermeyer JJ. Modification of lipid-related atherosclerosis risk factors by omega-3 fatty acid ethyl esters in hypertriglyceridemic patients. J Nutr Biochem 1993;4:706-12.
8. Bittolo-Bon G, Cazzolato G, Alessandrini P, Soldan S, Casalino G, Avogaro P. Effects of concentrated DHA and EPA supplementation on LDL peroxidation and vitamin E status in type IIb hyperlipidemic patients. In: Drevon CA, Baksaas I, Krokan HE, editors. Omega-3 fatty acids: Metabolism and biological effects. Basel: Birkhäuser, 1993:51-58.

9. Frankel EN, Parks E, Xu R, Schneeman BO, Davis PA, German JB. Effect of n-3 fatty acids-rich fish oil supplementation on the oxidation of low density lipoproteins. Lipids 1994;29:233-36.
10. Oostenbrug GS, Mensink RP, Hornstra G. Effects of fish oil and vitamin E supplementation on copper-catalyzed oxidation of human low density lipoprotein in vitro. Eur J Clin Nutr 1994; 48:895-98.
11. Suzukawa M, Abbey M, Howe PRC, Nestel PJ. Effects of fish oil fatty acids on low density lipoprotein size, oxidizability, and uptake by macrophages. J Lipid Res 1995;36:473-84.
12. Sirtori CR, Gatti E, Tremoli E, et al. Olive oil, corn oil, and n-3 fatty acids differently affect lipids, lipoproteins, platelets, and superoxide formation in type II hypercholesterolemia. Am J Clin Nutr 1992;56:113-22.
13. Fisher M, Upchurch KS, Levine PH, et al. Effects of dietary fish oil supplementation on polymorphonuclear leukocytes inflammatory potential. Inflammation 1986;10:387-91.
14. Fisher M, Levine PH, Weiner BH, et al. Dietary n-3 fatty acid supplementation reduces superoxide production and chemiluminescence in a monocyte-enriched preparation of leukocytes. Am J Clin Nutr 1990;51:804-808.
15. Vossen RCRM. Fatty acid modification and endothelial cell reactivity. Thesis. University of Maastricht 1993, ISBN 90-5278-070-6.
16. Demoz A, Willumsen N, Berge RK. Eicosapentaenoic acid at hypotriglyceridemic dose enhances the hepatic antioxidant defense in mice. Lipids 1992;27:968-71.
17. Thomas MJ, Thornburg T, Manning J, Hooper K, Rudel LL. Fatty acid composition of low-density lipoprotein influences its susceptibility to autoxidation. Biochemistry 1994;33:1828-34.
18. Whitman SC, Fish JR, Rand ML, Rogers KA. n-3 fatty acid incorporation into LDL particles renders them more susceptible to oxidation in vitro but not necessarily more atherogenic in vivo. Arterioscler Thromb 1994;14:1170-76.

ADMINISTRATION OF n-3 FATTY ACIDS TO HYPERTRIGLYCERIDEMIC PATIENTS REDUCES MONOCYTE TISSUE FACTOR ACTIVITY

Elena Tremoli, Susanna Colli, Mariagrazia Lalli, Sonia Eligini, Paola Maderna, Franco Pazzucconi, Patrizia Risé, and Claudio Galli
E. Grossi Paoletti Center, Institute of Pharmacological Sciences, University of Milan, Via Balzaretti 9, 20133 Milan, Italy

Introduction

TISSUE FACTOR BIOSYNTHESIS AND ITS BIOLOGICAL ROLE

Tissue factor (TF) is a membrane-bound glycoprotein that functions in the extrinsic pathway of blood coagulation by acting as a cofactor for factor VII [1,2]. TF binds the plasma serine protease factor VIIa and the resulting factor VIIa-TF complex acts as a catalyst for the conversion of factors IX to IXa and X to Xa, leading to the formation of thrombin [3].

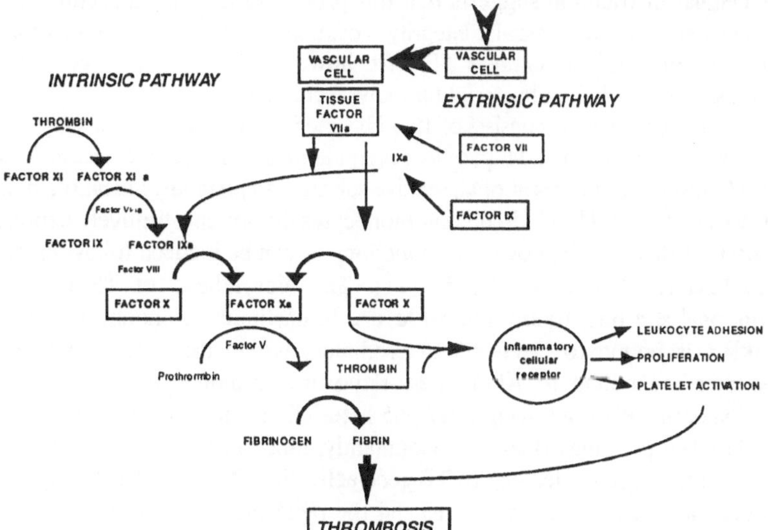

Figure 1. Central role of the tissue factor/factor VII complex in the blood coagulation pathway.

A. M. Gotto, Jr. et al. (eds.), Drugs Affecting Lipid Metabolism, 689–696.

Binding of factor VII to TF triggers factor VII-dependent coagulation through at least two mechanisms [4]. First, the binding of factor VII to TF facilitates factor VII activation; second, TF serves as cofactor for factor VIIa to activate factor IX and factor X. The functional activity of TF depends on its phospholipid environment. Association of TF apoprotein with either neutral or acidic phospholipids is required for activation of factor VII bound to TF [5]. Specifically, VIIa/TF complexes made with purified apoprotein reconstituted into phosphatidylcholine/phosphatidylserine vesicles readily activate factor X, whereas complexes made with the apoprotein reconstituted into vesicles containing phosphatidylcholine do not [6].

Regulation of the catalytic activity of the factor VIIa/TF complex is driven by at least two independent proteinase inhibitors, the TF pathway inhibitor TFPI [7,8], and the serpin antithrombin III [9,10]. TFPI has a negatively charged NH2 terminus, three Kunitz domains and a positively charged COOH-terminus. TFPI is thought to inhibit VIIa/TF in a two-step stoichiometric reaction. At first, factor Xa binds to reactive center arginine in the second Kunitz domain to give rise to Xa/TFPI complex with inhibited factor Xa activity. In the second step, the TFPI/Xa complex binds to VII/TF in a reaction in which the factor VIIa binds to a reactive center in the first Kunitz domain. The resultant quaternary Xa/TFPI/ VIIa/TF complex lacks VIIa/TF catalytic activity. It is important to note that these reactions operate at physiological concentrations of proteinases. TFPI, however, at concentrations far higher than those present in plasma, directly inhibits VIIa/TF catalytic activity. The regulation of VIIa/TF catalytic activity by antithrombin occurs with mechanisms different from those operating for TFPI.

TF is constitutively expressed in several tissues, such as brain, lung, and placenta and its cellular distribution suggests that this protein forms an hemostatic envelope that activates coagulation when vascular integrity is disrupted. Under normal conditions vascular cells do not constitutively express TF, that, however, can be expressed in response to different agonists, including bacterial lipopolysaccharide (LPS).

The human TF gene consists of 12.4 kbp and it is organized into six exons separated by 5 introns [2]. Activation of TF gene by several agonists induces the accumulation of 2.3 and 2.4 TF mRNAs as the result of alternative splicing. As previously mentioned, in contrast to extravascular sites, blood circulating monocytes do not constitutively express TF. The expression of this protein, however, in monocytes can be induced following exposure of cells to bacterial lipopolysaccharide [11]. The biosynthesis of TF is controlled at transcriptional and post-transcriptional levels. In unstimulated monocytes or endothelial cells, IκBα is bound to c-*rel*-p65 heterodimers within the cytosol, whereas *fos-jun* heterodimers are bound to AP-1 sites. Exposure of monocytes to LPS induces the dissociation of the IκBα, allowing c-*rel*-p65 heterodimers to migrate to the nucleus where they bind to their putative κB site. Concomitantly, functional interaction between different transcription sites occurs, leading to TF gene activation. TF mRNA is highly unstable due to the presence of AU-rich sequences and the rapid mRNA turnover is one of the rate limiting steps in the biosynthesis of TF protein. Interestingly, LPS has been shown, in addition to induce TF gene transcription, to stabilize TF mRNA transcripts [12]. In fact, in monocytes exposed to LPS maximal accumulation of TF mRNA transcripts occurs at 4 hours after the stimulus, a period of time corresponding to maximal expression of procoagulant activity (4-6 hours). Post-translational regulation of TF-surface expression involves the processes of disulfide bond formation, phosphorylation of the short cytoplasmic tail and N-glycosylation of 3 sites in the extracellular domain of the protein [13].

Monocyte TF activity has been shown to be increased in various animal models after endotoxin shock [14,15]. In addition, elevated levels of TF activity have been reported during extracorporeal circulation in patients undergoing aortocoronary bypass [16], possibly due to monocyte activation consequent to surgical maneuvers and during the outburst of unstable angina, as a result of lymphocyte activation from yet-undiscovered factor(s) [17]. Moreover TF has been found in the matrix of necrotic cores of atherosclerotic plaques [18], mostly associated with foam cells of monocyte/macrophage origin. Interestingly, cholesterol enrichment of macrophages has been shown to be associated with enhanced expression of TF [19], providing a link between lipids and the cell-mediated coagulation pathway.

N-3 FATTY ACIDS AND TF ACTIVITY OF MONOCYTES/MACROPHAGES

Epidemiological and interventional studies suggest that consumption of fish oil containing high concentrations of n-3 fatty acids confers protection against ischemic heart disease [20]. In addition it has been shown that n-3 fatty acids exert beneficial effects in animals and humans with atherosclerotic disease [21]. Some of the effects may be attributed to the activity of n-3 fatty acids on platelet activation, on plasma lipid levels, as well as on changes in the behavior of cells of the vessel wall. Interestingly, n-3 fatty acids have been shown to attenuate the proinflammatory potential of monocytes/macrophages. Indeed they reduce monocyte adhesion, chemotaxis, and cytokine and leukotriene synthesis [22].

In consideration of the potential role of TF expressed by monocytes/macrophages in atherosclerosis and thrombosis, it has been of interest to evaluate whether supplementation of n-3 fatty acids to humans might attenuate TF activity of monocytes. Indeed, administration of 1 g/Kg body weight of an n-3 ethyl ester concentrate to nonhuman primates subjected to carotid endoarterectomy has been shown to result in a dramatic impairment of mononuclear TF activity [23].

Patients and Methods

STUDIES IN HEALTHY SUBJECTS

Eight healthy subjects (4 males and 4 females, age range 23-39 years), were selected. The subjects received 3 capsules, 1 g each, containing n-3 fatty acid ethyl esters (Esapent, Pharmacia Carlo Erba, Milan Italy) for 18 weeks. The capsules contained 85% eicosapentaenoic (EPA) and docosahexaenoic (DHA) acids, ratio 0.9 to 1.5.

STUDIES IN PATIENTS WITH HYPERTRIGLYCERIDEMIA

Thirty patients with diagnosis of hypertriglyceridemia were selected among patients attending our lipid clinic. Patients selection was based on diagnosis of type IV hyperlipoproteinemia according to the World Health Organization criteria. None of the patients had clinical signs of atherosclerotic disease, nor they were hypertensive or diabetics. The study was placebo controlled for parallel groups. Patients were randomly assigned to receive either 3 g/day n-3 fatty acid ethyl esters or placebo (olive oil) for 24 weeks.

During these studies healthy subjects and patients were asked to maintain their usual diet and to refrain from consuming foods rich in n-3 fatty acids, as salmon herrings and tuna fish.

Monocyte Isolation and Stimulation

Blood, anticoagulated with 3.8% sodium citrate (9:1, v/v), was centrifuged at 150xg for 18 minutes to obtain platelet rich plasma. The residue was processed for mononuclear cell isolation using centrifugation on Ficoll-Paque as previously described [24]. Monocytes were purified by adhesion to plastic. For TF activity (TFa) determination, adherent monocytes were incubated for 4 hours at 37° C in 5% CO_2 humid atmosphere in the absence and in the presence of 10 μg/ml LPS. At the end of the incubation, cells were scraped off and subjected to three cycles of freezing and thawing.

Fatty Acid Measurements

Total phospholipids were isolated from lipid extracts by TLC, using hexane/diethylether/ acetic acid 80:20:1 v/v/v, as developing agents. The zones containing total phospholipids were scraped off. Fatty acid methyl esters were prepared by transmethylation using methanolic HCl. The methyl esters were separated by gas liquid chromatography on capillary columns (Supelcowax 10, Fused silica 30 m, 0.32 ID, 0.25 mm film) using programming temperature (140-210° C at 2.5/minute increments).

Assay of Tissue Factor Activity

Total cellular content of TFa was determined on disrupted monocytes by one stage clotting assay. Assay mixture contained 0.1 ml of cell lysates, 0.1 ml citrated pooled normal plasma, and 0.1 ml $CaCl_2$ 25 mM. Results were expressed in arbitrary units (U) by comparison to a standard curve of clotting times, obtained by serial dilutions of human placental thromboplastin.

Plasma Lipids

Plasma total cholesterol and triglycerides were determined by enzymatic techniques according to standardized procedures.

Results and Discussion

In a preliminary study, we administered to healthy subjects a moderate dose (3 g/day) of n-3 fatty acid as ethyl ester (85% EPA+DHA) for 18 weeks. During treatment, significant accumulation of n-3 fatty acids in plasma and in monocyte lipids was recorded (data not shown), concomitantly with reductions in plasma triglyceride levels (-22% after 18 weeks of treatment), and no effect on plasma cholesterol levels. Treatment with n-3 fatty acid ethyl esters significantly reduced TF activity of monocytes, both basal and LPS-stimulated (Table 1).

Table 1. Effect of n-3 fatty acid ethyl ester administration to healthy subjects on TF activity of adherent monocytes.

	TF Activity (U/μg protein)	
	Baseline	n-3 Treatment§
Unstimulated Monocytes	7.1 ± 1.1	2.0 ± 0.12*
LPS-Stimulated Monocytes	13.1 ± 1.8	2.6 ± 0.20*

The results represent the means ± SEM of values obtained in 6 subjects at each time point. * $p<0.001$ versus baseline, § treatment with n-3 fatty acid ethyl esters lasted for 18 weeks.

A double-blind placebo-controlled study was then performed in patients with hypertriglyceridemia. To this end 30 hypertriglyceridemic patients were assigned either to placebo treatment (3 g/day olive oil) or to n-3 fatty acid treatment (3 g/day n-3 fatty acid ethyl esters for 24 weeks. The results essentially confirmed those obtained in healthy subjects. In the placebo group, plasma levels of EPA and DHA remained unchanged (data not shown), whereas in patients who received n-3 fatty acid plasma levels of EPA and DHA significantly increased (Figure 2). Moreover, a significant reduction in basal and stimulated TF activity of monocytes from patients assigned to n-3 fatty acid treatment only was recorded (Figure 3).

These data indicate that n-3 fatty acid ethyl esters effectively reduce basal and LPS-stimulated TF activity of adherent monocytes both in healthy subjects and in patients with hypertriglyceridemia, thus reducing the contribution of these cells to localization of the fibrin network. The mechanism(s) underlying TF activity reduction after n-3 fatty acid intake is presently not known. Indeed, n-3 fatty acids, when incorporated into cellular membranes, alter the biosynthesis of eicosanoids, either by directly influencing the formation of arachidonate-derived products or being substrate for the biosynthesis of prostaglandins and hydroxy-fatty acids derived from EPA, which possess reduced biological activity compared with those derived from arachidonate. Another possibility is represented by the effect of n-3 fatty acids on cytokine generation by monocytes/macrophages. It has been reported that n-3 fatty acids effectively reduce IL-1 and TNF biosynthesis by monocytes [25]. Thus n-3 fatty acids reducing basal and stimulated TF activity in adherent monocytes may interfere with *in vivo* activation of thrombin generation, influencing positively the prothrombotic risk in hypertriglyceridemic patients.

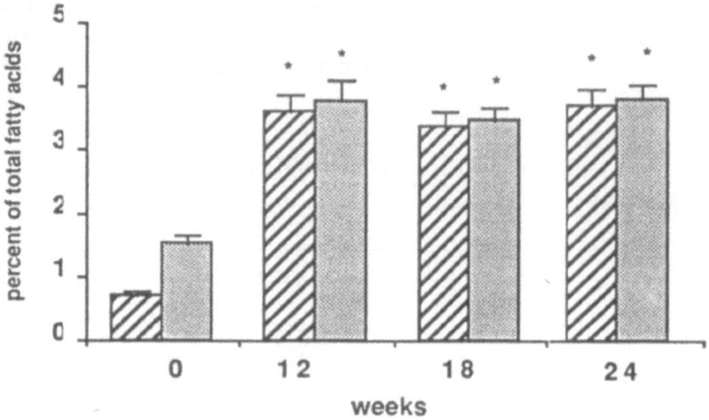

Figure 2. Fatty acid composition of plasma. Effect of 3 g/day n-3 fatty acid ethyl ester administration to hypertriglyceridemic patients (n=14). Values are means ± SEM. * $p < 0.001$ versus 0 weeks. ▨ EPA; ▩ DHA.

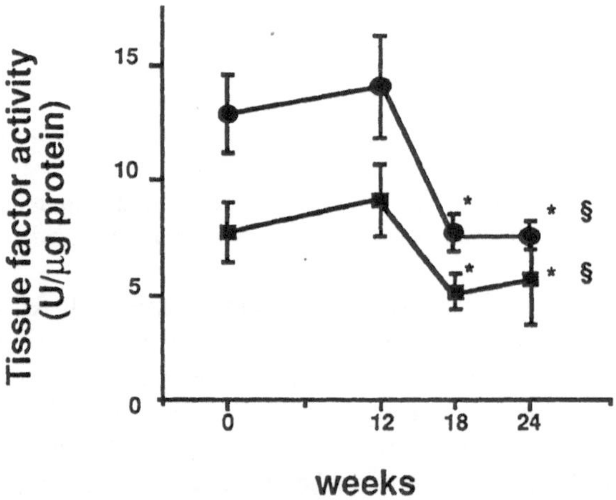

Figure 3. Effect of 3 g/day n-3 fatty acid ethyl ester administration to hypertriglyceridemic patients on TF activity of unstimulated (■) or LPS-stimulated (●) adherent monocytes. Data are the means ± SEM of individual values of 14 subjects at indicated times. * $p < 0.001$ versus time 0.

References

1. Nemerson Y, Bach R. Tissue factor revisited. Progr Hemost Thromb 1982;6:237-61.
2. Edgington TS, Mackman N, Brand K, Ruf W. The structural biology of expression and function of tissue factor. Thromb Haemost 1991;66:67-79.
3. Østerud B, Rapaport SI. Activation of factor IX by the reaction product of tissue factor and factor VII: Additional pathway for initiating blood coagulation. Proc Natl Acad Sci USA 1977;74:5260-64.
4. Edwards RL, Rickles FR. Macrophage procoagulant. Progr Hemost Thromb 1984;7:183-209.
5. Rapaport SI, Rao LVM. The tissue factor pathway: how it has become a "prima ballerina". Thromb Haemost 1995;74:7-17.
6. Neuenschwander PF, Fiore MM, Morrissey JH. Factor VII autoactivation proceeds via the interaction of distinct protease-cofactor and zymogen-cofactor complexes. J Biol Chem 1992;267:14477-82.
7. Rapaport SI. Inhibition of factor VIIa/tissue factor-induced blood coagulation: With particular emphasis upon a factor Xa-dependent inhibitory mechanism. Blood 1989;73:359-65.
8. Broze GJ, Girard TJ, Novotny WF. Regulation of coagulation by a multivalent Kunitz-type inhibitor. Biochemistry 1990;29:7539-45.
9. Lawson JH, Butenas S, Ribarik N, Mann KG. Complex-dependent inhibition of factor VIIa by antithrombin III and heparin. J Biol Chem 1993;268:767-70.
10. Rapaport SI. The extrinsic pathway inhibitor: A regulator of tissue factor-dependent blood coagulation. Thromb Haemost 1991;66:6-15.
11. Mackman N, Fowler BJ, Edgington TS, Morrissey JH. Functional analysis of the human tissue factor promoter and induction by serum. Proc Natl Acad Sci USA 1990;87:2254-58.
12. Brand K, Fowler BJ, Edgington TS, Mackman N. Tissue factor mRNA in THP-1 monocytic cells is regulated at both transcriptional and posttranscriptional levels in response to lipopolysaccharide. Mol Cell Biol 1991;11:4732-38.
13. Rickles FR, Hair GA, Zeff RA, Lee E, Bona RD. Tissue factor expression in human leukocytes and tumor cells. Thromb Haemost 1995;74:391-95.
14. Warr T, Rao LVM, Rapaport SI. The role of tissue factor (TF) in endotoxin-induced disseminated intravascular coagulation (DIC) in rabbits. Abstract. Thromb Haemost 1989;62:348a.
15. Edgington TS, Taylor F, Chang A, Morrissey JH, Blick K. Arrest of cellular coagulation in vivo by anti-tissue factor monoclonal antibody prevents lethal septic shock. Abstract. Thromb Haemost 1989;74:94a.
16. Kappelmayer J, Bernabei A, Edmunds LH, Edgington TS, Colman RW. Tissue factor is expressed on monocytes during simulated extracorporeal circulation. Abstract. Thromb Haemost 1993;69:1193a.
17. Neri Serneri GG, Abbate R, Gori AM, et al. Transient intermittent lymphocyte activation is responsible for the instability of angina. Circulation 1992;86:790-97.
18. Wilcox JN, Smith KM, Schwartz SM, Gordon D. Localization of tissue factor in normal vessel wall and in the atherosclerotic plaque. Proc Natl Acad Sci USA 1989;86:2839-43.
19. Lesnik P, Rouis M, Skarlatos S, Kruth HS, Chapman MJ. Uptake of exogenous free cholesterol induces upregulation of tissue factor expression in human monocyte-derived macrophages. Proc Natl Acad Sci USA 1992;89:10370-74.
20. Burr ML, Gilbert JF, Holliday RM, et al. Effects of changes in fat, fish and fibre intakes on death and myocardial infarction: Diet and reinfarction trial (DART). Lancet 1989;2:757-61.

21. Johnson BF, Daoud AS, Jarnolich J, Hosmer D, Johnson MH. Inhibition of atherosclerosis by cod liver oil in hyperlipidemic swine model. N Engl J Med 1986;315:841-46.
22. Tremoli E, Stragliotto E, Colli S, et al. Effects of n-3 fatty acids on monocyte functions. In: De Caterina R, Kristensen SD, Schmidt EB, editors. Fish oil and vascular disease. London: Springer Verlag, 1992:79-84.
23. Harker LA, Kelly AB, Hanson SR, et al. Interruption of vascular thrombus formation and vascular lesion formation by dietary n-3 fatty acids in fish oil in nonhuman primates. Circulation 1993;87:1017-29.
24. Colli S, Tremoli E. Multiple effects of dipyridamole on neutrophils and mononuclear leukocytes: Adenosine-dependent and adenosine-independent mechanisms. J Lab Clin Med 1991;118:136-45.
25. Endres S, Gorhani R, Kelley VE, et al. The effect of dietary supplementation with n-3 polyunsaturated fatty acids on the synthesis of interleukin-1 and tumor necrosis factor by mononuclear cells. N Engl J Med 1989;320:265-71.

INDEX

Medical Science Symposia Series

1. A.M. Gotto, C. Lenfant, R. Paoletti (eds.) and M. Soma (ass.ed.): *Multiple Risk Factors in Cardiovascular Disease.* 1992 ISBN 0-7923-1938-9
2. A.L. Catapano, A.M. Gotto, Jr., L.C. Smith and R. Paoletti (eds.): *Drugs Affecting Lipid Metabolism.* 1993 ISBN 0-7923-2232-0
3. T. Godfraind, S. Govoni, R. Paoletti and P.M. Vanhoutte (eds.): *Calcium Antagonists. Pharmacology and Clinical Research.* 1993 ISBN 0-7923-2259-2
4. D. Galmarini, L.R. Fassati, R. Paoletti and S. Sherlock (eds.): *Drugs and the Liver: High Risk Patients and Transplantation.* 1993 ISBN 0-7923-2307-6
5. P.M. Vanhoutte, P.R. Saxena, R. Paoletti, N. Brunello (eds.) and A.S. Jackson (ass.ed.): *Serotonin. From Cell Biology to Pharmacology and Therapeutics.* 1993 ISBN 0-7923-2518-4
6. A.G. Dalgleish, A. Albertini and R. Paoletti (eds.): *The Impact of Biotechnology on Autoimmunity.* 1994 ISBN 0-7923-2724-1
7. P.G. Crosignani, R. Paoletti, P.M. Sarrel, N.K. Wenger (eds.), M. Meschia and M. Soma (ass.eds.): *Women's Health in Menopause. Behaviour, Cancer, Cardiovascular Disease, Hormone Replacement Therapy.* 1994 ISBN 0-7923-3068-4
8. A.M. Gotto Jr., C. Lenfant, A.L. Catapano and R. Paoletti (eds.): *Multiple Risk Factors in Cardiovascular Disease.* 1995 ISBN 0-7923-3503-1
9. T. Godfraind, G. Mancia, M.P. Abbracchio, L. Aguilar-Bryan and S. Govoni (eds.): *Pharmacological Control of Calcium and Potassium Homeostasis. Biological, Therapeutical, and Clinical Aspects.* 1995 ISBN 0-7923-3604-6
10. A.M. Gotto Jr., R. Paoletti, L.C. Smith, A.L. Catapano and A.S. Jackson (eds.): *Drugs Affecting Lipid Metabolism. Risk Factors and Future Directions.* 1996 ISBN 0-7923-4167-8

KLUWER ACADEMIC PUBLISHERS – DORDRECHT / BOSTON / LONDON